ULTRASONIC ENERGY

Biological Investigations and Medical Applications

Edited by ELIZABETH KELLY

Preface

Biologic systems are characterized by complex organization at all levels of structure and ultrasonic energy can be employed to elucidate such organization of the various levels. For example, at low ultrasound intensities, the gross or microscopic features of soft tissue can be visualized by employing the acoustic reflection properties of tissue interfaces. Quantitative measurement of the ultrasonic absorption coefficients of tissues as a function of frequency and other parameters can disclose, at the macromolecular level, information on protein configurations and their incorporation into the biologic organization. Application of high-intensity ultrasound can result in *selective* modification of tissue and since this selective action can occur at the cellular level, ultrasound can be used to investigate and alter microscopic organization of tissue. Since tissue resembles liquids in regard to acoustic propagation properties, an adjunct to the biological investigations is the study of the physical phenomena accompanying the presence of ultrasonic fields in liquid or liquid-like media. The symposium held at the University of Illinois Allerton House, in June, 1962, included papers and/or discussion on these various aspects of the biophysics of ultrasound and the proceedings of that conference are included in this publication.

The application of ultrasonic energy has a vast potential in basic biologic research and in medicine. Unfortunately, the number of research scientists in this field is still comparatively small. The Physiology Branch of the Office of Naval Research should be commended for encouragement of research activity in this field not only by financial support of the present ultrasound symposia at the University of Illinois but also by contract support of basic research in this field.

The editor expresses her appreciation of the editorial assistance of Rosalie Eggleton and Melva Ponton.

ELIZABETH KELLY, *Editor*

Contents

1 Physical Principles Involved in the Action of Weak Ultrasound — 1
Wesley L. Nyborg

2 Biological Implications of the Action of Weak Ultrasound — 9
David E. Hughes

3 Some Aspects of Ultrasonic Cavitation — 23
Yoshimitsu Kikuchi, Hiroshi Shimizu, and Daitaro Okuyama

4 Ultrasonic Absorption by Biological Materials — 51
Floyd Dunn

5 Ultrahigh-Frequency Acoustic Waves in Liquids and Their Interaction with Biological Structures — 66
Floyd Dunn and Stephen A. Hawley

6 The Use of High-Intensity Ultrasound to Alter the Cellular Structure of the Anterior Pituitary — 77
Rolfs Krumins, Elizabeth Kelly, Francis J. Fry, and William J. Fry

7 Action of Intense Ultrasound on the Intact Mouse Liver — 85
Joseph C. Curtis

8 Morphology of Ultrasonically Irradiated Skeletal Muscle — 117
Reginald C. Eggleton, Elizabeth Kelly, Francis J. Fry, Ruth Chalmers, and William J. Fry

9 The Effect of Ultrasound in the Treatment of Cancer — 137
Karlheinz Woeber, M.D.

10 Biological Effects of Ultrasound on Neuromuscular Skeletal Systems — 150
Jerome W. Gersten, M.D.

11 Action of Ultrasound on the Internal Ear — 160
Michele Arslan, M.D., and O. Sala, M.D.

12 Destruction of Transplantable Ascites Tumors by Means of Intense Ultrasound 179
Toshio Wagai, M.D., and Yoshimitsu Kikuchi

13 Technical Developments of Focused Ultrasound and Its Biological and Surgical Applications in Japan 190
Katuya Yoshioka and Masuhisa Oka

14 Recent Developments in Ultrasound at the Biophysical Research Laboratory and Their Application to Basic Problems in Biology and Medicine 202
Francis J. Fry

15 Concepts of Electronic Design for Precision Ultrasonic Lesions 229
Gene H. Leichner

16 New Approaches to the Study and Modification of Biological Systems by Ultrasound 242
William J. Fry

17 Current Status of Ophthalmic Ultrasonography 260
Gilbert Baum, M.D., and Ivan A. Greenwood

18 The Use of Ultrasound to Record the Motion of Heart Structure 278
John M. Reid and Claude R. Joyner, M.D.

19 The Continuous Registration of the Movement of Heart Structure by the Reflectoscope Techniques — Methods of Registration 294
Carl Hellmuth Hertz

20 The Diagnostic Use of Ultrasound in Heart Disease 303
Inge Edler, M.D.

21 A Mirror System for Ultrasonic Visualization of Soft Tissues 322
Carl Hellmuth Hertz and Sven Olofsson

22 Registration of Movement of Cardiac Walls Using an Ultrasonic Reflection Procedure 327
Sven Effert, M.D., F. J. Deupmann, and J. Karytsiotis

23 Ultrasonic Diagnosis of Intracranial Disease, Breast Tumors, and Abdominal Diseases 346
Toshio Wagai, M.D., Ryoichi Miyazawa, Kazubumi Ito, and Yoshimitsu Kikuchi

24 An Ultrasonic Echoscope for Visualizing the Pregnant Uterus 365
G. Kossoff, W. J. Garrett, and D. E. Robinson

25 The Ultrasonic Tomograph and Its Use in Medical Diagnosis 377
Douglas Gordon, M.D.

Low-Intensity Ultrasound Research as Applied in Clinical Medicine 388
John H. Aldes, M.D.

1

Physical Principles Involved in the Action of Weak Ultrasound

WESLEY L. NYBORG
University of Vermont, Burlington, Vermont

Introduction by Dr. von Gierke

It is indeed a pleasure to open the first scientific session of this Symposium on Ultrasound in Biology and Medicine. Those of us who were here before are well aware of the unusual interest of these symposia. To those of you who are here for the first time, it may come as quite a surprise to hear about the extensive work in the ultrasound field, particularly that done here at the Biophysical Research Laboratory.

If some of you are wondering to what this very modern art design on the cover of the program refers, I think it depicts dancing molecules under the impact of ultrasonic energy. If some of you have a better explanation, we might consider this in the discussion. For the time being, I assume that this is more or less the theme of our first session – which is concerned with the physical action of ultrasound energy and its relation to the basic biological mechanism acting on the organisms. Regardless of the particular area of ultrasound in which one is interested, whether it is therapy, diagnosis, or basic biological applications, the first step in all of these areas is to find out how the energy is transported to the cells and/or interceptors and what the mechanism of action of this energy is. Our first papers, therefore, are devoted to these principal mechanisms.

In regard to the question on the cover, I think it probably suggests that things are very complicated and that we do not understand them at all. Perhaps I can now proceed to prove this point in my talk.

The subject of this talk is perhaps best indicated by pointing out what it does not include. The phenomena to be excluded are those associated with violent ultrasonically produced cavitation, attended by sudden collapse occurring in less than a sonic period. We consider here events which occur either (a) under conditions of high-amplitude sound where "collapse" cavitation is suppressed, or (b) under conditions where a form of "weak" cavitation, or bubble activity, takes place at relatively low sound levels.

I believe it is agreed that a variety of interesting and important effects takes place under conditions where collapse events do not occur. Thus Fry *et al.* (1951) have reported evidence against violent collapse-type cavitation when lesions are produced in nervous tissue. Goldman and Lepeschkin (1951) found residual effects in plant cells when cavitation was suppressed by superpressure. Rather recently, while I worked in collaboration with Dyer (1960) at Brown University and Hughes (1962) at Oxford University, it was found that a number of biological effects occur in situations where collapse cavitation is absent.

There are a number of instances in which sonically produced structural changes and rate changes in various processes are attributed to bubble activity but at amplitudes below threshold for collapse cavitation. (Roughly speaking, about 1-atm pressure amplitude is required for collapse.) It was shown by Frings (see Ackerman *et al.*, 1953) that paramecia are killed in the cavity of specially constructed small whistles provided that an air bubble is present, the pressure amplitude being about 0.1 atm. The contents of the cavity were found, upon observation during irradiation, to take part in a great deal of eddying which occurs near the air-liquid interfaces. This observation led to investigations by Kolb (1956) and Elder (1959) showing that these motions occur rather generally. Elder studied the motions which occur near a resonant gas bubble (resting on a solid boundary) set into vibration by an ambient sound field. When the bubble vibrates purely radially, the pattern is fairly simple; there is rough but useful theory available for this situation. When surface waves are established, as is commonly the case, the pattern is more detailed and is frequently asymmetric about an axis through the bubble normal to the boundary.

A number of experiments were carried out by the present author to determine what effects may be attributed specifically to sonically produced motions of this kind. It was found that thin layers of oil, grease, fluid paint, etc., loosely adhering on the boundary, are readily removed by the vibrating bubble. In addition, however, there is an attractive tendency which complicates the situation. Flakes or droplets of removed material return to the bubble, often completely covering its surface so that the bubble can no longer be seen.

In other experiments changes in the rates of certain kinds of reactions and processes were investigated. Figure 1, from a paper by Jackson, Gould, Adams, and me (1959), shows enhanced development of a photographic plate over an area surrounding the site of a vibrating resonant bubble, resting on the plate, in the presence of dilute developer. The frequency was 2000 cps; the pressure amplitude was of the order of 0.1 atm. The circular area directly under the bubble had no access to developer and hence is understandably of low photographic density. One may note an asymmetry in the development pattern around the bubble; this is probably to be explained by the action of an asymmetrical surface wave and its effect on the eddying.

Quite recently Gould (1961) completed an investigation of the effect of bubble-generated eddying on heat transfer. Heat was generated by a small resistance element embedded in plastic at a plane plastic-liquid interface. Transfer of heat from the element to the liquid was studied with and without excitation of a neighboring bubble resonant at 2000 cps. Significant changes were observed using pressure amplitudes up to about 0.1 atm; the heat transfer was found to be increased by factors up to ten when the bubble was set into vibration. We find it possible to fit approximate theory to the result and hence believe we are beginning to understand how surface processes in general may be affected by this kind of motion.

The bubble is an extremely effective (if somewhat temperamental) source of small scale circulation or microeddying. The reason for this effectiveness, according to theory, lies in the fact that the bubble acts as a "velocity amplifier" and gives rise to high gradients of velocity in its own vicinity. A related kind of eddying occurs near any obstacle such as a solid sphere suspended in a sound field. Theory indicates (Nyborg, 1958), however, that for a given pressure amplitude in a typical sound field the streaming associated with a resonant bubble may be greater by more than a factor of 10^6 than that near a solid fixed sphere of similar size. (It is true, however, that one should

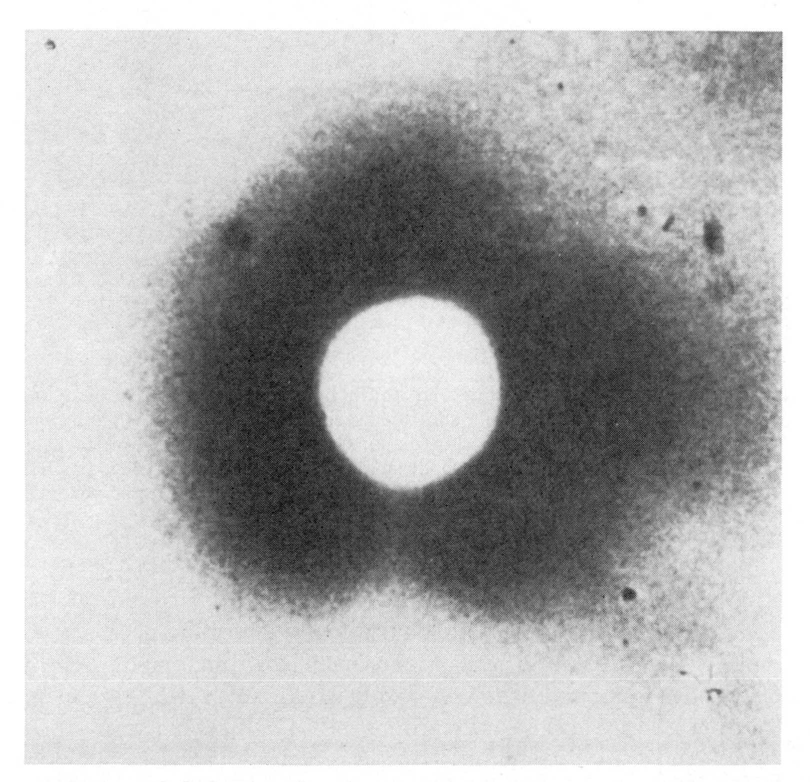

FIGURE 1. Enhanced darkening of a photographic plate in area surrounding a vibrating bubble (2 kc). Plate was immersed in dilute developer and exposed to light. White circular region shows where bubble rested on emulsion; developer did not reach this region. Accelerated development in ring just outside bubble attributed to sonically generated eddying; lack of radial symmetry probably a result of asymmetry in bubble surface vibration pattern. From reference 8.

be cautious about the latter theory; it is valid only if the amplitudes are not too high.)

It is frequently possible to obtain more reproducible results on effects of microeddying by using methods which do not depend on vibrating bubbles. Jackson (1960) showed that small scale circulatory motions occur in the region between the end face of a vibrating bar and a nearby opposing solid boundary (see Fig. 2). This source of motion has been used for studying effects on a variety of surface reactions and on electrochemical changes occurring at electrodes embedded in a plane plastic boundary (Nyborg and Seegall, 1959).

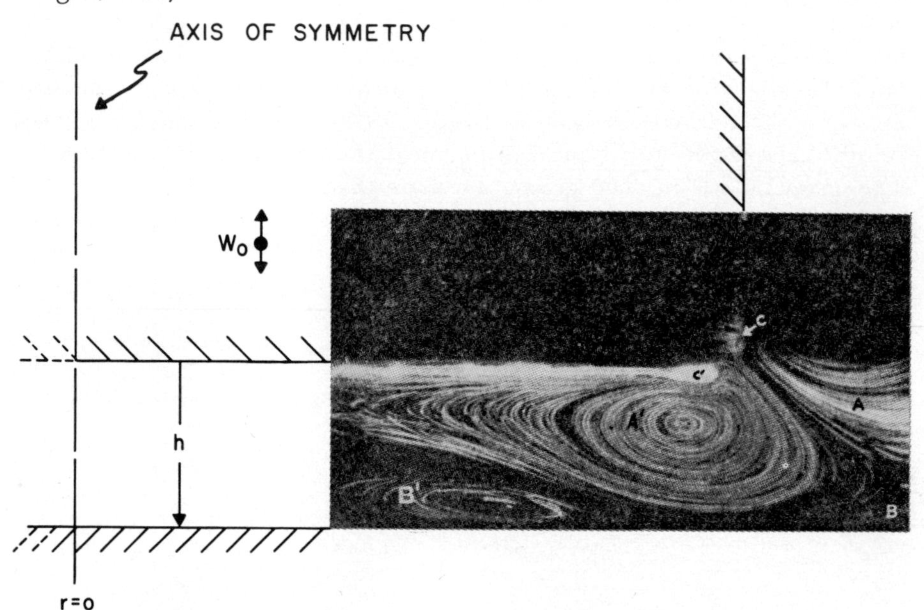

FIGURE 2. Streaming pattern generated in liquid between the end face of a longitudinally vibrating bar and a rigid plane a short distance from it. Line drawing shows outline of (half of) the bar and of the opposing plane. Circulation pattern is photographed by 120-sec exposures with light scattered from small suspended polystyrene particles which follow the flow. The lower end of the bar (diameter: 5.7 cm) vibrates vertically with velocity amplitude W_0, circulations occur in pairs labeled (A,A′), (B,B′) and (C,C′). From reference 11.

In some experiments with suspensions of biological cells and microorganisms (Hughes and Nyborg, 1962) a longitudinally vibrating needle protruded into a small flat cell containing the suspension. This arrangement permitted all parts of the suspension to be viewed during irradiation with 100 × magnification. By direct observation we determined that cell destruction (to be discussed in the paper by Dr. Hughes) was obtained in the absence of cavitation or bubble activity. Vigorous eddying occurred in the liquid near the needle and especially vigorously near its tip. We believe it is this motion which causes disintegration of the cells.

I would like to show now a film prepared at the University of Vermont with the assistance of Mr. Richard Paul. This film demonstrates the type of circulatory motions imparted to 100-μ polystyrene spheres suspended in a solution when a vibrating needle is inserted in the solution.

An aggregation tendency was also observed in the above mentioned treatment of cell suspensions. As time goes on, the cells apparently drift toward the vibrating object. This drift is superimposed on the circulation and tends to increase effectiveness of the sonic action; the cells move into the source region where they meet their destruction, thus making a localized source more efficient than it otherwise would be.

The sonically generated eddying near the tip of a vibrating needle is similar in scale to that near a vibrating resonant bubble. Approximate theory can be given for both situations. Examining the theory, one finds that typical speeds, shear rates, etc. achieved near a vibrating needle are also to be found near a bubble whose radial vibration amplitude is of the order of one-tenth its mean radius. Since a resonant bubble achieves such a vibration amplitude in a relatively weak sound field (in which the pressure amplitude may be 0.01 atm or less) it is reasonable to conclude cells can be broken in low amplitude sound fields due to the presence of resonant bubbles. Dr. Hughes will describe experiments in which this conclusion was borne out. In the experiments referred to, the sound was produced by dipping into a small sample of suspension the end of a vibrating bar (frequency: 20 kc) in which small holes had been drilled in order to encourage the growth of resonant bubbles. Biological effects were obtained with sonic amplitudes well below those required for production of collapse-type cavitation.

The following film was prepared at Brown University in collaboration with Dr. H. J. Dyer. The film demonstrates the effect of a vibrating needle, a few microns in diameter, brought in contact with the wall of a plant cell. The resultant motions inside the plant cells are discernible.

REFERENCES

1. Fry, W. J., D. Tucker, F. J. Fry, and V. J. Wulff (1951). J. Acoust. Soc. Am. *23*, 364.
2. Goldman, D. E., and W. W. Lepeschkin (1951). Research Report, Project NM 004 005.03.05, Naval Medical Research Institute, Bethesda, Md., 10 Dec.
3. Dyer, H. J., and W. L. Nyborg (1960). IRE Trans. Med. Electron. *ME-7*, 163.
4. Hughes, D. E., and W. L. Nyborg (1962). Science *138*, 108.
5. Ackerman, E., J. J. Reid, H. Kinsloe, and H. W. Frings (1953). WADC Tech. Rept. 53–82 (Jan.).
6. Kolb, J., and W. L. Nyborg (1956). J. Acoust. Soc. Am. *28*, 1237.
7. Elder, S. A. (1959). J. Acoust. Soc. Am. *31*, 54.
8. Nyborg, W. L., R. K. Gould, F. J. Jackson, and C. E. Adams (1959). J. Acoust. Soc. Am. *31*, 706.
9. Gould, R. K. (1961). Ph.D. Dissertation, Brown University.
10. Nyborg, W. L. (1958). J. Acoust. Soc. Am. *30*, 329.
11. Jackson, F. J. (1960). J. Acoust. Soc. Am. *32*, 1387.
12. Nyborg, W. L., and M. I. L. Seegall (1959). Proceedings Third International Congress on Acoustics, Elsevier Publishing Company, Amsterdam.

DISCUSSION

DR. KIKUCHI: Perhaps you have already explained this, but I am not quite certain if the particles demonstrated in the first movie were bubbles.

DR. NYBORG: No. They did look like bubbles, but they were polystyrene spheres suspended in a glycerin-water mixture.

DR. KIKUCHI: Is there some purpose for the use of glycerin?

DR. NYBORG: Only to provide a liquid mixture whose density matches that of the suspended solid particles.

DR. HERTZ: I would like to ask the frequency used in the last experiment.

DR. NYBORG: In the work with plant leaves we used either of two frequencies: 25 kc or 80 kc.

DR. HERTZ: Would you expect such effects in nondivergent fields?

DR. NYBORG: No, I would not. Theory for the eddying shows that it is the divergence of the field which is responsible for the motion. If the entire cell could be made to vibrate uniformly, that is, as a single body, one would expect no eddying at all. In our experiment the excitation is highly nonuniform in that only a small part of the cell wall is caused to vibrate, namely, that near the vibrating needle tip.

DR. HERRICK: What was the order of magnitude of temperatures measured in the plant cell experiments?

DR. NYBORG: Measurements of temperature were not made. Because of the nature of the motion (which is more like that near a small hydrodynamic point source than that in a plane wave), however, we would not expect much heat produced.

DR. VON GIERKE: Did you use media with different viscosities?

DR. NYBORG: The eddying near a vibrating needle has been observed with varying viscosities by using mixtures of glycerin and water. In gross observation little change is seen from varying viscosity over the range, say, from one to ten times that of water; theory indicates, however, that there really is a change occurring in the thin boundary layer adjacent to the needle surface. When the viscosity is much larger, changes in the eddying occur which are very obvious even in gross observation.

DR. WEISSLER: Did the eddying which we saw have anything to do with gas bubbles which may have been invisible in the movies?

DR. NYBORG: This is possible since with the plant cells we can't see any better than you can whether or not small bubbles are present; we have occasionally seen curious little motions in corners of cells which are rather difficult to explain. These might be caused by little bubbles that are covered over by plant tissues.

DR. W. J. FRY: Have you made calculations which would indicate the magnitude of the force involved, and have you compared the effects of sonically produced motion with those of motion produced by other means?

DR. NYBORG: From the theory we can estimate that velocity gradients are produced which are of the order of 10^4 to 10^6 sec^{-1}. From this one can, of course, calculate the viscous stress (viscosity $\times$ velocity gradient) in a medium of known viscosity. But as yet we do not know if this calculation would be a meaningful one for specifying the mechanical conditions to which the cells are subjected; thus, the cell breakage might depend more directly on some derivatives of the stress than on the stress itself. I have not experimented with other kinds of motion, and in respect to your second question, it is difficult to compare results from other fragmentation techniques used by other investigators. From a physicist's viewpoint it is alarming to discover that for none of the fragmentation methods is there definite information on what takes place when the cells or large molecules are broken. Even results from experiments based on relatively simple shear are not easy to interpret. Thus in experiments where suspensions are forced through capillaries, the shear stress varies across the cross-section, so that no definite statement is obtained concerning the stress required to cause the observed effect.

DR. VON GIERKE: Wouldn't you get some clues from streaming experiments, for example, by varying the tip diameter while holding the amplitude constant?

DR. NYBORG: Perhaps this can be done but up to now the situation has seemed too complex to yield very detailed data on cell constants, etc. from this type of experiment.

DR. W. J. FRY: About how large are typical streaming velocities here?

DR. NYBORG: Near the vibrating tip or near a resonant gas bubble, one expects from calculations that velocities may easily exceed 1 meter sec^{-1}. This is not very high but it is important to realize that this velocity occurs nearly up to the boundary, say, up to points only a few microns from it. To get the velocity gradient, we divide 1 meter sec^{-1} by that small boundary layer thickness to get values in the range mentioned.

DR. W. J. FRY: Apparently the motion is completely different from capillary flow. Would you compare it to turbulent flow?

DR. NYBORG: It is different from turbulent flow in that eddying is predictable, not chaotic. The boundary layer thickness is, however, possibly of the same order as that for high-speed turbulent flow.

DR. MACKAY: In the experiment with Dr. Hughes did the bubbles grow during the treatment? If so, did the rate of breakage increase during this growth?

DR. NYBORG: We let the bubbles grow first using a very weak sound field and then turned up the sound to the desired level. Then a number of events were found to occur: for example, surface waves are set up on the bubble as Willard showed some years ago; at moderate amplitudes the surface waves become very distorted and unstable; tiny "microbubbles" are sent off from the main bubble which are apparently associated with the surface activity—these attract each other and coalesce with great speed. Under typical conditions, all of these events, and possibly others, occur at once, and it has not been possible so far to separate out the effects of the separate processes.

DR. HERRICK: You mentioned weak fields. Can you give absolute values for the sound field amplitudes?

DR. NYBORG: The pressure amplitude varies from a little over 1 atm down to a few hundredths of an atmosphere. The upper limit is roughly the critical value for collapse cavitation.

DR. KOSSOFF: Do you expect any frequency dependence?

DR. NYBORG: In the sense that at higher frequencies one obtains the same velocity amplitude with a smaller displacement, a frequency dependence is to be expected. It turns out that the velocity of eddying at points near a boundary is expressed most directly in terms of particle velocity amplitude rather than particle displacement. Hence, at high frequencies we expect, in general, to get higher eddying speeds with the same displacement amplitude.

DR. KIKUCHI: In the cell disintegration experiments, how do you confirm the condition for bubble collapse?

DR. NYBORG: Actually we did not find it easy to do this by direct means to a large extent because the theory is not sufficiently advanced to explain all the observed events. However, we are quite sure that under our "weak cavitation" conditions, collapse did not occur since our pressure amplitude was significantly less than 1 atm. In addition, at a "critical" level *above* those corresponding to "weak cavitation," very marked changes occurred in the visual appearance of the cavitation field and in the noise generated from it. Chemical effects, which will be discussed in the paper by Dr. Hughes, begin to occur abruptly at the same "critical" level.

DR. VON GIERKE: Don't you think it is possible to define this whole area in a more quantitative way than it has been done so far? It is clear that the field, as such, is not described by just the frequency and intensity. One of the most important parts of your experiments is the curvature of the needle, because this determines the nonuniformity of the sound field. Now insofar as the reaction of this field with a particular particle is concerned, it is the diameter or size of the particle, combined with the curvature, and the frequency which determines this interaction, and so we always have these three parameters, and it appears to me that all of our experiments should be described in terms of such parameters. Don't you think we should be able to come to a more quantitative description of these effects?

DR. NYBORG: It certainly would be a definite improvement if more parameters of measurement were included.

DR. VON GIERKE: We could set up models for particular cases – for example, the reaction of stresses on this particular particle.

DR. NYBORG: To date, I haven't seen any reliable method for calculating the effects of stresses, either on cells or on large molecules.

DR. VON GIERKE: Yes, but at least you could compare your results on a semiquantitative basis.

Biological Implications of the Action of Weak Ultrasound

DAVID E. HUGHES [1]
University of Oxford, Oxford, England

Introduction by Dr. von Gierke

As Dr. Nyborg mentioned, he and Dr. David Hughes have collaborated on studies of biological cell disruptions initiated by application of low-intensity ultrasound. The mechanism of this cell disintegration is of great interest, both from the viewpoint of the physical characteristics of the sound field and in regard to the associated basic chemistry.

Two apparently unconnected fields in biology to which ultrasound is currently applied are: (1) the work of Dr. Fry and his associates on the modification of component cellular populations of tissue with either irreversible or reversible action without *direct* gross disruption of the individual cells and (2) so-called analytical morphology where an attempt is made to *directly* break open the cells by sound in order that enzymic or other constituents of isolated cell organelles may be examined and structure and function related one to another. It is with this latter application of ultrasound that I am primarily concerned. More recently, because of our additional interest in the metabolism and function of the inner ear, we have collaborated with J. Angell James of Bristol and studied the effect of ultrasound in the inner ear. We have also recently collaborated with Professor Guy Warwick at Guy's Hospital on the biochemical effects of focused ultrasound in the brain.

I have indicated that the first two fields mentioned, namely, (1) the modification of structure and function of cellular populations by ultrasound and (2) the chemical study of the internal constituents of the cells, are apparently unconnected, but I would like to stress that I believe that they are very much interconnected, as previously indicated by our chairman. The understanding of the effects of ultrasound both at the anatomical level and the cellular level

[1] Dr. Hughes's present address is Department of Microbiology, University College of South Wales and Monmouthshire.

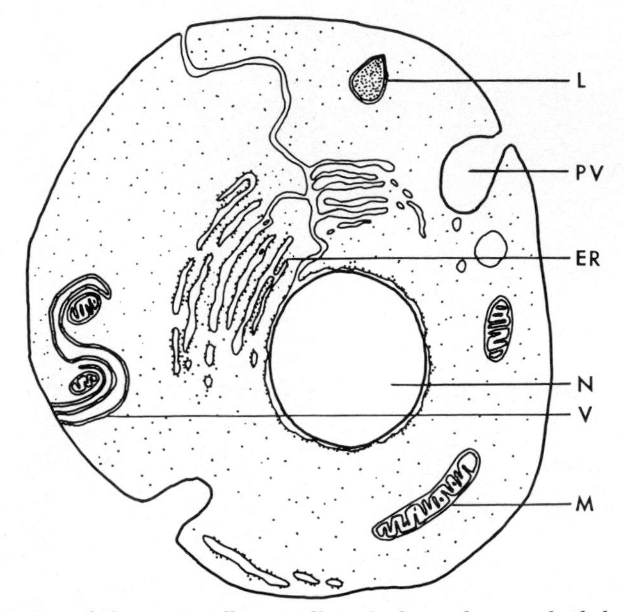

FIGURE 1. Diagram of the main cell organelles which can be seen both by electron and light microscopy and isolated from cells disintegrated by appropriate methods. The nucleus (N) contains enzymes concerned with nucleotide metabolism and several enzymes concerned with carbohydrate metabolism. The mitochondria (M) are the main energy producers of the cell while the disintegrated endoplastic reticulum (ER) (microsomal fraction) elaborates proteins. PV and V show pinocytotic and vesicular processes associated with water and solute transport. L represents a lipoidal inclusion. Photosynthetic organelles (chloroplasts) may be prepared from plant cells.

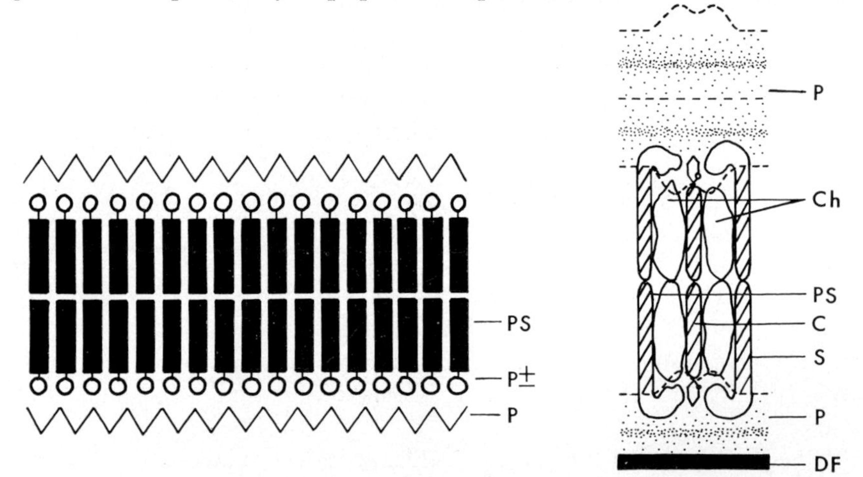

FIGURE 2. Diagram of molecular arrangement in unit membrane (Robertson, 1960). Such membranes are components of most of the cell organelles shown in Figure 1 and are found as well in microorganisms (Hughes, 1962a). Interconnected enzymic reactions such as oxidative phosphorylation depend on the orientation of phospholipid and protein in the membrane (Green, 1961). In most cells permeability is also controlled by the membranes. The detailed structure taken from Finean (1957) indicates a possible molecular arrangement. P, protein; P±, charged hydrophilic; Ch, cholesterol; PS, phosphorylserine; C, cerebroside; S, sphingomyolin; DF, difference factor; units of the lipid layer shown as dark rectangles in the diagram.

can only be brought about by fundamental research to discover the initial effect of the ultrasound, that is, the first detectable lesion. I am convinced that we can only detect such lesions by applying biochemical methods for the analysis of the effects of ultrasound in tissues and cells. Therefore, I would call this first detectable lesion a biochemical lesion from which the other lesions, such as the grosser anatomical ones detected by histological methods, follow.

Professor Nyborg and I have made preliminary experiments on biochemical lesions in some microorganisms, and I would like to discuss some of the results at this time. As you probably know, in the last 10 years there has been an almost complete revolution in the biochemical field which has resulted in an explosive growth in our knowledge of structure and function of animal cells. This has resulted from our ability to take cells apart and to keep the fragments more or less alive and working. Figures 1 and 2 give some details of cellular structure. It is possible by various methods to disrupt organisms such as yeast (Fig. 3) and to isolate the outside shell or hull, the mitochondria and microsomes. However, it has not yet proved possible to isolate the nuclei in such organisms as can be done with animal and plant cells. The isolated

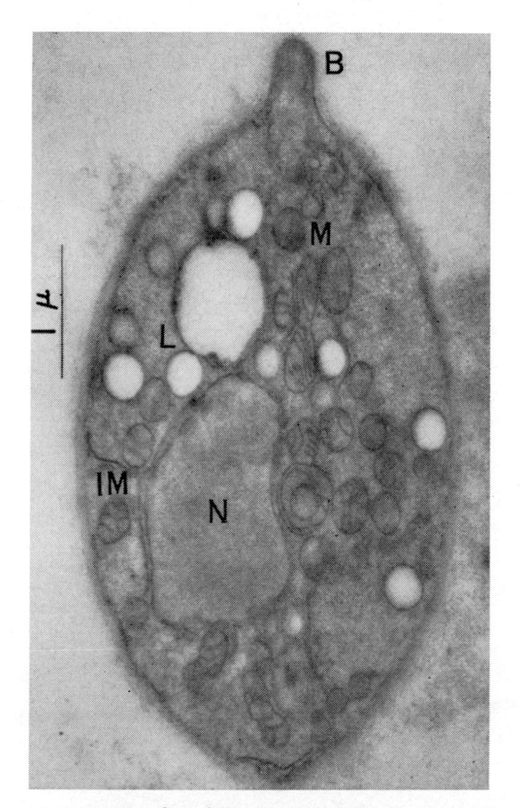

FIGURE 3. Electron micrograph of a thin section of yeast. In addition to the cell wall and plasma membrane, a nucleus, nuclear membrane, and mitochondria with crystae can be seen. B, bud; M, mitochondria; L, lipoidal inclusion; IM, internal membranes; N, nucleus. (Electron micrograph by courtesy of Dr. S. F. Conti, Department of Microbiology, Dartmouth Medical School.)

organelles can be studied as distinct biochemical entities and further disrupted in order to study their finer structure by electron microscopy. It is this approach that we label "analytical morphology." The bacteria, in addition to being smaller and less complicated in structure than yeast, are also much more difficult to break open in a controlled manner. However, finer fragments, prepared by general techniques in which ultrasound plays a part, are functionally similar to the larger cell organelles obtained from the higher organisms.

A typical micrograph of a bacterium (Fig. 4) shows that it possesses no distinct mitochondria or nucleus and that the cytoplasm is filled with small granules usually assumed to be ribosomes. The membrane which underlies the thick cell wall (plasma membrane) functions like a mitochondrial membrane in producing energy. In addition, it controls the permeability of the cell. The usual effect of high-power ultrasound on such cells is to reduce them to very small fragments (Hughes and Rodgers, 1960). These fragments are much finer than those observed as the result of other methods of dis-

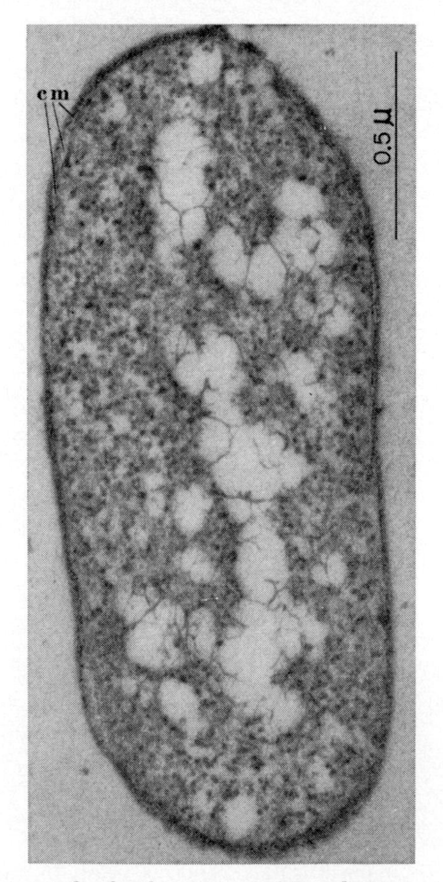

FIGURE 4. Electron micrograph of a thin section of *E. coli*. In contrast to the yeast shown in Figure 3, no distinct nuclear membrane or mitochondria are seen. cm, cytoplasmic membrane. (Electron micrograph by courtesy of Dr. S. F. Conti, Department of Microbiology, Dartmouth Medical School.)

integration. Such fine comminution of cell organelles has led to some confusion regarding the origin and function of granules which can be isolated by centrifugation of such preparations (Hughes, 1962a). One of the objects of our research has been to improve ultrasonic methods of disintegrating cells in order to reduce the gross comminution to gain an insight into the mechanism of cell disintegration by ultrasound. It seemed that this method offered chances of control which would make it possible to disintegrate the cell in a stepwise fashion, maintaining intact at each stage the structures revealed by electron microscopy.

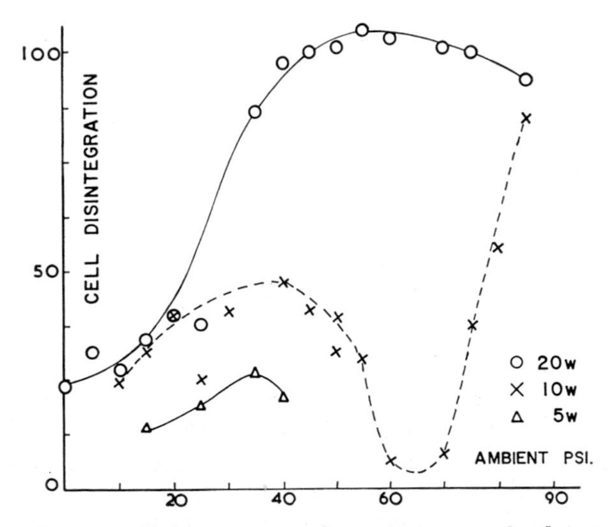

FIGURE 5. The effect of ambient pressure and power input on the disintegration of yeast (Neppiras and Hughes, 1964). A 1:6 (w/v) yeast suspension was treated in the apparatus shown in Figure 5 at varying ambient pressures and power input to the transducer. After 5 min the suspension was centrifuged for 10 min at 6000 g and total nitrogen estimated in the supernatent. Disintegration is expressed as per cent of the nitrogen released when all cells are disintegrated.

Figure 5, taken from a recent paper (Neppiras and Hughes, 1964), shows the effect of hydrostatic pressure at different sound intensities on cell breakage; the results agree fairly well with the prediction of the classical equations describing cavitation (Noltingk and Neppiras, 1950, 1951). Cavitation, when induced by the higher power levels and at high ambient pressures, appears to be more violent than at the lower powers and pressures. The effects of viscosity and surface tension also agree with the equations, that is, increasing viscosity and decreasing surface tension suppress cell breakage at a given power input (Hughes, 1962). Added nuclei in the form of various powders increased cell breakage only slightly where adequate access of air was present but increased breakage two- to threefold where access of air was limited (Table I). Solid nuclei-carrying air bubbles, such as diatomaceous earth, were the most effective in this respect. These observations confirm that cavitation is essential for cell breakage under these conditions.

TABLE I. THE EFFECT OF ADDED NUCLEI ON YEAST DISINTEGRATION.[1]

A 1:6 (w/v) yeast was treated with the output from a titanium probe for 4.5 min.[2] In Experiment A, 10 ml of suspension was treated in a tube 3.5-cm wide; in Experiment B, 10 ml of suspension was treated in a vessel 5-cm wide which allowed free access of air. In both cases, 0.1 g of powder was added. Disintegration was estimated by weighing the total solid released into the supernatent after centrifugation for 10 min at 6000 × g.

Powder added	*Temperature* °C	*Dry weight in super* *Experiment A*	*Experiment B*
None	17	14.8	45
Norite	19	17.6	47.5
Hyflo supercel	23	28.6	45
Powdered glass	23	28.3	51.5
Powdered glass [3]	23	26.1	–
Embacel	25	30.1	51

[1] Neppiras and Hughes, 1963.

[2] Sound intensity is difficult to define in this case since the system is one in which intense cavitation is taking place. Total sound output is of the order of 200 w.

[3] Powdered glass had been treated with a carbon tetrachloride solution of silicone and then heated at 100°C for 5 min to render it nonwettable.

The collapse or implosion of cavities has been predicted to be responsible for most of the biological effects of cavitation. Of these, free radical information which occurs toward the end of the collapse (Jarman, 1960) has been shown to be particularly injurious to biological material (Hughes, 1962). For instance, a crystalline enzyme, alcohol dehydrogenase, was found to be inactive after exposure to a cavitating solution for a period of only a few seconds. That this enzyme is more stable in cell extracts was shown to be due to the presence of natural free scavengers in the cells such as glutathione. Such compounds, if added to the purified enzyme, will protect it against the rapid inactivation due to free radical attack. Thus, there seems to be little doubt that, in certain cases, injurious effects associated with violent collapse-type cavitation are due to free radical attack. We became interested therefore in determining if such violent cavitation was, in fact, necessary for cell breakage. Experiments with various systems which produce different rates of free radical formation showed that there can be widely different rates of free radical formation in systems which produce similar levels of cell breakage (Hughes and Rodgers, 1960). Thus, free radical formation and cell breakage were independent (see also Grabar, 1958).

It was at this stage that we started to work with Dr. Nyborg, during his stay in England. Dr. Nyborg has already discussed some of the work concerned with the effect of shearing around bubbles, and I would like to discuss first this aspect of the research. As indicated in Figure 6, we measured the amount of cell breakage (as shown by the release of protein from cells) in the presence of bubbles formed at the base of a vibrating probe in which small holes had been drilled. The measurements were also made with a probe without holes. In addition, we measured the amount of free radical formation with this system, and, as you can see, this occurs suddenly at about an amplitude of 6.3 μ. At this stage, a sudden increase of noise was noticed, as well as the formation of discrete so-called cavitation streamers from the bubbles already on this probe. We are fairly convinced that it is at this stage that the violent collapse of bubbles occurs. The effects on DNA (MW $= 9 \times 10^6$) were also compared in this system. The figure also illustrates the different effects of liquid shear and free radical formation on the breakdown of polymeric DNA. Bubble activity, in the absence of free radicals, splits the DNA molecule across the backbone of phosphate-sugar linkages and reduces viscosity, whereas free radicals break the hydrogen bonding between nucleotides and thus increase the absorption at 260 mμ. The decrease in the viscosity was not accompanied by any increase of the absorption at 260 mμ of the DNA. Only when there was free radical formation was any increase at 260 mμ noted. These two graphs separate quite clearly what is tentatively suggested by the work of Doty (1958), who has shown that when the free radical scavengers are added during the ultrasonic treatment of DNA, there is no increase of 260-mμ absorption. It is surprising that the breakdown of DNA occurs so readily at the low amplitudes we used. These results demonstrate that both cell

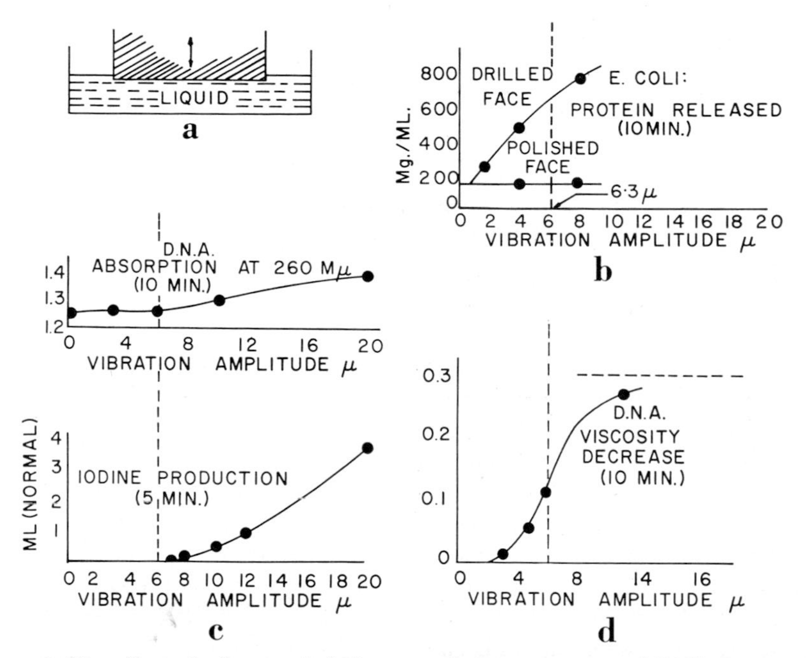

FIGURE 6. The effect of vibrating bubbles on cell disintegration and DNA denaturation (see Hughes and Nyborg, 1962). (a): cross-section of a 2-cm diameter brass probe drilled with fifty holes of 200-μ diameter and depth. (b): the disintegration of *E. coli* by drilled probe compared to the effect of a similar probe cut with a highly polished face. Disintegration was estimated by measuring the protein released from the cells into solution. (c): effect of vibration amplitude on: (1) DNA absorption at 260 mμ. The absorption of DNA is expressed as the optical density with a 1-cm light path and (2) free radical formation as measured by I_2 release from KI. (d): effect of vibration amplitude on viscosity of DNA solution expressed as a fractional decrease.

breakage and damage to a polymer such as DNA can occur at very low pressure amplitudes of sound. Such low pressures are not in the range associated with the typical collapse-type cavitation and its attendant phenomena, such as free radical formation. We suggest that the observed damage is caused by the shear stress set up by the rapid streaming around the vibrating bubbles. Such streaming (cavitation microstreaming) has been shown by Nyborg and his collaborators to bring about a number of physical and chemical changes (Elder, 1959).

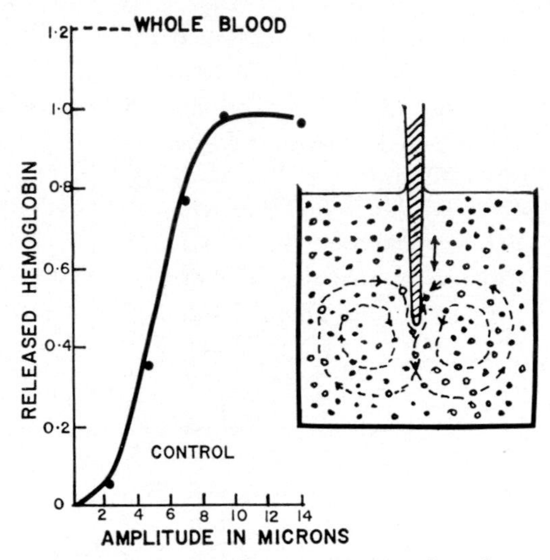

FIGURE 7. The effect of sonically induced streaming around a vibrating needle on human erythrocytes (from Hughes and Nyborg, 1962). A vibrating needle (end diameter: 15 μ) was driven at 85 kc/sec by a barium titanate cylinder. The needle was lowered into 0.1 ml of a 1:5(w/v) suspension in saline of freshly drawn erythrocytes. Hemoglobin was estimated spectrophotometrically in the supernatent after removing the cells by centrifugation.

In order to determine whether such streaming motions could cause damage to biological material, several types of material were tested with a vibrating needle designed to produce streaming in the absence of bubbles. Such liquid streaming was found to bring about the release of hemoglobin from suspension of erythrocytes (Fig. 7) without causing major damage to the cells as judged by light microscopy. A suspension of a typical bacterium, *E. coli*, was also found to be damaged, but very slowly when compared to the high-intensity treatments usually employed for these tougher organisms. It is noteworthy that the needle tip became coated with empty cells (Hughes and Nyborg, 1962). It was possible to produce various degrees of injury to the protozoan *Tetrahymena geleii* ranging from reversible inhibition of motility to complete destruction of visible cell structure. These effects depended directly on the amplitude of the sound.

There is also the possibility that internal streaming, which Dyer and Nyborg (1960) have demonstrated, may also produce damage before the catastrophic rupture of outer cell membranes. This is suggested by Figure 8 which shows time constants of the release into solution of various cell components from yeast treated in a 500-w cell distintegrator (Neppiras and Hughes, 1963).

The most striking feature is the release of some soluble enzymes and material such as small nucleotides very early on in the process. This suggests that damage to some permeability barrier occurs prior to rupture of the cell wall. In this connection, I should like to mention some very preliminary experiments which Professor Warwick and I carried out last year which showed that brain quickly lost its ability to extrude sodium when treated by focused ultrasound for short periods. These studies were performed on rat lobes which were irradiated for 2 to 5 sec with a focused 3 Mc source of 3000 w/cm^2. The tissue lost K^+ and gained Na^+ and water. Some such interference with Na^+ and K^+ transport could easily be caused by disorientation of the enzymic and structural makeup of the plasma membrane. For instance, it appears from the work of Whittam (1962) and others that membrane-bound ATPase or other enzymes (Hokin and Hokin, 1960) are concerned with Na^+ and K^+ transport. Interference with these enzymes in the membrane may affect permeability and the maintenance of ionic balance. Even stretching the membrane may do this. Such damage can only be satisfactorily studied by biochemical techniques; even electron microscopy is not subtle enough as yet to detect it. Most of the classical histochemical methods lack the specificity and

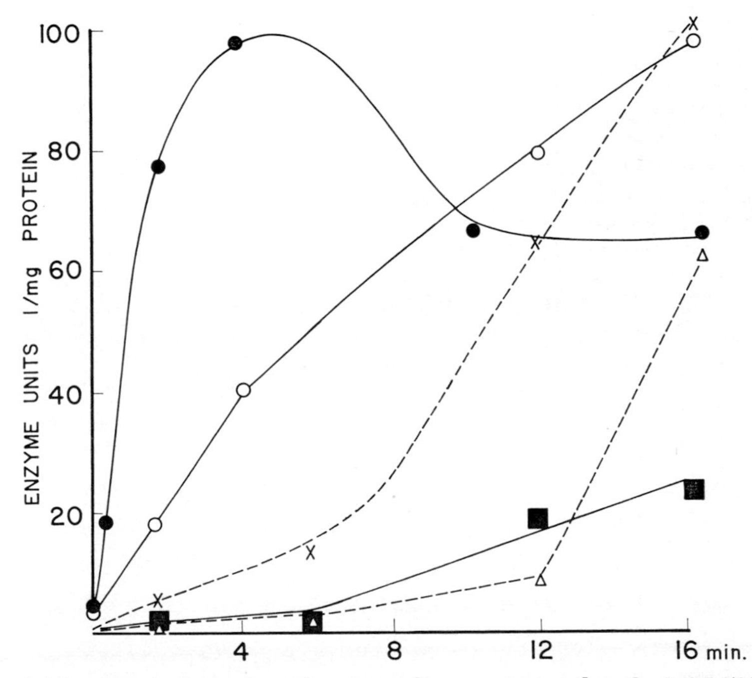

FIGURE 8. The release of protein and enzymes from yeast treated in the MSE 500-w cell disintegrator. Protein was estimated by the Folin reagent, alcohol dehydrogenase (Racker, 1949); succinic dehydrogenase, fumarase (Massey, 1955); aconitase (Green *et al.*, 1955). Enzyme activity is expressed in arbitrary units/mg protein. Protein, O———O; alcohol dehydrogenase, ●———●; aconitase, X— — —X; fumarase, △– – – – – –△; succinic dehydrogenase, ■———■.

resolution to detect anything but the consequences of the presence of the lesion, which may appear in a very much later stage.

To summarize, we have shown that the collapse stage of cavitation is not necessary for disintegrating cells, including bacteria. The experiments with vibrating bubbles and needles suggest that the streaming motions which they induce in the suspending liquid are sufficient to injure cells and, if sufficiently high sound pressures are employed, to disintegrate them. I have discussed briefly some collaborative experiments in which both physicists and biochemists have studied the physical mechanism of damage to cells by sonically induced cavitation. Some of our preliminary experiments and their biological implications have been mentioned in an attempt to persuade you that the first detectable lesions caused by ultrasonic energy will probably be an interruption of some vital dynamic chemical process. This I would like to call a "biochemical lesion." Such a process must underlie the more gross histological changes of the cells which are generally detected after some considerable time lapse. The term "biochemical lesion" has obvious analogs when applied to other biological areas; for example, this term has been used to describe the underlying phenomena in nutritional or genetic disorders. More subtle structural relationships at the molecular level are required to explain the disturbance beyond the biochemical lesion.

REFERENCES

Dyer, H. J., and W. L. Nyborg (1960). IRE Trans. Med. Electron. *ME-7*, 163.
Doty, B., B. B. McGill, and S. H. Rice (1958). Proc. Soc. Nat. Acad. Sci. U.S., *44*, 432
Elder, S. A. (1959). J. Acoust. Soc. Am. *31*, 54.
Finean, J. B. (1957). Acta Neurol. Psychiat. Belg. *5*, 462.
Grabar, P. (1958). Advances Biol. Med. Phys. *4*, 282.
Green, D. E. (1961). V Internat. Org. Biochem. Moscow. Reprint no. 176.
Green, D. E., S. Mü, and P. M. Kouhout (1955). J. Biol. Chem. *217*, 551.
Hokin, L. E., and M. I. Hokin (1960). Internat. Rev. Neurobiol. *2*, 99.
Hughes, D. E. (1962). J. Microbiol. Biochem. Eng. & Tech. *4*, 405.
Hughes, D. E. (1962a). J. Gen. Microbiol. *29*, 39.
Hughes, D. E., and W. L. Nyborg (1962). Science *138*, 108.
Hughes, D. E., and A. Rodgers (1960). Med. Electron., London, p. 347.
Jarman, P. (1960). J. Acoust. Soc. Am. *32*, 1459.
Massey, V. (1955). Methods in Enzymology *1*, 729.
Neppiras, E. A., and D. E. Hughes (1964). J. Biotech. & Bioeng. *6*, 247.
Noltingk, B. E., and E. A. Neppiras (1950). Proc. Phys. Soc. London., 63b.
Noltingk, B. E., and E. A. Neppiras (1951). Proc. Phys. Soc. London., 64b, 1032.
Racker, E. (1949). J. Biol. Chem. *184*, 313.
Robertson, J. D. (1960). Progress in Biophys. *10*, 343.
Whittam, R. (1962). Biochem. J. *83*, 29P.
Young, R. R., and E. Henneman (1961). Science *134*, 1521.

DISCUSSION

DR. W. J. FRY: Is there a point on those graphs where you would say effects are reversible?

Dr. Hughes: We have attempted to measure the viability of yeast and bacteria, but the measurements are unprecise compared with the measurements that we made of enzymes and other cellular material. We found no marked change in viability until the leakage of the more diffusible components is almost complete, when some permeability barrier must be ruptured fairly completely and the cells become nonviable. At this stage the process cannot be reversible.

Dr. W. J. Fry: Some of this is still reversible?

Dr. Hughes: We have indications that it may be, but this particular aspect has not yet been studied in detail.

Dr. W. J. Fry: You mentioned that you had a problem determining what fraction of the cells is affected; can't you carry out further studies to determine this?

Dr. Hughes: The work with bubbles and needles is on a scale which is considered by most biochemists to be at the ultramicro level; at the moment further refinement would not be possible. What we would like to have is an apparatus which is capable of treating larger volumes of cell suspension uniformly. Expressing enzyme activity as specific activity instead of total activity tends to discount the idea that just a small fraction of the cells are leaking. If this were so, then the protein and other constituents would come out at the same rate from the cells. We find differences between the rates of leakage and cell disappearance.

Dr. W. J. Fry: I see that you would get differential rates, but I'm not quite sure that I see how you eliminate the difficulties associated with the fact that you are working with a large population of cells. What part of the observed result is determined by cells breaking completely and what per cent is determined by cells leaking?

Dr. Hughes: Let's say that 20% of the cells were so weak that they broke completely during the first few moments; then the proportion of escaping components would be the same as when 40% or 100% were broken.

Dr. W. J. Fry: Let's say they started to leak.

Dr. Hughes: Oh, if they started to leak, then we should get such events as we actually find; that is, material appears in solution at different rates suggesting that everything doesn't come out at once.

Dr. W. J. Fry: Yes, I see that. But how do you decide that the time rate is related to the rate per cell or the fact that the cells are diffusing?

Dr. Hughes: This is one criticism of these kinds of results. However, the time constants for leakage and cell disappearance indicate that the leakage of smaller cell components is greater than that expected if only a few of the cells were broken completely.

Dr. W. J. Fry: By the way, what was the frequency of the sound applied in the brain studies and what sound dosage was given?

Dr. Hughes: It was 3 Mc, whereas most of the work I've described with cell suspensions is in the 20-kc range. The time of treatment was from a fraction of a second up to 5 sec of unpulsed sound at about 1 kw/cm^2. Effects due to heat cannot therefore be ruled out.

Dr. W. J. Fry: Do you make measurements to determine what changes you get if you heat the cells?

Dr. Hughes: Yes. A 5° rise in temperature in brain tissue could possibly produce the changes we find in sodium and potassium content.

Dr. W. J. Fry: Did you notice any gross change in the hydration of the cells? For instance, did you see a swelling?

Dr. Hughes: Yes, the measured edema is found a few minutes after treatment.

Dr. W. J. Fry: Is the animal then sacrificed?

Dr. Hughes: Yes, sacrificed almost immediately. We cut the lesion out as well as possible and estimate the wet and dry weight. Na^+ and K^+ are estimated by flame photometry.

Dr. W. J. Fry: You said you did electron micrograph studies. What were the results?

Dr. Hughes: In yeast and bacteria we detect no gross damage to the cells unless complete rupture of the wall occurs. Two mechanisms might be suggested for changes in permeability to be effective. One is by punching a hole through the membrane, and the other is by interfering with the transport mechanism itself which is controlled by orientation of membrane components. If the transport system is altered slightly, this itself might be reversible. Alternatively, if holes were made right through the membrane this would probably not be reversible. We have looked for holes through the membrane in the electron microscope but have not detected such changes even in badly leaking preparations.

Dr. W. J. Fry: I was thinking of the effects on mitochondria.

Dr. Hughes: Mitochondria might be better to use, and we have this in mind since they can perform work on ion transport and concentrate potassium against an electrochemical gradient.

Dr. Curtis: Have you attempted to see if you could alter this process of cell disruption by providing a source of chemical protection against radiation?

Dr. Hughes: Only by adding glutathione or some other sulphydryl compound like cysteine when we know we have high rates of free radical formation. Under these circumstances, the added reagent does not affect the rate of cell breakage. It does affect the rate of enzyme inactivation of those enzymes whose activity depends on S-S or SH linkages. Free radical scavengers do not affect the rate of inactivation of all enzymes since some of them are also inactivated by shearing (Hughes, 1962).

Dr. Curtis: I was thinking in terms of more subtle action which might be affected by force.

Dr. Hughes: We haven't been able to detect that. There is no doubt that the yeast breaks at the budding scar. This is a place where apparently the wall is not knit together, and there needs to be some further bonding by the action of compounds affecting disulphide bonds. We have not been able to detect the effect of these on the rates of breakage. We find that carbohydrates are released from the walls of yeast at a fairly constant rate (Hughes, 1962).

Dr. Carson: You mentioned the possibility of investigating the apparent change in the membrane. Could the physical change in the membrane be due to a strong shearing action?

DR. HUGHES: The effect of sound in causing a leakage of nucleotides is very much like the effect of adding detergents which are bound by the plasma membrane and appear to make it leaky. A violent stirring of the solution, which Dr. Nyborg found affected chemical reactions, would probably not affect the permeability of cells because these properties depend on active processes and not on diffusion alone. Active transport is connected with chemical reactions which are concerned with the breakdown and rebuilding of phosphate bonds inside the membrane. It is possible to interfere with these types of reactions and thus to affect transport both by chemical and physical methods.

DR. WOEBER: But are the leakages of this type very slow in normal cells?

DR. HUGHES: Oh, yes. For instance, growing or even dividing cells appear not to leak at all.

DR. WOEBER: Are these enzymes attacked quickly? Both in the intact cell and pure solution?

DR. HUGHES: No, the isolated crystalline enzymes are attacked very quickly, but in the intact cell the enzymes are not attacked quickly because of the free radical scavengers and other proteins which are also present in the cell.

DR. CARSON: One of the early slides was on the effect of pressure. Would you discuss in a little more detail the various parameters involved?

DR. HUGHES: Ambient pressure in the apparatus shown in Figure 6 is expressed as pounds per square inch with 15 lb as atmospheric pressure. The 20 w and the 10 w are the electrical power of the transducer. The amplitude was measured by means of a barium titanate zirconate crystal on the top of the transducer. It's interesting that we first noticed the differential leakage of material in these kinds of experiments. For instance, the nucleotides come out at low ambient pressures and before other major damage is detected. The alcohol dehydrogenase also comes out early and is all out after 6 min of treatment, whereas about 20 min are needed for full disruption when a total of 80% of cell protein is released.

DR. WEISSLER: What are the values of the sonic pressure at various points along there?

DR. HUGHES: The accurate translation of acoustic power from the input power was difficult because of the change in efficiency with ambient pressure. Estimation of this indicated an efficiency of about 30% at the cavitation suppression values which at atmospheric pressure is approximately 0.3 to 0.5 w/cm^2. This is discussed more fully elsewhere (Neppiras and Hughes, 1964).

DR. W. J. FRY: Do you feel you are changing the membrane or making changes inside the cell?

DR. HUGHES: I think there is good evidence that mechanisms concerned with permeability were affected very quickly during ultrasonic treatments of the cells. We know that these are bound in the membrane. As indicated by the leakage of nucleotides and enzymes, permeability is affected before any drastic breakage, which is indicated by the further leakage of other enzymes, especially those bound to the mitochondria, such as succinic dehydrogenase.

DR. W. J. FRY: Do you feel that this is all reversible?

DR. HUGHES: I think there is a good chance that the first changes in permeability are reversible. This might well explain the reversibility of lesions in nerve tissue which you observed in 1958 and Young and Henneman (1961) observed recently in nerve blocking. I think this might be found to be the first or underlying biochemical lesion.

DR. KELLY: What section of the rat brain did you use for your chemical studies?

DR. HUGHES: We treated either the left or right dorsal area, middle region of the anterior part of the cerebral hemisphere. A piece of tissue removed at the same time from the opposite lobe served as a control.

DR. KELLY: You did not study the adjacent area of the lesion?

DR. HUGHES: We studied the adjacent areas of the tissue because we wanted to know how well we were locating the lesion. In some experiments, we were not always able to cut out the lesion precisely. Of a total of five experiments, in three cases we did not excise the lesion very accurately and even in the other two cases there is some doubt that we excised the lesion precisely.

3

Some Aspects of Ultrasonic Cavitation

YOSHIMITSU KIKUCHI, HIROSHI SHIMIZU, and DAITARO OKUYAMA
Research Institute of Electrical Communication, Tohoku University, Sendai, Japan

Introduction by Dr. von Gierke

Our next speaker is Dr. Yoshimitsu Kikuchi of Sendai, Japan. As many of you know, Dr. Kikuchi, who is an electrical engineer, has worked on a variety of acoustic problems. His interests range from the physical aspects of acoustics, such as studies in the field of sonar, to medical applications, such as the use of ultrasound as a diagnostic tool. Later during this symposium, Dr. Kikuchi's colleague, Dr. Wagai, will talk to us regarding the medical work. Now, we are privileged to hear Dr. Kikuchi discuss his work in the field of ultrasonic cavitation.

1. INTRODUCTION

A number of research workers have been engaged in a study of ultrasonic cavitation for many years, but quantitative descriptions of the phenomena are so difficult that such descriptions are still unavailable. The present authors have also been investigating this phenomena for several years, as already indicated in the Third International Congress on Acoustics, and are convinced that a description of ultrasonic cavitation can be obtained by measurements of the variation of acoustic radiation resistance of the sound source into the cavitating medium (1). In the above referenced proceedings it is shown that ultimate acoustic outputs which cause cavitation, but do not cause any mechanical damage to the transducer, are very much dependent on radiation resistance characteristics measured in such liquids as water and other liquid media.

The extensive investigations carried out during the past 3 years have disclosed that the form of the variation of radiation resistance has a close and decisive connection with such phenomena as acoustic saturation or cavitation power. It may be said that no better method has been found, up to the present time, than the method proposed here for describing ultrasonic cavitation phenomena, insofar as the phenomena are related to the sound source.

Additional observations have been made, for both continuous wave radiation and pulsed radiation, of the effect on radiation resistance of the amount of dissolved air in the liquid medium, as well as the effect of the ultrasonic frequency. The radiation resistance always decreases considerably with the onset of cavitation. The first datum on this finding was reported by the present authors in 1959 (1, 2). In this paper, however, primarily the data obtained since that time will be discussed.

2. ANECHOIC WATER VESSEL FOR ACOUSTIC MEASUREMENTS

The water vessels used for acoustic measurements are anechoic containers, inside of which there are a number of wooden wedges covering the entire surface. If the frequency of the ultrasonic wave is as low as 20 kc, then the vessel must be as large as the one shown in Figure 1, which contains 1.2 tons of water. Figure 2 shows an automatic device for continuous degassification which was developed by the present authors in order to control the amount of dissolved air in the water at any desired value. The electric boiler heats the water to a specified temperature, and air bubbles are introduced into the heated water through a special device placed in the water in order that the dissolved gas concentration may quickly approach equilibrium at the desired temperature. After such treatment, the water passes through cooling vessels connected in cascade and then flows into the anechoic vessel after it has been cooled almost to room temperature. The cooling medium is the tap water itself which is to be degassified finally in the boiler. With this heat exchange, the heat efficiency of this device is excellent: with 8 kw of electricity the device can produce 150 l of degassified water per hour, even when it is adjusted for a very low air content, for example, as low as 5% of saturation at room temperature.

3. A CONVENIENT METHOD FOR MEASUREMENT OF AIR CONCENTRATION OF WATER

Figure 3 indicates the technique applied for measurement of dissolved air content of the water. A flask containing the sampled water is connected to a water-jet pump, to encounter a gradually decreasing pressure. When the initiation of a few air bubbles is observed inside the flask, the corresponding pressure value at this instant is the indication of the dissolved air concentration. The instant of bubble initiation can be determined very precisely if the sampled water in the flask is shaken once or twice and a weak ultrasonic vibration (approximately 1 cm/sec at 30 kc) is applied intermittently to the bottom of the flask during the observation. The accuracy of this method is sufficient for the present investigation.

4. TYPICAL CHARACTERISTICS OF RADIATION RESISTANCE AT HIGH SOUND LEVELS

Ultrasonic transducers used for the observation of radiation resistance characteristics are ferrite magnetostrictive vibrators with the radiation surface immersed directly in a liquid medium. Figure 4 indicates typical radiation resistance values obtained for an applied ultrasonic frequency of 28 kc, with water which has been degassed so that its dissolved air concentration

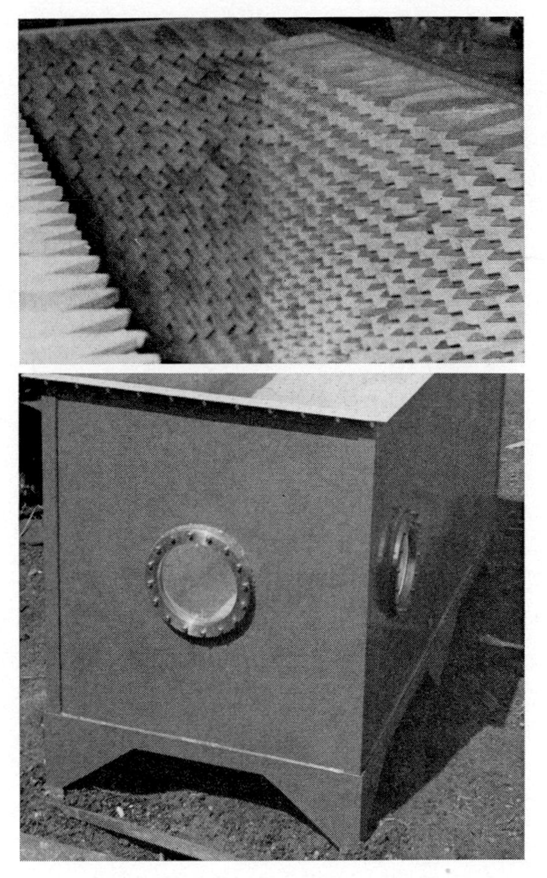

FIGURE 1. Anechoic water vessel.

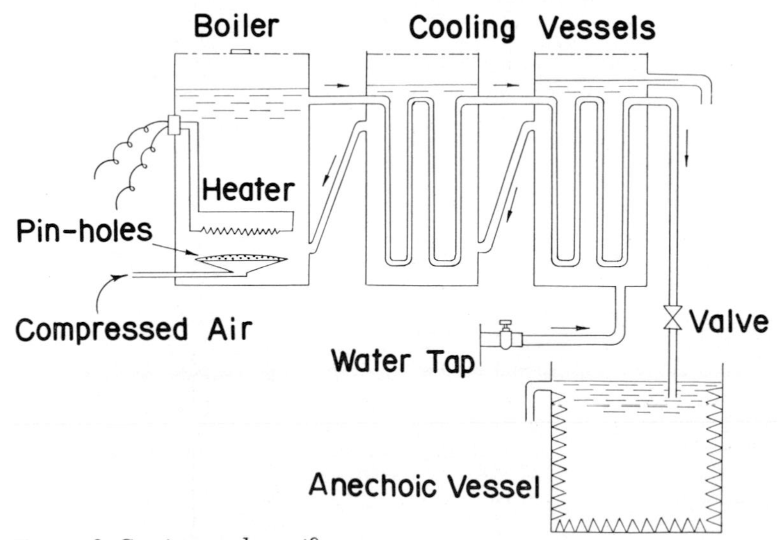

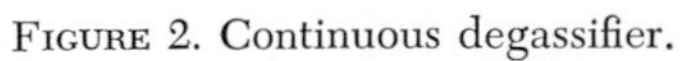

FIGURE 2. Continuous degassifier.

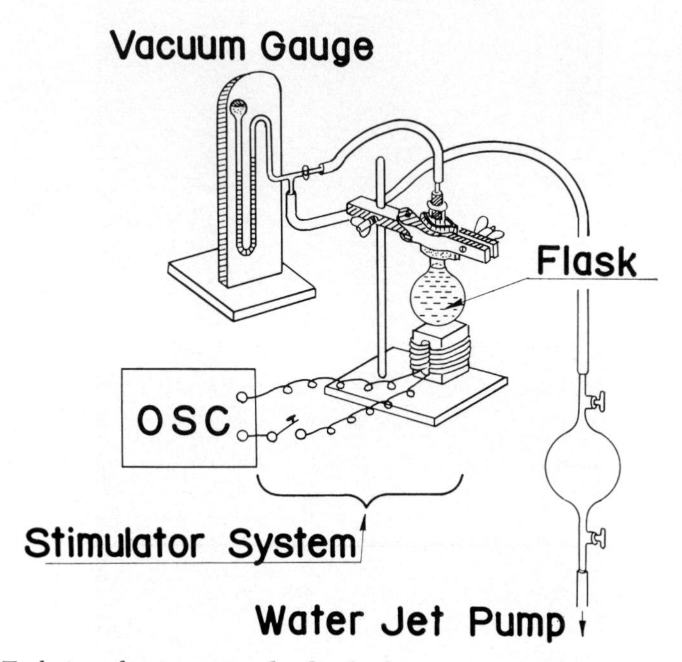

FIGURE 3. Technique for measuring the dissolved air concentration in water.

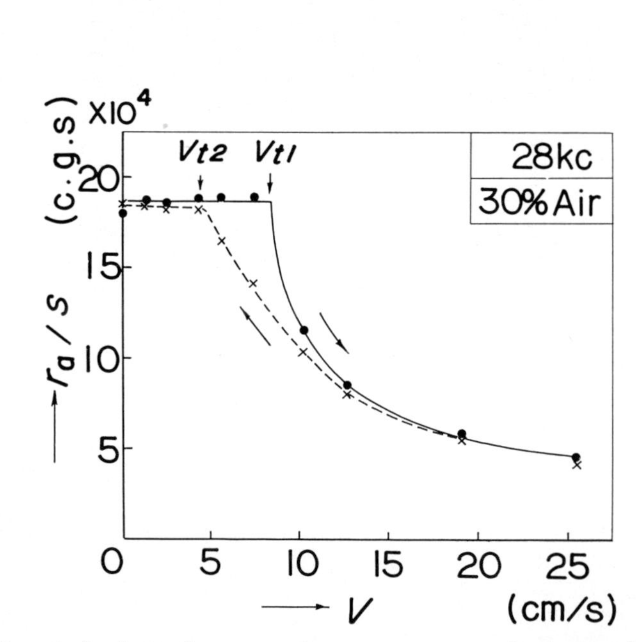

FIGURE 4. A typical relation between radiation resistance and vibrational velocity of a radiating surface. r_a, radiation resistance; S, area of radiating surface; v, vibrational velocity amplitude (r.m.s.), v_{t1}, first critical velocity; v_{t2}, second critical velocity.

is 30% of the nominal concentration in the saturated state at room temperature. The ordinate is the value of radiation resistance per unit area of the vibrating surface which oscillates in piston motion, and the abscissa is the vibrational velocity of the motion. With the increase of the vibrational velocity v,[1] the radiation resistance r_a begins to fall in a steep slope, so that its curve shows a definite change in slope or a sharp bend at a certain vibrational velocity, indicated by v_{t1}, which the present authors like to designate "critical velocity." At approximately this value of the velocity, the typical hissing noise of cavitation becomes audible, and oscillating small bubbles appear on the vibrating surface of the transmitter. With further increase of the vibrational velocity, the value of the radiation resistance approaches a value which is one-fifth to one-sixth of the starting value. When the velocity is decreased from this state of intense cavitation, a hysteresis appears in the characteristics (as shown by a broken line in Fig. 4) which returns to the original value at a certain velocity, indicated as v_{t2}, which is designated as "second critical velocity."

5. CAVITATION POINT

The same type of bend of the radiation resistance curve appears in almost every case, even when the conditions of observation are widely varied. Moreover, it is almost certain that this bend corresponds to the so-called cavitation point where cavitation either begins to appear or just vanishes. It is of interest to note there are very few methods which indicate the cavitation point so precisely as does this technique. The usual method is dependent on a graph of sound pressure amplitude vs driving current or voltage applied to the transducer, with the initiation of cavitation identified as the point at which the curve begins to deviate from a straight line. Generally, however, the departure point is not clear because the curve deviates gradually. In addition, such curves can exhibit a bend or change in slope when no cavitation exists since the change in slope can originate from the nonlinearities in the force factor and the internal mechanical resistance of the transmitter itself. In contrast, the method proposed here enables one to observe the sound pressure with reference to the vibrational velocity of the radiation surface. Therefore, the observation is independent of the internal characteristics of the transducer, and this independence may in part account for the very precise indication of the cavitation point.

6. DEFINITION OF RADIATION RESISTANCE

Radiation resistance was defined originally in relation to a phenomenon of infinitesimally small amplitudes as follows: denote $\bar{p}$ as a pressure averaged along the entire radiation surface, and S as the area of the surface; then, the reaction force F of the medium, acting on the surface, is expressed by Equation (1) as follows:

$$F = \bar{p}S. \tag{1}$$

This force is proportional to the alternating velocity, v, of the radiation surface so long as the physical nature of the acoustic medium does not vary with the

[1] v = vibrational velocity amplitude (r.m.s.).

increase of the sound pressure. The coefficient of this proportion is the radiation resistance, insofar as the radiation surface is large compared to the wavelength in the medium, and denoted usually by r_a, as shown in Equation (2).

$$r_a = \frac{F}{v} = \frac{\bar{p}}{v} S. \qquad (2)$$

When the vibration increases to such a large amplitude that the medium loses its linear nature, higher harmonic components appear in the sound pressure even when the vibrational velocity of the radiation surface is keeping its sinusoidal feature. The radiation resistance in this nonlinear state can be defined by the same equation, if the fundamental components of the sound pressure and the alternating velocity are always employed in the places $\bar{p}$ and v respectively. The vibrational velocity of the radiation surface is almost sinusoidal, so long as a magnetostrictive vibrator is used as a transducer in a liquid medium at its mechanical resonance. Consequently, Equation (2) seems to show that the radiation resistance r_a could be obtained by measuring only the averaged sound pressure $\bar{p}$. It is impossible, however, to measure the value of $\bar{p}$ without disturbing the sound field in front of the transducer. Therefore, a method was developed for measuring this value from the electrical side of an ultrasonic transducer. The details of this method were presented by the present authors at the Annual Meeting of the Acoustical Society of America (3) and may be briefly summarized as follows: when cavitation exists, the resulting variation of the acoustic radiation resistance r_a appears as a variation of a certain electrical value at the electric terminal of a transducer since the radiation resistance is the final loading on the transducer. The method is such that the variation of the electrical value which is directly related to the mechanical load is extracted quantitatively from other electrical deviations caused by nonlinearities of the transducer system, so that one can obtain the mechanical alternating values by the extracted variation of the electrical values.

7. RELATION OF ACOUSTIC POWER IN THE CASE OF CAVITATION

The acoustic power output of the transducer can be estimated from the radiation resistance characteristics measured as indicated above, with respect to various vibrational velocities of the surface. The acoustic power output P_a is as follows:

$$P_a = r_a v^2. \qquad (3)$$

A characteristic curve of the power output, represented by a thick line, is shown in Figure 5. In this case, the solid line curve in Figure 4 is employed as the characteristics of the resistance r_a in the equation. The power output is proportional to the square of the velocity in the range where the velocity is small. But in the range where the velocity exceeds the critical velocity v_{t1}, the power becomes approximately proportional to the velocity. This fact is of considerable interest and importance in regard to applications of ultrasonic energy.

The thin line in Figure 5 represents the characteristics of the averaged pressure $\bar{p}$, which can also be easily derived from the radiation resistance. After the initiation of cavitation the average pressure shows no further increase although the acoustic power output shows a continuous increase.

These facts give rise to an interesting question, namely, what are the characteristics of the power of sound waves which are located some distance from the sound source? Figure 6 shows the characteristic curve of sound

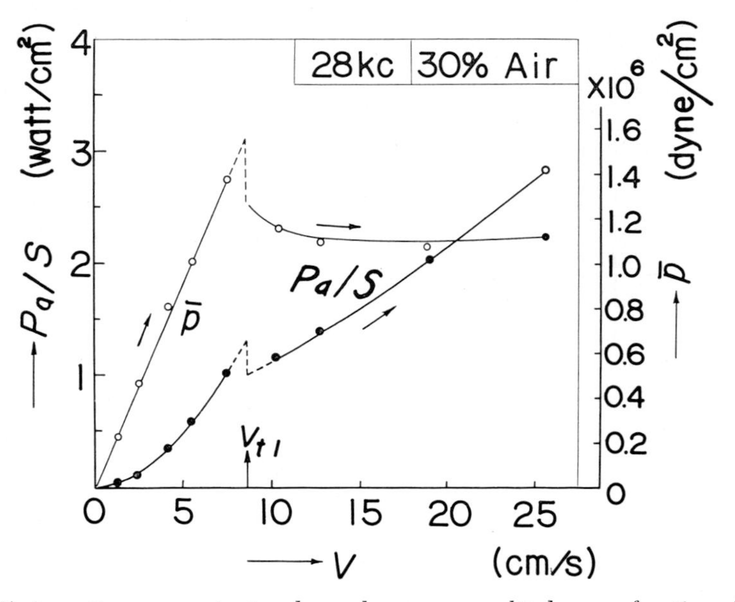

FIGURE 5. Acoustic power output and sound pressure amplitude, as a function of vibrational velocity. P_a, acoustic power output; S, area of radiating surface; $\bar{p}$, average sound pressure on the radiating surface; v, vibrational velocity amplitude (r.m.s.).

pressure p_1, which is the fundamental component of the sound wave observed at a certain distance from the transducer. The last two curves below this curve are the radiation resistance of the transducer and the averaged sound pressure on the radiation surface, respectively. These are measured simultaneously with the former. The curve of p_1 tends to a complete saturation after departure from a straight line at the cavitation point, which corresponds to the sharp bend in the middle curve. Both saturations of p_1 and $\bar{p}$ occur at approximately the same vibrational velocity, and both curves are nearly parallel to each other over the entire range. This fact suggests that even when intense cavitation exists in the medium of propagation, the usual law that the fundamental component of the sound pressure at a distance is determined by the fundamental component of the sound pressure on the surface of a sound source may still apply. Let us assume that this law is also applicable to the acoustic power relation, although some correction may be necessary since there is a certain change in the directional characteristics (1) of the transducer when it generates an intense cavitation. Then, the following equation is obtained:

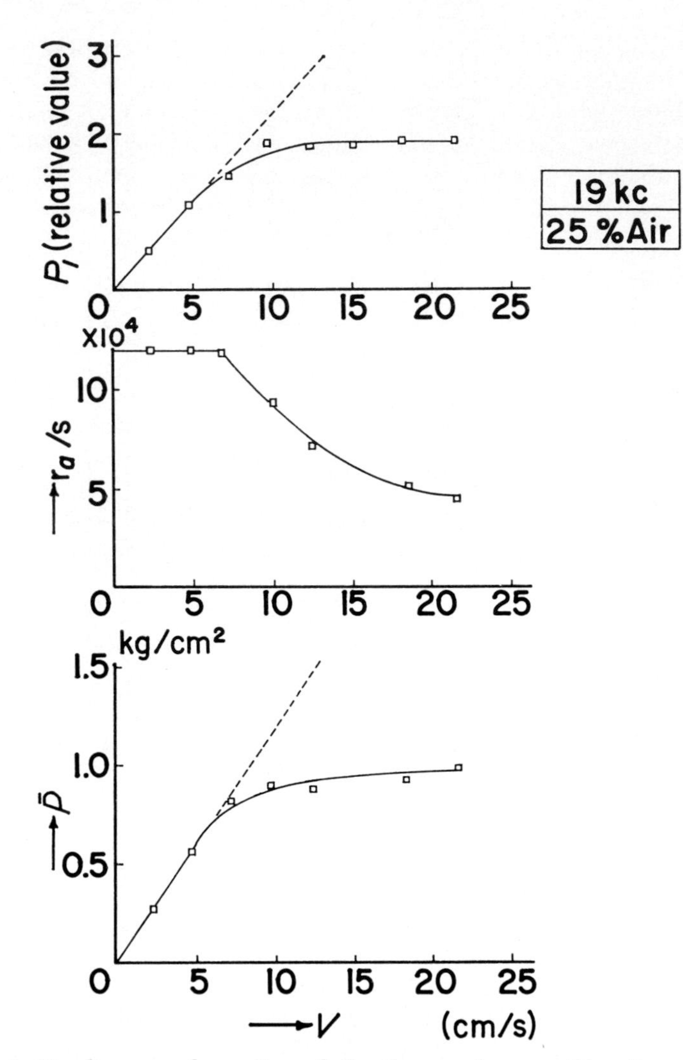

FIGURE 6. Simultaneous observation of the three major quantities. $\bar{p}$, average sound pressure on the radiating surface; p_1, fundamental component of observed sound pressure; r_a, radiation resistance; S, area of radiating surface; v, vibrational velocity amplitude (r.m.s.).

$$\frac{P_s}{S} = \frac{\bar{p}^2}{(r_a)_o/S}. \tag{4}$$

In this equation P_s is the power required for a sound source in order to produce a sound pressure p_1 at a distant point in the medium in case of no cavitation, and r_a with a subscript "zero" is the normal radiation resistance which does not decrease due to cavitation. As already indicated, however, the transducer radiates a power output P_a, which does not show a complete saturation. Then the mathematical difference between P_a and P_s, shown in Figure 7, must be the power consumed in the mechanism which generates the cavitation. From the standpoint of ultrasonic communication, this part of the power must be said to be a loss; but from the standpoint of cavitation use, this part is the useful power, as the power P_s propagates beyond the region of cavitation, although it might act as a catalyst to sustain the cavitation. In this particular case shown in Figure 7 the ratio of the useful power and the scattered power at the highest level is nearly one to one.

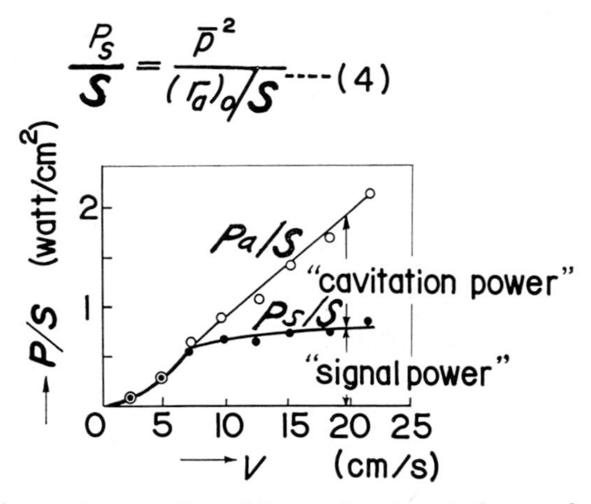

FIGURE 7. The difference between P_a and P_s as a function of vibrational velocity. P_s, power required of sound source to produce sound pressure p_1 (no cavitation); P_a, acoustic power output which the transducer radiates (cavitation present above a threshold value); $\bar{p}$, average sound pressure on the radiating surface; $(r_a)_o$, normal radiation resistance (weak vibration and no cavitation); S, area of radiating surface; v, vibrational velocity amplitude (r.m.s.).

8. CHARACTERISTICS WITH REGARD TO AIR CONCENTRATION OF THE WATER

Figure 8 shows the results obtained on radiation resistance characteristics for several kinds of water with varying amounts of dissolved air. The figure to the left shows the radiation resistance characteristics when the level of the vibrational velocity is increasing, and the figure to the right shows those when the level is decreasing. Each curve in both figures comes down to what is nearly a unique value, but each critical velocity v_{t1} or v_{t2} shifts its position toward smaller values with the increase of the air content. In Figure 9 the critical velocities are plotted with respect to air concentration of the water. The second critical velocity v_{t2} is always smaller than the first critical velocity v_{t1}.

9. CHARACTERISTICS WITH REGARD TO ULTRASONIC FREQUENCY

Figure 10 shows the frequency dependency of the radiation resistance measured in degassified water with an air concentration 29% of the saturation value. The critical velocity shifts its position toward larger values with the increase of frequency, and the extent of the decrease in resistance becomes larger with the decrease of frequency. The hysteresis, which is apparent as the driving level is decreased, has a tendency to become more prominent

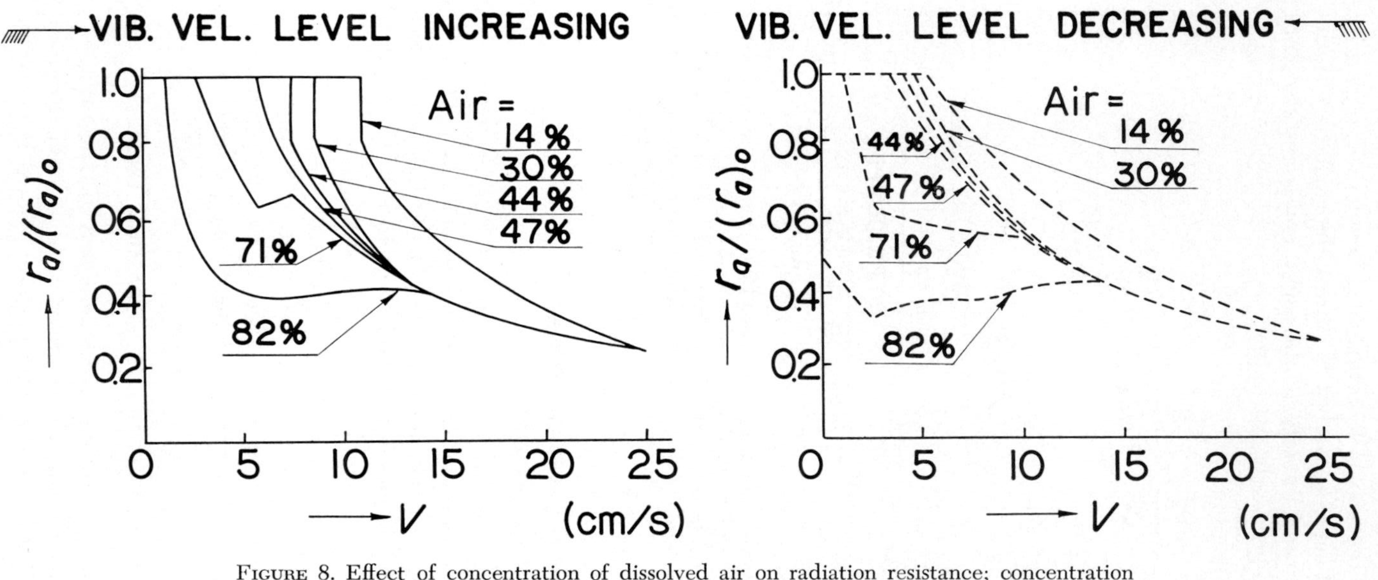

FIGURE 8. Effect of concentration of dissolved air on radiation resistance; concentration in relative percentage compared to the saturation value at room temperature. r_a, radiation resistance; $(r_a)_o$, normal radiation resistance (weak vibration and no cavitation); v, vibrational velocity amplitude (r.m.s.).

when the frequency is higher. Similar observations were made in nondegassified water with an air concentration 73% of the saturation value, as indicated in Figure 11. In comparison with Figure 10, although the critical velocities are less than those in the degassified water at every frequency, there is the same general tendency, that is, the higher the frequency, the larger the critical velocity. Figure 12 summarizes these results.

10. "SEEDING" OF CAVITATION NUCLEI

An interesting fact was found during the present experiments, namely, when the radiating surface was wiped with a finger immediately before the measurement of each point, the hysteresis between the curves for increasing driving level and for decreasing driving level disappears completely, as shown on the left in Figure 13. The figure to the right is a reference, showing the corresponding results obtained in the ordinary way.

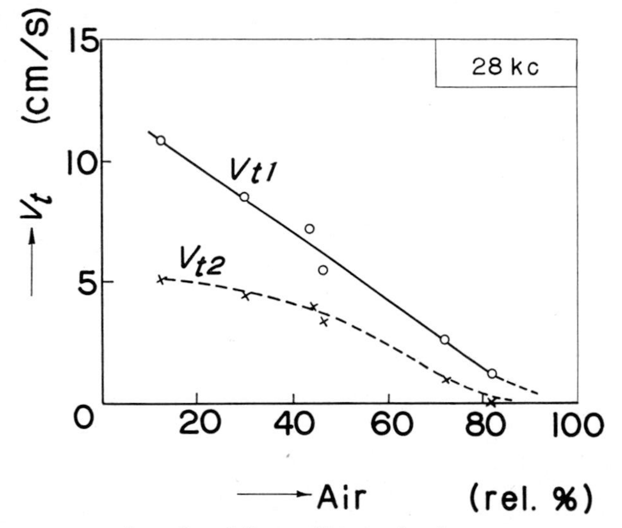

FIGURE 9. "First" and "second" critical velocities.

The present authors assume that the wiping of the radiation surface with a finger may correspond to the seeding of a number of groups of air molecules onto the radiation surface so that each group of the molecules may act as a nucleus of cavitation. In this respect, the words "seeding" and "nonseeding" are used in the figures as well as in the following description. It has been said that a number of nuclei are supplied continuously by each collapse of the cavities once a severe cavitation has occurred, and it is also said that the nuclei thus produced reduce the required sound pressure necessary to sustain the cavitation phenomenon. If this be true, then the same tendency for the reduction of sound pressure must occur during a period of increasing driving level when the supply of cavitation nuclei is sufficient. The proposed operation designated "seeding" may just correspond to this sufficient supply of the nuclei. The same observation was extended to the case of nondegassified water

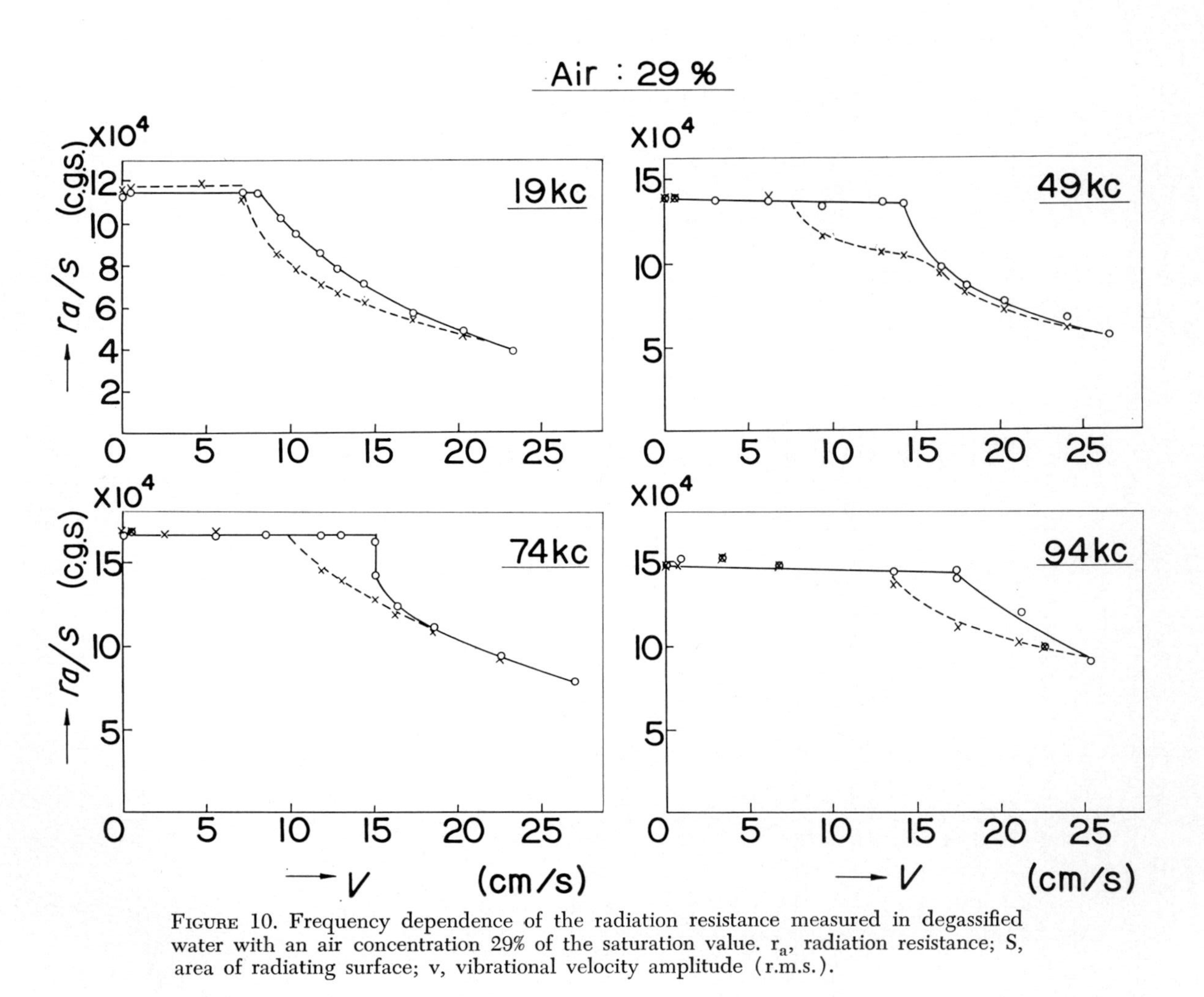

FIGURE 10. Frequency dependence of the radiation resistance measured in degassified water with an air concentration 29% of the saturation value. r_a, radiation resistance; S, area of radiating surface; v, vibrational velocity amplitude (r.m.s.).

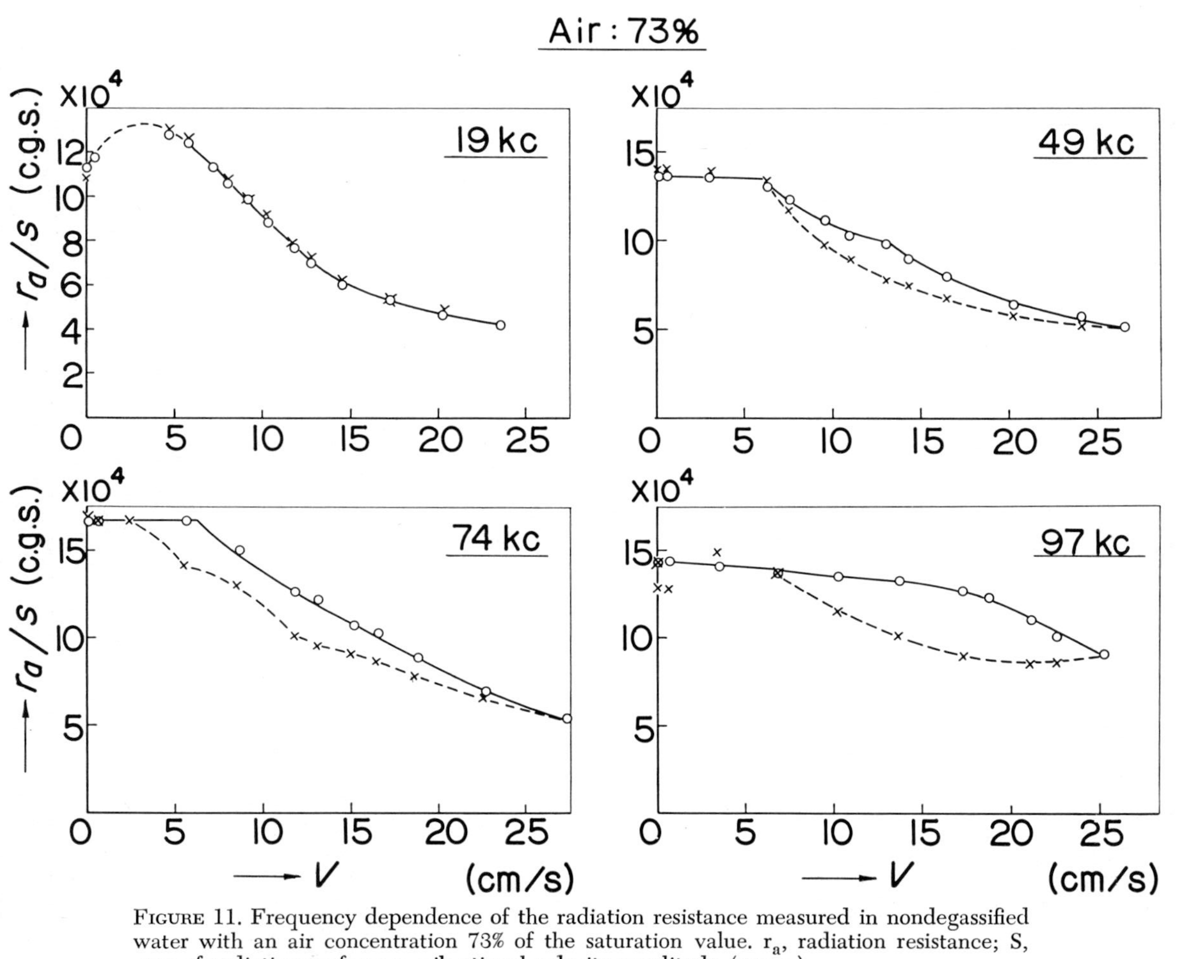

FIGURE 11. Frequency dependence of the radiation resistance measured in nondegassified water with an air concentration 73% of the saturation value. r_a, radiation resistance; S, area of radiating surface; v, vibrational velocity amplitude (r.m.s.).

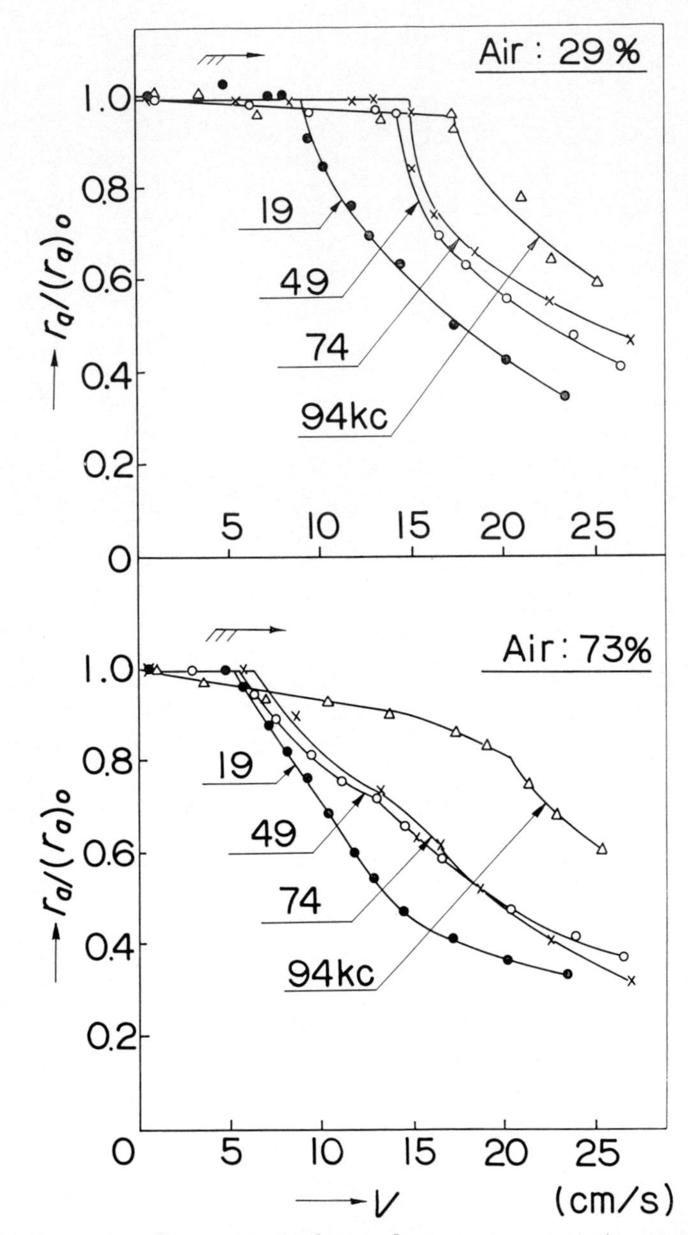

FIGURE 12. Frequency effect summarized. r_a, radiation resistance; $(r_a)_o$, normal radiation resistance (weak vibration and no cavitation); v, vibrational velocity amplitude (r.m.s.).

and also to the case of varying frequencies from 19 to 97 kc, and it was found that the "seeding" always destroys the hysteresis. It was also found that each characteristic curve in the case of seeding coincides quite well with each corresponding curve for decreasing driving level for the case of nonseeding.

It may be worthwhile to observe the characteristics of the averaged pressure $\bar{p}$ in relation to the operation of seeding. Figure 14 shows a comparison of the sound pressures at a certain high level of vibrational velocity in the case of

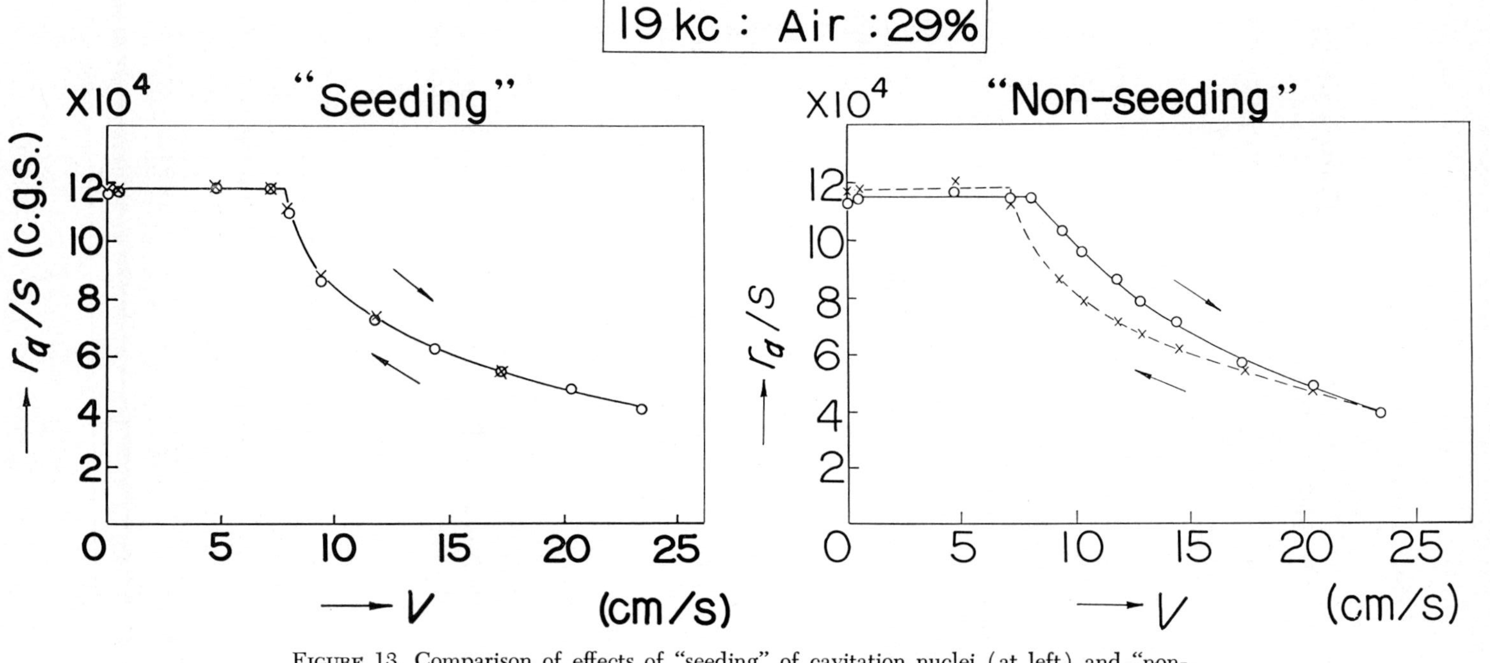

FIGURE 13. Comparison of effects of "seeding" of cavitation nuclei (at left) and "non-seeding" (at right). r_a, radiation resistance; S, area of radiating surface; v, vibrational velocity amplitude (r.m.s.).

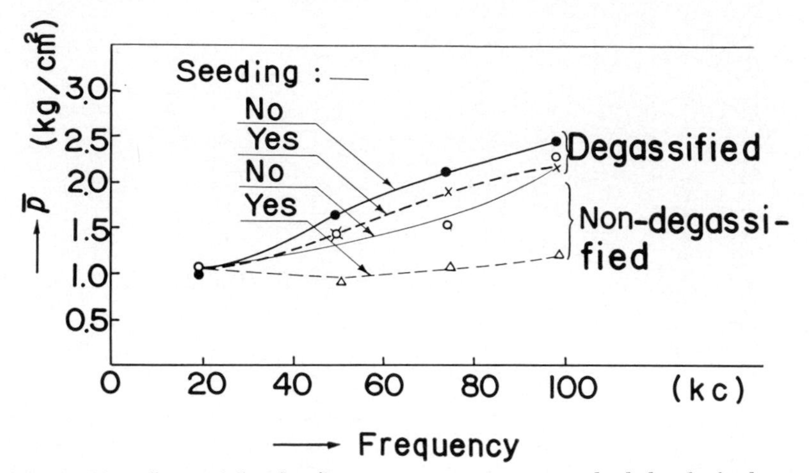

FIGURE 14. The effects of "seeding" on average pressure $\bar{p}$ at high level of vibration. $\bar{p}$, average sound pressure on the radiating surface.

seeding and nonseeding as observed in two kinds of water. The abscissa of this figure is the ultrasonic frequency in kc. The uppermost curve shown by a thick solid line is for nonseeding in degassified water with an air concentration 29% of the saturation value; the sound pressure increases with frequency and reaches a value of considerable magnitude at 97 kc. If seeding is applied, the second curve is obtained. The third and the fourth curves are those in non-degassified water, with nonseeding and seeding respectively; the effect of the seeding is the same as in the case of degassified water. It is of interest to note that the last curve is almost horizontal at a level of 1 kg/cm^2. This fact indicates that the sound pressure $\bar{p}$ in nondegassified water becomes independent of frequency when we apply the seeding operation to the radiation surface. It also means that the fundamental peak value of the sound pressure is in these cases about $\sqrt{2}$ times the atmospheric pressure. Another interesting finding is that at 19 kc the four types of sound pressure show almost no differences, irrespective of air concentration, seeding or nonseeding of the water.

11. RADIATION RESISTANCE IN THE CASE OF PULSED EXCITATION

All the previous data presented here were obtained for the case of continuous excitation. However, there are some transient phenomena of cavitation before reaching the stationary state of continuous cavitation, and sometimes there is a cavitationless period at the initial part of the transient when suitable conditions are employed. This fact is important not only for communication applications, but also for ultrasonic applications in general, because it may give rise to the introduction of new methods in this field. In this regard, a broad investigation was made of pulsed excitation, and the results are described in the following outline.

Pulsed excitation may be characterized by the parameters of pulse length and repetition period in addition to the three parameters already discussed for the case of continuous excitation, namely, (1) air concentration of the

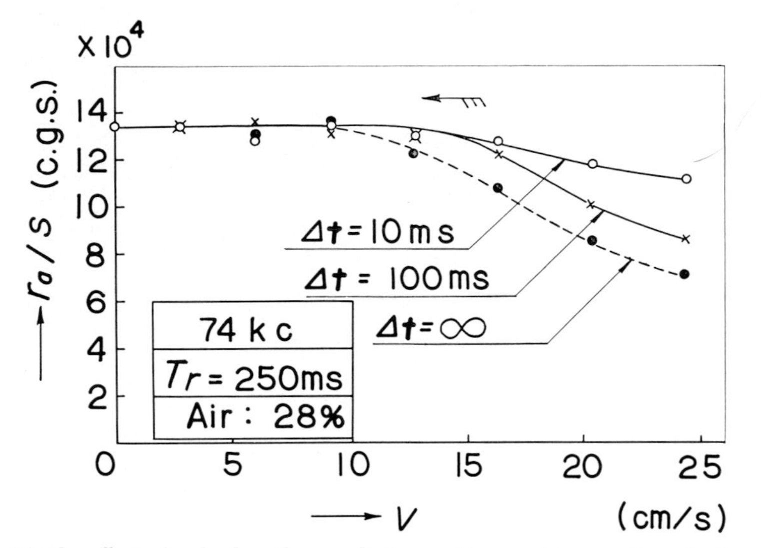

FIGURE 15. The effect of pulse length on radiation resistance. $\triangle$t, acoustic pulse length; r_a, radiation resistance; S, area of radiating surface; T_r, acoustic pulse repetition period; v, vibrational velocity amplitude (r.m.s.).

medium, (2) ultrasonic frequency, and (3) velocity amplitude of vibration of the transmitter surface.

Effect of Pulse Length

Figure 15 shows typical effects of variation of the pulse length which is indicated as $\triangle$t on each curve. It is quite obvious that the shorter the pulse length, the less the fall in radiation resistance, and the larger the critical velocity. These facts indicate that it is possible to obtain cavitationless radiation at higher levels when the pulse length is reduced.

In cavitationless radiation, both sound pressures, that is, the pressure on the surface and the distant field pressure are not saturated, and consequently higher pressures are available at both places, as indicated in Figure 16. When the pulse length is as short as 10 msec, the pressure $\bar{p}$ can rise to more than 3 atm without any tendency toward saturation, showing a clear contrast to the curve for continuous excitation, which is shown by the broken line. The sound pressure in a distant field p_1 has the same feature as shown in the figure below.

Effect of Repetition Period

In Figure 17 a characteristic phenomenon is shown with respect to the repetition period. The parameter T_r is the repetition period, and the abscissa $\triangle$t is the pulse length. The vibrational velocity is kept constant, at almost the highest available level with this apparatus. In the present case cavitationless radiation persists for a pulse-length duration as long as 50 msec if the repetition period is as long as 500 msec, but it persists for only several msec if the repetition period is as short as 30 msec.

Effect of Frequency

In Figure 18, which shows the effect of frequency, the upper curve represents the top curve of the former figure (Fig. 17). If the repetition period is

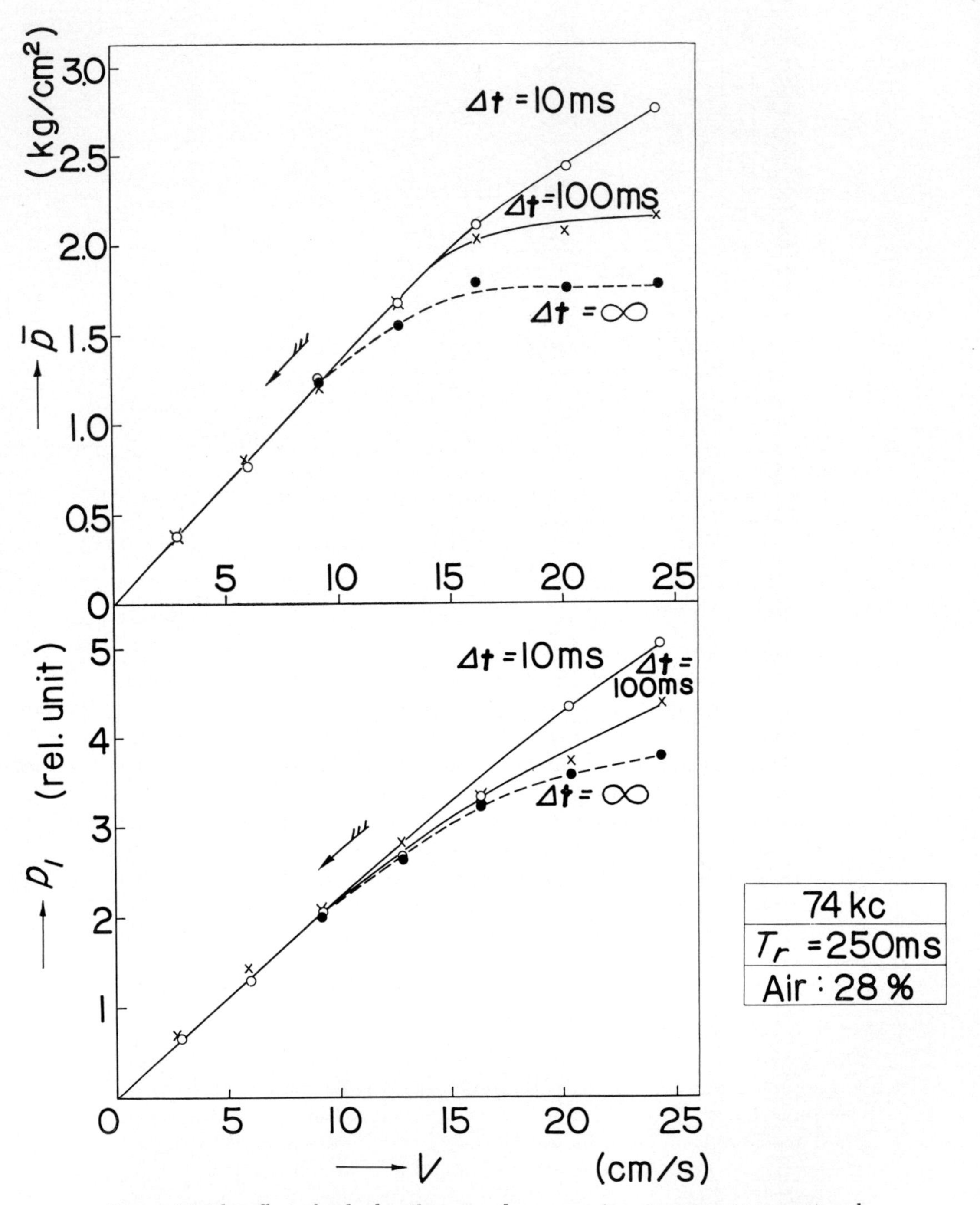

FIGURE 16. The effect of pulse length on sound pressure characteristics. Δt, acoustic pulse length; p_1, fundamental component of observed sound pressure; $\bar{p}$, average sound pressure on the radiating surface; T_r, acoustic pulse repetition period.

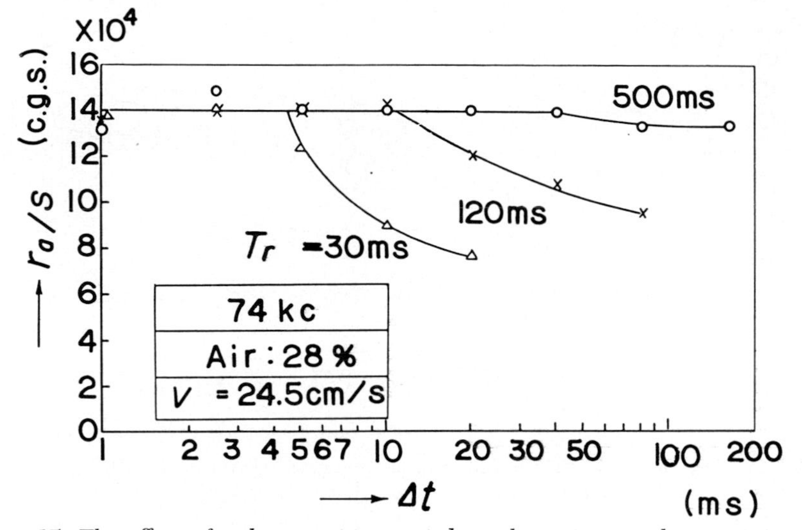

FIGURE 17. The effect of pulse repetition period on the resistance characteristics with respect to pulse length. T_r, acoustic pulse repetition period; Δt, acoustic pulse length; r_a, radiation resistance; S, area of radiating surface.

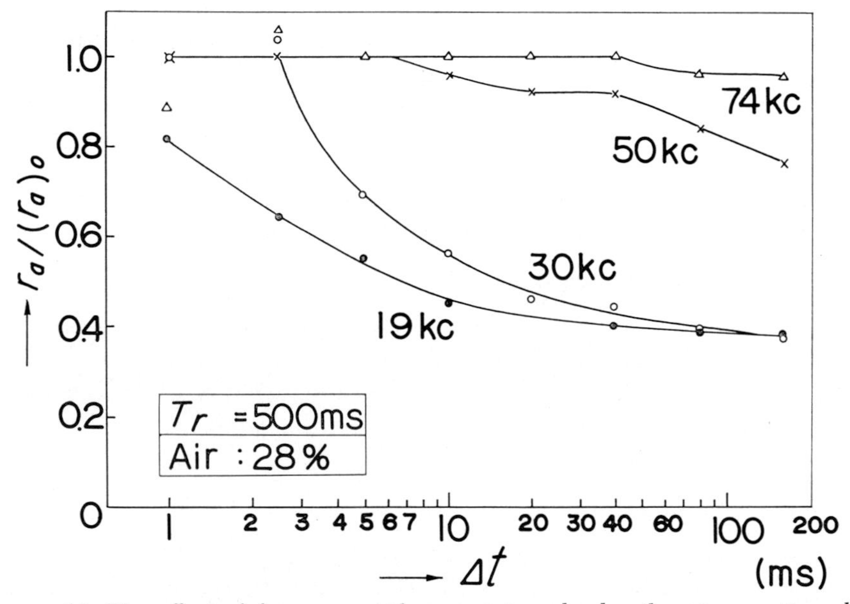

FIGURE 18. The effect of frequency with respect to pulse length. Δt, acoustic pulse length; r_a, radiation resistance; $(r_a)_o$, normal radiation resistance (weak vibration and no cavitation); T_r, acoustic pulse repetition period.

kept constant at 500 msec, as the frequency is lowered, the range of cavitationless radiation is confined within the shorter pulse lengths.

Effect of Air Concentration

Air concentration is the last, but not the least, parameter of cavitation phenomena, not only for the case of continuous excitation but also for the present

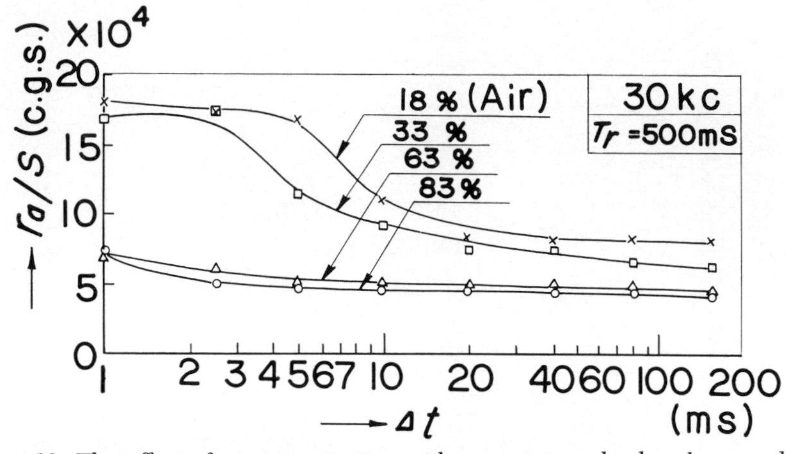

FIGURE 19. The effect of air concentration with respect to pulse length. r_a, radiation resistance; S, area of radiating surface; $\triangle$t, acoustic pulse length; T_r, acoustic pulse repetition period.

case of pulsed radiation. A typical characteristic of the effect is shown in Figure 19. The cavitationless radiation becomes limited within the ranges of shorter pulse lengths with an increase of air concentration, and finally the range goes away to the left beyond this figure. The ultrasonic frequency in this particular case is 30 kc, the level of the vibrational velocity is at its highest value, and the repetition period is 500 msec. When the repetition is more frequent, the ranges are more limited. If lower levels are employed for the velocity, the ranges for cavitationless radiation become wider with respect to each parameter stated above. Figure 20 shows typical characteristics at 30 kc.

12. EFFECT OF SURFACE ROUGHNESS

A rough surface seems to give a stable adhering area for air molecules which can act as cavitation nuclei. Observations have, however, shown that this effect exists only for a particular range of air concentration, even when such observations are made for range of roughness CLA values (center-line-average) between 0.37 and 9.1 μ.

13. EFFECT OF SURFACE EROSION

On the other hand, surface erosion results in some interesting phenomena. Vibrators with polished radiation surfaces were immersed in either nondegassified or degassified water to generate continuous intense cavitation, and repeated observations were made on the degree of erosion and the characteristics of the radiation resistance. Nondegassified water showed little change throughout a 16-hr excitation, although the surface was quite eroded at the end of the experiment, as shown in Figure 21. The photograph on the left side shows the entire view of the radiation surface, while the right side shows a microscopic view of the surface; a dense distribution of erosion pits, 0.2 mm in average depth, is evident. In contrast, for degassified water (nonseeded) characteristics such as are shown in Figure 22 were obtained. The top curve

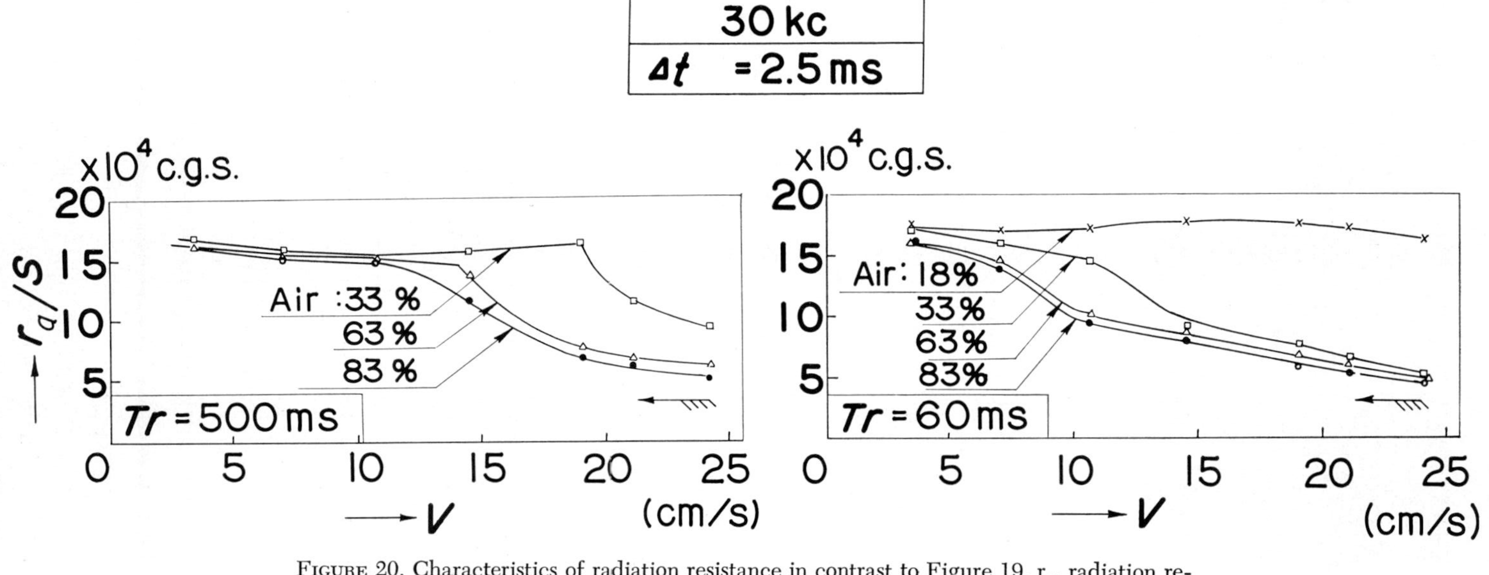

FIGURE 20. Characteristics of radiation resistance in contrast to Figure 19. r_a, radiation resistance; S, area of radiating surface; v, vibrational velocity amplitude (r.m.s.); Δt, acoustic pulse length; T_r, acoustic pulse repetition period.

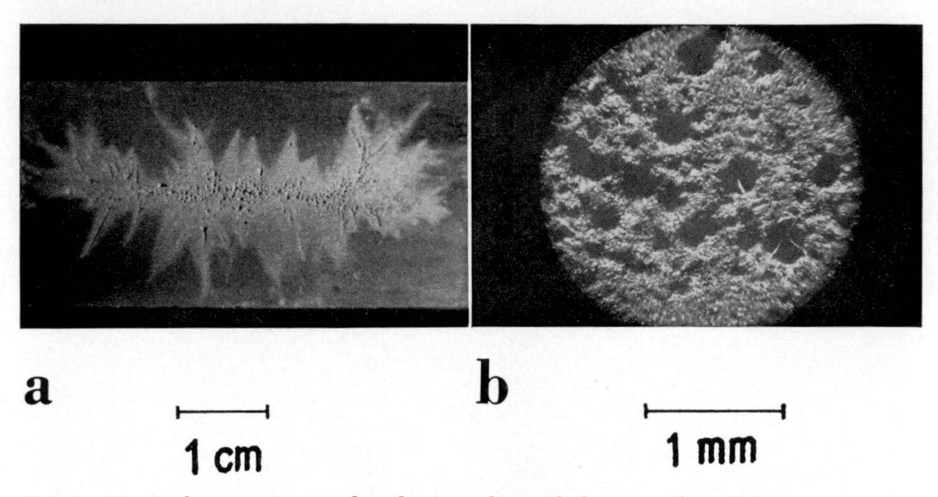

FIGURE 21. Surface erosion produced in nondegassified water after 16-hr excitation. a. Overall view of radiating surface. b. Enlarged view of the radiating surface.

shows characteristics measured before the erosion experiment; the second curve, that measured after 30-min excitation, the third, that of 2 hr, etc. and the bottom curve, that of a 16-hr excitation. For these curves it is evident that the critical velocity approaches lower values with an increase of erosion and that the degree of the resistance fall becomes larger and larger.

14. EFFECT OF SURFACE DEGASSIFICATION

These phenomena give rise to speculation whether air molecules may be trapped in the erosion pits, supplying sufficient cavitation nuclei. To confirm this assumption, a series of experiments was carried out in which the radiation surface was degassified in order to destroy air molecules on the surface. The ferrite vibrator with an eroded surface was immersed in well-degassified water, and the entire setup was placed in a low pressure bell jar for 30 hr, followed by 2 hr of ultrasonic excitation of large amplitude. Following this degassification, the characteristics were again measured under atmospheric pressure, and it was found that the original characteristics of the curve were restored almost completely. But once the surface was dried in air, the characteristics were almost the same as the bottom curve. As a result of these experiments, it may be said, therefore, that the fall of radiation resistance in association with erosion is not directly due to the extreme roughness of the eroded surface, but is due to the supply of cavitation nuclei, as set forth in the assumption. Air molecules may adhere more easily to erosion pits than to a surface of average roughness.

15. EXPERIMENTS IN OTHER LIQUIDS

Similar observations were made in other liquids, such as transformer oil, mobile oil, and castor oil. In these liquids, which are more viscous than water, several unusual phenomena are found, especially in castor oil, in which the effect of surface degassification is rather peculiar. When the vibrational ve-

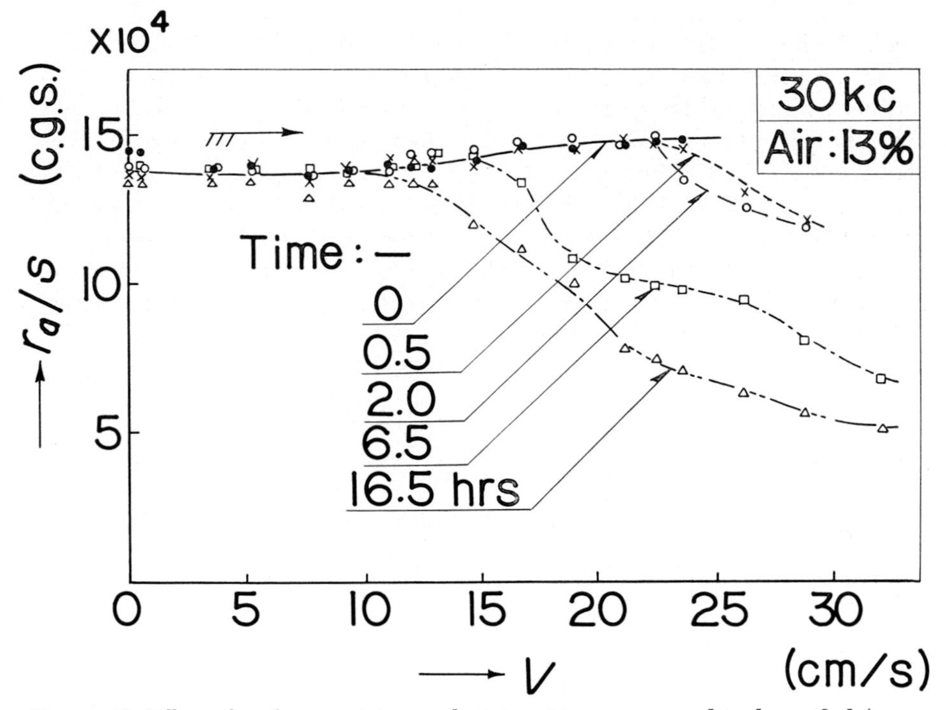

FIGURE 22. Effect of surface erosion on radiation resistance measured in degassified (non-seeded) water. r_a, radiation resistance; S, area of radiating surface; v, vibrational velocity amplitude (r.m.s.); Time, duration of acoustic irradiation.

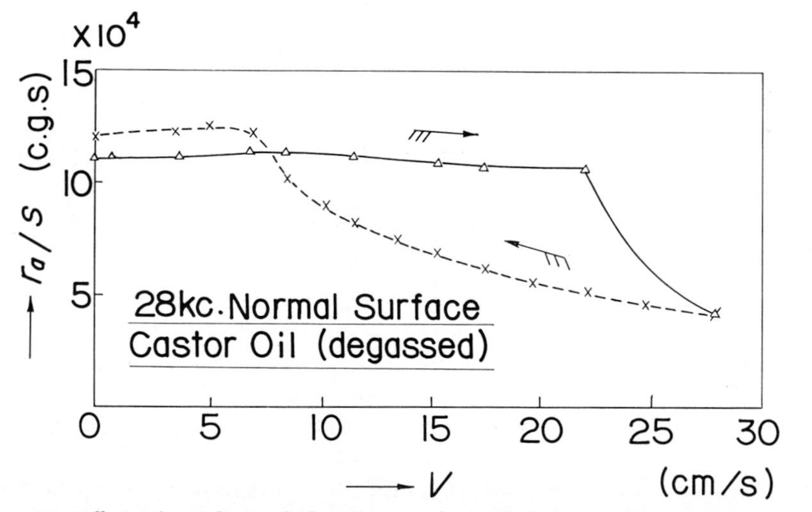

FIGURE 23. Effect of nondegassified surface in degassified castor oil. r_a, radiation resistance; S, area of radiating surface; v, vibrational velocity amplitude (r.m.s.).

locity of a well-polished ferrite surface is increased in degassified castor oil and then decreased, characteristic curves are obtained as shown in Figure 23. The solid line is the curve corresponding to the case of increasing driving level, and the broken line is that corresponding to the case of decreasing driving level. The hysteresis is considerably larger than that in water. When the process of surface degassification is accomplished by the same method as described with regard to water, the cavitation point increases remarkably, and the curve shows no fall until the level of the velocity exceeds 28 cm/sec, as shown by a solid line in Figure 24. But once the transmitter is excited to a level where cavitation is induced, the characteristic relation obtained for decreasing driving level completely changes feature, as shown by the broken line which is much the same as the curve obtained without surface degassification. Moreover, this low resistance character never returns to the original characteristics shown by the solid line, unless the ultrasonic radiation is suspended for a considerably longer period of time, or a new surface degassification is again applied.

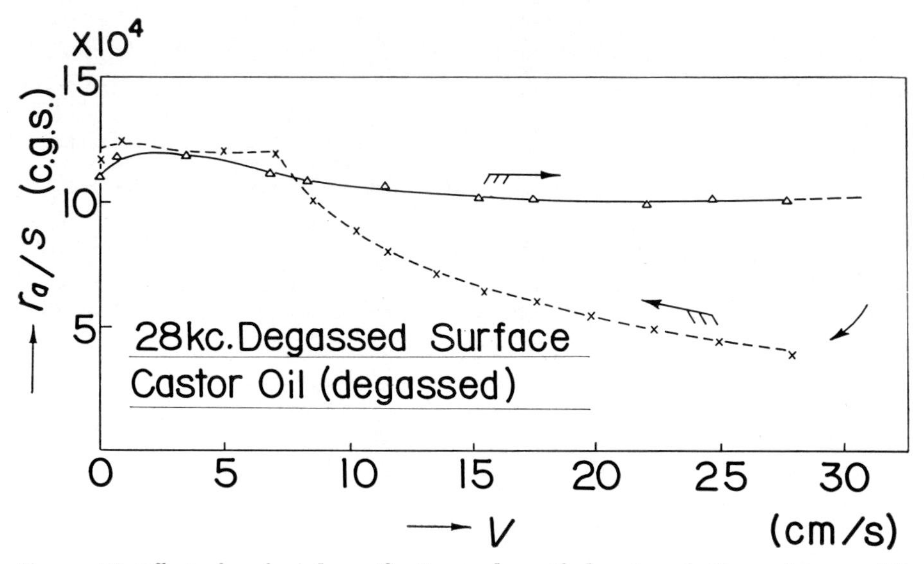

FIGURE 24. Effect of surface degassification in degassified castor oil. Curve shows no fall until level of velocity exceeds 28 cm/sec. r_a, radiation resistance; S, area of radiating surface; v, vibrational velocity amplitude (r.m.s.).

16. CONCLUSION

In summary, in the preliminary sections of the present report, a simple interpretation of radiation resistance at high sound levels in terms of important aspects of cavitation phenomena is presented; the quantities which appear in the formulas are sound-field pressure, pressure averaged over the transmitter surface, acoustic power, cavitation power, and also the so-called cavitation point. Next, detailed data are given showing the resistance characteristics as measured in water with various air concentrations, from the degassified state to a nearly saturated state. For these observations, several important parameters were varied so that the data might cover a wide range of applications. The range of ultrasonic frequencies was from 19 to 97 kc, and the range of the velocity amplitude of the radiating surface was sufficient to include a value as large as 25 cm/sec in r.m.s. value. In every case, the radiation resistance shows a sharp fall when cavitation occurs and finally decreases to a value as small as one-fifth or one-sixth the starting value.

In addition, equipment for continuous degassification of water is illustrated, together with a proposal for a simple method for rapid measurement of the air concentration of water.

A method designated as "seeding" for supplying artificial cavitation nuclei is also described and some interesting findings are indicated. Of particular interest is the complete disappearance of cavitation hysteresis which generally appears between the increasing and the decreasing driving level cases when "nonseeding."

The midsection of this paper includes outlines of various results obtained from observations made for the case of pulsed radiation. The five parameters in this case were: pulse length, pulse repetition period, ultrasonic frequency, velocity amplitude of the radiation surface, and air concentration of the medium. One of the important findings from the pulsed radiation studies is the disclosure of quantitative criteria between the various parameters describing limits for cavitationless radiation.

Following this, the roughness and erosion characteristics of the transmitter surface are discussed in relation to the radiation resistance. It is concluded that the roughness and erosion per se do not appreciably affect the cavitation phenomena, but the air molecules lodged in the erosion pits have evident effect on the phenomena. In the last section of the paper a brief description of a peculiar phenomenon observed in degassified castor oil is given, although further observations are necessary in order to analyze the data.

REFERENCES

1. Kikuchi, Y. (1961). Recent Results of Research and Development in the Field of Ultrasonics in Japan, Proc. of the 3rd ICA, Stuttgart, 1959, 1193–1206.
2. Kikuchi, Y., and H. Shimizu (1959). On the Variation of Acoustic Radiation Resistance in Water Under Ultrasonic Cavitation, J. Acoust. Soc. Am. *31*, 1385–86.
3. Kikuchi, Y., H. Shimizu, and D. Okuyama (1962). A Method for Measuring Acoustic Radiation Resistance of a Transducer Generating Intense Ultrasonic Cavitation, ASA Ann. Meeting, May 23–26, New York City, N.Y.

DISCUSSION

DR. W. J. FRY: I was wondering whether you made estimates of the percentage of gas that is in the water in the dissolved state and in the bubble state. One might interpret the percentage in the bubble state to explain the observed effect of frequency. In other words, what percentage of gas is in the dissolved state, and does the variation of the threshold particle velocity essentially measure the amount of gas in this state? — that is, the free gas influences the compressibility and thus modifies the radiation resistance.

DR. KIKUCHI: Yes. I made measurements of gas content which was in dissolved state, and I consider that such changes in compressibility of the liquid at the radiation surface cause the radiation resistance to decrease. The bubble phenomena have been observed by looking in the very close vicinity of the irradiating surface. As I have reported in the proceedings of the Third International Congress, the bubbles begin to appear on the surface and accumulate step by step, so that with the lapse of 5 msec or more, the bubbles grow to a certain volume. This is the phenomena on the surface, or just above the surface. If the water is not degassified, the small bubbles flow into the medium in such a manner that the distribution of bubbles is not uniform in the near field. I think that Professor Fry's suggestion about the threshold velocity, however, is not applicable in this case of ultrasonic cavitation.

DR. W. J. FRY: The effect of frequency appears to suggest that the dissolved vs free gas content may be changed. Is it possible to make any quantitative correlations in this regard?

DR. KIKUCHI: The major portion of the effect of frequency on the radiation impedance is not dependent on the relative amount of free and dissolved gas in the water nor on the surface distribution of the bubbles.

DR. W. J. FRY: The effects would certainly be directly related to the medium in contact with the vibrating surface.

DR. KIKUCHI: [The following statement was inserted during the editing procedure at Dr. Kikuchi's request.] There was some discrepancy in the terminology on "bubble state" as used in this discussion between Dr. Fry and myself. I thought at the time of discussion that the term "bubble state" referred to the bubbles produced by the cavitation. No appreciable bubbles exist in the water before the cavitation point. In answer to the statement of Dr. Fry, I would like to reply, "Yes, that is the point I have stated in my paper, and this statement should also be applied to the foregoing discussions."

DR. VON GIERKE: Are you measuring radiation resistance or acoustic impedance?

DR. KIKUCHI: Radiation resistance, the resistive part of the radiation impedance.

DR. HUGHES: Was your transmitter always large compared to the wavelength?

DR. KIKUCHI: In almost all cases the surface dimension is two or three times the wavelength. But in cases of smaller ratios, I expressed the radiation resistance variation by using the theoretical value as a reference.

DR. VON GIERKE: When you indicate a pressure, such as the pressure across the membrane or the pressure in the far field, is this only that part of the pressure which is in phase with the particle velocity or is this the total pressure?

DR. KIKUCHI: Total pressure in your sense, and it is designated $\bar{p}$ across the membrane and p_1 for the distant field pressure. The positions at which p_1 measurements were made were far from the cavitation region.

DR. VON GIERKE: In that case I should expect such an effect as Dr. Fry mentioned to be reflected mainly in the complex impedance at the surface and not only at a distance, because the near field properties—and this is actually what you refer to—would be reflected in the total impedance.

DR. KIKUCHI: I am now measuring the reactive part of the radiation impedance. As a matter of fact, up to the present time this measurement shows little change. But insofar as this broad concept is concerned, I am convinced that this radiation resistance should be primarily considered in regard to cavitation applications.

DR. W. J. FRY: You showed a curve of output power vs particle velocity. Was there any linear relation between output power and the square of the particle velocity of bubble surface values? I wondered whether this linear range was predictable from the values of the radiation resistance. In other words, did you find that you could correlate these two things? I've forgotten exactly how you measured the output power in that case.

DR. KIKUCHI: The power is the product of the radiation resistance measured and the square of the radiation surface velocity measured.

DR. VON GIERKE: I have another question in this connection. If this (Fig. 7) is your power curve, you called this a power in the medium and this your decavitation power? I don't think this term "cavitation power" is too well chosen because it is not the power which is locked in that was used in cavitation. This power is still in the medium. As you said, most of it is in the harmonics. And I wonder how much of this power is actually used for producing the cavitation and how much is still in the liquid medium to be propagated in harmonics.

DR. KIKUCHI: Well, this part is the cavitation part, including higher harmonics and subharmonics. And this is the fundamental part which propagates beyond the cavitation range. And from the standpoint of communication, this part is usable.

DR. VON GIERKE: Is it usable for linear transmission?

DR. KIKUCHI: Yes.

DR. VON GIERKE: How much power is lost and is actually transmitted into the cavitation?

DR. KIKUCHI: This includes harmonics. If you are interested in cavitation power consumed, you must measure the total power consumed in the harmonics. But we did not do this.

DR. VON GIERKE: You don't know whether this is a large percentage of this other part or a small percentage?

DR. KIKUCHI: Almost equal at the higher level of –

DR. VON GIERKE: No, you see it is almost equal here, but much of this part here is still in the liquid. And how much has been consumed by producing the bubbles?

DR. KIKUCHI: That is a problem of time of the consumption. A time rate must be set. The harmonics part propagates anyway by the sound speed so it cannot be consumed in the cavitation region. So how do you define the differentiation of the cavitation power consumed and that propagated as a harmonics component?

DR. VON GIERKE: This power here is from the metal, and you can measure the power in the first harmonic, the power in the second harmonic, until you reach this point and you have the power in all harmonics. And then the difference in this power and this power is the power that you have in cavitation.

DR. KIKUCHI: Yes, that is a very interesting problem, but so far as my proposed method is concerned, such harmonics cannot be measured from the electrical terminal. You must use some acoustic measurement by using microphones, and so forth. In that case the accuracy must be confirmed quite precisely after several painstaking calculations. That is a different problem from mine.

Ultrasonic Absorption by Biological Materials

FLOYD DUNN
Biophysical Research Laboratory, University of Illinois, Urbana, Illinois

Introduction by Dr. Carstensen

The next paper, to be presented by Dr. Floyd Dunn, concerns the propagation characteristics of ultrasound in biological materials. It is obvious that characteristics such as speed of sound and absorption coefficients must be quantitatively known in order to apply logically this form of energy to the alteration and examination of tissue. Ultimately, these parameters determine the design of the equipment since they are intimately concerned with such details as size of focus and depth of penetration of the ultrasound. Finally, such studies may add to our basic knowledge of tissue structure since the magnitude of the ultrasonic absorption is partly dependent on configuration of the macromolecular structure.

A. INTRODUCTION

Interest in ultrasonics as an experimental tool for analysis of biological systems and as an agent useful in medical diagnosis and therapy continues to increase. A comparison of the papers published in the proceedings of the previous symposium (1) with those of the present symposium reveals that great strides have been made in the application of ultrasonic techniques to biological research and to medical practice. Also revealing, in such a comparison, is the apparent decrease in interest in the elucidation of the physical mechanisms involved when high-frequency acoustic waves interact with living systems. The impression is obtained from publications in the recent literature that the fundamental acoustic properties of biological materials are known and that the problems arising in applications of ultrasound to biophysical and medical problems are merely those in technique. This, unfortunately, is not true since relatively little is known and understood of the physical mechanisms attending the propagation of high-frequency acoustic waves in biological structures. It is axiomatic that these physical mechanisms implicit in the interaction of ultrasound and biological systems must be determined to provide information basic to the full utility of this form of energy. An important adjunct to the understanding of the fundamental physical mechanisms is a deep insight into the absorption processes occurring when materials are exposed to high-frequency acoustic energy.

This paper reviews experimental data (published in the technical literature) concerned with the dependence of the ultrasonic absorption coefficient upon acoustic field variables, namely, frequency and wave amplitude, and state variables, namely, temperature and concentration which are important for understanding basic processes of absorption. Several tissues, namely, refractive media of the eye and lung, which exhibit absorption properties greatly different from most soft tissues, that is, fat, muscle, liver, nerve, etc., are discussed separately. A brief statement describing the absorption coefficient of bone is also included. No formal theory is presented for explaining the observed dependencies of the ultrasonic absorption coefficient; however, the apparently successful interpretation of the unusual acoustic absorption properties of lung is mentioned briefly. Allusion is made to several dependencies of the absorption coefficient upon specific physical variables where they appear to resemble those of known mechanisms arising from the interaction of ultrasound and nonbiological materials.

B. FREQUENCY DEPENDENCE

The literature is replete with data regarding the dependence of the ultrasonic absorption coefficient upon the acoustic frequency. A tabulation of the ultrasonic absorption and velocity data has been compiled by Goldman and Hueter (2). Figure 1, taken from their paper, is a graphical representation of the acoustic amplitude absorption coefficient per wavelength for several mammalian tissues in the frequency range from approximately 200 kc to 10 Mc. The scatter of the data, exhibited by the bands or broad shaded regions,

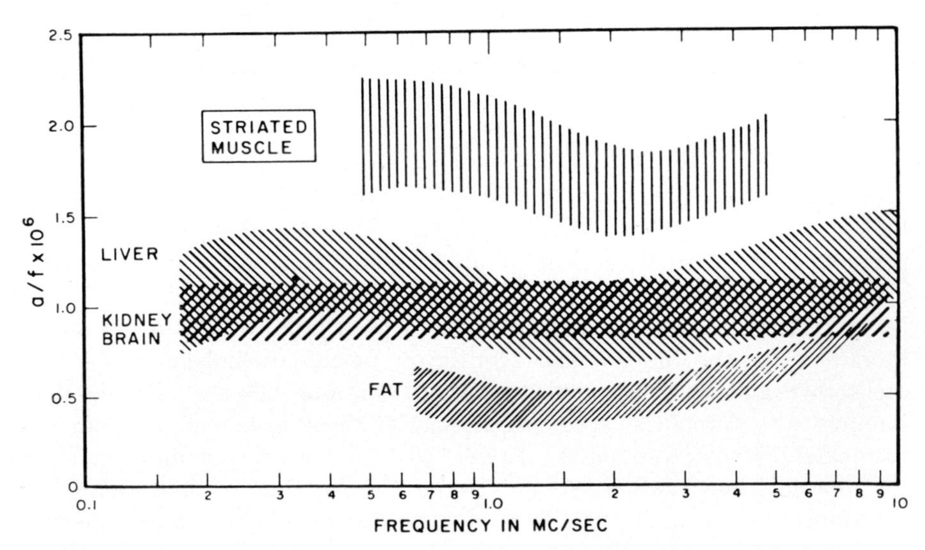

FIGURE 1. Acoustic amplitude absorption coefficient (in db/cm) per wavelength vs frequency for several mammalian tissues (after Goldman and Hueter).

results from the attempt to include all measurements (available at that time) by numerous investigators employing different experimental techniques. The appearance of the bands of Figure 1 is not wholly surprising since many investigators neglect to give complete specifications of their experimental procedure and/or a description of the state of the specimen used. For example, it is known that the measurements represented in Figure 1 were performed at different temperatures. However, it is not possible to determine from the literature the temperatures employed by the investigators reporting the data. (The influence of temperature upon the absorption coefficient is discussed in the next section.) It is, however, possible to discern several relatively simple relationships. For example, the absorption per wavelength, α/f, is generally constant over the frequency range considered. For fat, α/f, increases slightly in the frequency range from 1 to 10 Mc. The experimental results for striated muscle and liver appear to exhibit a minimum in the neighborhood of 2 Mc.

Another way of presenting absorption data, which may be useful in the elucidation of mechanisms, is illustrated in Figure 2, prepared by Hueter (3). Here, the logarithm of the absorption coefficient is plotted as a function of the logarithm of the sound frequency, and the slopes of the resulting

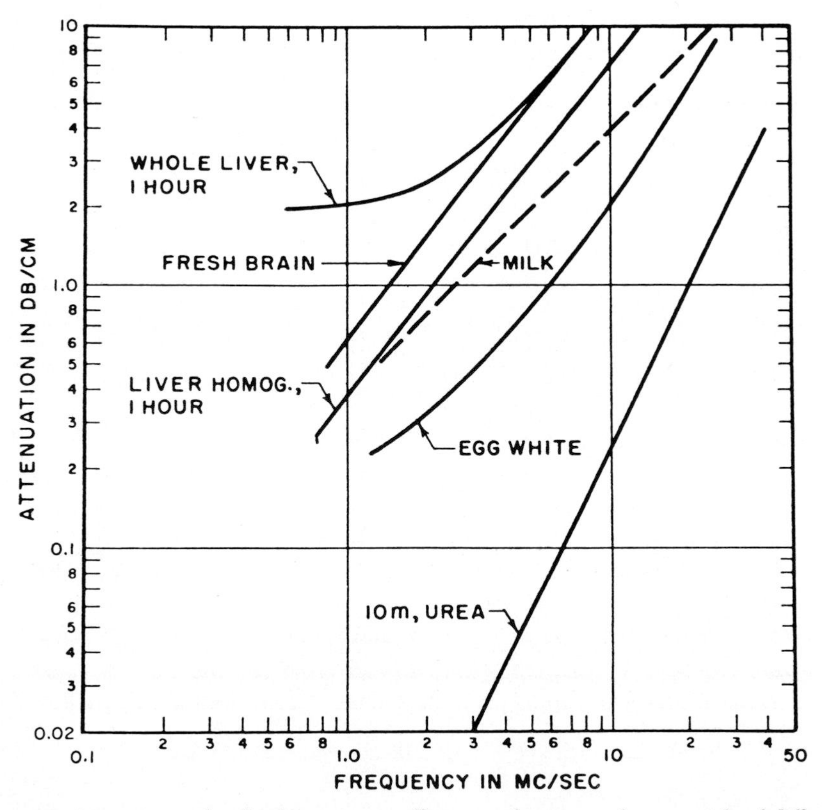

FIGURE 2. Acoustic amplitude absorption coefficient vs frequency for materials of different biological complexity (after Hueter, 1958).

curves are examined (the slope is the exponent on frequency upon which the magnitude of the absorption coefficient depends). Figure 2 shows several materials of increasing biological complexity and illustrates correspondingly more complicated behavior. The 10-molar urea solution exhibits a slope of 2 indicative of classical viscous absorption for which

$$\alpha/f^2 = \text{constant.} \qquad (1)$$

Classical viscous absorption results from the fact that liquids exert a finite resistance to shearing forces such that changes in density are not in time phase with changes in pressure (4).[1] Homogenized milk, a suspension of fat particles and hydrated casein complexes, exhibits a slope of nearly unity from approximately 1 to 40 Mc. Behavior of this type cannot be explained in terms of simple viscosity or scattering theories. The curves for the absorption coefficients of egg albumin, brain tissue, liver, and striated muscle (not shown in Fig. 2) exhibit slopes between 1 and 2 in the neighborhood of 1 Mc and approaching a slope of 2 at higher frequencies. Hueter (3) has suggested that this type of frequency dependence can be described for specific muscle preparations by a double relaxation process in which the bulk (volume) viscosity of the tissue possesses a relaxation frequency near 40 kc and the shear viscosity possesses a relaxation near 400 kc. Although it is conceded that this is an oversimplification of a complicated process, it will be shown below that the temperature dependence of the acoustic absorption coefficient lends support to this view.

C. TEMPERATURE DEPENDENCE

To the writer's knowledge, only two studies dealing with the dependence of the ultrasonic absorption coefficient of biological materials upon temperature have been reported. The absorption coefficient of the spinal cord of young mice (approximately 24 hr after birth) has been measured in vivo by Dunn (5) at the sound frequency of 1 Mc, employing the transient thermoelectric method (4). Figure 3 is a graphical representation of the acoustic intensity absorption coefficient vs temperature where it is seen to increase from 0.034 cm^{-1} at 2°C to 0.25 cm^{-1} at 45°C. The positive temperature coefficient of absorption eliminates shear viscosity as a possible mechanism. However, this variation does resemble the temperature dependence of the absorption coefficient of high-viscosity liquids above the main relaxation frequencies of the liquid (6). Thus, the monotonic increase in the absorption coefficient as a function of temperature (at 1 Mc) of the spinal cord of young mice is considered to lend support to Hueter's (3) suggestion, discussed above, that a double relaxation process occurs wherein both the bulk viscosity and the shear viscosity relax out at frequencies well below the frequency of measurement.

Carstensen, Schwan, and co-workers have carried out an extensive study

[1] For a comprehensive discussion of acoustic absorption mechanisms relative to biological materials and of methods of determining absorption coefficients experimentally see W. J. Fry and F. Dunn in "Physical Techniques in Biological Research," W. L. Nastuk, ed. (Academic Press, New York, 1962), Vol. IV, Chap. 6, p. 261.

on the ultrasonic properties of blood and its components (7). It was determined that the absorption properties of blood are determined largely by the protein content, and the absorption coefficient was shown to be directly proportional to the protein concentration, whether in solution or contained within cells. Figure 4 shows their ultrasonic absorption data for hemoglobin solutions as a function of temperature at three acoustic frequencies. The negative temperature coefficient suggests that shear viscosity plays a significant role in the absorption mechanism.

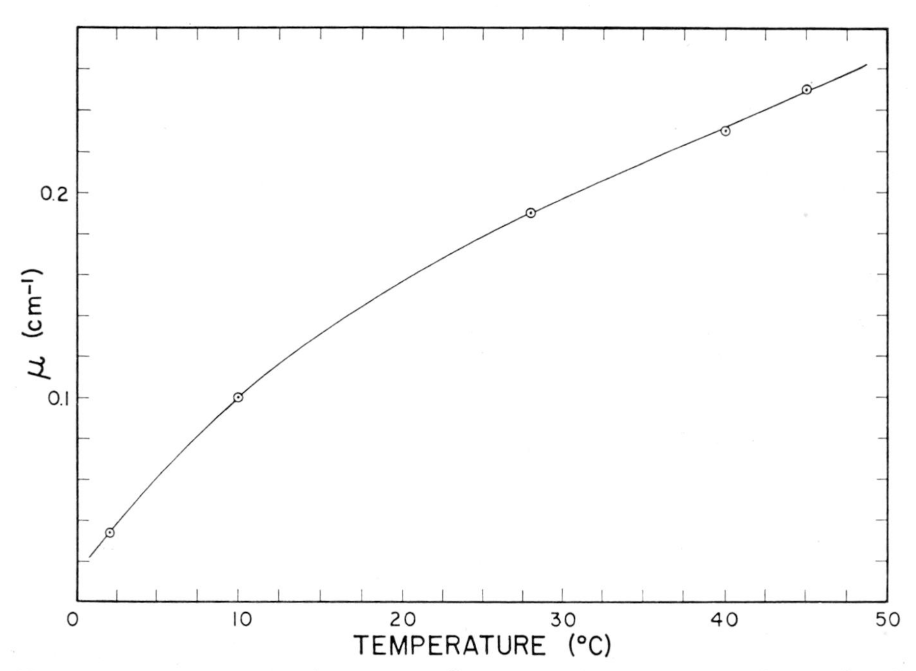

FIGURE 3. Acoustic intensity absorption coefficient vs temperature at 1 Mc for spinal cord of young mice (after Dunn).

The temperature dependence of the absorption coefficient, particularly that for young mouse spinal cord, illustrates the necessity for complete specification of the state of specimens when reporting experimental results. The data for the young mouse cord shows that a sevenfold increase in the absorption coefficient occurs in the temperature range from 0 to 45°C. Although the rate of change of the positive temperature coefficient appears to exhibit a marked decrease in the neighborhood of the normal temperature of adult mammals, namely, 37°C, it must be recalled that these measurements represent only one species and one tissue structure. Other specimens may exhibit even more pronounced temperature dependencies.

D. CONCENTRATION DEPENDENCE

The dependence of the ultrasonic absorption coefficient upon the concentration of tissue components in solution has been referenced in the previous section, and it is interesting to compare, as Hueter (3) has done, the absorption in brain tissue reported by numerous investigators with the absorption of concentrated solutions of red cells, as shown in Figure 5. The curve through the nerve tissue data is drawn with a slope of 1.3 (that is, $\log \alpha / \log f = 1.3$) which is also the average slope found for concentrated red cells (7). The figure illustrates that nerve tissue behaves very much like a concentrated aggregate of protein with the absorption increased by approximately a factor of two, perhaps due to the protein-protein interactions associated with the formation of tissue structure.

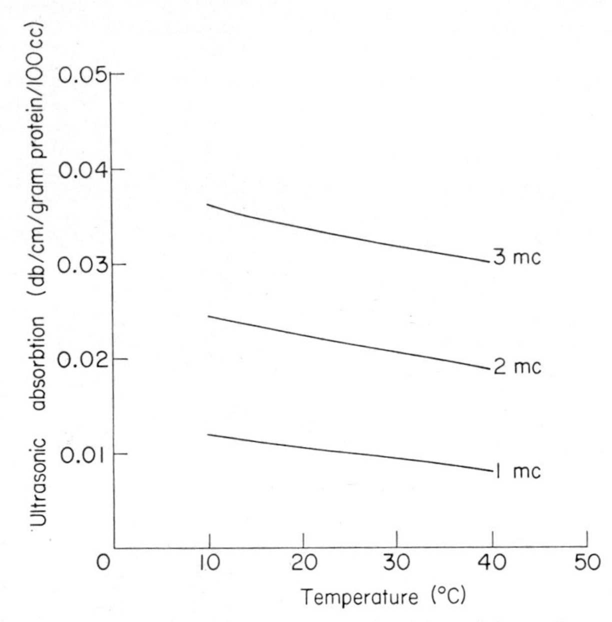

FIGURE 4. Ultrasonic absorption vs temperature for hemoglobin solutions at three frequencies (after Carstensen *et al.*).

E. AMPLITUDE DEPENDENCE

The transient thermoelectric method employed in obtaining the value of the absorption coefficient as a function of temperature of the young mouse spinal cord (see Section C) included exposure of each specimen to different acoustic intensity levels of incident sound energy (5). Thus, the method made data available on the dependence of the acoustic absorption coefficient upon the sound amplitude. The procedure (4, 8) used consisted of placing small thermocouples in the tissue, exposing the specimen to a pulse of sound of known amplitude, and observing the initial time rate of temperature change associated with the phase of the response due to absorption of sound in the body of the material surrounding the thermocouple junction. The relation describing quantitatively these events is

$$\left(\frac{dT}{dt}\right)_o = \left(\frac{\mu}{\rho C_p}\right) I, \quad (2)$$

where $\left(\frac{dT}{dt}\right)_o$ is observed initial time rate of change of temperature, I is the

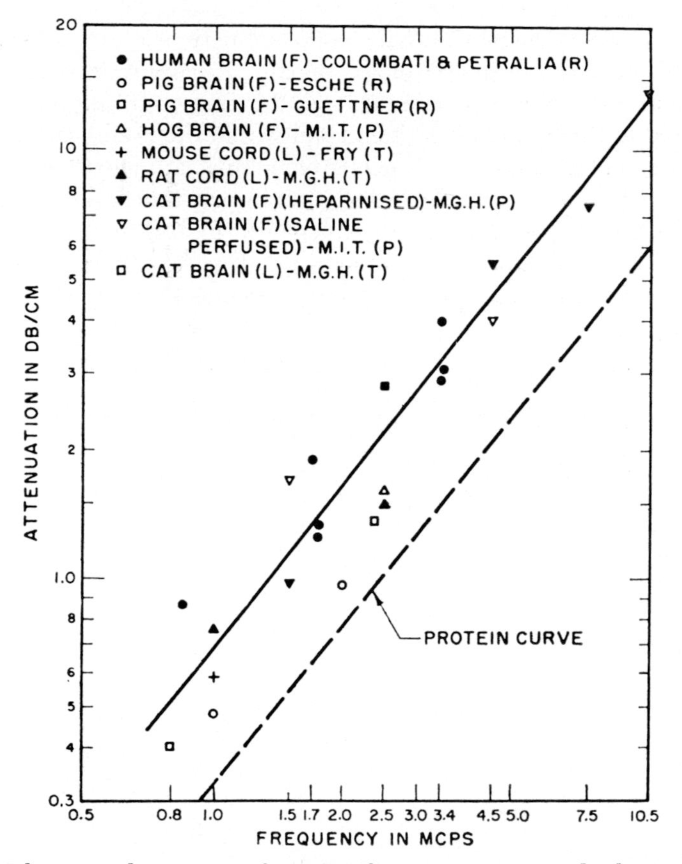

FIGURE 5. Ultrasonic absorption vs frequency for nervous tissue and solution of 85% red cells from human blood (after Hueter, 1958).

known acoustic intensity incident on the tissue, μ is the acoustic intensity absorption coefficient per unit path length ($\mu = 2a$), and ρC_p is the heat capacity per unit volume of the tissue. Equation 2 states that for the quantity $\mu/\rho C_p$ constant, the initial time rate of change of temperature $\left(\frac{dT}{dt}\right)_0$ is a linear function of the acoustic intensity. Figure 6 shows that in the range of incident acoustic intensities from a few watts per square centimeter to nearly 200 w/cm^2 and at three base temperatures of the animals, this linear relationship indeed obtains. On the assumption that the heat capacity per unit volume, ρC_p, is not dependent upon the intensity, it can be concluded that in the range of intensities employed here, the absorption coefficient is independent of the intensity of the incident wave for the experimental preparations of this study, that is, the type and preparation of tissue employed.

Concerning the lack of dependence of the absorption coefficient of nerve tissue upon the sound intensity in these experiments, the following statements can be made. The propagation distance from sound source via degassed mammalian saline to tissue was approximately 5 cm. This distance is sufficiently short in the saline so that the initially monochromatic waves produced by the vibrating element (X-cut quartz plate) remain virtually monochromatic during propagation to the specimen; that is, the energy transferred from the fundamental to the harmonics, which results from the nonlinear equation of state of the liquid medium (4), is negligible in this path length at the highest intensities employed. Thus, the wave incident on the tissue is essentially undistorted from the initial single frequency form. On the assumption that the coefficients in the equation of state of tissue are approximately the same as those of water, and since the propagation distance in the tissue is relatively short (approximately 0.5 mm), the transfer of energy from the incident fundamental wave to its harmonics is negligible within the specimen.

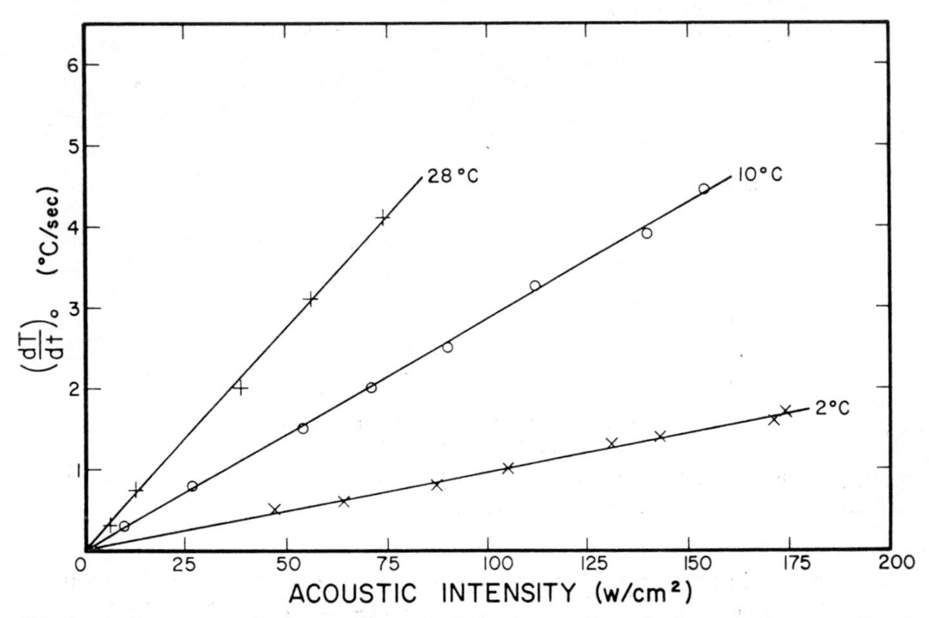

FIGURE 6. Time rate of change of temperature in spinal cord of young mice produced by absorption of 1 Mc sound vs incident acoustic intensity at three temperatures (after Dunn).

F. ABSORPTION IN BONE

Bone represents a tissue component possessing acoustic propagation properties greatly different from those of the soft tissues discussed in the previous section. Hueter (9, 2) has measured the acoustic absorption coefficient of fresh human skull in the frequency range from 0.6 to 3.5 Mc at temperatures between 25 and 30°C. These measurements show that the absorption coefficient of bone exhibits a frequency squared dependence upon frequency of the classical viscous type to approximately 2 Mc with a transition to a lower power frequency dependence at higher frequencies. The acoustic amplitude absorption coefficient per unit path length in bone is of the order of 1 cm^{-1} at 1 Mc, approximately an order of magnitude greater than that of most soft tissues at the same temperature and frequency.

G. ABSORPTION IN REFRACTIVE MEDIA OF THE EYE

Because of the capability of ultrasonic visualization methods for *seeing* structures within the eye not possible by any other ophthalmic instruments, it is essential that data describing the acoustic propagation characteristics of the various media of the eye be available. To the writer's knowledge, the only work of this type reported in the literature is that of Begui (10). He determined the ultrasonic absorption coefficients of the aqueous and vitreous humors at 30 Mc and that of the lens at 3 Mc. The specimens were obtained from excised, fresh calf eyes. At 30 Mc and 27.5°C, the aqueous and vitreous humors both exhibit an acoustic amplitude absorption coefficient of 0.35 cm^{-1}. Since this is approximately 50% greater than the absorption coefficient of dilute salt solutions, it suggests that the absorption coefficients of the humoral materials of the eye possess a viscous type dependence upon frequency; that is, the absorption coefficient increases as the square of the frequency.

The lens exhibits a value of 0.7 cm^{-1} for the acoustic amplitude absorption coefficient at 3 Mc and 28°C. Since the lens contains a relatively high concentration of protein, it may be assumed, in the absence of further information, that the frequency dependence of the absorption coefficient of the lens will resemble that of other tissue for which the absorption appears to be dominated by the protein content (see Section D). In view of this, it may be assumed that the absorption coefficient of the lens varies approximately with the first power of the frequency.

Investigators (11) currently using ultrasonic methods for diagnosing disorders of the human eye feel that the absorption values given by Begui are too large. The following statements are offered as possible explanations. The difference may result from comparison of eyes of different animals. Indeed, Begui observed that the viscosity of the intraocular fluid of calf eyes is greater than the values normally stated for that of human eyes. Further, the specimens used by Begui were stored at temperatures in the neighborhood of 0 to 5°C and were used for measurement purposes within a time interval of 10 days. Diagnostic procedures are, of course, performed in vivo. Autolysis of the stored specimens may have occurred, although it is not immediately apparent that under these conditions the absorption coefficient should increase.

H. ABSORPTION IN LUNG TISSUE

The acoustic amplitude absorption coefficient of excised dog lung containing residual air has been determined by Dunn and Fry (12) at 0.98 Mc and 35°C. The very large value obtained, 4.7 cm^{-1}, is more than an order of magnitude greater than the absorption coefficient of dry oxygen or nitrogen at STP. In order to account for the absorption greatly in excess of that exhibited by soft tissue structures (namely, a factor of fifty greater), a model based upon the gross structure of lung tissue is employed to permit calculations. The model considers the lung to be composed of a uniform distribution of spherical gas bubbles imbedded in a liquid-like medium of high viscosity. The gas within the bubbles is considered to have the physical properties of air at STP. The imbedding medium is considered to have physical properties similar to water, with the exception of the shear viscosity which is taken to be 150 poises. The population of the bubbles is chosen to be consistent with the measured density of the specimen. This requires a packing of the bubbles approximately midway between hexagonal closest packing (each sphere touched by twelve neighboring spheres) and cubic closest packing (each sphere touched by six neighboring spheres). The bubble radius was chosen as a weighted average of the dimensions of the gaseous structures of lung.

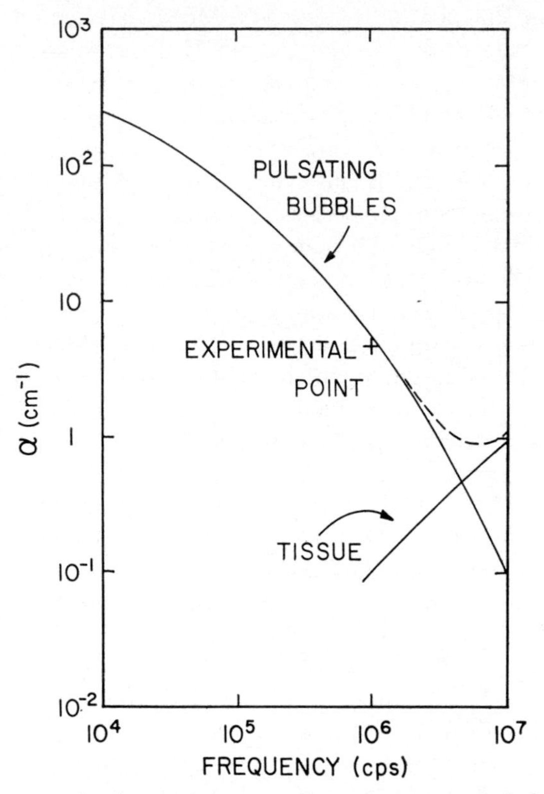

FIGURE 7. Acoustic amplitude absorption coefficient per unit path length in lung vs frequency for bubble radius of 0.3 mm (after Dunn and Fry).

The incident sound energy excites the bubbles to pulsate, and the bubbles dissipate energy by radiating spherical sound waves. Figure 7 shows the experimentally determined point and the results of calculations for bubbles of 0.3 mm radius based on this loss mechanism. The agreement between the experimentally determined value and the model is considered sufficiently good to lend support to the view that the mechanism of ultrasonic absorption in lung tissue at 0.98 Mc is primarily the result of reradiation of sound waves by pulsating gaseous structures.

It is reasonable to assume that the tissue (the high-viscosity liquid-like imbedding material) also contributes to the total absorption of lung. Assuming a value of 0.1 cm^{-1} at 1 Mc for the absorption coefficient of the tissue and a linear increase with frequency, the curve labeled "TISSUE" of Figure 7 results. If it is assumed further that the total absorption coefficient, a_T, is the arithmetic sum of that due to pulsating bubbles, a_b, and that due to tissue, a_t, that is,

$$a_T = a_b + a_t, \tag{3}$$

then the dashed curved of Figure 7 results and, for the numerical values chosen, predicts a minimum value for the absorption coefficient occurring at approximately 6 Mc with a value of $a_T = 0.9\ \text{cm}^{-1}$.

The samples used in this study contained approximately one-third the average resting respiratory air of normal lung. If it is assumed that inflation of the lung to normal respiratory level has the effect of increasing the bubble radius (without altering the bubble population), then the acoustic absorption coefficient decreases, as shown in Figure 8.

I. CONCLUDING REMARKS

This paper reviews the results of selected experimental investigations which yield information regarding the dependence of the ultrasonic absorption coefficient of biological structures (in the absence of cavitation) upon important physical parameters. It is seen that the state of knowledge in this area remains primitive as regards the understanding of the interaction of sound and tissue.

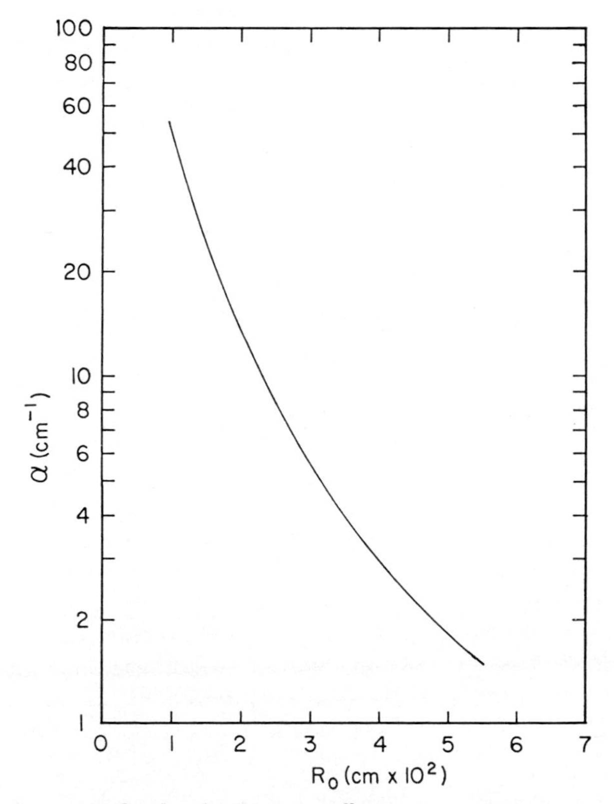

FIGURE 8. Acoustic amplitude absorption coefficient per unit path length in lung vs bubble radius at 1 Mc (after Dunn and Fry).

While this field of endeavor appeared ready to flourish during the past decade, there appears to be a prevailing lack of interest at present. Additional experiments are desperately needed to add information to the body of knowledge already accumulated. In this regard, the author urges investigators to report all pertinent information describing the state of the specimen and the complete set of physical parameters as well as the final result obtained during the experimental procedure.

REFERENCES

1. Kelly, E., ed. (1957). "Ultrasound in Biology and Medicine" (American Institute of Biological Sciences, Washington, D.C.).
2. Goldman, D. E., and T. F. Hueter (1956). J. Acoust. Soc. Am. *28*, 35.
3. Hueter, T. F. (1958). WADC Tech. Rept. 57–706.
4. Fry, W. J., and F. Dunn (1962). *In* "Physical Techniques in Biological Research," W. L. Nastuk, ed. (Academic Press, New York), Vol. IV, Chap. 6.
5. Dunn, F. (1962). J. Acoust. Soc. Am. *34*, 1545.
6. Litovitz, T. A., and T. Lyon (1954). J. Acoust. Soc. Am. *26*, 577.
7. Carstensen, E. L., K. Li, and H. P. Schwan (1953). J. Acoust. Soc. Am. *25*, 286.
8. Fry, W. J., and R. B. Fry (1953). J. Acoust. Soc. Am. *25*, 6.
9. Hueter, T. F. (1962). Naturwissenschaften *39*, 21.
10. Begui, Z. E. (1954). J. Acoust. Soc. Am. *26*, 365.
11. Baum, G., and I. Greenwood, private communication.
12. Dunn, F., and W. J. Fry (1961). Phys. Med. Biol. *5*, 401.

DISCUSSION

DR. MACKAY: How was the value of shear viscosity of the lung tissue chosen, that is, of the imbedding medium, in the pulsating bubble theory?

DR. DUNN: The value chosen, 150 poises, is an average value for soft tissue determined by Dr. von Gierke and co-workers. (See von Gierke *et al.*, J. Appl. Physiol. *4* [1952], 886.)

DR. CARSTENSEN: How were the absorption measurements in the lung tissue made?

DR. DUNN: Determinations were made of the fraction of the incident acoustic energy reflected from the lung specimen and that propagated through the specimen. A transient-type thermoelectric detector was used to investigate the "standing wave" pattern in the field between the sound source and the specimen. The density of the specimen was determined and these data, together with an appropriate analysis, yielded the reflection coefficient. The specimen was then placed between the source and the detector, and a measure of the intensity of the sound wave after traversing the sample was obtained. The absorption coefficient per unit path length was then determined from a knowledge of the energy reflected at the two lung-saline interfaces, the thickness of the sample and the acoustic intensity detected by the probe, assuming an exponential dependence of the intensity upon the thickness of the specimen.

DR. KIKUCHI: Are the bubbles resonant at the frequency at which the measurements were made?

DR. DUNN: No. The resonant frequency of the bubbles was near 10 kc and the measurements were made near 1 Mc. You might recall that the bubbles are considered to be imbedded in a medium having a viscosity more than 10,000 times that of water.

DR. MACKAY: What is the the Q of the bubble?

DR. DUNN: The bubble has a rather low Q. One can get some idea of this from the bandwidth of Figure 7.

DR. NYBORG: How did you determine the resonant frequency of the bubbles?

DR. DUNN: We made use of expressions for the resonant frequency and the dissipation parameters given by Devin (J. Acoust. Soc. Am. *31* [1959], 1645; see also reference 4 of paper). Loss mechanisms due to thermal, viscous, and radiation dissipation are considered. All three were included in the preparation of Figure 7; however, at the frequency of 1 Mc the thermal and viscous parameters are negligible in comparison with the radiation parameter.

DR. NYBORG: How was the bubble population determined?

DR. DUNN: The density of the lung samples was determined, and the bubble radius was chosen to be an average value of the gaseous structures within the lung. The bubble population then had to be consistent with these values. It is interesting to note that the surface area of lung tissue computed from the values used in this analysis agrees rather well with the accepted values obtained by other methods.

DR. KIKUCHI: Did you consider the possibility of gas bubbles being produced as a result of the acoustic irradiation?

DR. DUNN: The mathematical model does not consider this. However, the experimental arrangement was such that only a small fraction (a maximum of 0.2%) of the gas within the specimen could be dissolved by the surrounding liquid.

DR. KIKUCHI: Have you considered the effect of a distribution of bubbles of many different radii?

DR. DUNN: No, we have not. A second approximation model might consider the lung as a distribution of spherical and cylindrical pulsating gaseous structures.

DR. HERIC: The postulated loss mechanism would not exist in neonatal lung. Did you make measurements on such specimens?

DR. DUNN: No. However, one of the animals had a pneumonitis at the time the lung was excised, and this specimen yielded an increased density by approximately 100% and a decreased absorption coefficient by approximately 25%.

DR. GORDON: I wish to make two points. First, the ultrasonic absorption coefficient of bone is very difficult to measure and equally difficult to use when attempting to determine proper dosages for radiation. This is due to the fact that bone in situ has very irregular surfaces and scattering may be more important than absorption. Therefore, attenuation may be a more appropriate concept for bone. Our experience shows that the apparent attenuation by bone is greater than the published values of absorption. Second, the difference between absorption of live tissue and excised or dead tissue is very great. It is questionable whether absorption measurements on excised tissue are of practical value for determining sound intensity values to be used on living specimens.

Dr. Dunn: Regarding the first point, the difficulties in making absorption measurements in bone certainly exist. The values presented in the talk were obtained by Hueter. In order to avoid the problems just raised, that is, to have specimens of relatively simple geometrical shapes, he machined pieces of skull bone into discs from which scattering was negligible.

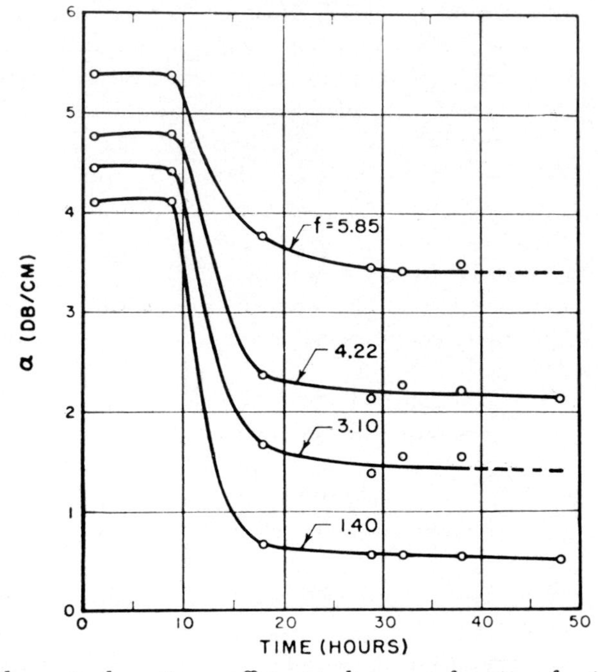

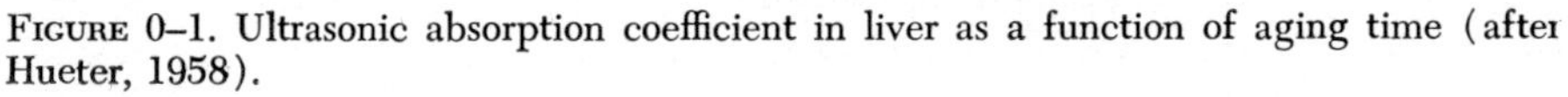
Figure 0–1. Ultrasonic absorption coefficient in liver as a function of aging time (after Hueter, 1958).

The second point is a very important one, and this was alluded to at the end of the talk. Professor Fry has measured the absorption coefficient in cat brain in vivo and in excised fresh slabs by inserting small thermocouples and observing the time rate of change of temperature and has obtained very close agreement.

The measurements of the absorption coefficient of the spinal cord of young mice were made in vivo. The young mouse was specifically chosen for this study because it is essentially poikilothermic and as such can be carried through temperature cycles from approximately 0 to 40°C without producing permanent changes.

Dr. von Gierke: I wish to question reports of the difference in absorption of dead tissue and live tissue. Our measurements show no remarkable difference, that is, the general spread of the biological data from one preparation to another was probably larger than could be attributed to the change from live to dead. Do you know of a good set of data dealing with the same type of tissue under the same conditions which illustrates a transition from live to dead tissue?

DR. DUNN: Figure 0–1, prepared by Hueter, shows the absorption coefficient of liver, which has a very homogeneous structure and exhibits little variation from species to species, as a function of time post mortem at four frequencies. The 1-hr in vitro values are nearly identical with in vivo values. It is seen that virtually no changes occur in the absorption coefficient until about 9 hr post mortem at which time it decreases and levels off at approximately 20 hr post mortem. The decrease in the absorption coefficient varies from approximately a factor of eight at 1.40 Mc to less than a factor of two at 5.85 Mc. These measurements were made at 25°C, but the tissue was maintained at 10°C between measurements. Since 9 hr are required for the absorption properties to begin changing, it is quite likely that many in vitro measurements are made within this time period.

Ultrahigh-Frequency Acoustic Waves in Liquids and Their Interaction with Biological Structures

FLOYD DUNN and STEPHEN A. HAWLEY
Biophysical Research Laboratory, University of Illinois, Urbana, Illinois

Introduction by Dr. Carstensen

One of the outstanding characteristics of the ultrasound symposia held at the University of Illinois is the opportunity to have a relaxed discussion about current progress in research. Consequently, we have the opportunity of learning some possible new approaches to problems, or occasionally, we may hear about some recent research results that look very promising. I know that Dr. Floyd Dunn has recently been doing work with biological materials in the several-hundred-megacycle frequency region, and although he did not plan to give a talk on this topic during the symposium, I have persuaded him to discuss his recent experiments in this field.

A. INTRODUCTION

Research recently carried out at this laboratory has produced methods for generating and detecting acoustic waves in liquids in the kilomegacycle frequency region. Associated studies of the interaction of these ultrahigh-frequency sound waves with biological systems are just beginning. This paper discusses the techniques for generating and detecting uhf acoustic waves in liquids and includes a brief description of an experiment illustrating that interesting possibilities lie ahead.

B. METHODS OF GENERATING UHF SOUND IN LIQUIDS

Two methods of exciting quartz plates to propagate uhf sound in liquids have been employed (1).

The first method can be described as standard as far as the transducer is concerned in that the piezoelectric radiator, a thin X-cut quartz plate electroded on both major faces, is supported by clamping on the periphery. The radiating face is in contact with the liquid medium under investigation and the opposite face is terminated by a material of low characteristic acoustic impedance. The radiating face is held at ground potential and the opposite face is electrically connected to the oscillator via one or more inserted short sections of coaxial transmission line and 50-ohm cable, as illustrated in Figure 1. The inserted sections are designed to produce an impedance match between the 50-ohm line and the quartz plate assembly. For example, in the case of a single insert, the characteristic impedance of the coaxial section is designed, as is common practice, to be the root-mean-square of the input impedance of the transducer assembly, and that of the 50-ohm line and its length is chosen as an odd multiple of a quarter wavelength of the wave in the section.

Quartz plates having fundamental thickness modes of vibration of 4, 12, 15, 18, and 30 Mc, with diameters ranging from ¼ to ¾ in, have been employed. These have been operated at the odd harmonics to nearly 2 kMc. That is, for the 4-Mc plate operated at 1948 Mc, the highest operating frequency attempted thus far, the 487th harmonic is excited. The pulse lengths employed,

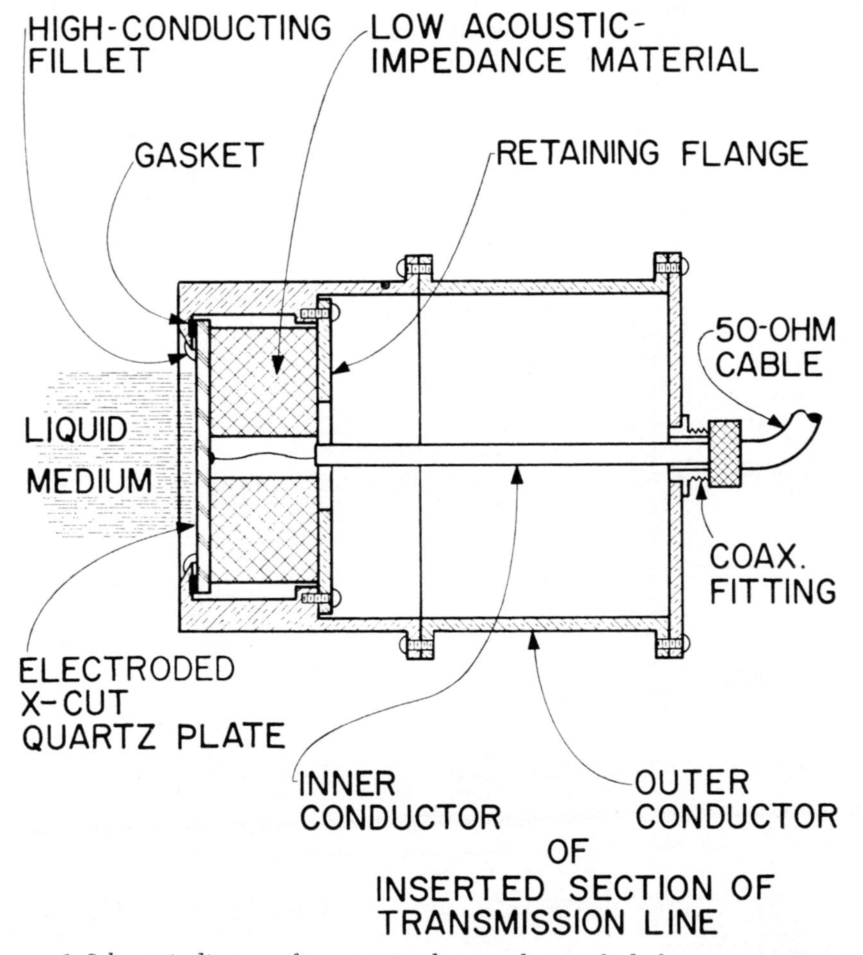

FIGURE 1. Schematic diagram of transmission line coupling method of exciting X-cut quartz plate.

namely, 0.1 sec, result in the establishment of steady-state conditions in the vibrating element.

A second method of exciting the quartz plate utilizes a resonant electromagnetic cavity. Here, the electroded quartz plate is placed in the reentrant structure of a cylindrical cavity, as shown in Figure 2. The design of the cavity follows from established engineering principles (2), taking due account of the fact that the relative dielectric constant of the piezoelectric material is considerably greater than unity. Accordingly, a cavity transducer was designed and fabricated to resonate at 820 Mc, the 205th harmonic of the 4-Mc quartz plate. Excitation was accomplished by coupling the 50-ohm rf transmission line to the fundamental mode of the magnetic field of the

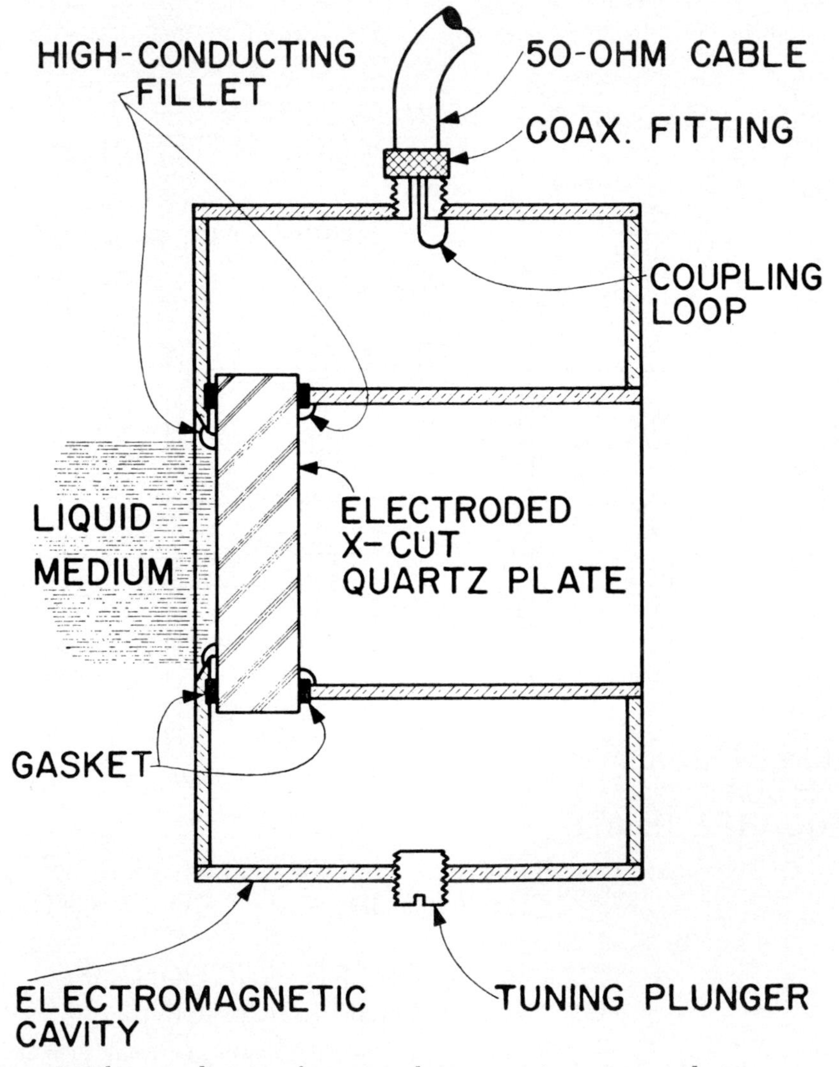

FIGURE 2. Schematic diagram of resonant electromagnetic cavity transducer.

cavity via a small wire loop from the center conductor of the transmission line to ground. A threaded plug was provided, enabling alteration of the cavity volume, for final tuning adjustment. The Q of the cavity, when the quartz plate radiates acoustic waves into a liquid having a value of $\rho C \simeq 1.5 \times 10^5$ g/cm^2 sec, is approximately forty implying a half-power frequency width of approximately 20 Mc. Thus only a few odd harmonic frequencies of the 4-Mc quartz plate can be excited to generate appreciable acoustic power in the liquid by the fixed-dimension cavity employed here.

Both methods are capable of producing sound amplitudes of sufficient intensity in liquids to be detected with ease. The fixed-dimension cavity method, however, has the inherent disadvantage of being restricted by the electromagnetic Q of the unit to a narrow frequency range of operation.

It is possible to solder the quartz plate, having vacuum-deposited gold or silver electrodes on the major faces, directly to the metallic members of either type of transducer, thereby eliminating the gaskets and electrically conducting fillets illustrated in the figures.

C. METHOD OF DETECTING UHF SOUND IN LIQUIDS

A miniature copper-constantan thermocouple probe is employed to detect the uhf acoustic waves (1). The probe, illustrated in Figure 3, is made by etching commercially available 0.0005-in-diameter wire in acid in the vicinity of the junction (to reduce the original diameter), and fabricating the thermocouple by a welding technique in which a condenser is discharged through a circuit containing the thermocouple elements (3).

The structure of the assembled unit is such that little distortion occurs in translation through viscous fluids. A particular advantage of the detector lies in the microscopic volume occupied by the junction. Thermocouples with a maximum dimension of the junction of 5 μ (approximately 10-Ω resistance) are readily constructed. This does not represent the minimum size for such probes, and procedures for fabricating smaller junctions are currently being developed.

For the determination of acoustic absorption coefficients at ultrahigh frequencies, the following procedure is used (4-6): The quartz plate, in contact with the liquid, is excited electrically, at an odd harmonic, to produce a single acoustic pulse with rectangular envelope of 0.1-sec duration. As a result of this relatively short acoustic pulse, the action of the viscous forces brought into play by the relative motion between the thermocouple wires and the imbedding liquid produces a transient temperature rise in the immediate neighborhood of the thermocouple junction. The resulting transient thermal emf produced in the thermocouple circuit is a measure of the acoustic intensity in a plane wave field in the neighborhood of the junction. The transient thermal emf is fed into a DC amplifier which in turn is fed to the vertical deflection plates of an oscilloscope. The thermocouple response, which is directly proportional to the acoustic intensity in the neighborhood of the junction, is observed as the deflection of the electron beam spot from its initial equilibrium position. The deflection of the oscilloscope beam spot is observed for varying distances between the source and probe (this measurement being made with a micrometer having a least count of 0.00001 in). The points are plotted on semilog paper and a straight line of best fit is drawn through the set of points. The acoustic intensity absorption coefficient per unit path length is then readily computed from a knowledge of the slope of this line, assuming that the intensity decreases exponentially with increasing distance from the source.

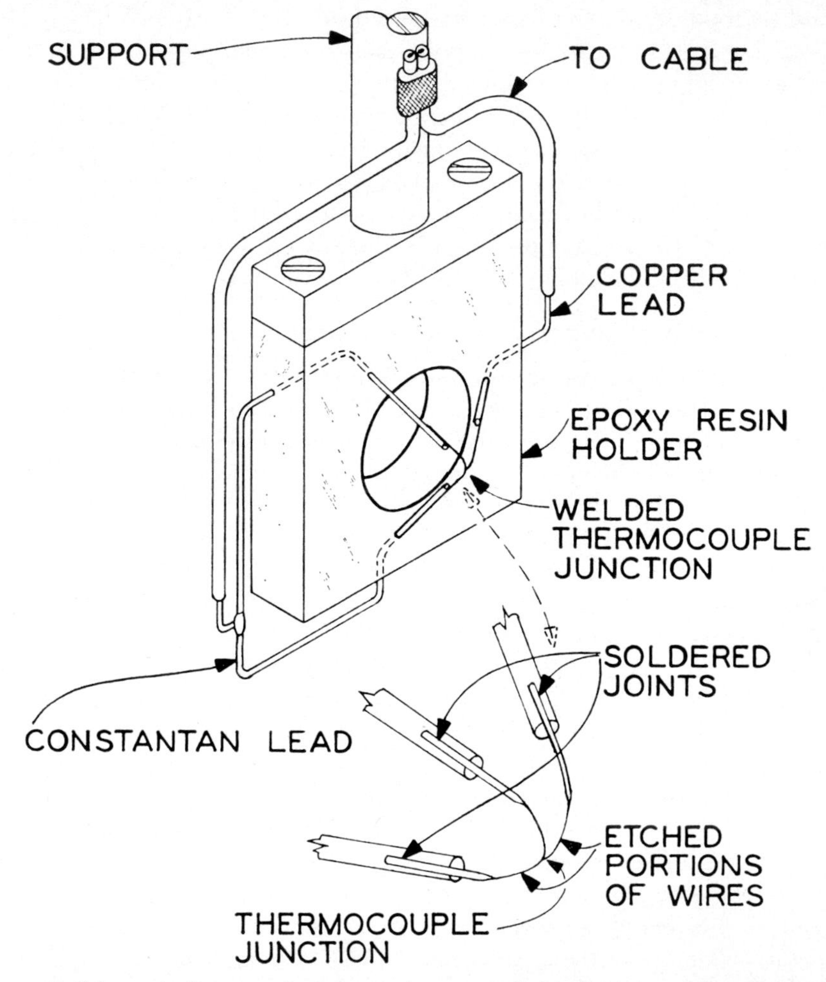

FIGURE 3. Schematic diagram of miniature thermocouple for detecting uhf acoustic waves in liquids.

D. ULTRAHIGH-FREQUENCY ACOUSTIC ABSORPTION MEASUREMENTS

The transient thermoelectric method has been used to study the uhf behavior of the acoustic absorption coefficient of several liquids. For all of the measurements reported below, the acoustic intensity ranges from the 10^{-3} to 10^{-2} w/cm^2 and the temperature rise in the liquid varies from 10^{-2} to 10^{-1}°C.

Figure 4 shows the absorption data obtained by the method described above for castor oil at 30°C together with data obtained by other methods (7–10). It is seen that the agreement between the five independent investigations is generally good. The curve drawn through the plotted points has a slope of 1.66. The dashed line is the computed Stokes viscous absorption for castor oil. The measured values lie below the Stokes values throughout the frequency range above 1 Mc. Figure 5 shows the absorption data for cottonseed oil at 26°C obtained by the method discussed in this paper and by the pulse method (8). It is seen that cottonseed oil behaves as a true Stokes liquid in the frequency range of measurement from 3 to 100 Mc. Figure 6 shows absorption data for Dow-Corning silicone fluid 710 at 26°C to nearly 2 kMc determined by the transient thermoelectric method. The point at 1 Mc was also determined by another method (11). The dashed curve is the Stokes absorption. Assuming negligible velocity dispersion, the data fits very closely a single relaxation process centered at approximately 40 Mc.

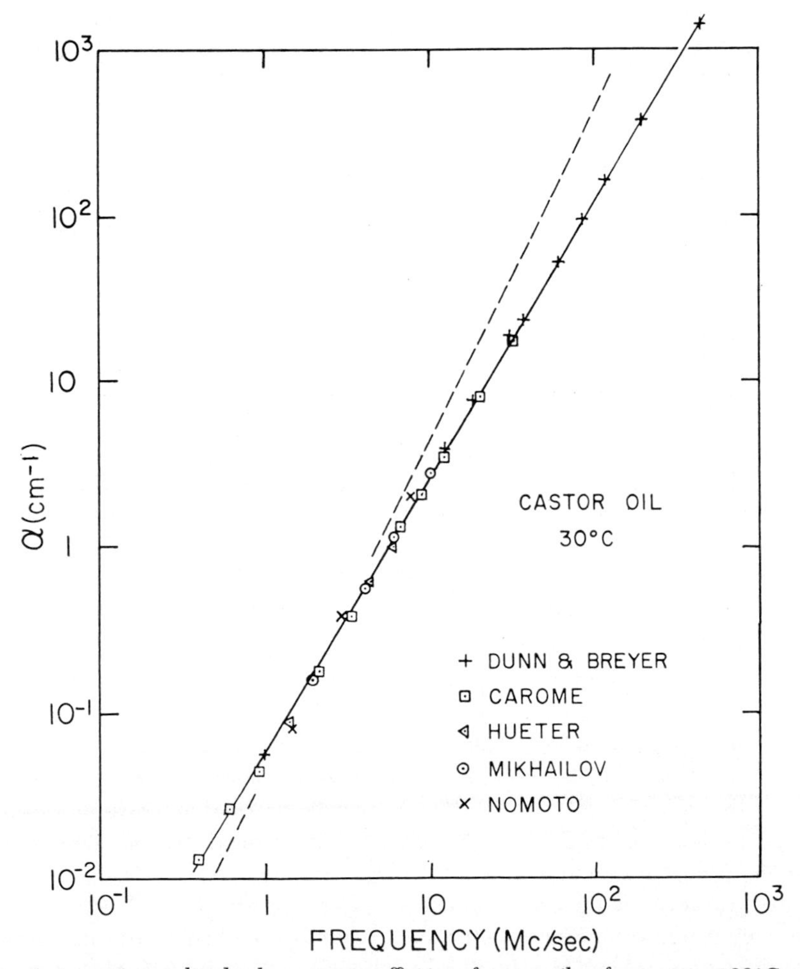

FIGURE 4. Acoustic amplitude absorption coefficient of castor oil vs frequency at 30°C.

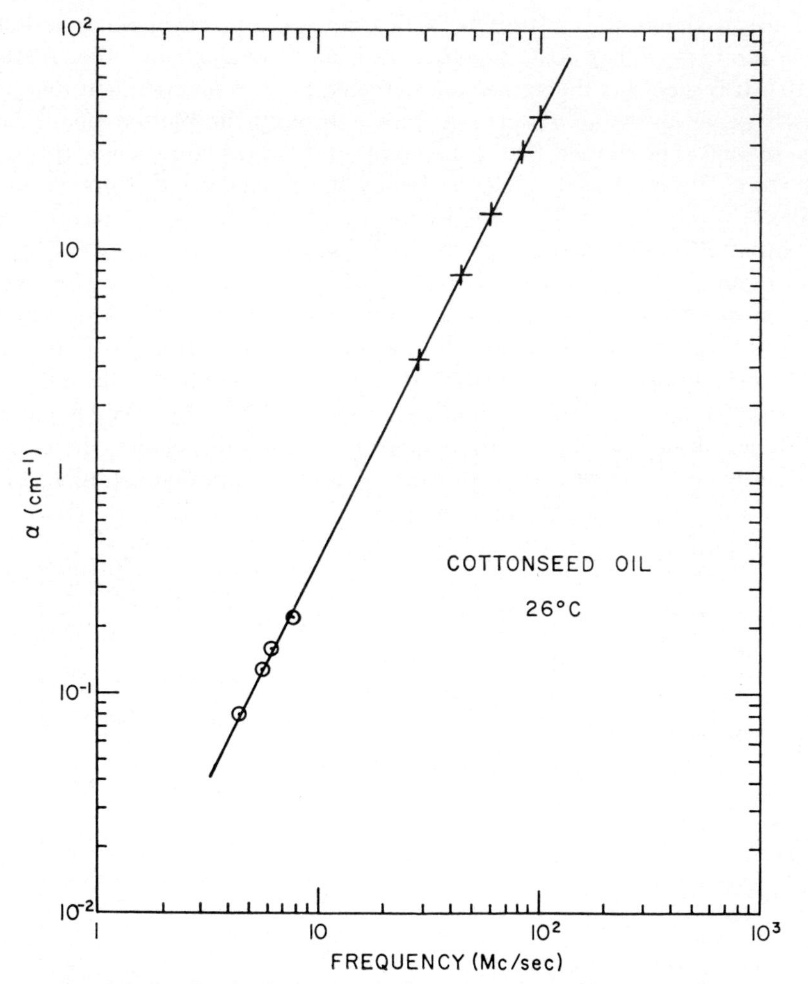

FIGURE 5. Acoustic amplitude absorption coefficient of cottonseed oil vs frequency at 26°C. +, Dunn and Breyer; O, Mikhailov (7).

E. EXAMPLE OF THE INTERACTION OF UHF ACOUSTIC WAVES WITH BIOLOGICAL STRUCTURES

Rotifers (12), small polynucleated aquatic animals several hundred microns in length, were suspended in physiological saline on the surface of the quartz plate of the type of transducer illustrated in Figure 1 (that is, the transducer was arranged to radiate vertically upward). At room temperature, and with no sound present, the specimens attach their (lower) extremity to the surface of the quartz plate and adopt a nearly vertical posture undergoing undulating-like dances in an approximately 60° conical volume. The animals were exposed to single ultrasonic pulses ranging from 0.1-sec to several minutes duration at acoustic intensities of the order of 10^{-3} w/cm² in the frequency range from 200 to 600 Mc. It was observed that only in relatively narrow frequency bands in the neighborhoods of 270 and 510 Mc were these

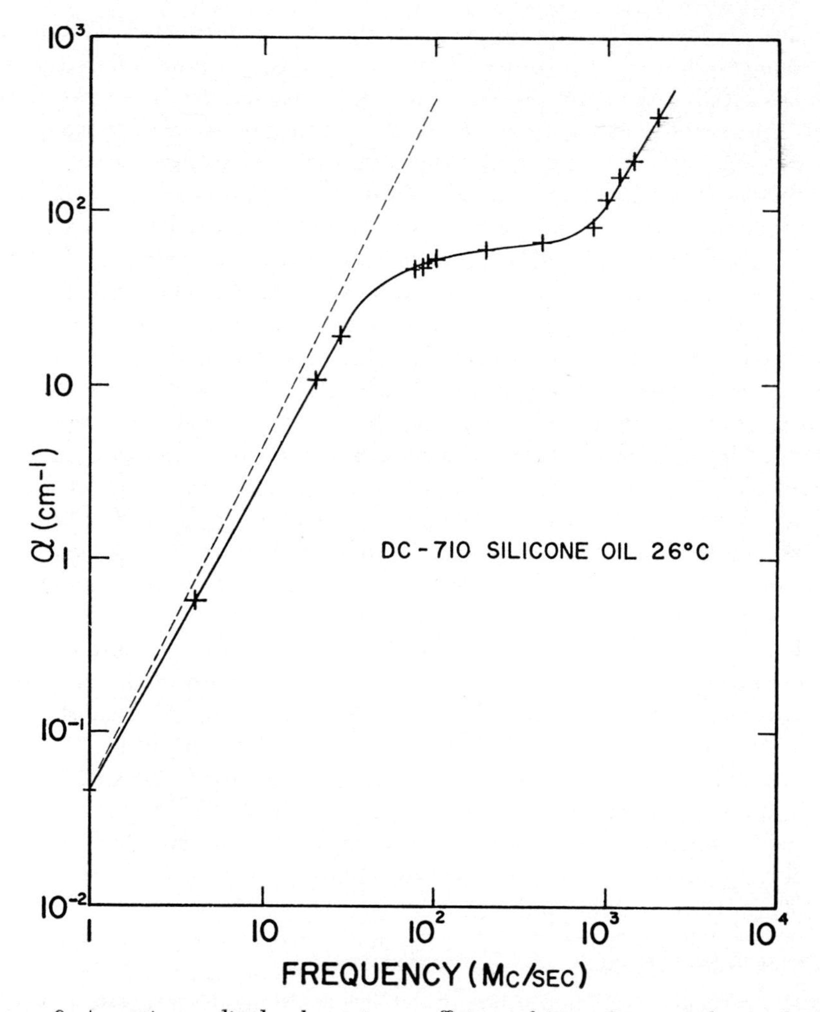

FIGURE 6. Acoustic amplitude absorption coefficient of Dow-Corning silicone fluid vs frequency at 26°C.

characteristic activities altered. The nature of the change in activity was virtually complete cessation of all movement. The animal, still attached to the quartz plate, assumed a globular configuration and remained dormant. Upon cessation of short acoustic pulses (3 to 30 sec), the specimen recovered the characteristic activity. Numerous rotifers were studied in this manner and any single specimen could be carried through repeated acoustic cycles, throughout the frequency range investigated, without apparent damage. Pulse durations of the order of several minutes led to apparent irreversible damage as viability did not return.

These observations illustrate a unique interaction between sound waves at approximately 270 and 510 Mc and the in vivo rotifer. Although the nature of the interaction is at present unknown, the following statements can be made. Injury produced in rotifers (and other biological structures) at lower frequencies (below 1 Mc) has been attributed to cavitation present during ultrasonic exposure (13). However, the thresholds of cavitation at the frequencies employed in the present study are considerably in excess of the sound intensities produced, namely, in the vicinity of 10^5 w/cm^2 (5). This fact, together with the finding that the suppression of rotifer activity occurs in particular frequency bands, should eliminate cavitation as the mechanism of interaction. In the absence of more specific information, let it be assumed that the acoustic intensity absorption coefficient per unit path length in the rotifer is the same as the average value observed for the mammalian central nervous system, namely, approximately 0.2 cm^{-1} at 1 Mc, and that it increases linearly with frequency. This leads to an estimate of the time rate of temperature rise in the rotifer of approximately 3×10^{-2}°C/sec. It is seen that for acoustic exposure durations as long as 10^2 sec, the maximum temperature developed in the animal, in the absence of thermal conduction, is but several degrees above room temperature and this is not sufficient to be considered seriously, for the rotifer thrives at temperatures in excess of 35°C (14). The greatest temperature developed in the saline containing the specimen was of the order of 30°C, that is, a temperature increase of approximately 5°C. The absorption of sound in the imbedding liquid is sufficiently great, as is the path length in the chamber, such that standing waves of large amplitude are not produced. That this is not important in the alteration of the activity of the rotifer was verified by the observation that changing the acoustic path length had no observable effect upon the experimental results.

As the observed effect appears in the neighborhood of 270 and 510 Mc, two frequency regions nearly integrally related, it is tempting to consider a resonance phenomenon as playing a role in the interaction. However, considerably more work will have to be accomplished before the verity of this suggestion can be established.

F. CONCLUDING REMARKS

The techniques for generating and detecting uhf acoustic waves in liquids appear to have reached a degree of sophistication enabling them to be employed in investigations of biological systems. However, such applications are currently in a very early and primitive stage. This laboratory plans to conduct additional experiments in this area. The experiment described in the previous section illustrates that interesting results may be forthcoming.

REFERENCES

1. Dunn, F., and J. E. Breyer (1962). J. Acoust. Soc. Am. *34*, 775.
2. See, for example, T. Moreno, "Microwave Transmission Design Data" (McGraw-Hill Book Company, Inc., New York, 1948), Chap. 13, p. 210.
3. Hawley, S. A., J. E. Breyer, and F. Dunn (1962). Rev. Sci. Instr. 33, 1118.
4. Dunn, F. (1960). J. Acoust. Soc. Am. *32*, 1503.
5. Fry, W. J., and F. Dunn (1962). *In* "Physical Techniques in Biological Research," W. L. Nastuk, ed. (Academic Press, New York), Vol. IV, Chap. 6.
6. Fry, W. J., and R. B. Fry (1954). J. Acoust. Soc. Am. *26*, 311.

7. Wuensch, B. J., T. F. Hueter, and M. S. Cohen (1956). J. Acoust. Soc. Am. *28*, 311
8. Mikhailov, I. G. (1958). Soviet Phys. – Acoustics 3, 187.
9. Nomoto, O., T. Kishimoto, and T. Ikeda (1953). Bull. Kobayasi Inst. Phys. Res. 2, 72.
10. Carome, E. F., John Carroll University, Cleveland, Ohio, private communication.
11. Del Grosso, V. A., U.S. Naval Research Laboratory, Washington, D.C., private communication.
12. See for example, R. W. Pennak, "Fresh-Water Invertebrates of the United States" (Ronald Press, New York, 1953), Chap. 8.
13. Goldman, D. E., and W. W. Lepeschkin (1952). J. Cell. Comp. Physiol. *40*, 255.
14. Finesinger, J. E. (1926). J. Exp. Zool. *44*, 63.

DISCUSSION

DR. VON GIERKE: Have you tried focusing the sound waves at these very high frequencies?

DR. DUNN: We have not attempted to focus since all materials, including any materials from which lenses could be fabricated, absorb sound energy at a very high rate at these microwave frequencies. However, at these frequencies a very interesting situation occurs. Consider the sound source to be approximately 1 cm in diameter. Since the absorption coefficient of all liquids is very high at these frequencies, the measurements are always made with the probe a very short distance from the quartz plate; that is, the distance from the probe to the sound source is very small by comparison with the diameter of the source. With the probe on the axis of the quartz plate, contributions to the intensity at the probe position from the periphery of the sound source are negligible by comparison with those from the axial region. Thus, we have, possibly for the first time, what may be described as an infinite acoustic source, as viewed by the probe positioned on or near the axis of the source.

DR. VON GIERKE: You have, then, a solid acoustical transmission line between two electrical surfaces.

DR. DUNN: Yes. I should point out that while our work has resulted in the generation and detection of the highest frequency acoustic waves in liquids attained thus far, namely, up to 2 kMc, other investigators have measured the absorption and speed of sound in quartz bars at frequencies as high as 24 kMc (see for example E. H. Jacobson, in "Quantum Electronics," C. H. Townes, ed. [Columbia University Press, New York, 1960], p. 468).

DR. HERRICK: Why do you use a thermocouple in preference to a very fine thermistor as the acoustic detector?

DR. DUNN: Primarily because we have the technology for fabricating thermocouple detectors as small as 5 μ and the possibility of fabricating them as small as 1 μ. The smallest thermistor elements currently available are larger than 50 μ. In principle, they could be made smaller, but there are many technical problems involved. Your suggestion is a good one since the thermistor should provide an acoustic detector of considerably greater sensitivity than that of the thermocouple.

DR. BELL: Do you anticipate problems associated with heating the biological materials at these high frequencies?

DR. DUNN: We do not anticipate any great problems because of the following. If we assume a value 0.2 cm^{-1} as an average value for the acoustic intensity absorption coefficient per unit path length of biological materials at 1 Mc and assume further that this increases linearly with frequency, then at 1000 Mc the absorption coefficient has a value of 200 cm^{-1}. The highest acoustic intensities that we have been able to produce thus far are approximately 0.1 w/cm^2; however, the rotifer experiments were carried out at intensities of the order of 10^{-3} w/cm^2. For the highest intensities currently available, at 1000 Mc, this implies a time rate of temperature rise, in the absence of thermal conduction processes, of less than 10°C/sec. Since thermal conduction would serve to limit the temperature rise and the rotifer experiments indicate that events occur within time intervals less than 1 sec, it appears that results of more than routine interest are produced without appreciable heating of the biological specimen.

The Use of High-Intensity Ultrasound to Alter the Cellular Structure of the Anterior Pituitary

ROLFS KRUMINS, ELIZABETH KELLY, FRANCIS J. FRY, and WILLIAM J. FRY
Biophysical Research Laboratory, University of Illinois, Urbana, Illinois

Introduction by Dr. Carstensen

The next paper concerns a topic of basic biological interest, namely, the possible use of high-intensity ultrasound to control hormonal functions of the body by means of its effect on the pituitary gland. The paper will be presented by Elizabeth Kelly.

This preliminary report is concerned with the degenerative and regenerative processes occurring in the anterior pituitary gland as a result of ultrasonic irradiation. In order to study such processes by histological techniques, ultrasonic lesions of a variety of sizes and geometric configurations were produced in different positions in the anterior pituitary of cats and the resultant cellular changes were studied for sacrifice times from 1 hr to several months. The initial purpose of this research was the investigation of the possibility of using high-intensity ultrasound to produce selective effects, temporary and permanent, on the cellular composition of the anterior pituitary gland.

Figure 1 shows the stereotaxic apparatus used to support the cat in position in preparation for ultrasonic irradiation, the attached x-ray cassettes used in taking roentgenograms to identify landmarks on the sella turcica and the coupling pan which supports the transmitting liquid. A portion of the cat's skull is removed in order to maintain a precise focus and accurate control of the dosage for the sound beam within the brain. Degassed mammalian Ringer's solution is used as the liquid coupling agent between the sound transducer and the brain tissue. The sound source is lowered into the liquid in the coupling pan, and irradiation is accomplished through the intact dura mater. The sound is produced by a single X-cut quartz crystal and focused with a lens to produce a high-intensity beam at a frequency of 4 Mc/sec. The dosage of ultrasound applied to produce the cellular changes was uniformly high, but some variation of the level was utilized as one parameter for con-

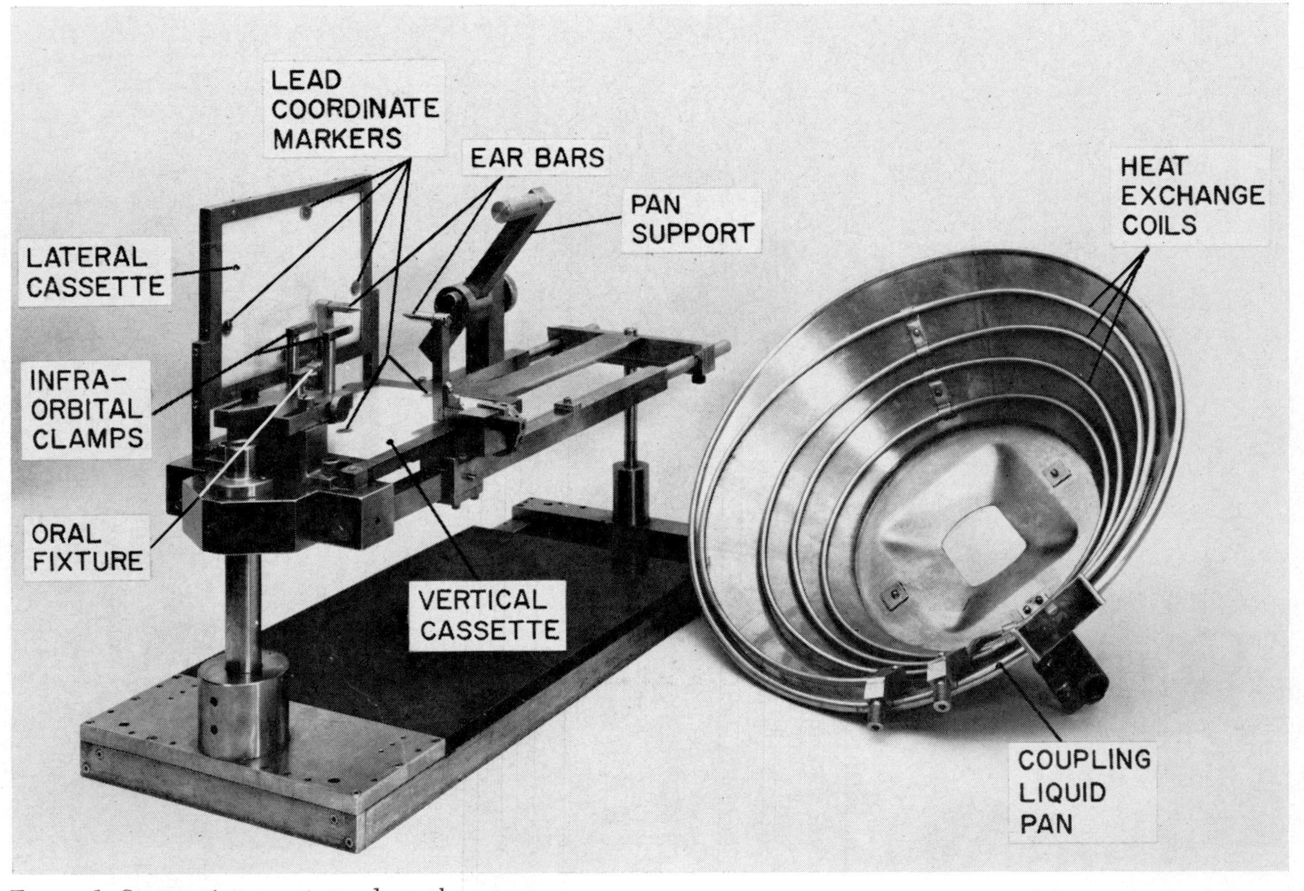

FIGURE 1. Stereotaxic apparatus and attachments.

trolling the effect of the irradiation on the cellular structure. Details of the irradiation dosages will not be discussed in this presentation except to indicate that for the average ultrasound dosage applied, the particle velocity amplitude was approximately 600 cm/sec. This corresponds to approximately 90 atm pressure amplitude[1] for the focused field. The lesions were produced by a series of closely spaced ultrasonic exposures (0.2 to 0.3 mm separation). The irradiation time for a single exposure was also used as a variable to control the effects on the cellular structure but was, in general, close to 0.5 sec.

The cytological studies were made on the hypophyses of cats sacrificed at times varying from 1 hr to 3 months after ultrasonic irradiation. The two groups of pituitary cells considered in this paper fall under the general classification of chromophiles, namely, the acidophils (alpha cells) and basophils (beta and delta cells). These two groups are of considerable importance and are concerned with the function of various hormones such as ACTH, TSH, corticotrophin, and somatotrophin (1). Figure 2 shows a Gomori-stained transverse section of the anterior pituitary of a normal cat—the cytoplasm of the acidophils appears red, that of the basophils blue. Consideration of Figure 2 appears to indicate a greater concentration of acidophils in the lateral areas with the basophils more restricted to the central area. Such an arrangement would agree with the observations of Dawson regarding the location of the different types of cells of the anterior pituitary gland of the cat (2).

Figure 3 shows a gallocyanin-stained tissue section of the anterior pituitary of a normal cat—the nuclei of the various cells are stained blue with only a very light staining of the cytoplasm. The DNA and RNA of the nucleus are affected by this stain, as well as the RNA of the cytoplasm. The normal tissue of this figure can be compared to that of Figure 4 which shows a gallocyanin-stained transverse section of the pituitary of a cat sacrificed 3 days after irradiation. The tissue at the base of this figure illustrates a so-called thermal lesion (the thermal lesion extends dorsal to the base on the left side), that is, a lesion produced primarily by a transfer of heat from the bone surrounding the pituitary. (The ultrasonic absorption coefficient of bone is much greater than that of soft tissue.) The most striking effect of the thermal lesion is the almost complete absence of cells. Such thermal lesions can be prevented by placing the focus of the sound beam more dorsally in the structure, but it is of interest to study such lesions and compare them with ultrasound lesions that are not complicated by direct heat transfer. For example, in the tissue section illustrated in this figure, the "ultrasound" lesion is apparent dorsal to the thermal lesion at the base of the gland, but, in contrast to the thermal lesion, it exhibits only slight changes with the gallocyanin stain. In this regard, it is of interest to compare Figure 5, which shows a magnified view of the normal or unirradiated area of the gland shown in Figure 4, with Figures 6 and 7 which show, at the same magnification, the ultrasound lesion regions and the thermal lesion region of the same gland. In the unirradiated area

[1] Expressed in terms of intensity for a plane wave, this pressure amplitude would correspond to an intensity of 2700 w/cm ^{2}.

(Fig. 5) the nuclei of the cells are quite distinct, with some indication of the surrounding cytoplasm. In the ultrasound lesion area (Fig. 6) the nuclei are a little swollen and the cytoplasm shows vacuolization and there is some depletion in the number of cells. However, in the thermal lesion area (Fig. 7) it is evident that the effect of the heat has been quite drastic, with an almost total depletion of nuclei. Since all of these sections were stained with gallocyanin, which reacts with nucleic acid, it would appear reasonable to conclude that in the case of the thermal lesion the nucleic acids were affected by the thermal energy. The Feulgen test, which is a specific for DNA, yielded a negative result indicating that essentially no DNA remained in the thermal lesion area.

Figure 8 shows a tissue section of the pituitary gland of the same cat just described, but the stain applied is Gomori. As indicated previously, after application of this stain, the acidophils appear red, and the basophils blue. The nuclei of the cells are also stained. If one now examines the thermal lesion area, which appeared almost devoid of cells when stained with gallocyanin, it is evident that there is a considerable cell population. In addition, in the upper area of the gland the extent of the ultrasound lesion is more clearly defined, although in the gallocyanin stain it was only just detectable. Figure 9 illustrates a magnified view of the normal or unirradiated region of this Gomori-stained tissue section, while Figures 10 and 11 respectively show at the same magnification the ultrasound lesion and thermal lesion regions. It is quite evident that in the ultrasound lesion area, the secretion granules are greatly depleted and those that are still present are not as deeply stained as previously. Many of these cells are undergoing degeneration, but the nuclei are present in the scattered acidophils. By contrast, for the thermal lesion, the secretion granules are now deeply stained but no nuclei are present. The blood vessels still contain blood elements.

Summarizing the data for this cat, it can be concluded that with a sacrifice time of 3 *days* and for the specific ultrasound dosage applied, it is possible to distinguish two types of lesions. In the "thermal" lesion, the nuclei are destroyed, while the cytoplasm appears intact. In the ultrasound lesion, the nuclei are relatively unaffected, while a large percentage of the secretion granules are depleted.

Figure 12 (gallocyanin stain) demonstrates a series of lesions, with normal pituitary tissue between the affected areas.[2] A greater dose of ultrasound was used than that applied to produce the lesions demonstrated in the previous figures, and the cat was sacrificed after a 7-day interval. If the lesions in this figure are compared with that of the previous gallocyanin-stained lesions, it is immediately evident that the destruction in the ultrasound lesion is much greater than in the previously illustrated ultrasound lesions. Further, there is no sharp demarcation between the thermal lesion and the ultrasound lesion. Figure 13 represents a Gomori stain of the same region shown in Figure 12, and here again it is evident that the destruction is extreme. One does not

[2] The torn area is a result of a mechanical break of the tissue due to poor fixation.

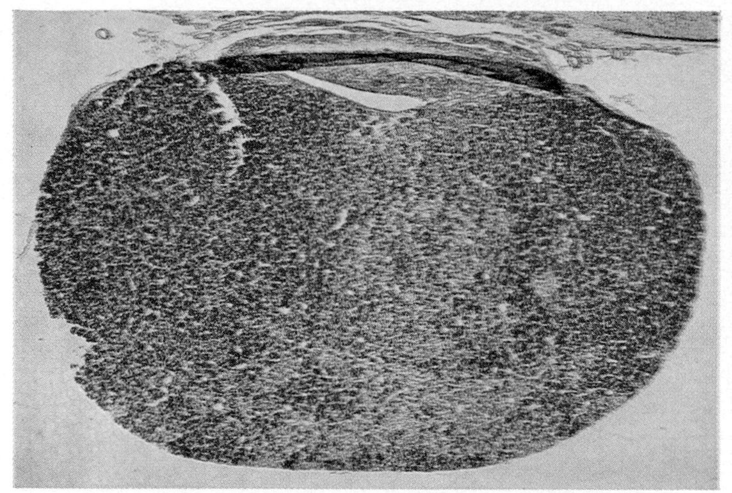

Figure 2

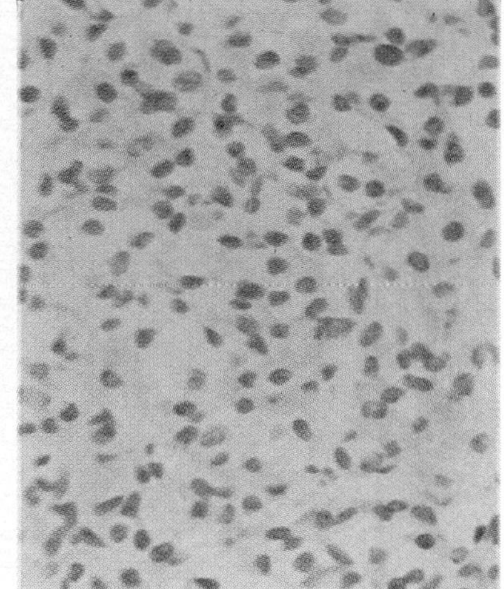

Figure 5

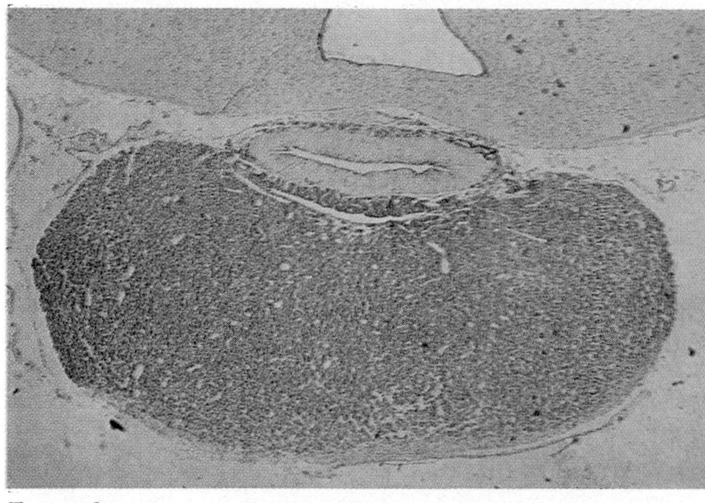

Figure 3

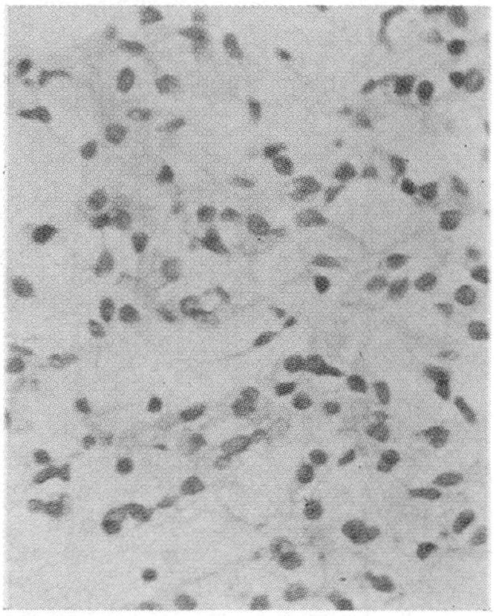

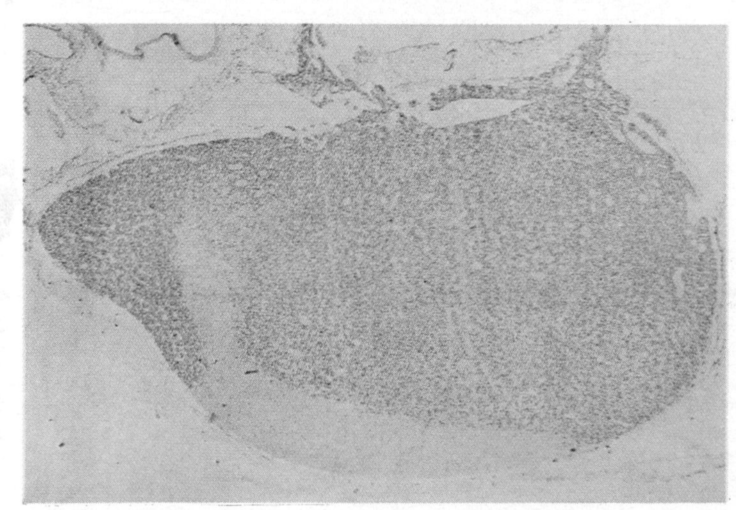

Figure 4

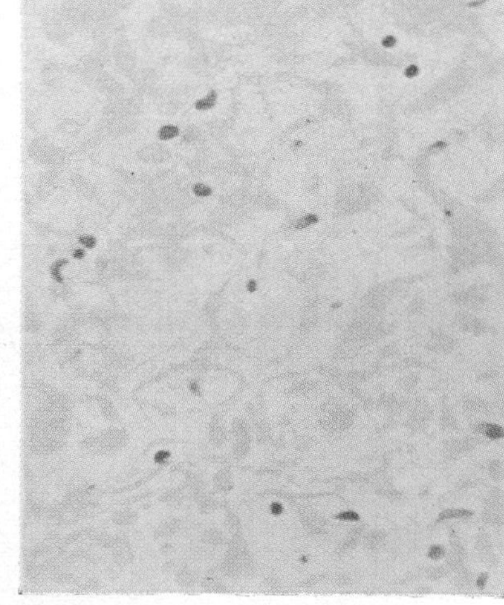

Figure 7

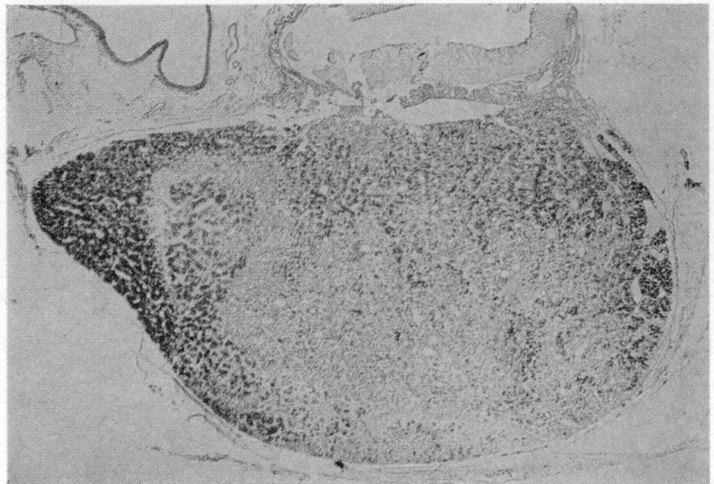

FIGURE 8

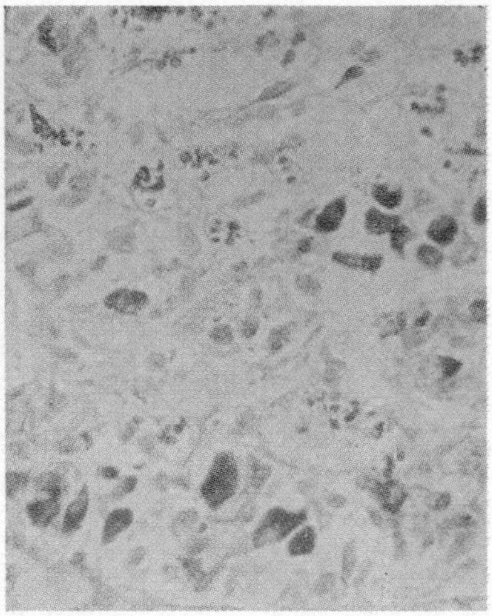

FIGURE 11

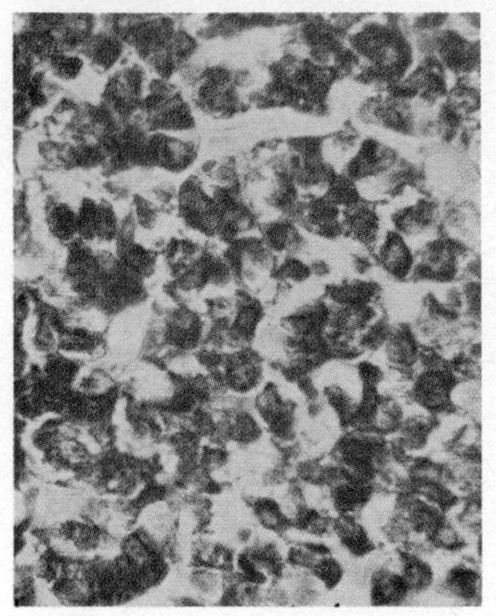

FIGURE 9

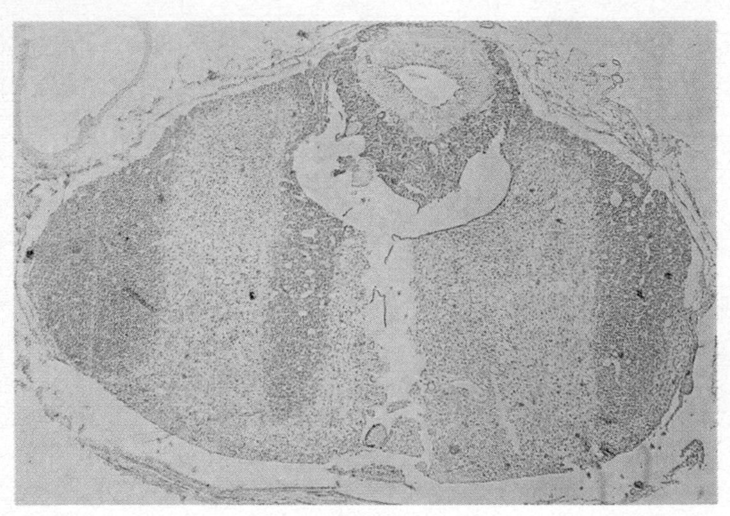

FIGURE 12

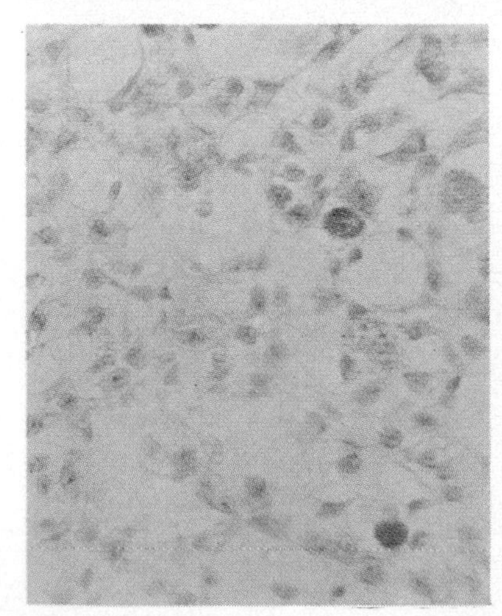

FIGURE 10

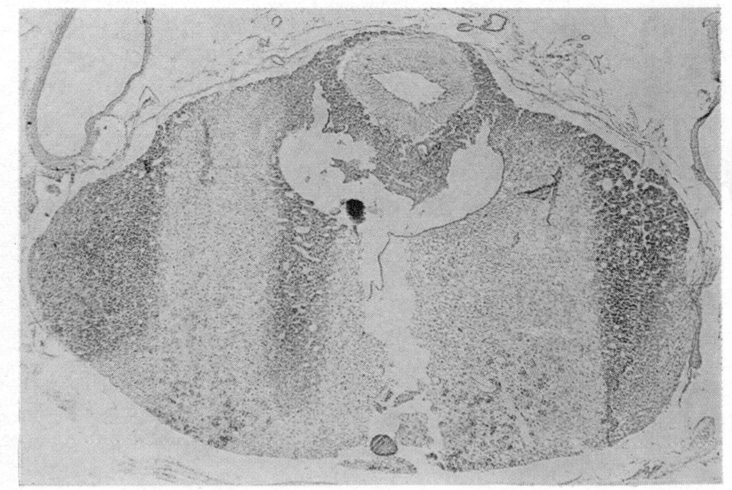

FIGURE 13

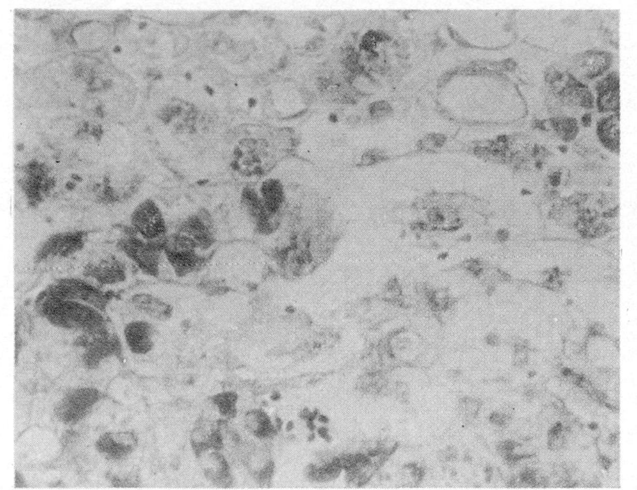

FIGURE 14

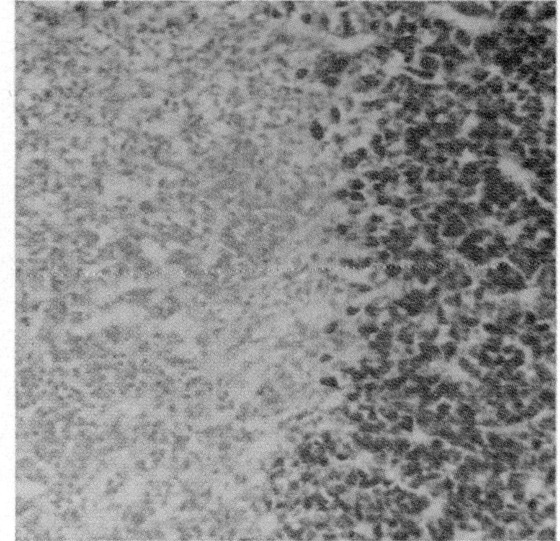

FIGURE 17

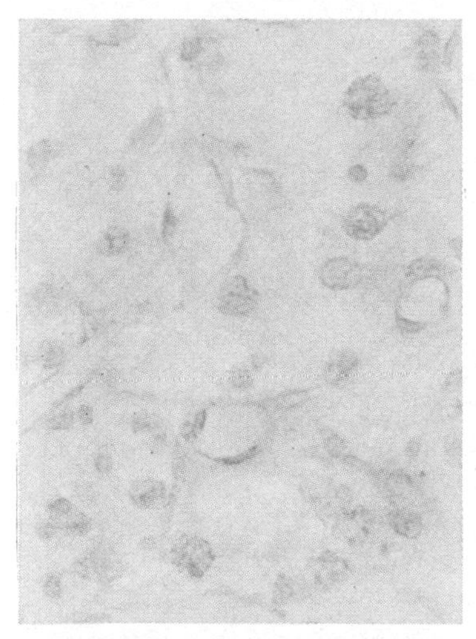

FIGURE 15

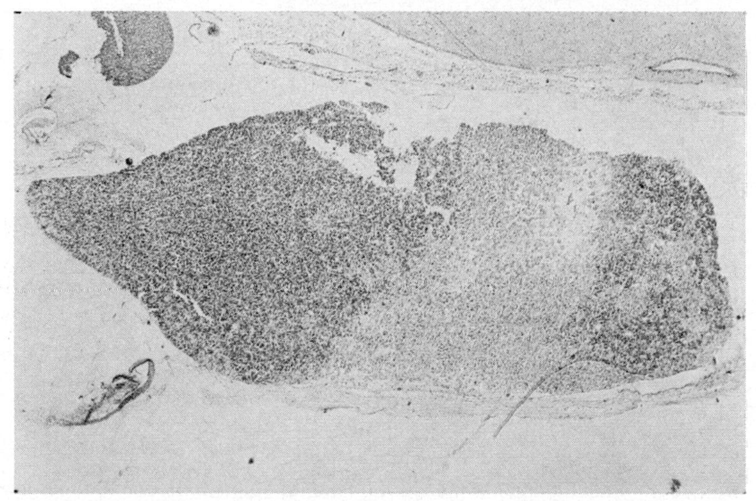

FIGURE 18

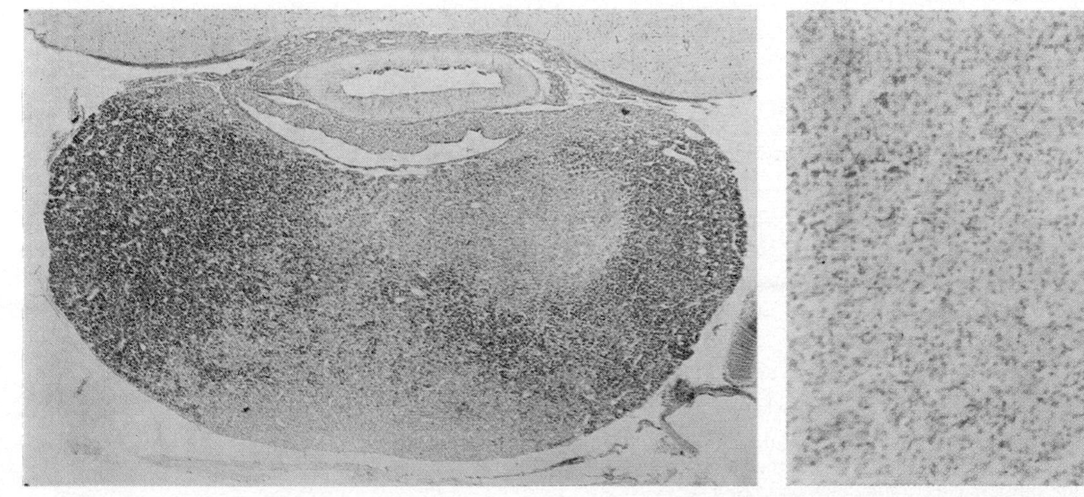

FIGURE 16

FIGURE 19

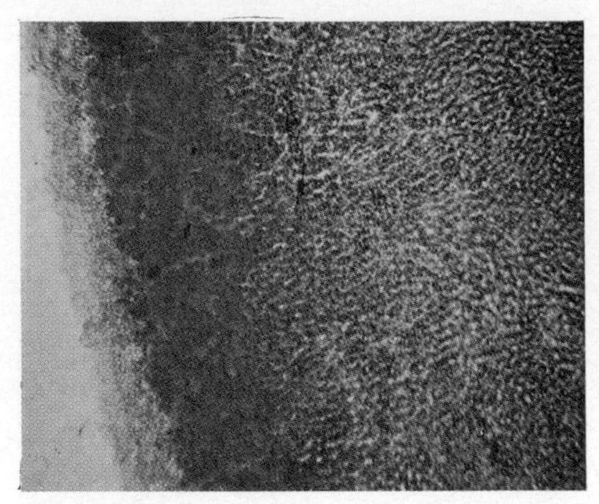

FIGURE 20

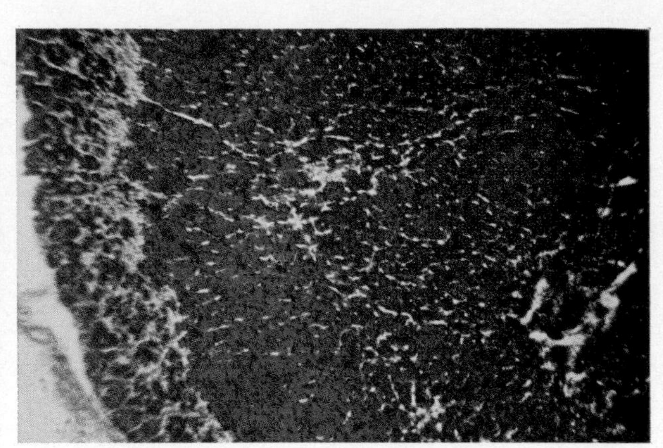

FIGURE 21

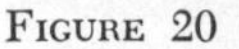

FIGURE 2. Transverse tissue section of anterior pituitary of normal cat — Gomori stain.

FIGURE 3. Transverse tissue section of anterior pituitary of normal cat — gallocyanin stain.

FIGURE 4. Transverse tissue section of anterior pituitary of cat sacrificed 3 days after ultrasonic irradiation of a portion of the gland — gallocyanin stain.

FIGURE 5. Magnified view of unirradiated region of anterior pituitary section shown in Figure 4 — gallocyanin stain.

FIGURE 6. Magnified view of ultrasonic lesion region of anterior pituitary section shown in Figure 4 — gallocyanin stain.

FIGURE 7. Magnified view of thermal lesion region of anterior pituitary section shown in Figure 4 — gallocyanin stain.

FIGURE 8. Transverse tissue section of anterior pituitary of same cat illustrated in Figure 4 — Gomori stain.

FIGURE 9. Magnified view of unirradiated region of anterior pituitary section shown in Figure 8 — Gomori stain.

FIGURE 10. Magnified view of ultrasound lesion region of anterior pituitary section shown in Figure 8 — Gomori stain.

FIGURE 11. Magnified view of thermal lesion region of anterior pituitary section shown in Figure 8 — Gomori stain.

FIGURE 12. Transverse tissue section of anterior pituitary of cat sacrificed 7 days after ultrasonic irradiation of separate regions of the gland — gallocyanin stain.

FIGURE 13. Transverse tissue section of anterior pituitary of same cat illustrated in Figure 12 — Gomori stain.

FIGURE 14. Magnified view of thermal lesion region of anterior pituitary section shown in Figure 13 — Gomori stain.

FIGURE 15. Magnified view of ultrasound lesion region of anterior pituitary section shown in Figure 13 — Gomori stain.

FIGURE 16. Transverse tissue section of anterior pituitary of cat sacrificed 21 days after ultrasonic irradiation of a portion of the gland — Gomori stain.

FIGURE 17. Magnified view of border between ultrasonically irradiated region and normal region of anterior pituitary section shown in Figure 16 — Gomori stain.

FIGURE 18. Transverse tissue section of anterior pituitary of cat sacrificed 3 months after ultrasonic irradiation of a portion of the gland — Gomori stain.

FIGURE 19. Magnified view of ultrasound lesion region of anterior pituitary section shown in Figure 18 — Gomori stain.

FIGURE 20. Tissue section of adrenal gland of normal cat — sudan III stain.

FIGURE 21. Tissue section of adrenal gland of cat sacrificed 3 months after ultrasonic irradiation of a portion of the anterior pituitary — sudan III stain.

see intact secretion granules in the ultrasound lesion as was evident in Figure 8. At the base of the slide, however, some secretion cells are evident. Figure 14 is a magnified view of the base region. The secretion cells are quite prominent but they do not exhibit nuclei. Also evident are the blood cells and the fibrous reticulum. Figure 15 shows a magnified view of the ultrasound lesion. The majority of the gland cells are gone, and a high macrophagic activity is underway. In some regions, free debris, fragments of cytoplasm and cell nuclei are stained.

The ultrasound lesions demonstrated in the upper areas of Figures 12 through 15 are due to the ultrasonic energy per se and are not complicated by extraneous heating, for example, heat transfer from bone. However, these lesions differ considerably from the ultrasound lesions demonstrated in Figures 4 through 11. It is evident, therefore, that depending on the dosage, ultrasound may produce a variety of effects on the cellular structure of the anterior pituitary gland, ranging from partial depopulation to complete destruction.

The sacrifice times (interval between irradiation and sacrifice) for the two experimental cats discussed above were comparatively short (3 and 7 days). Figure 16 demonstrates a high-intensity ultrasound lesion in which the sacrifice time was considerably longer, namely, 21 days. The predominantly blue stain of the lesion region indicates a general absence of acidophil cells since a Gomori stain was applied (compare with Fig. 2). A region of particular interest is the upper right-hand area, since in a normal cat the acidophil population would predominate in this area (2). Figure 17 is a magnified view of part of this area which includes the boundary between the unirradiated and the lesion zones. The absence of acidophil cells within the lesion area is quite striking. Preliminary evidence indicates that the basophils are regenerated cells. The same type of result, namely, the predominance of basophils in the region of the lesion was observed in cats sacrificed 30 days and 3 months after irradiation. For example, Figure 18 shows a Gomori-stained transverse tissue section of a pituitary of a cat sacrificed 3 months after irradiation. Again, the lesion region is stained predominantly blue, and a magnified view of this region (Fig. 19) indicates almost a complete absence of acidophil cells. If ultrasonic energy can be applied to selectively depress the acidophil population, the results would be of tremendous medical significance since the acidophils are associated with the production of growth hormone.

In addition to the histological studies of the pituitary glands of the irradiated cats, such studies were made on the adrenals, thyroids, and ovaries. A number of physiological tests were made on the animals during the intervals following irradiation. These latter included a study of the effects of the pituitary lesions on: (1) estrus cycle — as indicated by the vaginal smear test, (2) thyroid metabolism — as indicated by the cholesterol levels in the blood, and (3) sugar metabolism — as indicated by blood sugar levels and insulin tolerance levels. All of these studies are still in the preliminary stages so the results will not be discussed in detail at this time. However, it is of some interest to indicate here the results of some of these tests on the cat whose pituitary sections show a predominance of basophil cells in the lesion region 3 months after irradiation. The plasma cholesterol levels and the volume of urine output were normal. The histological studies of the thyroid and ovaries did not indicate any gross changes, except for an abnormal flatness of the epithelial cells of the thyroid and an indication of abnormally enlarged follicles in the ovary. The histological changes in the adrenal gland, however, were more drastic. Figure 20 shows a tissue section of normal adrenal gland stained for fat distribution with Sudan III. The various layers of the adrenal can be clearly distinguished, namely, the capsule on the outer edge, the glomerulosa zone, and the outer and inner fasciculata zones. The red stain represents fat deposits. Figure 21 illustrates a tissue section of the adrenal of the cat sacrificed 3 months after irradiation. It is quite apparent that considerable change has taken place in the amount and distribution of fat. The same layers are evident, the capsule, the glomerulosa, and the fasciculata (the blue area in the center is a portion of the medulla), but the most striking change is the tremendous increase in fat in the fasciculata zone. The fat is

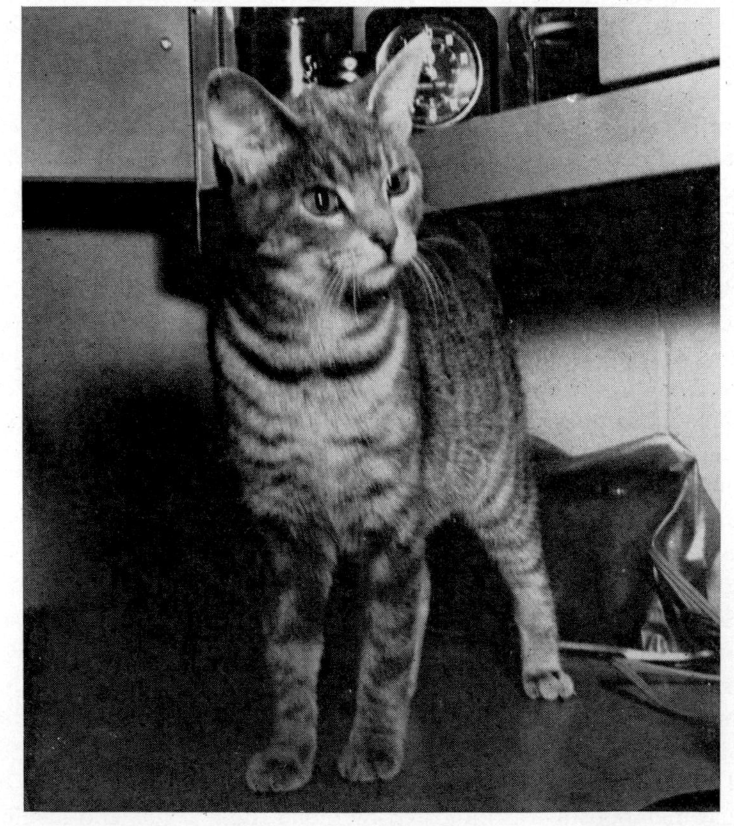

FIGURE 22. Photograph of cat which exhibited abnormal fat distribution within the fasciculata zone of the adrenal gland (see Fig. 21) following ultrasonic irradiation of a portion of the anterior pituitary. Picture taken on day of sacrifice, 3 months following the irradiation.

now heavily distributed over both areas of this zone and is also present in the glomerulosa. There is also an increase of connective tissue.

It is of interest to note that, in general, the cats appeared undisturbed by the pituitary irradiation after their initial recovery from the operative procedure. For example, Figure 22 is a picture of the cat that exhibited the abnormal fat distribution in the adrenal glands. This picture was taken on the day of sacrifice, and the cat was alert and healthy.

REFERENCES

1. Ezrin, C., H. E. Swanson, J. G. Humphrey, J. W. Dawson, and F. M. Hill (1959). The cells of the human adenohypophysis in thyroid disorders. J. Clin. Endocrinol. & Metab. *21*, *8*, 958–966.
2. Dawson, A. B. (1956). Some evidences of specific secretory activity of the anterior pituitary gland of the cat. Am. J. Anat. *78*, 347–405.

DISCUSSION

Dr. Carstensen: The information on regeneration of basophil cells would appear to be of great significance. Can you distinguish the regenerated area quite clearly?

Dr. Kelly: In the long-term cats, such as those sacrificed after 1- and 3-month intervals, the regeneration appears quite distinct. Connective tissue growth and basophil regeneration can be seen in the lesion area. In the case of cats sacrificed after shorter time intervals, such as 10 and 14 days, mitotic activity is evident in the lesion area.

Dr. Gordon: Ultrasound has been used previously to irradiate the anterior pituitary of carcinoma patients. I am a radiologist and, therefore, not intimately concerned with the results of such studies, but it is my general impression that this method has had some clinical success.

Dr. Kelly: Evidently the studies to which you are referring are concerned with complete destruction of the pituitary gland by ultrasound, that is, a hypophysectomy. It is relatively simple to perform ultrasonic hypophysectomies on experimental animals. The approach in this study, however, is to use the ultrasound to produce selective effects on the cellular components rather than to accomplish simple destruction.

Dr. Weissler: It is interesting that the pathology of the thermal lesion is different than that of the ultrasound lesion. Do you know what the relative temperatures were in the thermal lesion area and in the ultrasound lesion area?

Dr. Kelly: We did not make any temperature measurements. However, in previous studies at the Biophysical Research Laboratory concerned with the use of ultrasound for investigations of the central nervous system, temperature measurements were made in the irradiation area. Perhaps Professor Fry would care to comment on the result of those studies.

Dr. W. J. Fry: In the brain, for temperature rises of 18°C in white matter and 10°C in gray matter, we did not produce thermal lesions, although the usual ultrasonic selective lesion effects were produced. I would guess, therefore, that the temperature rise in the thermal lesion areas of the pituitary were certainly more than 20°C.

DR. CURTIS. Are these pituitary lesions the result of both heat and ultrasound, that is, are they combined lesions?

DR. KELLY: The lesions in the base, which we have called thermal lesions, are certainly dependent on the combined effects of direct heat transfer from the bone and ultrasound. It is convenient to distinguish them as thermal lesions since the lesions in the upper area are not complicated by direct heating, although heating is also involved. The essential point is that the effects on the cellular population for the two types of lesions are quite different. Of course, the effects are dependent also on the dose of ultrasound. With sufficient intensity, complete destruction can take place in the ultrasound lesion area.

DR. KIKUCHI: You could have avoided the problem of heat transfer from the bone by controlling the doses so that there was time for the heat to dissipate.

DR. KELLY: We knew that the heating of the bone could be avoided, but we did not make any attempts in that direction because we found it of interest to compare the histological results for the so-called thermal lesions and ultrasound lesions.

7

Action of Intense Ultrasound on the Intact Mouse Liver

JOSEPH C. CURTIS[1]
Brown University, Providence, Rhode Island

Introduction by Dr. Carstensen

The next paper is concerned also with the use of ultrasound to produce cellular changes in biological tissue. In this case the tissue of interest is the liver.

Recent reports of biological applications of intense ultrasound (1–13) indicate that ultrasonic techniques have considerable potential in basic and applied neurology, tissue visualization, and experimental biology. The realization of this potential will depend largely upon how well the underlying mechanisms of ultrasonic action are understood. While the literature on the biological effects of ultrasound is extensive (14–16), relatively few attempts have been made to relate the effects of intense ultrasound upon intact tissues to such basic mechanisms. The most elaborate studies to date are those dealing with the central nervous system (1–9). The investigations reported here are concerned with the effects of intense ultrasound of 1-Mc frequency upon the liver of the intact mouse. These studies were made: (1) to determine what changes are produced in the intact liver by focused ultrasound when administered continuously or pulsed, and (2) to find out how the observed effects are related to the intensity, duration, and, in the case of pulsed irradiation, the temporal distribution of the acoustic energy.

The findings of a dosage study and a description of the cytological changes produced by intense ultrasound are reported here.

Our present understanding of the mechanisms involved in the localized destruction of tissue by intense ultrasound is based primarily upon the studies of Fry *et al.* (17–20) and those of Hueter, Ballantine, and associates (9, 21, 22). Dunn and Fry (20) have shown that while the frequency of incidence of paralysis produced by ultrasound in precooled one-day-old mice is dependent upon the initial tissue temperature, it is not dependent upon the attain-

[1] Dr. Curtis' present address is Biology Department, Clark University, Worcester, Massachusetts.

ment of a critical temperature. Their study, which has involved a broad range of doses, indicates that the action of ultrasound upon the central nervous system is predominantly mechanical in nature. Based upon a similar study, Hueter, Ballantine, and Cotter (21) have proposed a "temperature-dependent mechanical effect originating at weak points of the tissue structure." Their observations that a much greater intensity was required at 2.5 Mc to obtain the same effect produced at 1 Mc suggested an effect that was not predominantly thermal in origin. Since the absorption coefficient α increases with frequency, a greater effect would be expected at the higher frequency if injury were due primarily to heating.

While a number of investigators (23–27) have described effects of ultrasound upon liver, few have studied the effects of intense ultrasound in terms of the dosage parameters. Bell (27) found that focused ultrasound produced lesions selectively at the surface of an irradiated lobe in the mouse, these lesions most often being localized at that surface farthest from the sound source. He demonstrated that similar lesions could be produced by direct exposure of the liver to focused light. However, the extent of the injury caused by these different agents appeared to be comparable only when a much greater temperature rise was produced in the liver treated with focused light. A comparison of the effect of precooling animals upon the extent of injury produced by focused light with the extent of injury produced by ultrasound further indicated that the destructive effects of these two physical agents are not identical. Whereas the liver injury produced by focused light could be inhibited by precooling the mice, that caused by ultrasound could not. Bell (27) suggested that "the heating action of ultrasound works synergistically with its other actions" to produce the observed biological effects.

An attempt has been made in the studies reported here to determine the relative importance of several possible mechanisms in producing liver injury. The results may be considered in the light of the following questions: (1) How is the frequency of occurrence of hepatic lesions such as those described by Bell (27) related to the duration and intensity of focused ultrasound of 1-Mc frequency? (2) How is the probability of such lesions related to the time distribution of the acoustic energy when administered as a series of pulses of short duration, the intensity and total amount of acoustic energy administered remaining constant? (3) What are the cytological changes in the mouse liver which has been exposed to either continuous or pulsed ultrasound over the threshold range of doses? What differences in the nature and amount of injury exist between livers continuously irradiated for relatively long periods and those exposed to series of short duration pulses of ultrasound, the total energy administered being constant?

MATERIALS AND METHODS

The ultrasonic generator was built by personnel of the Metals Research Laboratory of the Division of Applied Mathematics of Brown University. A frequency of 1 Mc was used throughout this study. Silver-plated quartz crystals with a surface area of 6.63 cm^2 were used as transducers. The sound was focused by means of a planoconcave polystyrene lens with a focal distance of

6.0 cm and a radius of curvature of 2.25 cm. The ultrasonic generator consisted of an oscillator, power amplifier, pulse modulator, and crystal matching-network. For continuous transmissions, operation of the oscillator was controlled by an electric timer. For pulsed transmissions, the modulator provided pulse durations ranging from 0.001 to 1.0 sec and pulse periods ranging from 0.1 to 30 sec.

White mice of the inbred BUB and BUA strains maintained at Brown University were used in these studies. BUB mice weighing between 30 and 32 g were used in the dosage study. Mice of both BUB and BUA strains were used for temperature measurements in irradiated liver. Animals were sacrificed 24 hr after irradiation in the dosage study and the left lateral lobe and left caudal lobes were examined for the presence of a necrotic lesion produced by the focused ultrasound. When a lesion existed, it was generally of macroscopic dimensions and readily visible, being at the surface of the irradiated lobe. In cases where the existence of a necrotic lesion was uncertain, the irradiated tissue, along with a piece of an unirradiated lobe, was fixed in Bouin's fluid for examination with the light microscope. For the dosage studies reported here, serial sections were prepared and stained with hematoxylin and eosin. The choice of the presence or absence of a necrotic lesion 24 hr after irradiation as a suitable criterion for the dosage study was based upon the observation in previous studies that irreversible cell injury was characterized by a well-defined necrotic zone by this time.

The experimental arrangement is similar to that described by Bell (28) at the last symposium held here (Fig. 1). The quartz crystal is mounted at one end of an aquarium tank and a sound-absorbing cell containing castor oil and steel wool is mounted at the other end. The focusing lens is mounted on the face of the crystal holder a distance of 0.25 in in front of the quartz crystal.

In preparation for irradiation, the hair is shaved off the abdomen of the mouse and the animal is anesthetized with veterinary Nembutal and placed in a plastic chamber with an open window which permits direct exposure of the abdomen and underlying liver to the ultrasound. This chamber, in turn, is secured to a positioning system and partially immersed in a tank of degassed water, which serves as the coupling medium between the transducer and the mouse. Because the outline of the left lateral lobe can be seen through the translucent skin, the mouse can be positioned so that the left lobe is at the site of the focal region of the sound beam. The skin of the abdominal region is wet with a detergent to minimize the possibility of entrapped air bubbles.

The acoustic power output is routinely measured with a Siemen's Sonotest soundmeter. The crystal driving-voltage is monitored with a vacuum tube voltmeter. Copper-constantan thermocouples made of 0.001-in wire are used to determine the dimensions of the focal region of the sound beam. Although the thermocouple technique of Fry (29) has been employed for calibration of the focused ultrasound, this method is not used routinely because of the greater ease of the radiation pressure method. The dimensions of the focal region are determined by scanning the sound field with the thermocouple in directions along the axis of the sound beam and along the two coordinates at right angles to the beam. An example of measurements made at right angles

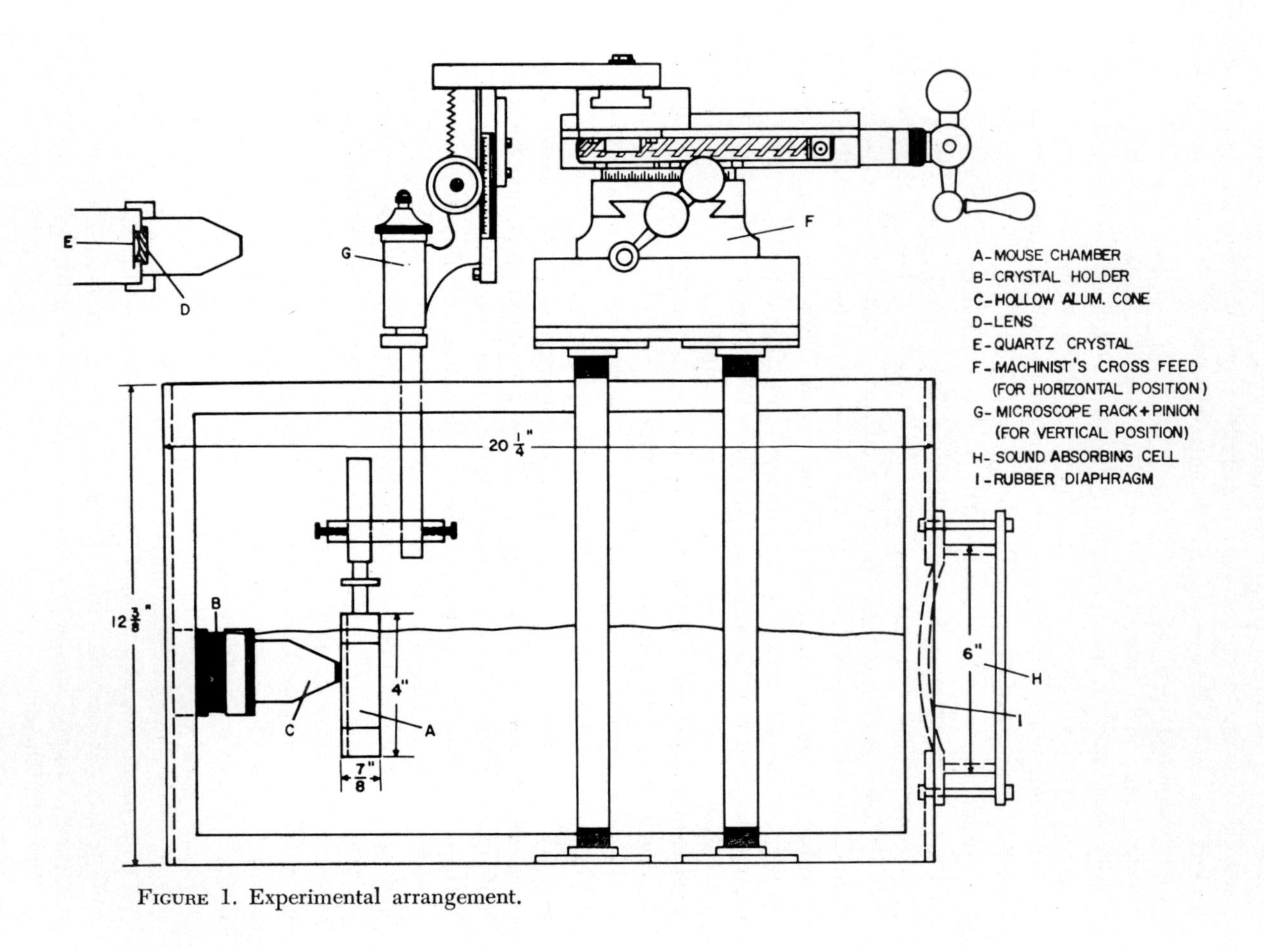

FIGURE 1. Experimental arrangement.

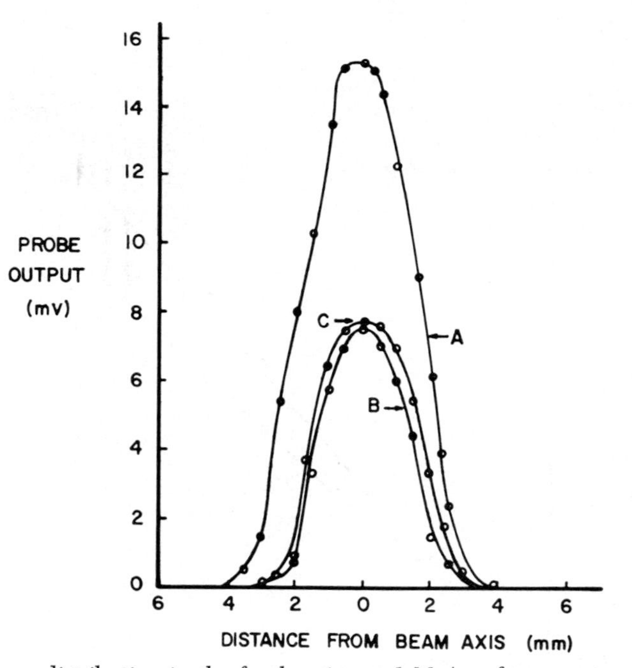

FIGURE 2. Energy distribution in the focal region at 1-Mc/sec frequency as determined by lateral scans. A, through the horizonal plane of the beam axis; B, 2.7 mm above; C, 2.7 mm below.

to the beam (1) through the horizontal plane of the beam axis and (2) at a distance of 2.7 mm above and below this plane is shown in Figure 2. The dimensions of the main lobe of the focused beam are dependent upon the focal distance and aperture of the focusing lens and upon the wavelength (30). The focal distance of the lenses used is 6.0 cm, the radius of the lens, 1.45 cm, and the wavelength, 1.5 mm. The radius of the focal region is 3.75 mm. The acoustic power output of both unfocused and focused sound has been measured with the radiation pressure meter and output in both cases appears linearly related to the square of the crystal driving-voltage over the range of intensities employed in this study (Fig. 3). All doses expressed in watts in this report refer to the acoustic power delivered to the focusing lens.

Thermocouples made of 0.001-in copper-constantan wires with a junction diameter of less than 0.005 in were used to measure the temperature changes produced in the liver by focused ultrasound. Temperature changes in irradiated tissue were measured initially in two different ways – first, by inserting the thermocouple in the liver prior to irradiation, and second, by inserting the thermocouple immediately following irradiation. The latter method was adopted for all measurements reported here because vascular injury was produced by the thermocouple, significantly affecting the removal of heat from the region exposed to ultrasound.

A number of histological and cytological techniques were employed in the microscopic examination of cell injury. Hematoxylin and eosin preparations were made routinely for general histological detail. The periodic acid-Schiff

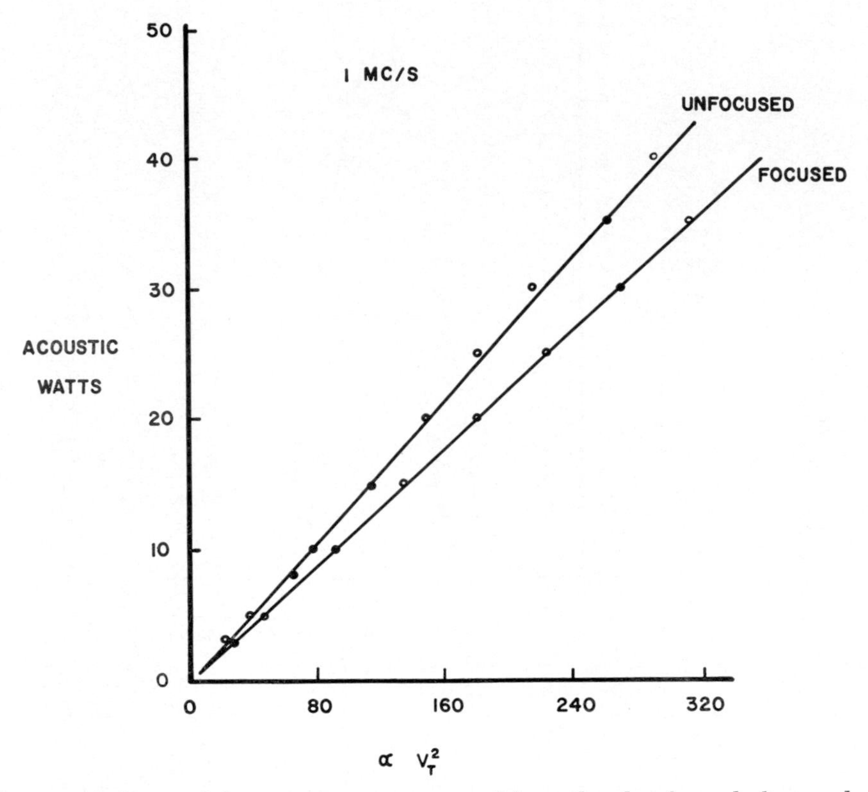

FIGURE 3. Relation of the acoustic power output of focused and unfocused ultrasound of 1-Mc/sec frequency, as measured with the Siemen's Sonotest soundmeter, to the crystal driving-voltage, V_T.

technique was employed on tissues fixed in Rossman's fluid to detect changes in the glycogen content of hepatic cells. Tissues fixed in Serra's fluid for 1 hr were treated according to the Feulgen method for the demonstration of deoxyribonucleic acid. Tissues similarly fixed were stained with methylene blue according to Singer's (34) method to demonstrate the nucleic acids in liver cells, sections incubated in ribonuclease serving as controls for observations of ribonucleic acid. Mitochondria were fixed and stained according to Regaud's method. Foot's silver-impregnation technique and Masson's trichrome stain were used to study connective tissue fibers.

Mice treated with ultrasound were given tail vein injections of 0.2 ml of 10% India ink or Thorotrast in 0.9% saline at different times after irradiation to determine (1) whether hepatic lesions produced by ultrasound were infarctive and (2) whether there was any selective effect with regard to the type of cell injury occurring at threshold dose levels. Since the macrophages of the liver sinusoids phagocytize most of the Thorotrast injected into the blood (31), evidence of phagocytic activity by cells lining sinusoids in noninfarcted lesions would suggest a selective destruction of the hepatic cells by ultrasound. India ink or Thorotrast was injected at times ranging from 1 min after irradiation to 30 days later. The animals were sacrificed 30 min after receiving an injection. This interval allowed sufficient time for most of the injected particles to be removed from the blood by the macrophages.

DOSAGE STUDY

A dosage study involving single doses of ultrasound was made to relate the frequency of incidence of hepatic lesions to the intensity and duration. Between 25 and 35 animals were exposed to each dose of ultrasound in an experiment in which the acoustic power was 35 w and the duration of the irradiation varied from 2.0 to 4.5 sec. The percentage of animals with liver necrosis 24 hr after irradiation is shown in Figure 4. Treatment of the data by the probit method yielded a probability of 0.95 for a larger X^2, indicating that the

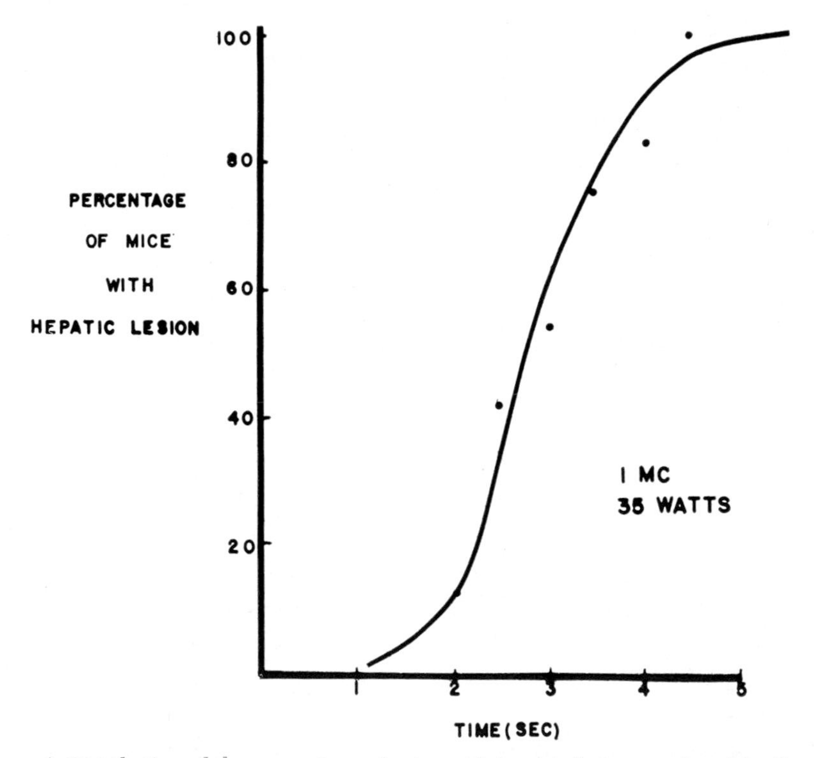

FIGURE 4. Distribution of the percentage of mice with hepatic lesions produced by focused ultrasound as a function of the duration of irradiation at a constant acoustic intensity.

experimental results are well described by the expected curve shown in Figure 4. When positive identification of a necrotic lesion was not possible by gross observations 24 hr after treatment, the irradiated tissue was fixed and serial sections were examined with the light microscope.

Similar numbers of animals were exposed to single doses of ultrasound at different intensities, the duration of irradiation remaining constant, namely, 15 sec. The distribution of the number of animals with hepatic lesions is plotted as a function of the acoustic power output of the unfocused sound beam (Fig. 5). A value of P of 0.85 was obtained by probit methods.

An extensive study was made of the frequency of occurrence of hepatic lesions produced by focused ultrasound as a function of the duration of irradiation at acoustic power levels of 5, 10, 15, 25, and 35 w to determine how the frequency of lesion occurrence depends upon these two dosage parameters. The 10, 50, and 90% frequency values obtained at these power levels are plotted in terms of the reciprocal of the exposure time and the power output. The results (Fig. 6) suggest that, for a given frequency of lesion occurrences, a linear relationship exists between the intensity and the reciprocal of the exposure time over the range of acoustic power levels from 5 to 30 w. This range corresponds to a range of average focal intensities from approximately 10 to 60 w/cm². As determined by linear regression analysis of the probits, a

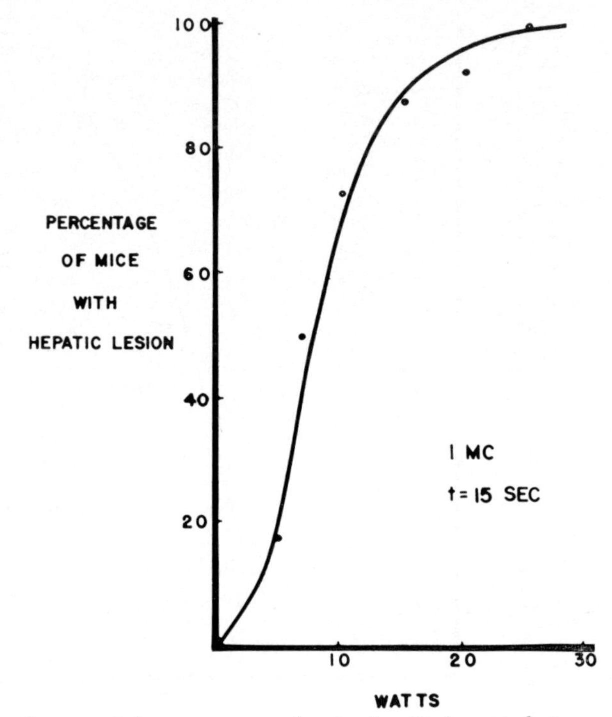

FIGURE 5. Distribution of the percentage of animals with hepatic lesions as a function of the acoustic intensity (expressed as acoustic power output of the unfocused ultrasound) at a constant exposure time of 15 sec.

value of P of less than 0.01 was obtained for the 50% frequency regression line, where the dosage relationship may be most accurately determined. Thus, the frequency of occurrence of hepatic lesions resulting from a single exposure to ultrasound appears to be describable in terms of an $I \times t$ dose law over this range of intensities.

It was not possible on the basis of the data obtained in this study to determine whether the predominant effect of ultrasound was a thermal one. A technique similar to that described by Barth and his associates (32) was used in an attempt to resolve this question. A dosage study involving pulsed ultrasound was made in order to determine how the frequency of occurrence of

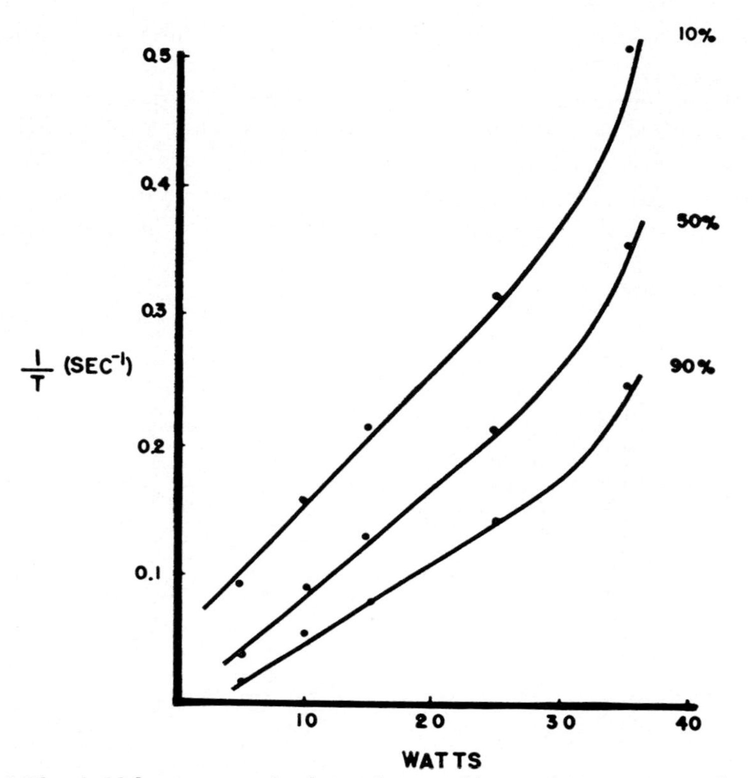

FIGURE 6. Threshold dosage region for the production of hepatic lesions in mice. The 10, 50, and 90% frequencies of lesion incidence are plotted as a function of the acoustic power output and the reciprocal of the exposure time.

hepatic lesions was related to the time distribution of the acoustic energy. In this study, the liver of the intact mouse was exposed to a series of short pulses of ultrasonic energy, the pulse duration being either 0.1 or 0.2 sec, the total exposure, 30 sec. The range of intensities was the same as that in the CW study. The period of time over which the acoustic energy was administered was varied at each intensity level. Evaluation of the dosage data was based on treatment of groups of 20 or more experimental animals. As in the previous experiment, the animals were sacrificed 24 hr after irradiation and the irradiated liver examined grossly for a necrotic lesion. If it was not possible to determine by macroscopic observation whether a necrotic lesion had been produced, the irradiated tissue was fixed and serial sections were studied with the light microscope. The percentage of animals with lesions obtained for each dosage may be plotted in terms of the duty factor in order to relate the occurrence of injury to the time distribution of the acoustic energy (Fig. 7). The frequency distribution of animals with hepatic lesions appears strongly dependent upon the rate at which the ultrasound is pulsed. The dependence is directly related to the ultrasonic intensity. The curves in Figure 7, derived by the probit method, were found to be well described by the experimental data obtained in this study. A given frequency of lesion incidence was found to be describable in terms of a linear relationship between the logarithm of the reciprocal of the duty factor and the intensity over most of the dosage range (Fig. 8).

This dependence of the frequency of lesion incidence upon the duty factor suggested that heating or other second order effects play a predominant role in the production of such lesions. Measurements were therefore made of the temperature rise in intact livers exposed to ultrasound as a function of the two parameters — intensity and duty factor — the total exposure remaining con-

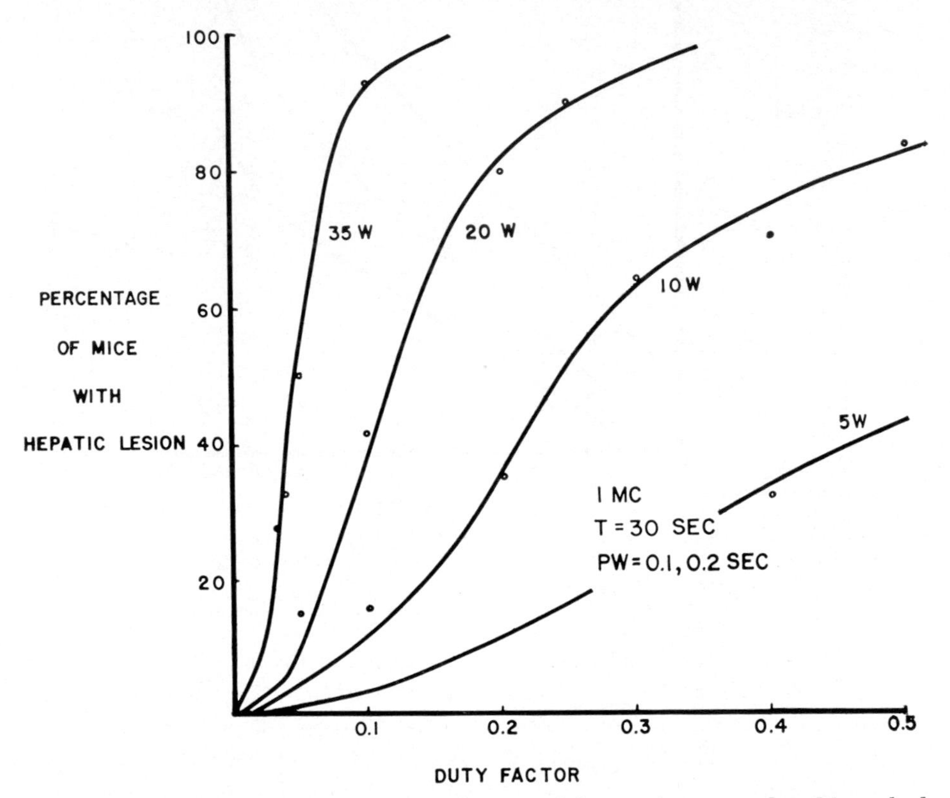

FIGURE 7. Distribution of the percentage of mice with hepatic lesions produced by pulsed ultrasound as a function of the duty factor. Distribution curves derived by probit analysis of data at power levels of 5, 10, 20, and 35 w. Constant exposure time: 30 sec.

stant. Temperature measurements were made in six or more animals for each ultrasonic dosage, using copper-constantan thermocouples made of 0.001-in wire. The mean temperature rise for each dosage is plotted as a function of the duty factor in Figure 9.

Heating of the liver during ultrasonic irradiation was also studied in terms of whether blood circulation was normal or impaired. Temperature rises in the irradiated livers of anesthetized animals killed by a blow to the head just prior to irradiation were compared to those in the treated livers of control anesthetized animals. The occurrence of higher temperatures in livers of animals irradiated with pulsed ultrasound immediately after sacrifice as opposed to those produced in controls similarly irradiated suggested that the circu-

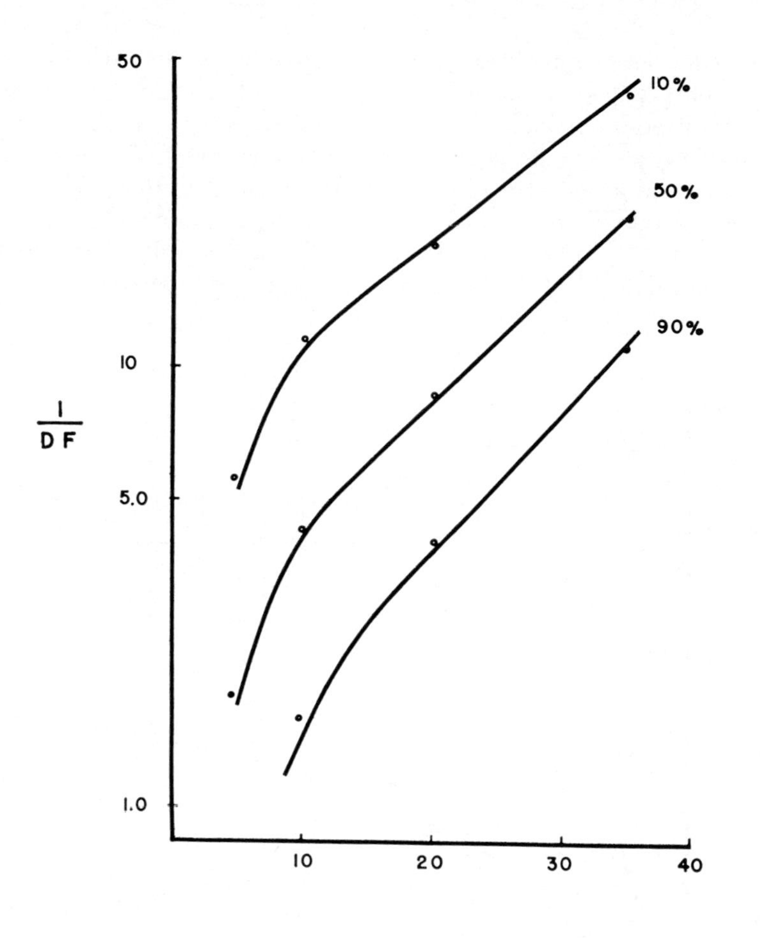

FIGURE 8. Threshold dosage region for the production of hepatic lesions in mice by pulsed ultrasound of 1-Mc/sec frequency. The 10, 50, and 90% lesion incidences are plotted in terms of the log $\left(\frac{1}{D\ F}\right)$ and the acoustic power output.

lating blood played a major role in removing heat from the irradiated tissue. Pulsed ultrasound (power level: 20 w; duty factor: 0.1; total exposure: 30 sec) produced a mean temperature rise of 10°C in livers of animals sacrificed just before irradiation, as opposed to only a 3°C rise in the livers of control anesthetized animals (Fig. 9).

CYTOLOGICAL STUDY

Microscopic examination of the cellular and tissue changes produced by ultrasound was carried out in conjunction with the dosage studies. More than 400 animals were exposed to threshold and "subthreshold" doses of either continuous or pulsed ultrasound as determined in the above study and sacrificed at times varying from immediately after irradiation to 30 days later. The term "subthreshold" is arbitrarily assigned to those dosages which produce the frank lesions manifest 24 hr after irradiation in less than 10% of the experimental animals. The irradiated liver, together with a piece of an unirradiated lobe, was fixed, imbedded, sectioned, and stained for examination with the light microscope. The purpose of this study was threefold: (1) to describe the nature and extent of cell injury associated with threshold doses of continuous and pulsed ultrasound; (2) to determine whether any selective action of ultrasound was associated with threshold doses of pulsed ultrasound; and (3) to determine whether any effects were observed in livers exposed to subthreshold doses of pulsed ultrasound and, if so, to compare these effects with those typical of threshold doses.

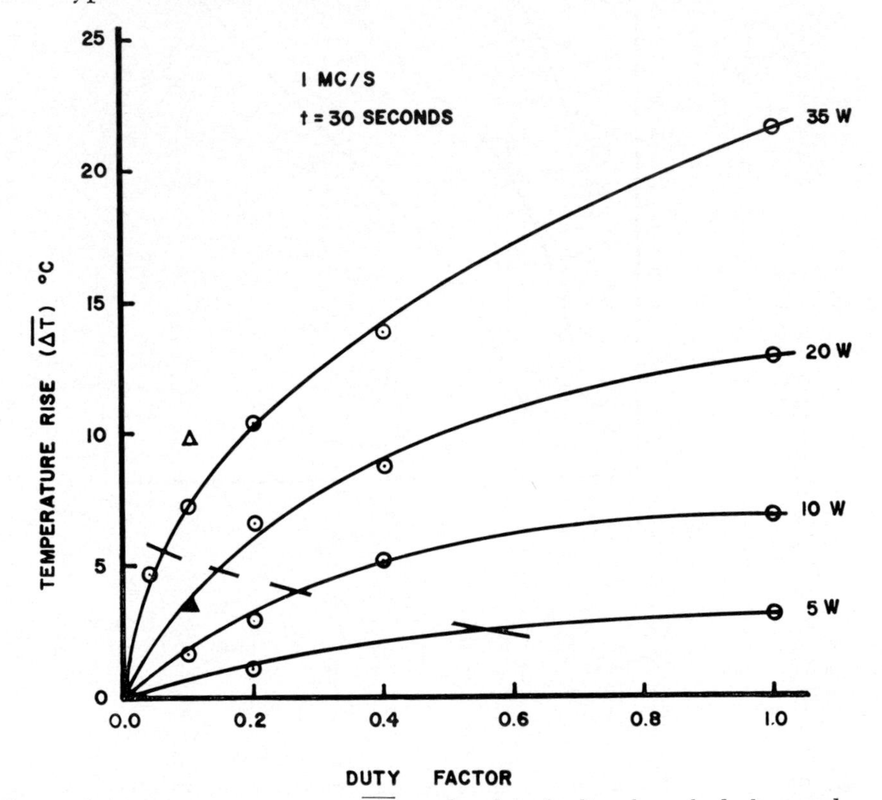

FIGURE 9. Mean temperature rises, $\overline{\triangle T}$, produced in the liver by pulsed ultrasound as a function of the duty factor at power levels of 5, 10, 20, and 35 w; t = 30 sec. △, the mean temperature rise in animals sacrificed just prior to irradiation; ▲, the mean temperature rise in control animals exposed to the same dose of ultrasound (dose: 20 w; duty factor: 0.1; total exposure: 30 sec).

Immediately after irradiation at the higher dosage levels employed in this study, the liver injury was similar to that described by Bell (27). Sinusoids were distended and congested with swollen red blood cells (Fig. 10). Cell injury was evidenced by cytoplasmic vacuolation, glycogen disruption, swollen mitochondria, and pyknotic nuclei. The disruption of the RNA and DNA of hepatic cells was indicated by the marked reduction in cytoplasmic basophilia and in the intensity of the Feulgen reaction of the nuclei of injured cells. A distortion of the normal appearance of parenchymal cell plates was occasionally observed near the surface of the lesion after exposure to such doses. This distortion was characterized by a marked degree of red blood cell-packing in sinusoids at the center of the lesion (Fig. 11).

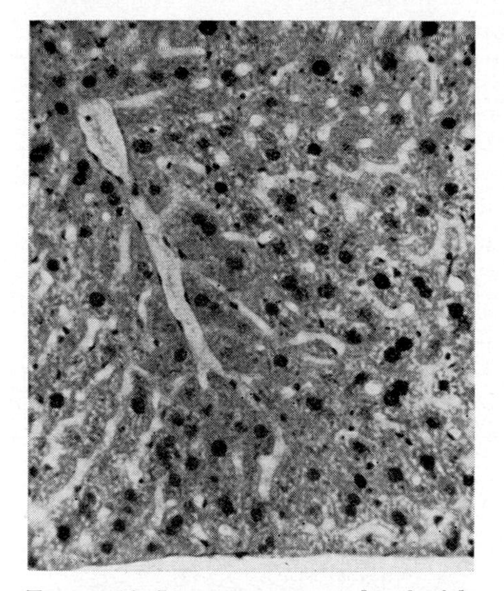

FIGURE 10. Liver injury immediately following ultrasonic irradiation. Sinusoids are distended and engorged with red blood cells. H & E.

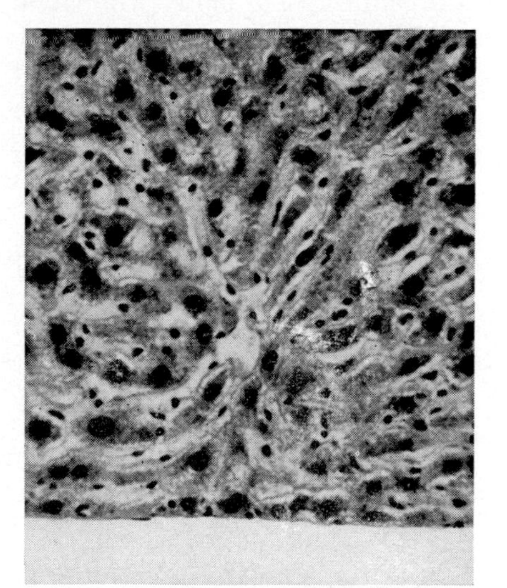

FIGURE 11. Distorted parenchymal cell cords immediately after irradiation. H & E.

Immediately after irradiation, the boundary of the damaged region, while appearing well defined macroscopically, was not so readily apparent in terms of the cytological changes. A gradation of cellular changes extended radially from the center of the lesion at the lobe surface to surrounding regions of undamaged tissue. The most profound changes were found in parenchymal cells in this central region of the lesion at the lobe surface. The cytoplasm of these cells was full of small vacuoles, giving a honeycomb appearance. Mitochondria were generally either not visible at all, or appeared only as slightly stained, enlarged, spherical, or vesicular bodies. A gradual increase in the number of mitochondria was noticeable, extending from this central area radially. A similar gradation existed with respect to the amount of disruption of the glycogen of parenchymal cells. Where the damage was greatest, the glycogen no longer appeared granular and was not distributed throughout the cytoplasm as in the unirradiated cells; rather, it often appeared concentrated in one end of the parenchymal cells, presumably due, in part, to the action of the fixative. Such a picture, in contrast to the normal one, indicated that the ultrasound had produced a rapid breakdown of cytoplasmic organization.

During the first hour following irradiation, there often was a disappearance of glycogen from injured hepatic cells. However, in large infarctive lesions, considerable glycogen remained in hepatic cells in the central portion of the damaged tissue. This appeared due to the vascular occlusion and to coagulative heating effects caused by the ultrasound. In smaller lesions, injured parenchymal cells contained little or no glycogen at this time (Fig. 12).

Lesion size and the degree of infarctive injury were related to the intensity, and, in the case of pulsed irradiation, to the pulse rate, when the duration of irradiation was constant. Infarctive lesions were generally produced by ultrasound when acoustic power levels of 20 w or greater and single exposures of 5 sec or longer were used. Similar lesions were usually produced by pulsed ultrasound when these power levels were used in conjunction with duty cycles of 10% or greater and 30-sec exposures. The extent of vascular injury was demonstrated by the perfusion of irradiated livers with India ink – the infarcted areas, not penetrated by the ink, being sharply outlined by the surrounding undamaged tissue, which was readily perfused (Fig. 13).

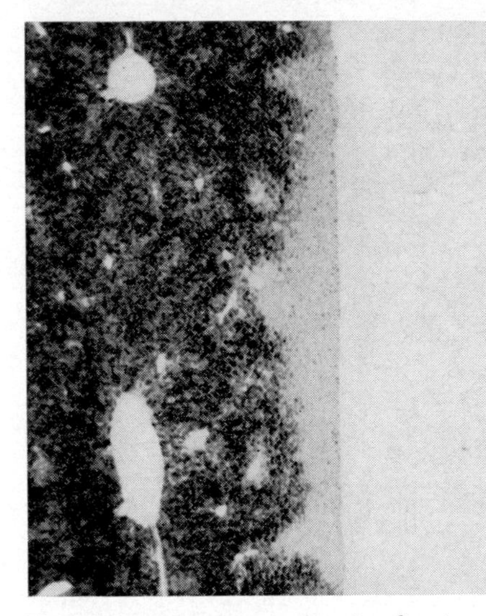

FIGURE 12. Liver injury 30 min after irradiation. Marked loss of glycogen from injured hepatic cells at the surface of the liver. Periodic acid-Schiff.

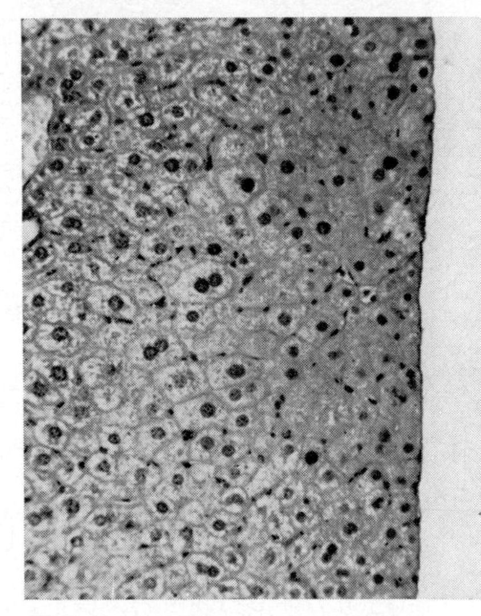

FIGURE 13. Cell injury about a central vein near the dorsal surface of the left lateral lobe of the liver 30 min after pulsed irradiation. Injured cells appear swollen and possess a fine granular cytoplasm. H & E.

In approximately 3% of the mice exposed to threshold doses, injury at the surface of the liver was accompanied by hemorrhagic lesions which occurred in an irregular manner within the irradiated lobe. While gas bubbles were not in evidence in the lesions localized only at the lobe surface, they were frequently seen in regions of hemorrhagic injury, suggesting that the latter injury is associated with a degassing effect.

Infarctive lesions were seldom observed immediately after treatment with pulsed ultrasound at dosages involving power levels of 10 w or less and exposures of 30 sec. In the absence of such vascular injury, the disruptive effects of ultrasound frequently appeared limited to parenchymal cells, and in numerous instances, such injury was localized to centrolobular regions adjacent to the surface of the liver (Figs. 15, 16) (Fig. 14: normal hepatic cells). Such localized injury was observed in histological preparations by 30 min after irradiation. Injured cells appeared swollen and possessed a granular cytoplasm. One hr after irradiation, little or no glycogen was demonstrable in injured hepatic cells about central veins near the surface of the liver (Fig. 16). The sinusoids were not occluded by red blood cells and the sinusoidal endothelium appeared intact. A similar centrolobular localization of cell necrosis was observed 24 hr after treatment with pulsed ultrasound (Fig. 17).

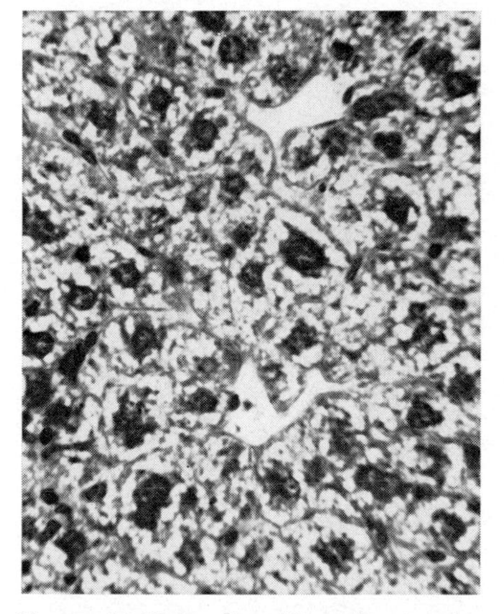

FIGURE 14. Unirradiated liver showing the normal appearance of hepatic cells about a central vein. H & E.

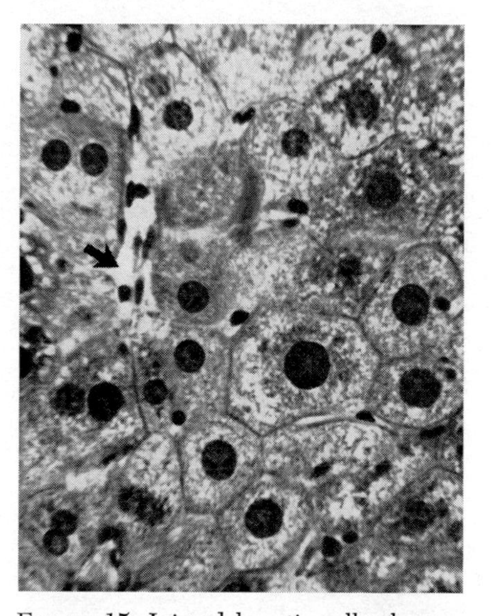

FIGURE 15. Injured hepatic cells about a central vein near the surface of the liver after pulsed irradiation. Hepatic cells have granular cytoplasm. Sinusoids and central vein (arrow) are not congested with red blood cells. Same animal as in Figure 14. H & E.

The appearance of these noninfarctive lesions shortly after irradiation suggested the possibility that ultrasound at certain dosage levels selectively destroyed the parenchymal cells of the liver. A technique similar to that described by Bell (28) was employed to determine whether endothelial elements survived the effects of ultrasound in regions of parenchymal cell necrosis. Small amounts of Thorotrast or India ink were injected into the tail vein of experimental animals at times ranging from immediately after irradiation to 24 hr later. Such materials are normally phagocytized by the macrophages which are located along the sinusoids of the liver (Fig. 18); hence, evidence of such activity by these cells in hepatic lesions would suggest that the ultrasound selectively destroys the parenchymal cells. The presence of numerous macrophages loaded with Thorotrast in regions of parenchymal cell necrosis 24 hr after pulsed irradiation clearly demonstrated that portions

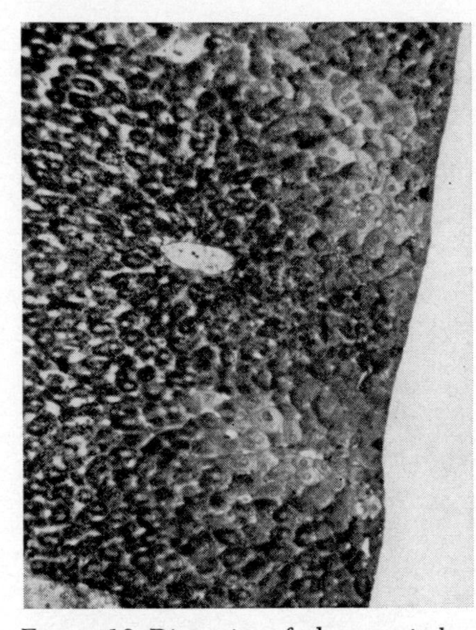

FIGURE 16. Disruption of glycogen in hepatic cells appears localized about central veins near the surface of the liver. One hr after pulsed irradiation. Periodic acid-Schiff.

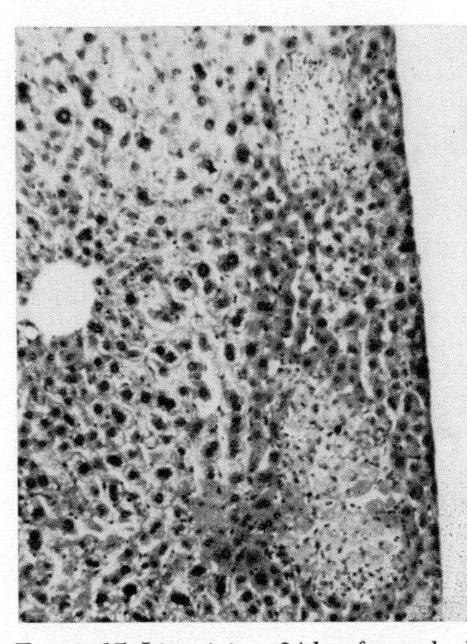

FIGURE 17. Liver injury 24 hr after pulsed irradiation. Necrosis localized to centrolobular regions near the surface of the liver. H & E.

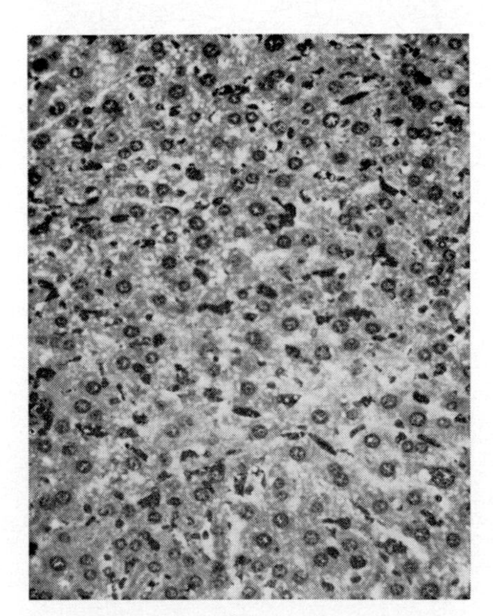

FIGURE 18. Macrophages of the sinusoids of unirradiated liver 30 min after the injection of India ink. H & E.

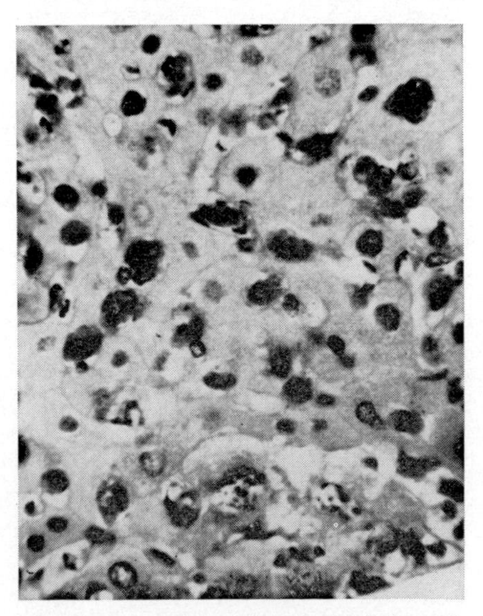

FIGURE 19. Macrophages loaded with Thorotrast in region of hepatic cell necrosis produced by pulsed ultrasound. Twenty-four hr after irradiation. H & E.

of these lesions were not infarcted and suggested the selective destruction of parenchymal cells. However, the comparatively greater numbers of macrophages containing Thorotrast in such lesions, as opposed to the numbers in comparable unirradiated regions, suggested that macrophages not originally present in these lesions became lodged in the vascular spaces of such noninfarctive necrotic zones. Twenty-four hr after irradiation, some of the phagocytically active macrophages in these vascular spaces appear to line the sinusoids, suggesting that they were originally present in these areas and apparently survived the irradiation (Fig. 19). However, the necrotic appearance of many endothelial cells at this time and the lack of a viable sinusoidal endothelium in similar lesions at later times indicated that there was apparently little selectivity in terms of cell destruction in those lesions which were manifest 24 hr after irradiation.

Infarctive lesions appeared blanched at 6 to 12 hr after irradiation. In general, the sequence of degenerative and reparative events associated with infarctive hepatic lesions was the same for threshold doses of both continuous and pulsed ultrasound. A more detailed description of these events may be found elsewhere (27). These lesions had two predominant features at later times. First, they became circumscribed by a fibrotic capsule by 5 days after irradiation (Fig. 20). Second, the necrotic hepatic cells, as Bell (27) has previously reported, remained intact as long as 15 days after irradiation. A similar fibrotic encapsulation and persistence of necrotic tissue were also typical of microscopic lesions, which occasionally consisted of isolated regions of cell destruction. These small lesions were similarly localized at the surface of the irradiated liver. In only a few instances were lesions found 24 hr after irradiation in which the normal lobular arrangement appeared disrupted. The parenchyma was dissociated and the resulting spaces were engorged with red blood cells (Fig. 21). The intact necrotic cells, few in number, were dispersed in these spaces and directly exposed to the blood, suggesting that a dissolution of injured parenchymal cells and sinusoidal endothelium had occurred.

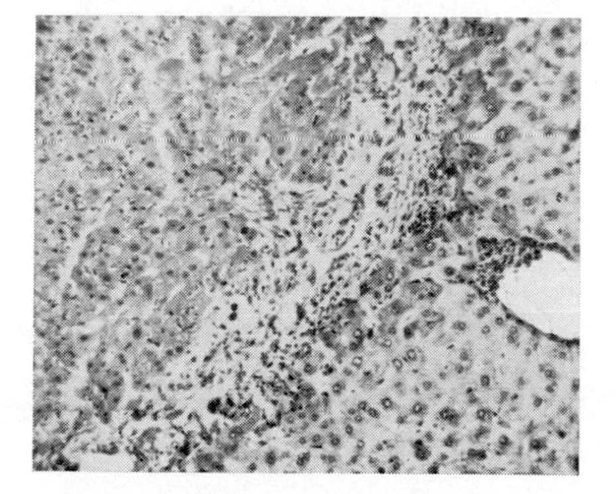

FIGURE 20. Necrotic lesion 5 days after ultrasonic irradiation. Necrotic hepatic cells appear intact. Fibrotic tissue has formed at the periphery of the lesion. H & E.

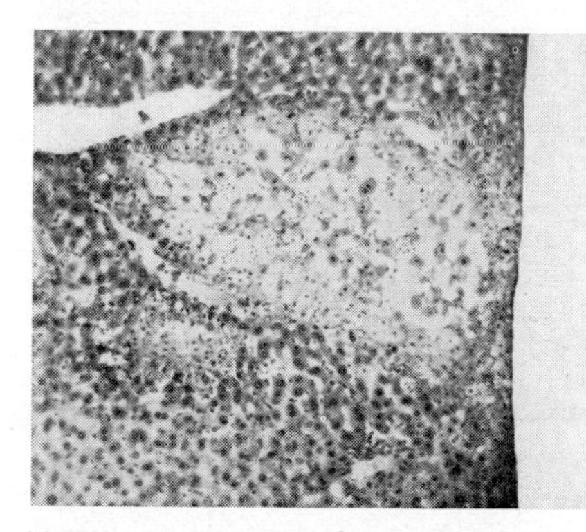

FIGURE 21. Necrotic lesion 24 hr after pulsed irradiation. A dissociation of the injured parenchyma and endothelium has occurred. H & E.

Changes in the liver treated with subthreshold doses of pulsed ultrasound were studied in mice sacrificed serially up to 30 days later. Although necrotic lesions were found only infrequently 24 hr after irradiation, hepatic injury was observed in approximately 50% of the mice sacrificed 10 and 30 days later. Five days after irradiation, hepatic cells and the sinusoidal endothelium appeared abnormal. Injured hepatic cells were often noticeably smaller than normal cells. The cytoplasm of injured cells was homogeneous, lacking the irregularly clumped basophilic component typical of the cytoplasm of unirradiated hepatic cells. Endothelial cells were detached from the surfaces of hepatic cells and appeared round in contrast to their normal flattened shape (Fig. 22). Ten days after irradiation, injured hepatic cells often contained little or no glycogen (Fig. 23). This absence of glycogen from hepatic cells appearing sublethally injured was also typical of liver injury 30 days after irradiation. While some of the hepatic cells in the irradiated tissue appeared necrotic at these times, no large necrotic mass circumscribed by fibrotic tissue, such as that typically found 5 days after larger doses of ultrasound, was observed. No comparable changes were observed in the liver of control animals. Sinusoids were not occluded and regions of such injury did not appear to be infarcted. Viable macrophages in such lesions were demonstrated by the injection of Thorotrast. These preliminary observations of the effects of subthreshold doses suggest that intense ultrasound when administered as a series of short pulses sufficiently spaced in time produces cell injury quite different from that typical of the infarctive lesions caused by threshold doses of continuous and pulsed ultrasound.

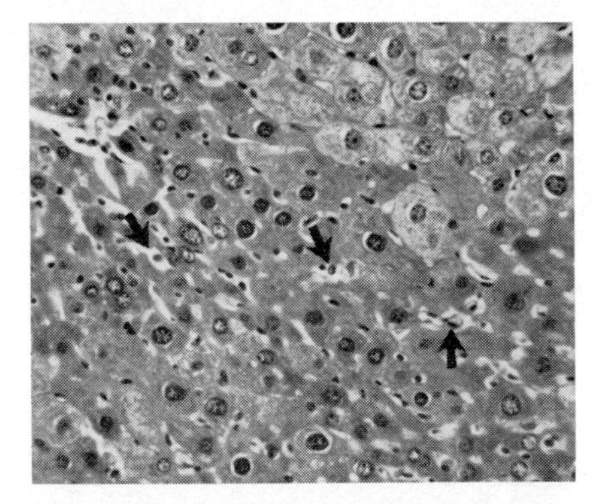

FIGURE 22. Liver injury 5 days after pulsed irradiation at subthreshold dosage level. Endothelial cells (arrows) have rounded up and appear detached from surfaces of hepatic cells. H & E.

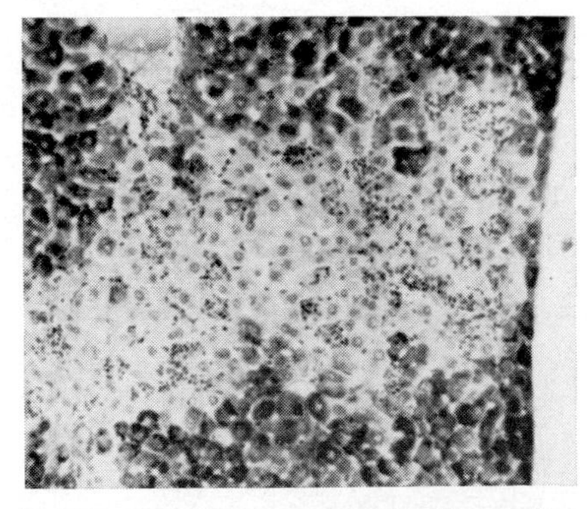

FIGURE 23. Liver injury 10 days after pulsed irradiation at subthreshold dosage level. Leucocytic activity about individual necrotic cells. Most of the hepatic cells, although containing little glycogen, appear to have survived the irradiation. Periodic acid-Schiff.

DISCUSSION

The changes produced in the intact liver of the mouse by focused ultrasound depend upon the amount of acoustic energy to which the tissue is exposed and the rate at which this energy is administered. When this rate is sufficiently high, irreversible changes in the form of cell destruction and vascular injury are visible immediately after irradiation. Such injury is typical of those ultrasonic doses which produce a significant temperature rise above normal body temperature. As Bell (27) has previously reported, the injury produced by focused ultrasound in the liver of the intact mouse is generally localized at the surface of the irradiated lobe which is farthest from the transducer.

No selective action of ultrasound upon tissue elements or cells was demonstrable in a study involving single exposures of from 2- to 40-sec duration over the range of average focal intensities from 10 to 70 w/cm^2. Endothelial cells, as well as parenchymal cells, are destroyed by focused ultrasound at such dosage levels. The nonselective nature of tissue destruction and the predominant localization of such destruction to the surface of the irradiated liver suggest that the injury typical of such dosages is dependent upon a selective heating effect at this surface.

If heating were responsible for this localized injury, then the dosage would be expressible in terms of an $I \times t$ dose law. While this law does not appear to describe the dose relationships over the entire range of intensities studied, it seems to hold for that range of average focal intensities from approximately 10 to 60 w/cm^2. Thus, the distribution of animals with hepatic lesions appears describable by a dose dependence wherein the intensity of the ultrasound is inversely proportional to the exposure time. The deviation from this relationship at higher intensities suggests that some effect of ultrasound other than that predominating over this range becomes important.

The relative importance of the heating action of ultrasound in the production of liver injury was studied by administering a given amount of acoustic energy at different rates by means of pulsed irradiation. Heating effects may be minimized by making the time interval between pulses sufficiently long. Thus, if the tissue destruction observed in the liver were due primarily to heating, the distribution of animals with hepatic lesions would depend greatly upon the duty factor, a measure of the rate at which the ultrasonic energy is administered, when the intensity and total acoustic energy is constant. As shown in Figure 7, the distribution of animals with hepatic lesions produced by pulsed ultrasound is strongly dependent upon the pulse rate when the total exposure and intensity are constant. Temperature measurements made in the liver for each dosage show that a range of mean temperatures from 37.0 to 42.5°C corresponds to the threshold region. In other words, this range of temperatures corresponds to that range of dosages which produce hepatic lesions in 10 to 90% of the animals treated.

Fry (1, 17–19) and Bell (27) have reported the destructive effects of intense ultrasound upon the spinal cord and liver, respectively, in precooled animals wherein the maximum temperatures developed during irradiation were well below normal body temperature. Their findings in hypothermic animals suggest that a thermal effect is not the primary cause of such injury. In the study reported here, however, a comparison of the frequency of lesion incidence (Fig. 7) with the corresponding mean temperature rises (Fig. 9) reveals that the percentage of animals with liver injury is closely related to the temperature changes produced in the liver when the initial body temperature is approximately 34.5°C. While mean temperature rises of from approximately 2 to 3°C were associated with those dosages which produced lesions in 10% of the animals irradiated, mean temperature rises of from 6 to 8°C were typical of dosages producing hepatic lesions in 90% of the treated mice.

The mean temperature rises corresponding to those dosages which produce lesions in 50% of the irradiated animals are indicated by the line intersecting each temperature curve (Fig. 9). The finding that the mean temperature rises typical of dosages producing this percentage of lesions are different for different intensities seems to suggest that such injury may not be dependent upon the attainment of a critical temperature level. Such a finding would suggest an effect of ultrasound other than one of thermal origin. If the production of such hepatic lesions were primarily due to a mechanical action of ultrasound, it should be possible to produce such lesions with pulsed ultrasound under conditions wherein little or no tissue heating occurs. However, since the mean temperature of the untreated liver of anesthetized mice is 34.5°C, pulsed ultrasonic irradiation, which produces hepatic lesions such as those described in the dosage study reported here, is always accompanied by a rise in the temperature of the irradiated liver. Such injury has not been observed after treatment at dosage levels that do not produce a temperature rise in the liver. Although it can not be concluded that tissue heating is the only cause of liver injury, it is evident that the probability of producing these lesions is strongly related to the measurable temperature rise occurring in the irradiated liver.

The development of much higher temperatures in the intact liver of anesthetized animals sacrificed just prior to irradiation as compared to those produced in the livers of anesthetized control animals indicates that the circulating blood plays a significant role in the removal of heat from the irradiated tissue when the ultrasound is pulsed. In a study of focal lesions in the brain of the cat, Basauri and Lele (9) found that the probability of lesion occurrence was greater in animals in which cranial circulation was temporarily arrested than it was in animals with normal circulation. Their findings that both the size and the probability of occurrence of focal lesions in the cat brain are dependent upon the tissue temperature suggest that such lesions are primarily thermal in origin.

Lesion size in the liver of the mouse varies considerably at any given dosage level. This probably involves the uncertainty of the positioning procedure, that is, the difficulty of aligning the liver so that the focal region is always traversing the same part of the left lateral lobe. When the lesions produced by pulsed ultrasound are small, the injury may be localized to a number of isolated regions. The distribution of such injury often appears related to the lobular arrangement of the hepatic parenchyma (Figs. 15, 16).

Thirty min after irradiation, little or no disruption of endothelial cells or vascular occlusion is apparent in such microlesions (Figs. 13, 15), which distinguishes them from the larger infarctive lesions (Fig. 10). However, both the small lesions with localized injury and the larger solid lesions occur at the surface of the irradiated liver and become isolated from surrounding undamaged tissue by the formation of fibrotic tissue at the periphery of the lesion. The necrotic parenchyma generally remains intact, and the cell boundaries persist long after irradiation in these lesions. This is probably due primarily to thermal effects, that is, the destruction of the cellular proteolytic enzymes and the isolation of the destroyed tissue from the circulating blood.

The disruption of the lobular arrangement of hepatic cells and the dissociation of injured cells are observed in approximately 3% of the irradiated animals. Such disruption is characteristic of the hemorrhagic lesions which infrequently accompany the surface lesions produced in livers by ultrasound at high threshold dose levels. This disruptive injury is generally distributed across the exposed lobe and is associated with gas bubbles which are visible after irradiation, suggesting that such injury is related to degassing effects. The appearance of the mechanically disrupted cells in such regions is quite different from that of the cells in the lesions localized at the lobe surface. Thus, the latter injury does not appear to be attributable to the cavitation effect.

A dissociation of parenchyma is observed only infrequently in livers exposed to low threshold doses of pulsed ultrasound. There is no evidence of gas bubble formation or of a mechanical disruption of hepatic cells in this injury such as that mentioned above. Twenty-four hr after irradiation, the hepatic cells in such microscopic lesions localized at the lobe surface appear necrotic and dissociated from one another. The large spaces in these lesions are filled with blood which is in direct contact with injured hepatic cells (Fig. 21). The absence of an intact endothelium suggests that a dissolution of endothelial cells has occurred.

A gradation of effects, then, in terms of the amount and the degree of localization of hepatic injury, has been observed over the threshold range of dosages for pulsed ultrasound. The extent of injury ranges from the gross infarctive lesions to the noninfarctive microscopic lesions, which, in some cases, consist of isolated regions of cell destruction. The variation in the appearance of these lesions 24 hr after irradiation is probably attributable to whether the parenchyma and endothelium have been exposed to high temperatures and, also, whether the damaged tissue has been isolated from the circulation. Lesions characterized by marked cell disruption and distension of occluded sinusoids immediately after irradiation and, subsequently, by fibrotic encapsulation and the persistence of the necrotic parenchyma, are typical of high threshold dosages and corresponding high mean temperature rises. The serial-time study of lesions produced by low threshold doses, that is, ones which result in little vascular occlusion immediately after irradiation, suggests that the injured tissue undergoes a more rapid autolysis than that of the larger lesions.

The localization of injury to the surface of the liver is typical of the threshold range of doses for CW and pulsed ultrasound, suggesting that the effect or effects of ultrasound which result in demonstrable lesions at 24 hr after treatment are common to both types of irradiation. Not only is the ultrasonic energy selectively absorbed at the lobe surface, but apparently, energy absorption processes may be further localized to the central, rather than the periportal, regions of hepatic lobules near the surface of the liver.

Since both the degree of localization of tissue destruction and the extent of tissue heating are dependent upon the rate at which ultrasonic energy is administered, it is possible that selective heating occurs in the centrolobular regions adjacent to the surface of the irradiated liver. For CW irradiation and for pulsed irradiation involving high pulse rates, lesions encompassing a volume of tissue consisting of a number of lobules would appear continuous because regions in which critical temperature levels are attained would overlap. With sufficiently long intervals between pulses, much of the energy dissipated to heat would be carried away by the circulating blood, and temperature dependent effects of ultrasound would be localized at those sites where the energy is selectively absorbed.

Cell injury is observed at 30 min after irradiation in livers exhibiting such localized effects. Hepatic cells in centrolobular regions are swollen, the cytoplasm granular in appearance. The striking difference in appearance between hepatic cells disrupted by pulsed ultrasound, as in these localized lesions, and those destroyed by the direct application of heat suggests that the destructive effects of pulsed ultrasound may not be entirely explicable in terms of thermal effects. In heat-killed cells, the cytoplasm is coagulated into large irregular masses. In liver treated with pulsed ultrasound at threshold dosage levels which minimize heating effects, the cytoplasmic content of hepatic cells is disintegrated, its granular appearance suggesting that macromolecular aggregates normally present have been reduced to ones of much smaller dimensions (Fig. 15). The microstreaming phenomena produced in plant cells exposed to ultrasonic vibrations which were recently reported by Dyer and Nyborg (33) suggest one mechanism by which such a disintegration of cytoplasmic structure may occur.

As early as 30 min after pulsed irradiation at low threshold dosage levels, injured hepatic cells possess little or no RNA, DNA, or glycogen that is demonstrable by histochemical methods. While cell vacuolation is typically found 1 hr after irradiation in regions peripheral to an infarctive lesion, little or none is associated with the localized cell injury typical of threshold dosages at this time. The absence of vascular injury and of parenchymal cell vacuolation in livers where the injury appears localized to hepatic cells in centrolobular regions suggests that the vacuolation typical of the larger infarctive lesions is due to anoxic conditions resulting from the vascular injury.

The examination of the phagocytic activity of liver macrophages in microscopic lesions produced by threshold doses of pulsed ultrasound provides little evidence of any selective destruction of hepatic cells. In the few instances where a dissociation of hepatic parenchyma was observed in microscopic lesions 24 hr after irradiation, little or no intact sinusoidal endothelium remained in the disrupted tissue, suggesting that the endothelial cells may be more easily damaged by the action of ultrasound than the hepatic cells.

The liver of the mouse has been exposed to subthreshold doses of pulsed ultrasound, examined 24 hr later, and the animals sacrificed 5, 10, and 30 days after irradiation. Liver injury was macroscopically detected at the later times in animals in which no injury was grossly visible 24 hr after irradiation. At 5 days, injured cells often appear smaller than undamaged hepatic cells, and, as a result, the cords of cells in affected regions are distorted, and the cells elongated (Fig. 22). Ten and 30 days after irradiation, the lesions consist predominantly of abnormal, but apparently surviving, hepatic cells, some necrotic cells being seen in the center of such lesions. Sublethally damaged cells have a relatively homogeneous cytoplasm in which little glycogen (Fig. 23) or basophilia attributable to RNA is demonstrable. While the endothelial cells in regions of such injury are often rounded up and appear detached from the parenchymal cells, the sinusoids are not occluded by red blood cells as is typical of the injury found immediately after treatment with larger doses of ultrasound. In a few instances, a dissociation of injured hepatic tissue is apparent (Fig. 24). In such lesions, the injured hepatic cells possess considerably less cytoplasmic RNA than undamaged cells in adjacent areas.

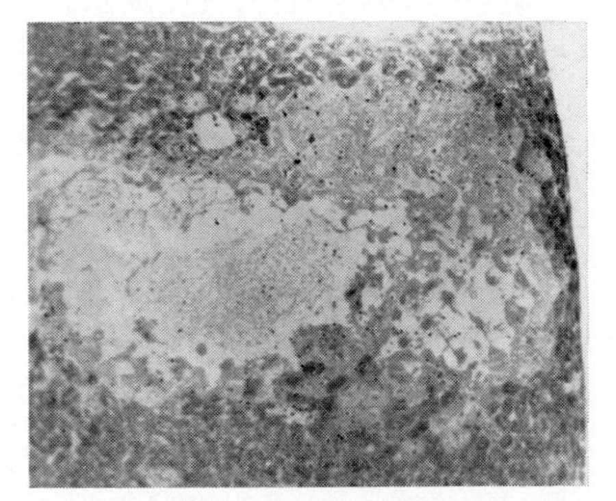

FIGURE 24. Liver injury 10 days after pulsed irradiation at subthreshold dosage level. A dissociation and a lysis of parenchymal and endothelial cells are apparent. Reduction of basophilia of cytoplasm of injured hepatic cells. Methylene blue-Singer.

Pulsed ultrasound at subthreshold dosage levels, then, produces cell injury which is not characterized immediately after irradiation by the marked disruption of cellular content which is typical of threshold doses. At such subthreshold dosage levels, heating effects are minimized. Thus, it appears that focused ultrasound, in the absence of tissue heating, produces a subtle form of cell injury which becomes apparent in histological preparations at much later times than that which is accompanied by demonstrable tissue heating. This latent response will be studied further in an attempt to determine how cells appearing sublethally injured long after irradiation have been altered.

REFERENCES

1. Fry, W. J. (1958). Intense ultrasound in investigations of the central nervous system, *in* "Advances in Biological and Medical Physics," C. A. Tobias and J. H. Lawrence, eds. (Academic Press, New York), Vol. VI, pp. 281–348.
2. Fry, F. J., H. W. Ades, and W. J. Fry (1958). Production of reversible changes in the central nervous system by ultrasound. Science *127*, 83–84.
3. Fry, W. J. (1958). Unsolved problems in acoustics – biological and medical acoustics. J. Acoust. Soc. Am *30*, 387–393.
4. Fry, W. J., R. Meyers, F. J. Fry, D. F. Schultz, L. L. Dreyer, and R. F. Noyes (1958). Topical differentia of pathogenetic mechanisms underlying Parkinsonian tremor and rigidity as indicated by ultrasonic irradiation of the human brain. Trans. Am. Neurol, Assn., 16–24.
5. Fry, W. J., and F. J. Fry (1960). Fundamental neurological research and human neurosurgery using intense ultrasound. IRE Trans. Med. Electron. *ME-7*, 166–181. Reprinted in Proc. Biomed. Eng. Symposium (San Diego, 1961).
6. Fry, W. J., and F. Dunn (1962). Ultrasound: analysis and experimental methods in biological research, *in* "Physical Techniques in Biological Research," W. L. Nastuk, ed. (Academic Press, New York), Vol. IV, Chap. 6, pp. 261–394.
7. Fry, W. J. (1962). Present and future applications of ultrasonics in bio-medicine. Proc. Inst. Radio Engrs. *50*, 1393–1404.
8. Fry, W. J., and R. Meyers (1962). Ultrasonic method of modifying brain structure(s), 1st Internat. Symposium on Stereoencephalotomy. Confinia Neurologica *22*, 315–327.
9. Basauri, L., and P. P. Lele (1962). A simple method for production of trackless focal lesions with focused ultrasound: statistical evaluation of the effects of irradiation on the central nervous system of the cat. J. Physiol. *160*, 513–534.
10. Baum, G., and I. Greenwood (1958). The application of ultrasonic locating techniques to ophthalmology. A.M.A. Arch. Ophthal. *60*, 263–279.
11. Howry, D. H. (1957). Techniques used in ultrasonic visualization of soft tissues, *in* "Ultrasound in Biology and Medicine," E. Kelly, ed. (American Institute of Biological Sciences, Washington, D.C.), pp. 49–65.
12. Dunn, F., and W. J. Fry (1959). Ultrasonic absorption microscope. J. Acoust. Soc. Am. *31*, 632–633.
13. Bell, E. (1959). A new approach to some problems in experimental embryology through the use of ultrasound, *in* "Proceedings of the First National Biophysics Conference," H. Quastler and H. J. Morowitz, eds. (Yale University Press, New Haven).
14. Grabar, P. (1953). Biological actions of ultrasonic waves, *in* "Advances in Biological and Medical Physics," J. H. Lawrence and C. A. Tobias, eds. (Academic Press, New York), Vol. 3.
15. Obolensky, G. (1957). Diverses actions des ultra-sons en biologie. Ann. Biol. *33*, 465–521.
16. Bauer, A. W. (1957). Ultrasonic research: progress during the past three years. Brit. J. Phys. Med. *20*, 151–158.
17. Fry, W. J., V. J. Wulff, D. Tucker, and F. J. Fry (1950). Physical factors involved in ultrasonically induced changes in living systems: I. Identification of non-temperature effects. J. Acoust. Soc. Am. *22*, 867–876.
18. Fry, W. J., D. Tucker, F. J. Fry, and V. J. Wulff (1951). Physical factors involved in ultrasonically induced changes in living systems: II. Amplitude dura-

tion relations and the effect of hydrostatic pressure for nerve tissue. J. Acoust. Soc. Am. *23*, 364–368.
19. Fry, W. J. (1953). Action of ultrasound on nerve tissue – a review. J. Acoust. Soc. Am. *25*, 1–5.
20. Dunn, F., and W. J. Fry (1957). An ultrasonic dosage study: functional end-point, *in* "Ultrasound in Biology and Medicine," E. Kelly, ed. (American Institute of Biological Sciences, Washington, D.C.), pp. 226–258.
21. Hueter, T. F., H. T. Ballantine, Jr., and W. C. Cotter (1957). On the problem of dosage in ultrasonic lesion making, *in* "Ultrasound in Biology and Medicine," E. Kelly, ed. (American Institute of Biological Sciences, Washington, D.C.), pp. 131–155.
22. Lele, P. P. (1962). A simple method for production of trackless focal lesions with focused ultrasound: physical factors. J. Physiol. *160*, 494–512.
23. Bejdl, W. von (1951). Der Einfluss des Ultraschalls auf das Glycogen der Leberzelle und auf die kupfferschen Sternzellen. Acta Anatomica *11*, 444–460.
24. Hug, O., and R. Pape (1954). Nachweis der Ultraschallkavitation im Gewebe. Strahlentherapie *94*, 79–99.
25. Jankowiak, J., J. Hasik, Cz. Majewski, and R. Markowski (1958). Influence of ultrasound on some histological and histochemical reactions in the liver of the rat. Am. J. Phys. Med. *37*, 135–142.
26. Southam, C. M., H. Beyer, and A. C. Allen (1953). The effects of ultrasonic irradiation upon normal and neoplastic tissues in the intact mouse. Cancer *6*, 390–396.
27. Bell, E. (1957). The action of ultrasound on the mouse liver. J. Cell. Comp. Physiol. *50*, 83–103.
28. Bell, E. (1957). Some changes in liver tissue which survives irradiation with ultrasound, *in* "Ultrasound in Biology and Medicine," E. Kelly, ed. (American Institute of Biological Sciences, Washington, D.C.), pp. 203–225.
29. Fry, W. J., and R. B. Fry (1954). Determination of absolute sound levels and acoustic absorption coefficients by thermocouple probes – theory and experiment. J. Acoust. Soc. Am. *26*, 294–317.
30. Hueter, T. F., and R. H. Bolt (1955). Sonics (John Wiley and Sons, New York), p. 267.
31. Benacerraf, B., G. Biozzi, B. N. Halpern, and C. Stiffel (1957). Physiology of phagocytosis of particles by the R.E.S., *in* "Physiopathology of the Reticulo-endothelial System," B. N. Halpern, ed. (Charles C. Thomas, Springfield, Ill.).
32. Barth, G., H. Erlhof, and F. Streibl (1950). Über den wirkungsmechanismus biologischer Ultraschallreaktionen. II. Impulsversuche mit Ultraschallhämolyse. Strahlentherapie *81*, 129–134.
33. Dyer, H. J., and W. L. Nyborg (1960). Ultrasonically-induced movements in cells and cell models. IRE Trans. Med. Electron. *ME–7*, 163–165.
34. Singer, M., and G. B. Wislocki (1948). The affinity of syncytium, fibrin and fibrinoid of the human placenta for acid and basic dyes under controlled conditions of staining. Anat. Rec. *102*, 175–193.

DISCUSSION

Dr. Carstensen: One of your slides shows the surface of the liver with two blood vessels in evidence, and there appears to be a lesion around each of these vessels. Would you show that slide again and tell us how the liver was irradiated?

Dr. Curtis: The ultrasound has traveled from left to right through the liver shown in Figure 16. The disruption of glycogen in hepatic cells appears localized to regions around the central veins of lobules at the dorsal surface of the left lateral lobe; the animal was sacrificed 1 hr after irradiation.

Dr. Carstensen: Was the whole area irradiated more or less uniformly?

Dr. Curtis: It would be difficult to determine the uniformity of the sound field in the intact animal. However, since the diameter of the focal region is ten times greater than the distance between sites of disruption in Figure 16, I am reasonably certain that the apparently undamaged tissue surrounding these areas has been exposed to ultrasound.

Dr. Carstensen: Is it fair to say that there may have been a local destruction because of the presence of the blood vessels? Was such localized destruction commonly found or was this more or less of an isolated situation?

Dr. Curtis: If the localized injury were due to the presence of blood vessels alone, I would expect to find such injury about all blood vessels across the entire width of the liver exposed to the ultrasound. For threshold doses, however, we generally find such an effect localized to areas adjacent to the dorsal surface of the liver. This suggests that such localized disruption is related to (1) an action of ultrasound which occurs selectively at or near tissue interfaces and (2) differences in the physical properties of different parts of the liver. Such differences would most likely be associated with the lobular arrangement of the liver parenchyma. For example, such differences might be related to the distribution of the supporting connective tissue in the mouse liver. Most of this connective tissue is found in the periportal region of the lobule about the hepatic portal veins, considerably less extending into the mid- and centrolobular regions. I would like to point out that when we find very minimal amounts of injury, we do not always find this pattern of centrolobular disruption. A shallow necrotic lesion may extend continuously along the dorsal surface (Fig. 12). The localization of cell injury to centrolobular regions adjacent to the surface of the liver is most frequently encountered when the ultrasound has traversed a relatively thin part of the lobe.

Dr. W. J. Fry: In brain and other tissues, we observe that after irradiation at dosages higher than those required to produce a minimum effect, a so-called island formation occurs. This region is presumably more drastically affected than the periphery so that it appears morphologically intact for a much longer period of time than the boundary region of the lesion. I wonder whether you have observed this pattern of destruction in the liver?

Dr. Curtis: Are you referring to the fact that the action of ultrasound in the brain appears greater at the center of the lesions?

Dr. W. J. Fry: I refer to the fact that a region of the central nervous system irradiated at a dosage level above the minimum required for destruction of neural elements exhibits a normal appearance for a considerable time after exposure, whereas the periphery, where the dosage grades off, appears drastically changed in a relatively short time after exposure. We have interpreted this to mean that the dissolution of the tissue structure in the part of the lesion removed from the periphery must be initiated by the invasion of agents from the boundary. This invasion may require several days.

DR. CURTIS: While it is true that the normal lobular arrangement of hepatic cells in the center of lesions is generally undisturbed, these cells appear necrotic within several hours after irradiation. Immediately after irradiation, there is a zone of graded cell injury at the periphery of the lesion; 6 hr later, this zone has been replaced by a narrower zone of degenerating cells between the necrotic lesion and the surrounding undamaged tissue.

DR. KELLY: How do changes in the DNA content of hepatic cells irradiated with subthreshold doses compare with those observed in tissues irradiated at higher doses? Do you have any quantitative data on the effect of subthreshold doses of ultrasound on the DNA content of hepatic cells?

DR. CURTIS: Two hr after irradiation, there is little or no DNA, as revealed by the Feulgen method, in hepatic cells of lesions such as those just described. Such marked changes are not produced by subthreshold doses. No attempt has been made to quantitatively study the effects of subthreshold doses upon the DNA content of the hepatic cell. In our histochemical study, a reduction of the Feulgen-reactive DNA has been observed shortly after irradiation in hepatic cells exposed to such doses.

DR. KELLY: Are you carrying out a dosage and serial-time study of cell injury caused by such doses and attempting to relate the effect of ultrasound on DNA and RNA to these variables?

DR. CURTIS: We are irradiating the livers of mice with subthreshold doses and sacrificing these animals at different times after irradiation in order to follow the cellular changes associated with the sublethal injury we have observed 30 days later. Gross observations of the intact liver at earlier times give no clues as to the chronology of events which have taken place in livers which exhibit histological evidence of such injury 30 days after irradiation. Realizing the hazards involved, we hope to construct a dynamic picture of the cellular changes produced by subthreshold doses of pulsed ultrasound by making observations on the irradiated livers of series of animals sacrificed at different times after treatment.

DR. BELL: In the experiments in which you injected Thorotrast to determine whether the cells, particularly of the endothelial system, were still viable, how long after irradiation did you inject the Thorotrast?

DR. CURTIS: Thorotrast was injected at times ranging from immediately after irradiation to 30 days later. The animals were routinely sacrificed 30 min after receiving the injection to allow sufficient time for the Thorotrast to be removed from the blood by the phagocytic cells. Thus, our earliest observations were made 30 min after irradiation. Thorotrast, as you probably know, is the trade name for a 25% stabilized colloidal thorium dioxide preparation (Testagar & Co., Detroit, Mich.).

DR. BELL: Do you find Thorotrast in macrophages in the lesions produced by sublethal dosage levels, regardless of the time after irradiation?

DR. CURTIS: Phagocytically active macrophages have been observed in sinusoids in regions of sublethal hepatic cell injury at all times studied to date.

DR. BELL: Do you have any other evidence regarding the viability of cells in lesions which you see as long as 30 days following irradiation? These are very interesting lesions that you are able to produce by series of short exposures.

DR. CURTIS: Our evidence of the viability of hepatic cells in such lesions is based upon histological observations in preparations stained with hematoxylin and eosin, and those treated according to the periodic acid-Schiff method and the Feulgen method for the demonstration of the glycogen and DNA, respectively.

DR. BELL: Have you detected Thorotrast in the cells?

DR. CURTIS: As I mentioned earlier, we find evidence of viable macrophages which have taken up the Thorotrast at times ranging from shortly after irradiation up to 30 days later in regions where hepatic cells appear sublethally injured as evidenced by the reduced glycogen and DNA content of these cells. However, there appear to be fewer macrophages containing Thorotrast in these areas than in adjacent undamaged areas.

DR. BELL: Have you looked at this material later than 30 days?

DR. CURTIS: We have recently obtained material at 60 and 90 days after irradiation but have not yet looked at the histological preparations.

DR. VON GIERKE: Does the data which you have presented on the dose dependence of hepatic lesion production indicate that you get the same temperature rise independent of the other variables? Also, have you estimated the temperature rise that is produced by subthreshold doses?

DR. CURTIS: Your first question can best be answered by comparing the dependence of lesion frequency and of mean temperature rise upon the duty factor as shown in Figures 7 and 9, respectively. The line intersecting each temperature curve in Figure 9 represents the mean temperature rises obtained at dosages which produce lesions in 50% of the irradiated animals. The mean temperature rises associated with the percentage appear directly related to the intensity—at higher intensities, the mean temperature rise is greater. This seems contrary to what one would expect if the injury were due primarily to heating, that is, the mean temperature rises would be the same for those dosages corresponding to a given frequency of lesion incidence. However, a comparison of the duty factors corresponding to a 50% lesion incidence at the different intensities reveals that the duty factor does not vary inversely with the intensity in a linear manner, but, as shown in Figure 8, varies exponentially with it. In other words, while the mean temperature rises corresponding to this lesion frequency are greater at the higher intensities than the lower ones, the rate at which acoustic energy is delivered to the liver is actually greater at the lower intensities. This apparent contradiction, I believe, may possibly be explained in terms of the relative effectiveness of ultrasound of high intensity, as opposed to that of lower intensities, in disrupting the blood circulation in the irradiated liver.

DR. VON GIERKE: My second question was whether you had estimated the temperature rise involved in the case of subthreshold dosages.

DR. CURTIS: Temperature rises of less than 2°C have been obtained in connection with the subthreshold dosages employed in this study.

DR. KIKUCHI: In regard to the temperature measurements, isn't there the possibility that the heat is dissipated by the thermocouple itself?

DR. CURTIS: This is a possibility and the extent to which this may occur will depend upon the dimensions and design of the thermocouple. We mount our copper-constantan thermocouples on a glass rod which has been drawn out to a fine tip at one end. The two thermocouple wires are attached to the glass rod so that the junction is beyond the tip of the rod. We use a glass support because of its poor heat-conducting properties and place the junction beyond the tip of the rod to minimize any heat dissipation by the thermocouple holder. Earlier we had used the method of mounting the thermocouple junction at the tip of a hypodermic needle but found such thermocouples to be less sensitive to small temperature changes than the ones we are now using.

DR. KIKUCHI: The focal region of the ultrasound is quite small so that the temperature rise must be very localized. What were the dimensions of the wire?

DR. CURTIS: The diameter of the wire is 0.001 in. The soldered junction is approximately 0.004 in (0.1 mm) in diameter which is small in comparison to the diameter of the focal region (7.5 mm). However, the temperature rises obtained at the lower threshold doses may not be a true indication of the localized temperature rises since lesions resulting from such doses often are smaller than the focal region, the dimensions of areas of localized disruption approaching those of the thermocouple.

DR. F. J. FRY: When you cut off the blood circulation, was the dose required to produce evidence of a lesion considerably less than that required in the usual situation?

DR. CURTIS: We have not made a study to determine how the amount of injury produced in the liver by ultrasound is affected by temporarily blocking the blood circulation during irradiation.

DR. F. J. FRY: Do you sacrifice the animal before irradiation?

DR. CURTIS: Yes, in this experiment the mice received a lethal blow just prior to irradiation. Temperature measurements were made in the livers of animals so sacrificed and in those of anesthetized animals serving as controls. The animals in both groups received the same dose of ultrasound. The mean temperature rise in the irradiated livers of the animals sacrificed just prior to irradiation was almost three times as great as that in livers of the controls.

DR. CARSTENSEN: You have mentioned that at some dose levels there was evidence of an action that was more or less centered around the central veins near the surface of the liver.

DR. CURTIS: Yes, the appearance of such localized injury is shown in Figure 16.

DR. CARSTENSEN: This localization would seem to be in opposition to the temperature differences you find.

DR. CURTIS: Any attempt to explain these localized effects must take into account the microcirculation of the liver, since our results indicate that the blood plays an important role in the removal of heat from areas exposed to pulsed ultrasound. A possible explanation is that while the ultrasound at high intensities may irreversibly alter the lobular circulation, irradiation at lower intensities may have only a temporary effect upon the circulation. It must also be kept in mind that the dimensions of the regions of such localized injury often approximate, or, may be smaller than, the size of the thermocouple.

DR. LIBBER: Have you tried irradiating hypothermic or hybernating rodents?

DR. CURTIS: No, I haven't done this, but Dr. Bell (see introduction) performed such an experiment upon precooled mice.

DR. KELLY: Did the subthreshold studies involve a range of doses?

DR. CURTIS: We have used acoustic power outputs of 15 w or less in conjunction with pulse rates that would give us a very low probability of producing the necrotic lesions used as criteria in the dosage studies described in this report.

DR. NYBORG: I believe you indicated in previous discussions that the lesions produced at the higher intensity levels occur quite often at the dorsal surface of the irradiated lobe. I have two questions about that. First, do you have further information as to why the injury occurs at this site? Second, do you have the same localization with the subthreshold irradiation?

DR. CURTIS: The localization of injury along the surface of the liver is often less striking at the lower doses. Some variability is encountered in this regard because our procedure of irradiating the liver in the intact mouse makes it difficult to always be certain that we're irradiating through the same thickness of liver. It is apparent at all dose levels that the localization of injury to the dorsal surface is less striking when the focused ultrasound traverses the liver near the edge of a lobe where it is relatively thin. An example of the distribution of the injury produced by a subthreshold dose is shown in Figure 23. The direction of the irradiation is from top to bottom in this figure.

DR. BELL: Therefore, it is substantially localized to the surface of the lobe further from the transducer?

DR. CURTIS: While the zone of injury does extend from the surface into the lobe, it doesn't have the shape typical of the necrotic lesions produced by higher doses, namely, that of a spherical segment.

DR. NYBORG: Do you have any further information as to why this localization occurs? I remember that you've done a number of experiments on this.

DR. CURTIS: We have attempted to determine whether the amount of injury occurring at the dorsal surface of the liver is affected by the physical state of the liver. The turgidity and the elastic stress in the tissue can be increased by perfusing an abnormal amount of blood into the liver – the liver of the mouse is a very distensible organ. The results to date, while preliminary, suggest that the amount of injury selectively produced at the dorsal surface of the liver by ultrasound is strongly affected by changes in the turgidity of the liver produced by varying its blood volume. We are attempting to refine our perfusion technique in order to quantitatively study this effect.

Dr. F. J. Fry: Figure 20 shows the edge of a lesion where the tissue is more or less unaffected as well as an adjacent region of fairly extensive damage at the lesion periphery and a central region which appears to have less damage. Now, if I'm not mistaken, the tissue is not damaged in the area adjacent to the lesion shown in Figure 20.

Dr. Curtis: Yes, the hepatic cells in the region adjacent to the necrotic lesion do not appear damaged.

Dr. F. J. Fry: There appears to be a bank of extensive damage next to this unaffected region. The action of the ultrasound appears to have been most destructive at the periphery of the lesion.

Dr. Curtis: The region that I think you're referring to is the zone at the periphery of the necrotic tissue where fibrogenesis is occurring.

Dr. F. J. Fry: Does this zone surround the whole lesion?

Dr. Curtis: Yes, a fibrotic capsule forms about the lesion between 3 to 6 days after irradiation, not only at the internal boundary of the lesion, but at the surface of the lobe as well.

Dr. Bell: I think one ought to say a word about the phenomenon of sound reflection at the dorsal surface of the liver. This represents a zone of an enormous impedance barrier for the sound as it passes through the lobe which is divided up and capsulated by connective tissue. There could very well be an air space behind the lobe.

Dr. Herrick: What are the dimensions of the focal region in relation to the size of the liver lobe? How uniform is your sound field?

Dr. Curtis: The dimensions of the focal region are such that it extends the entire width of the left lateral lobe. An example of the distribution of acoustic energy in the focal region, as determined by making lateral scans with a thermocouple, is shown in Figure 2.

Dr. Carstensen: It is essentially a pencil of sound rather than a sharp focal region.

Dr. Weissler: Going back to your observation of greater damage in the distended liver, could this be due to the same sort of thing that caused an increase of effect with pressure that Dr. Hughes reported this morning? Dr. Hughes showed that as he increased the pressure above atmospheric, there was a maximum effect. In fact, many people have found that pressures of perhaps 2 or 3 atm, depending upon the ultrasonic intensity, produce a maximum effect. Perhaps your finding of a greater damage at higher pressure is dependent on this sort of effect?

Dr. Hughes: I think you have to be careful in attempting to explain such an effect, because it is possible that the first result is concerned with an alteration in the nature of the cavitation collapse rather than an increase in pressure on the cells.

Dr. Curtis: In view of our histological studies, I do not believe that the injury localized at the surface of the liver can be attributed to a cavitation mechanism. Only infrequently, at the higher intensities, do we find such injury accompanied by a more destructive type of cell injury in which there is evidence of cavitation. The two types of injury differ in many respects.

DR. BELL: By inflating the liver with an excess of blood one would be exposing a much larger volume of blood to high-intensity ultrasound and would therefore be causing a considerably greater damage to the blood and blood cells. From the general appearance of these lesions, which indicates that they are infarctions, the blood that is irradiated apparently stays there so that if a larger volume of blood is irradiated, a larger lesion would probably be the result.

DR. CURTIS: I do not believe that the size of these lesions can be attributed simply to infarctive effects since the preliminary observations mentioned in regard to the variation of lesion size as a function of the distended state of the liver were made immediately following the irradiation of isolated livers. It still remains a question in my mind whether this localized injury can be entirely explained in terms of selective heating at the surface of the liver. In distended livers the surface dimensions of the lesions are much greater than in normal livers, namely, the diameter of the lesion at the surface is much larger than the diameter of the focal region. This increase in the dimensions of the lesion at the lobe surface is often not accompanied by a comparable increase in the depth to which the lesion penetrates into the lobe. If such injury were due only to the establishment of a high-temperature gradient at the lobe surface, one would expect heat transfer to occur as rapidly into the liver lobe as along its surface. The fact that in many cases this does not appear to be the situation suggests that this localization may be due, in part, to a mechanical effect of ultrasound along the surface of the liver. A mechanical action seems to be indicated by the alterations in cytoplasmic structure observed shortly after exposure of the liver in the intact mouse to low threshold doses of pulsed ultrasound.

DR. KELLY: Did you indicate that glycogen also disappeared in connection with subthreshold doses? Have your subthreshold studies included observations at a number of different times after irradiation?

DR. CURTIS: A rapid loss of glycogen from hepatic cells, such as that typical of lesions produced by threshold doses of ultrasound, has not been observed after the administration of subthreshold doses. However, little or no glycogen was demonstrable in the hepatic cells of lesions found 10 and 30 days after exposure to the latter doses. An example of such injury is shown in Figure 23. We have made observations immediately following irradiation and 24 hr, 5, 10, and 30 days later.

Morphology of Ultrasonically Irradiated Skeletal Muscle

REGINALD C. EGGLETON, ELIZABETH KELLY, FRANCIS J. FRY, RUTH CHALMERS, and WILLIAM J. FRY

Biophysical Research Laboratory, University of Illinois, Urbana, Illinois

Introduction by Dr. Herrick

The history of the application of physical agents to medicine has not been a happy one partly because such agents have been applied in some instances before their basic action on the biological system was thoroughly understood. A most encouraging aspect of this meeting is the emphasis on understanding the basic mechanisms involved in the observed effects of ultrasound. The next paper concerns the application of electron microscope techniques in order to determine the effects of ultrasound on muscle. It will be presented by Dr. Eggleton.

Studies involving the use of ultrasound as a research tool to produce differential and controlled changes in biological tissue are of particular interest to this laboratory. The research program has included an investigation of the use of high-intensity ultrasound to produce functional changes in striated skeletal muscle (1, 2). In the present study, the morphological ultrastructure of ultrasonically irradiated skeletal muscle is being investigated with the aid of the electron microscope. It is hoped eventually to relate structural changes with corresponding functional changes and possibly with basic muscle mechanisms.

Although the ultrasound equipment used in these experiments was designed primarily for the production of focal lesions in the CNS, it was readily adapted to the requirements of this study. This equipment consists of a single-beam focusing transducer driven at 4 Mc by a feedback-controlled amplifier. More detailed descriptions of the equipment will be given later in this symposium by F. J. Fry and G. H. Leichner of this laboratory. Sound pressure amplitudes in the range of 50 atm were applied to the muscle for periods of the order of 0.8 sec. A beam-width characteristic of the transducer was 0.6 mm to the half-power point. The specimen thickness was approximately 1 mm.

Because there are many systems of muscle nomenclature, perhaps it is appropriate first to describe the terms used here. Figure 1 shows a portion of three myofibrils. Note the sarcomere between two "Z" bands. The "A" band is the dark area, and the "I" band is the light area. The "H" zone is the lighter portion of the "A" band, and the "M" line is in the center of the "H" zone. It is generally thought that the protein, myosin, occupies the "A" band and is composed of filaments 100 A in diameter and that the protein, actin, is the principal ingredient of the "I" band which is composed of 50-A-diameter filaments. The actin presumably extends into the "A" band, giving rise to a zone of overlap. Note further that the sarcomere is of the order of 2 μ long and 0.5 μ in diameter.

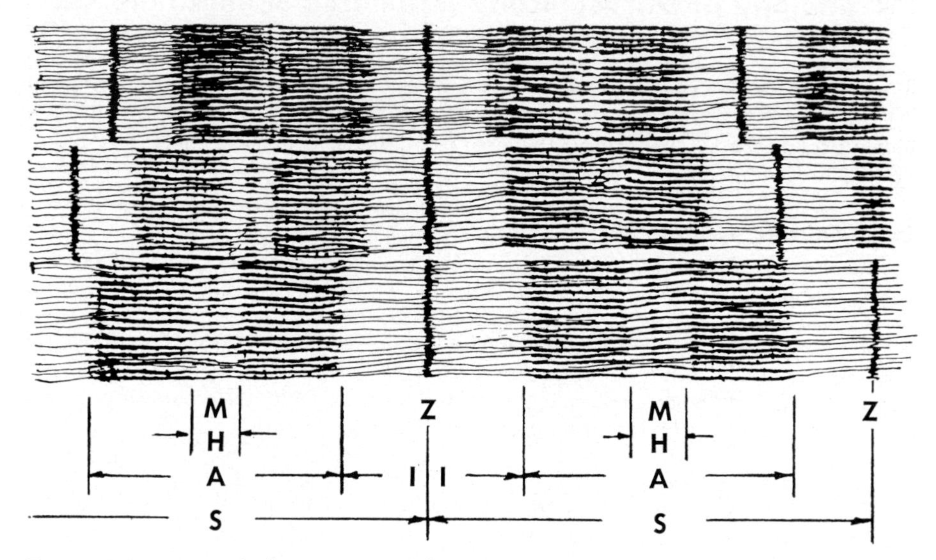

FIGURE 1. Diagram of ultrastructure of frog sartorius muscle showing nomenclature used in this paper.

It has been found that ultrasound lesions in muscle are, as might be predicted, relatively complex. One of the more interesting phenomena observed is the loss of band structure within the lesion. It is very common to find along the edge of the lesion, as shown in Figure 2, a normal-appearing fiber next to a fiber in which the band structure is destroyed. Longitudinal filaments about 100 A in diameter can be seen in this area. The filaments appear to be continuous rather than discontinuous as might be predicted from the Huxley-Hanson model (3). It is further noted that this change in band structure usually occurs at the fiber boundary. This observed condition cannot be explained in terms of sound or heat temperature gradients across the small (0.1 μ) gap between fibers.

To understand the changes caused by high-intensity ultrasound, it is first necessary to have more information on the effect of heat on muscle since ultrasound causes heating of the tissue. Accordingly, several series of excised frog

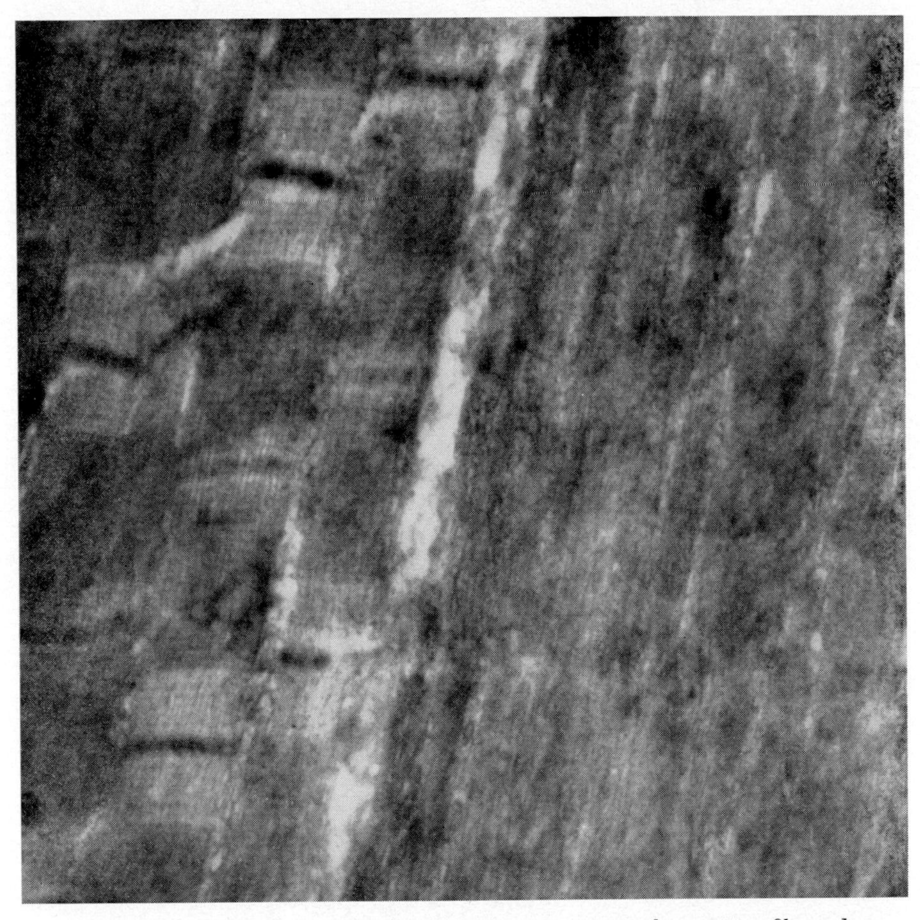

FIGURE 2. An ultrasonically irradiated muscle showing a normal-appearing fiber adjacent to a fiber in which the band structure is destroyed.

sartorius muscles were immersed in heated Ringer's solution that ranged in temperature from 35 to 55°C. In one series, the muscles were immersed in the heated Ringer's solution for a period of 2 min. In other experiments, a hcat exposure of 15 sec was used. As a means of following dimensional changes in the muscle during the various processing procedures, three fine silk threads were tied in the edge of the muscle in such a configuration that both lateral and longitudinal changes could be determined (Figs. 3, 4). The muscles were held at about 20% stretch during the heat exposure and subsequent fixation and dehydration procedures.

All muscles were fixed in veronal-buffered osmium tetroxide solution, dehydrated in graded alcohols, and imbedded in methacrylate. Some of the imbedded specimens were sectioned into 25 slices and mounted on microscope slides with a water base mounting medium (Fig. 5). The mounted sections were scanned under the light microscope and selected areas were dissected out of the specimen slice and secured to a mounting tip using dental wax

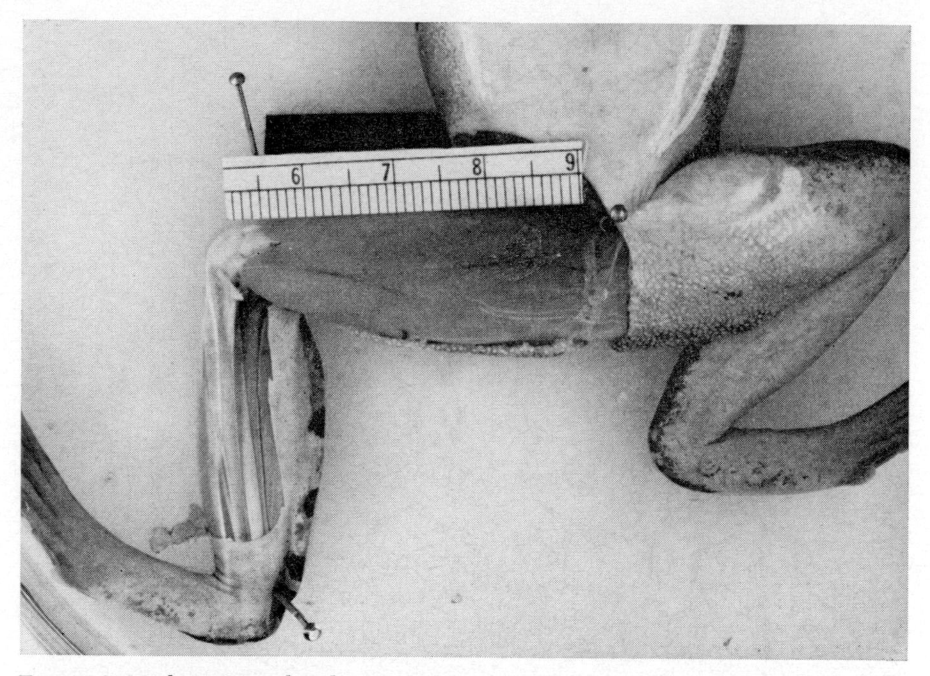

FIGURE 3. Markers were placed in the edge of the sartorius muscle so that dimensional changes could be followed through the processing of the muscle. Dimensions were recorded for various postural configurations.

(Figs. 6, 7). The selected specimen area was sectioned in a Porter-Blum microtome for examination in the electron microscope.

It was immediately evident upon a cursory examination of the sections of heat-treated muscles that the band structure appeared normal in specimens subjected to temperatures up to about 40°C. Muscles exposed to temperatures of about 45°C or higher contained no normal bands. Between these two temperatures there was a gradual transition in the percentage of the muscle fibers with normal bands. The structure shown in Figure 8 is typical of a muscle subjected to 43.25°C. Note that the bands have disappeared, but the longitudinal filaments are still intact. A small percentage (5 to 10%) of the volume of this specimen contained rather normal-appearing bands as shown in Figure 9. Figure 10 is an example of the most intact part of 43.75°C muscle as found in this particular specimen. An occasional isolated sarcomere can be seen. The longitudinal filaments are generally present, but the myofibrils are not always distinct. It should be noted that in any given heat-treated muscle there is a spectrum of effects. In the series of micrographs shown in Figure 11 (a 43.75°C muscle), myofibrillar structure is clear in #1 but is not present in #4. Mitochondria are present in all cases and appear normal morphologically although no measurements were made to determine their condition. It was also noted that the change in ultrastructure was accompanied by a change in the gross appearance of the muscle from a translucent to an opaque white.

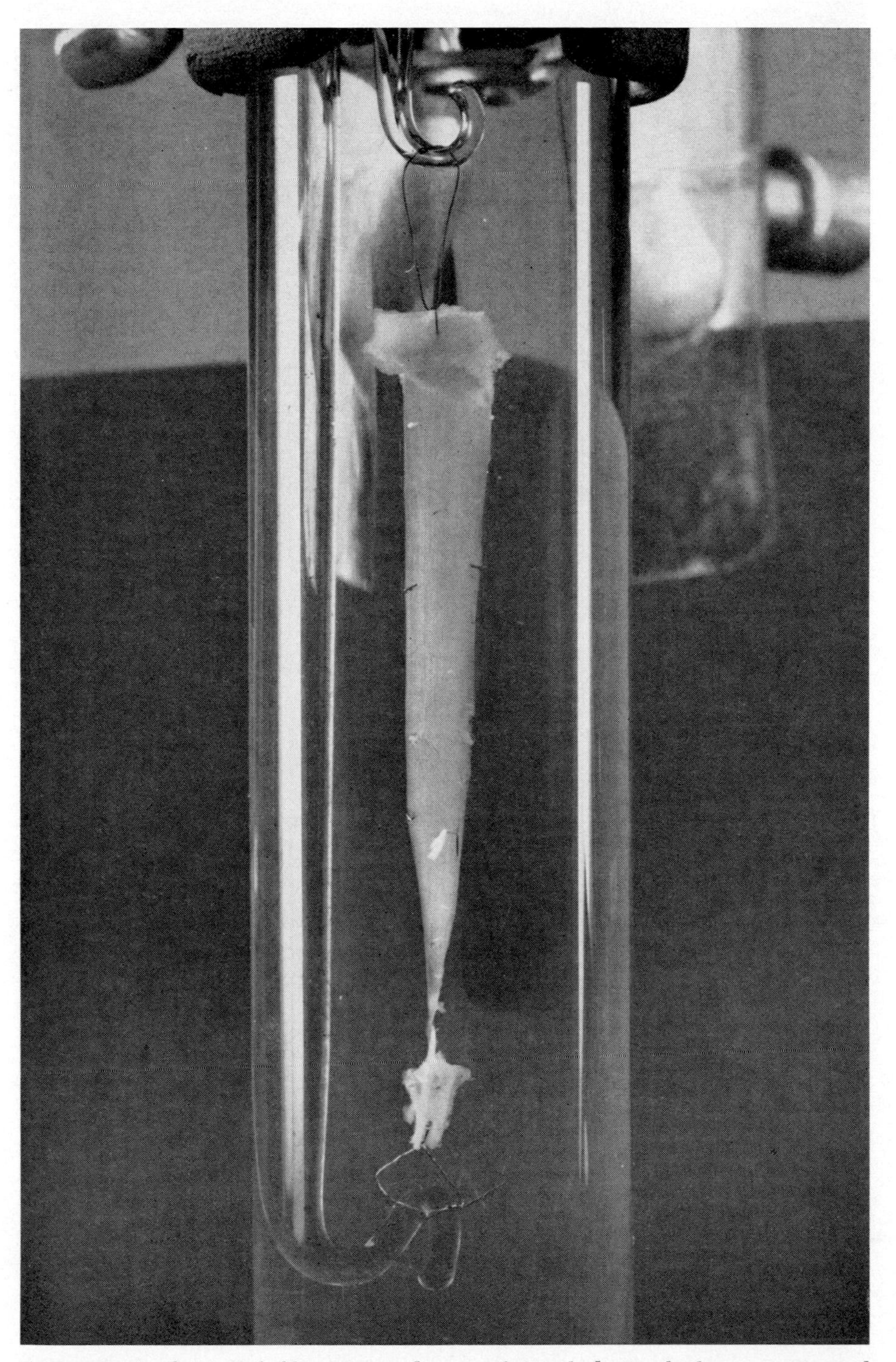

FIGURE 4. Muscles were held at various degrees of stretch during the heat exposure and subsequent fixation and dehydration procedures.

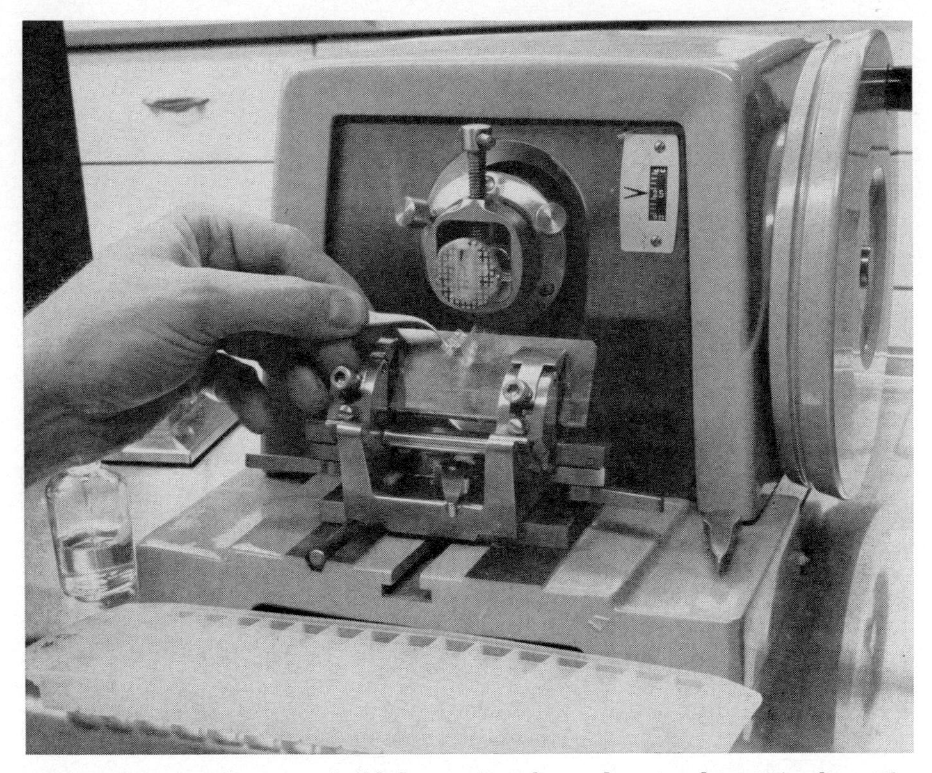

FIGURE 5. The muscles were imbedded in methacrylate and sectioned into 25-μ slices. The mounted slices could be scanned under the light microscope for areas of interest.

A corresponding series of pictures of muscle cross-sections is shown in Figure 12. Note that in #1, the myofibril is still clearly defined by the sarcoplasmic reticulum, the filaments are in a systematic array, and there are no large interstitial spaces in this part of the muscle. Succeeding pictures show increasing amounts of disorder with large interspaces present. In #4 there is no myofibrillar structure and many filaments are indistinguishable against a general background of debris. At higher temperatures the conditions shown in #4 become more prevalent. Also, at the higher temperature there is abnormal band structure such as that shown in Figure 13. This muscle was immersed for 2 min in a Ringer's bath which had been heated to 50°C. The fact that the muscle was unrestrained may explain the short sarcomere length, although not all unrestrained heat-treated muscles have contracted sarcomeres. The important features to be noted are the presence of the transmyofibrillar bridges and the general form of the myofibril. This is typical of perhaps 10 to 25% of this muscle. No longitudinal filaments are discernible in this muscle.

More than one mechanism is involved in the effect of heat on muscle. The following observations are noted: (1) Loss of band structure is evidence of damage to muscle and may result from various nutritional deficiencies (4)

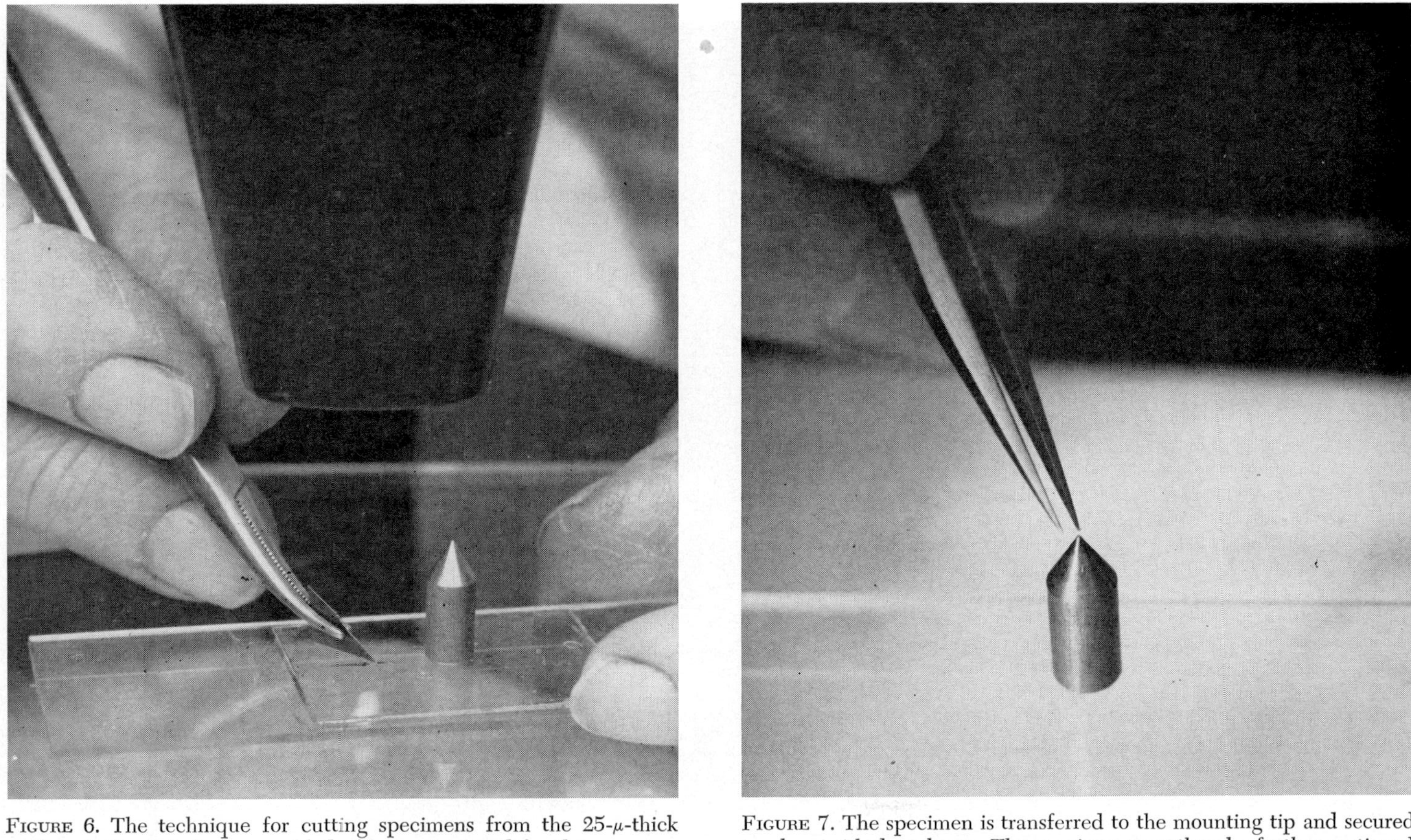

FIGURE 6. The technique for cutting specimens from the 25-μ-thick sections is illustrated. A razor blade fragment is used for this purpose.

FIGURE 7. The specimen is transferred to the mounting tip and secured in place with dental wax. The specimen may then be further sectioned in the ultramicrotome.

as well as from heat and ultrasound. This loss of structure apparently is a property of the fiber, that is, all myofibrils within a fiber lose their bands while the fibers on either side may be quite normal in appearance (4). (2) Fibers toward the outside of the heat-treated muscle are more likely to retain their band structure than are central fibers. (3) The time constant for the

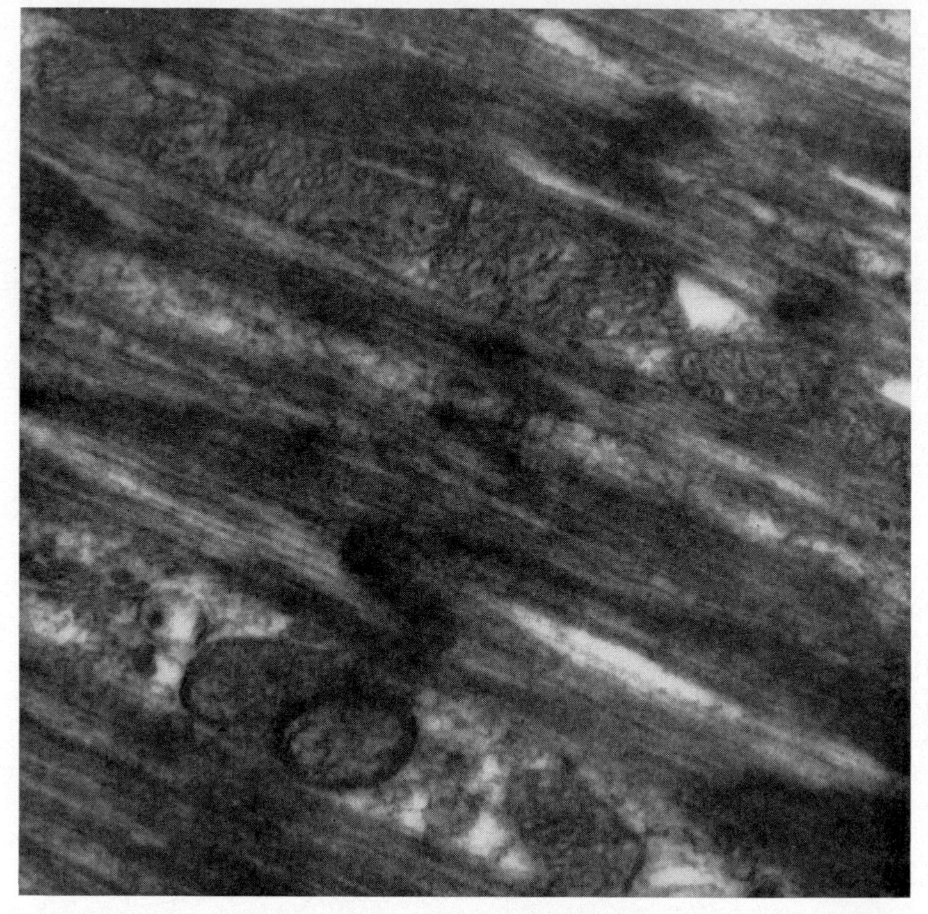

FIGURE 8. Structure typical of muscle subjected to 43.25°C. Bands have disappeared, but the longitudinal filaments are still intact.

primary action of heat on muscle would seem to be short—possibly less than 15 sec. (4) The lengths of the sarcomere "A" band and "I" band do not change significantly for muscles (held at 20% stretch) exposed to temperatures up to approximately 43°C. (5) The center-to-center distance of the filaments measured in the "H" zone are about the same for muscles exposed to various temperatures up to approximately 46°C. Filaments have not been found in muscles heated above 46°C. (6) A type of damage to the muscle is observed in which band structure is destroyed but longitudinal filaments remain intact.

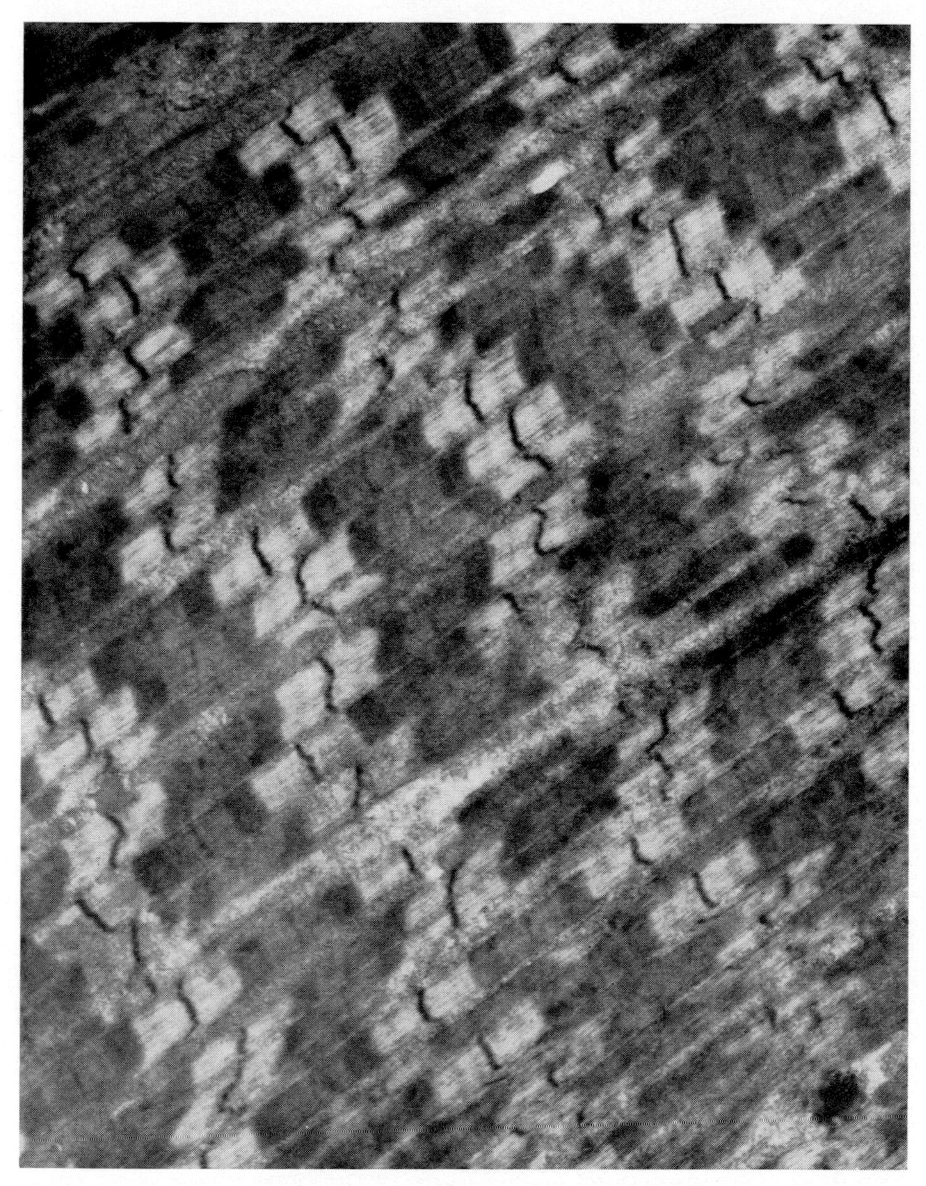

FIGURE 9. A small percentage of the muscle heated to 43.25°C shows normal appearing band structure.

One hypothesis which is being considered to explain these observed changes is that some agent already present within the muscle fiber is responsible for the loss of band structure. This agent, after the release by any one of several "stimuli," might diffuse along the fiber affecting all the myofibrils within it but does not readily diffuse across the sarcolemma into adjacent fibers. Perhaps the myosin of the "A" band is mobilized by this agent to provide a means for the myosin to diffuse into the "I" band where it combines

FIGURE 10. Muscle heated to 43.75°C is illustrated showing the most intact structure in this particular specimen.

with the actin to form an actomyosin complex, thus resulting in the general appearance shown in Figure 14.

It was reported by Jensen (5) in 1914 that frog sartorius muscle exhibits reversible and irreversible heat contraction. The reversible heat contraction takes place between 37 and 39°C and the irreversible thermal rigor takes place between 39 to 45°C. Later, Mirsky (6), in working with myosin isolated from frog muscle, found myosin denatures in two distinct steps. He found a pronounced change in solubility occurring at 37°C. As the myosin is heated to temperatures over 39°C, a second change takes place; beginning at about 41°C, the gel draws together into a number of firm opaque clumps. As previously noted, the authors of this paper found what appears to be a two-step

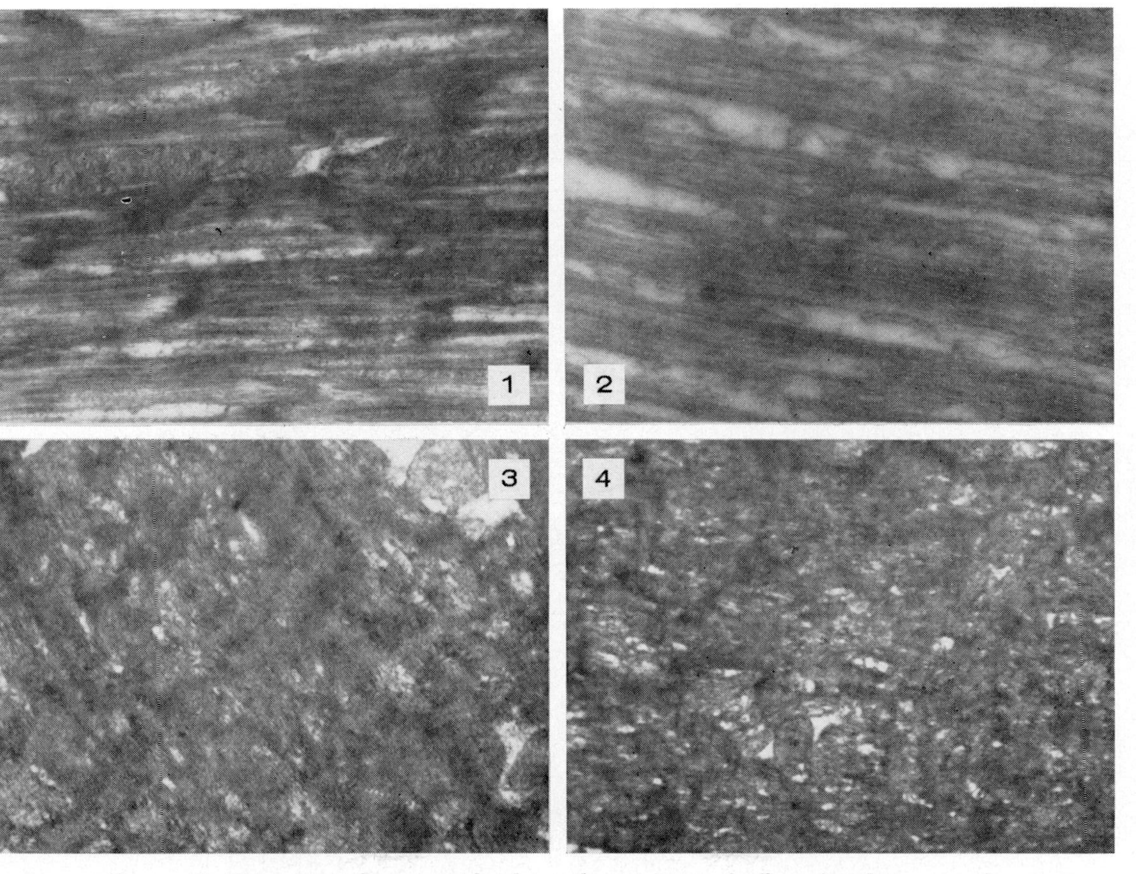

FIGURE 11. This series of micrographs shows the spectrum of effects found in a muscle heated to 43.75°C. The micrographs are arranged in order of increasing amounts of destruction of muscle ultrastructure: 1, least evidence of destruction; 2, 3, intermediate level of destruction; 4, complete destruction.

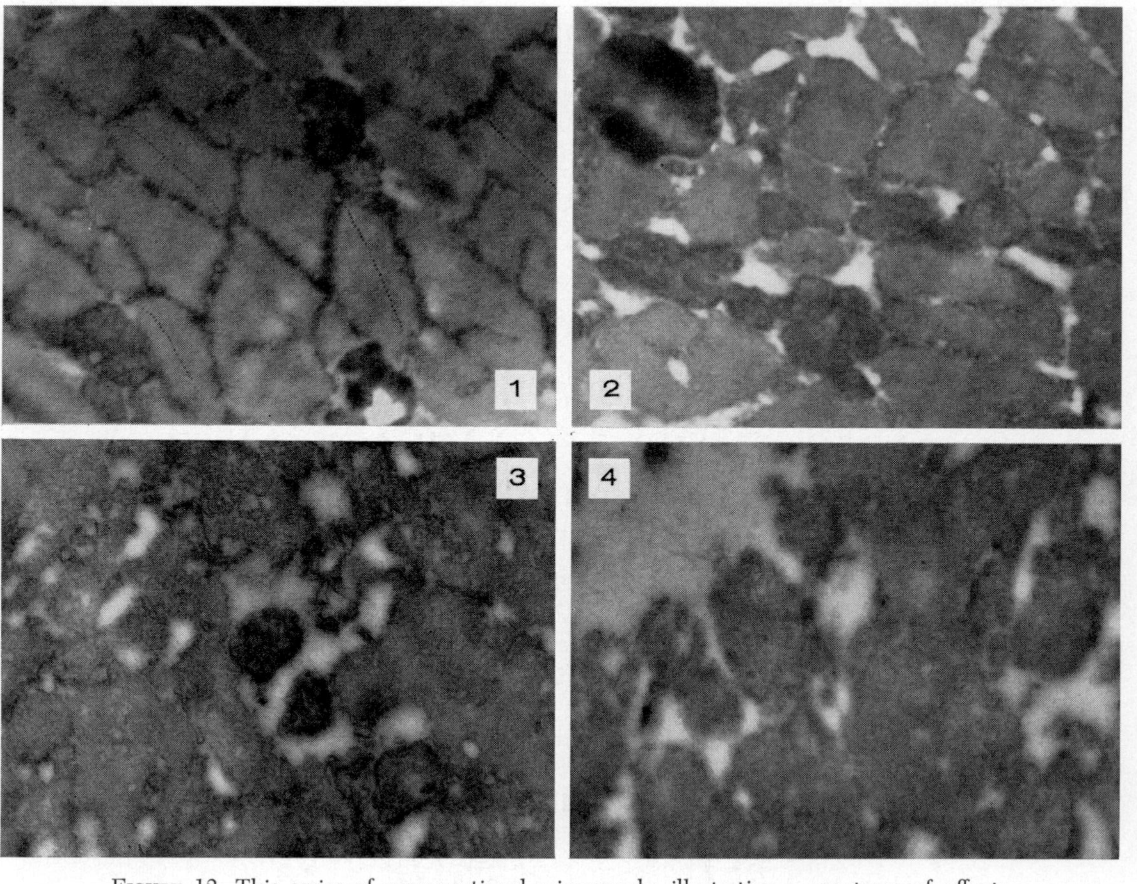

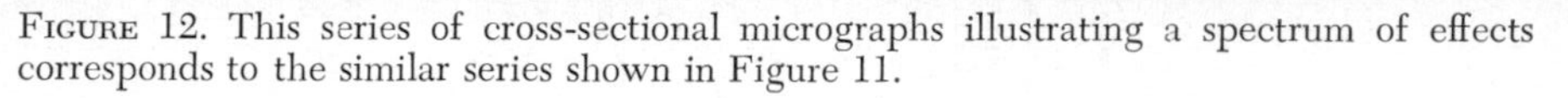

FIGURE 12. This series of cross-sectional micrographs illustrating a spectrum of effects corresponds to the similar series shown in Figure 11.

change in ultrastructure of the frog muscle exposed to high temperatures. In the temperature range of 40 to 44°C it was found that the band structure disappears leaving 100-A-diameter longitudinal filaments clearly visible while in the temperature range from 44 to 46°C, the filaments are found to disappear.

Another type of damage to muscle which has been observed and reported on by previous authors (7) is noted again here because it plays a part in the general configuration of the ultrasound lesion. Figure 15 shows a single fiber damaged by mechanical stretching of the fiber, and Figure 16 shows the same type of damage produced by ultrasound. It appears that the myofibrillar bun-

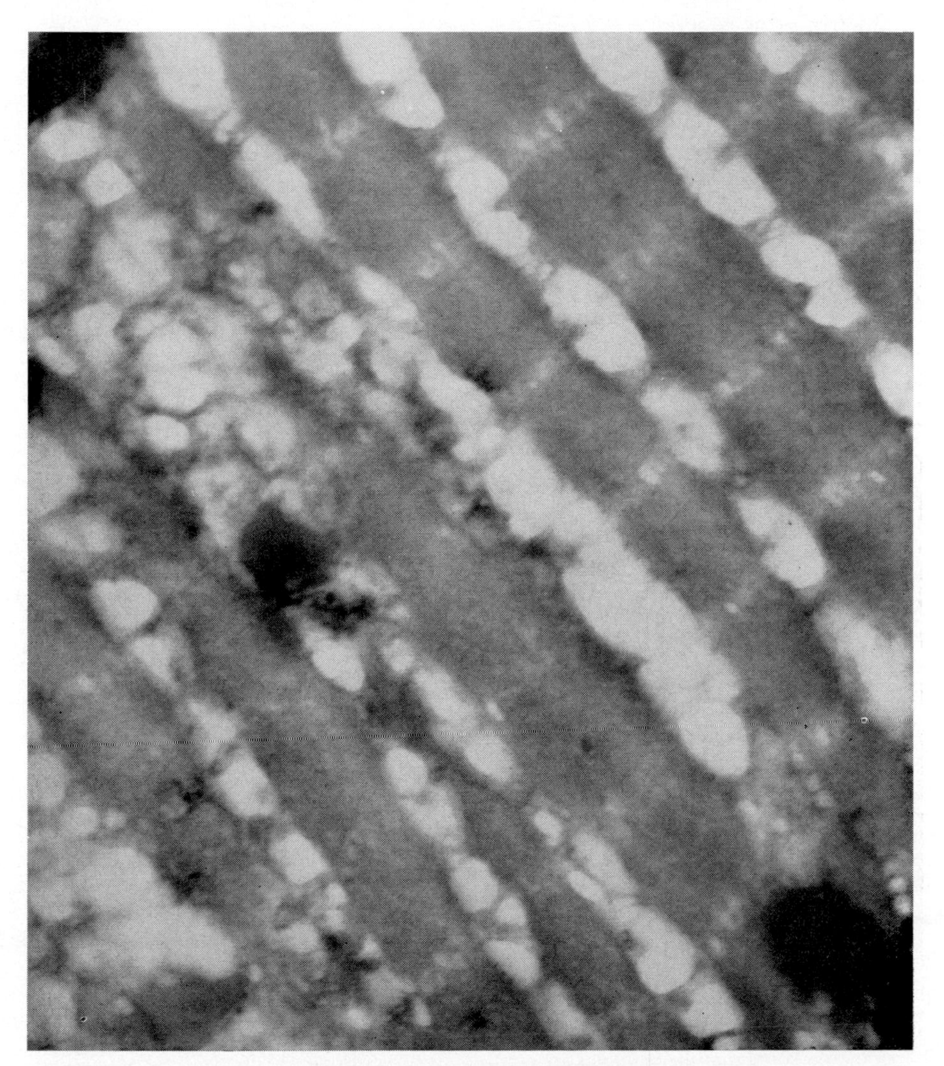

FIGURE 13. Muscle immersed for 2 min in Ringer's bath heated to 50°C is illustrated. Transmyofibrillar bridges and remnants of band structure are in evidence.

dle is under stress and is in equilibrium with the constraining force of the sarcolemma. The breaking strain of the sarcolemma is considerably greater than that of the myofibrillar bundles, thus when the sarcolemma is stretched, the adhering bundles stretch with it until the breaking stress of the bundles is exceeded. When this occurs, the structural part of the bundles (the filaments) apparently contracts and forms a series of compact masses at distributed sites within the sarcolemma, and the medium which surrounds the filaments in the intact fiber now fills the spaces between the compact masses. The area of these compact masses can be measured and the volume estimated. The values obtained may be compared with the estimated volume of intact fiber based on measurements outside of the damaged area and before the fiber was damaged. Table I shows some examples of these volume changes which result from this process.

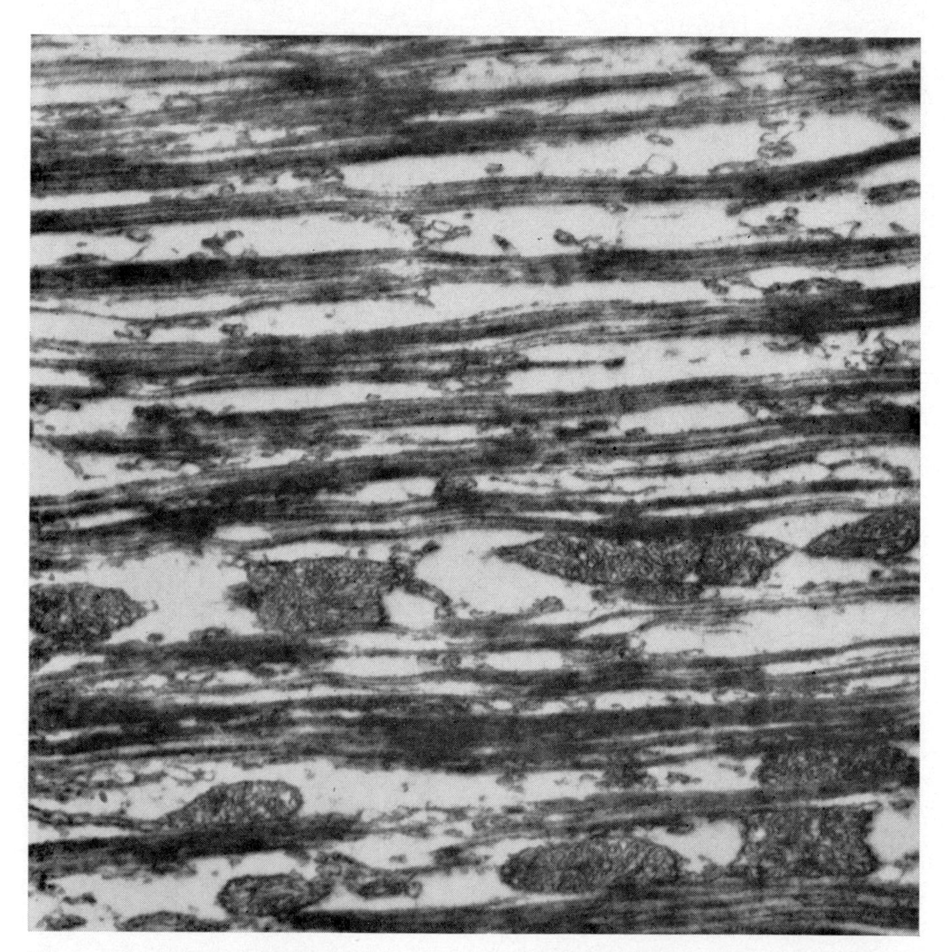

FIGURE 14. Electron micrograph of frog sartorius muscle exposed to 42°C bath for 15 sec. It should be noted that the filaments are continuous for a distance in excess of the sarcomere length.

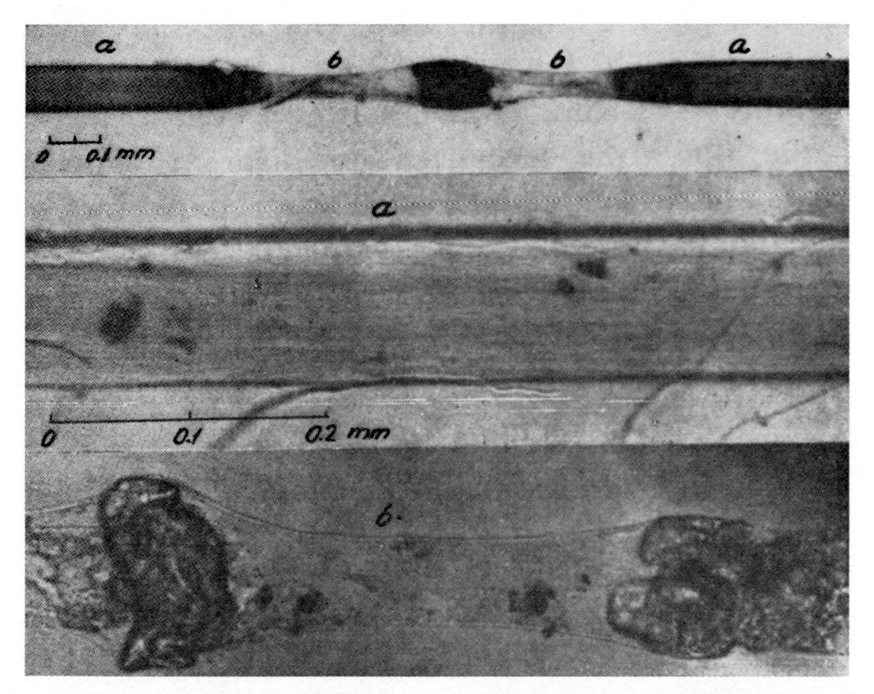

FIGURE 15. Photomicrographs of fibers damaged by mechanical stretching of the fiber (after Buchthal, 1951). a, undamaged fiber; b, empty sarcolemma tube.

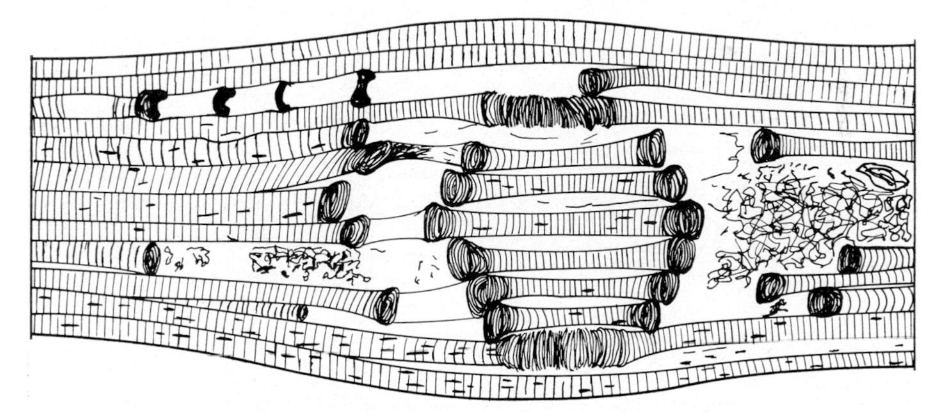

FIGURE 16. Damage produced by ultrasound similar to the damage illustrated in Figure 15. Sketch based on microscopic observations.

Another process which may be contributing to the structure of the ultrasonic lesion in muscle is "heat fixation." Biologists have long used heat as a means of fixing tissue. Focused ultrasound causes a rapid increase in temperature within the central part of the muscle and is calculated to be about a 46°C rise above 19°C ambient temperature for the sound levels used here. The gross configuration of the high-level focused ultrasound lesion in muscle is

TABLE I. VOLUME CHANGES IN MUSCLE FIBERS RESULTING FROM BREAKS IN THE MYOFIBRILLAR BUNDLES.

Muscle no.	*Estimated volume undamaged*	*Measured volume damaged*	*Ratio* V_o/V_i
1.	$3.35 \times 10^6 u^3$	$2.25 \times 10^6 u^3$	1.5
2.	$4.26 \times 10^6 u^3$	$2.06 \times 10^6 u^3$	2.0
3.	$5.15 \times 10^6 u^3$	$2.72 \times 10^6 u^3$	1.9
4.	$8.18 \times 10^6 u^3$	$1.96 \times 10^6 u^3$	4.1

characterized by an island of relatively intact tissue surrounded by a moat within which there is extensive tissue damage. It seems reasonable to suppose that the structure within the central island has been preserved due to heat fixation. This conclusion is supported by the observation of an *immediate* opacity change in the tissue. In the island, the sarcomere length is consider-

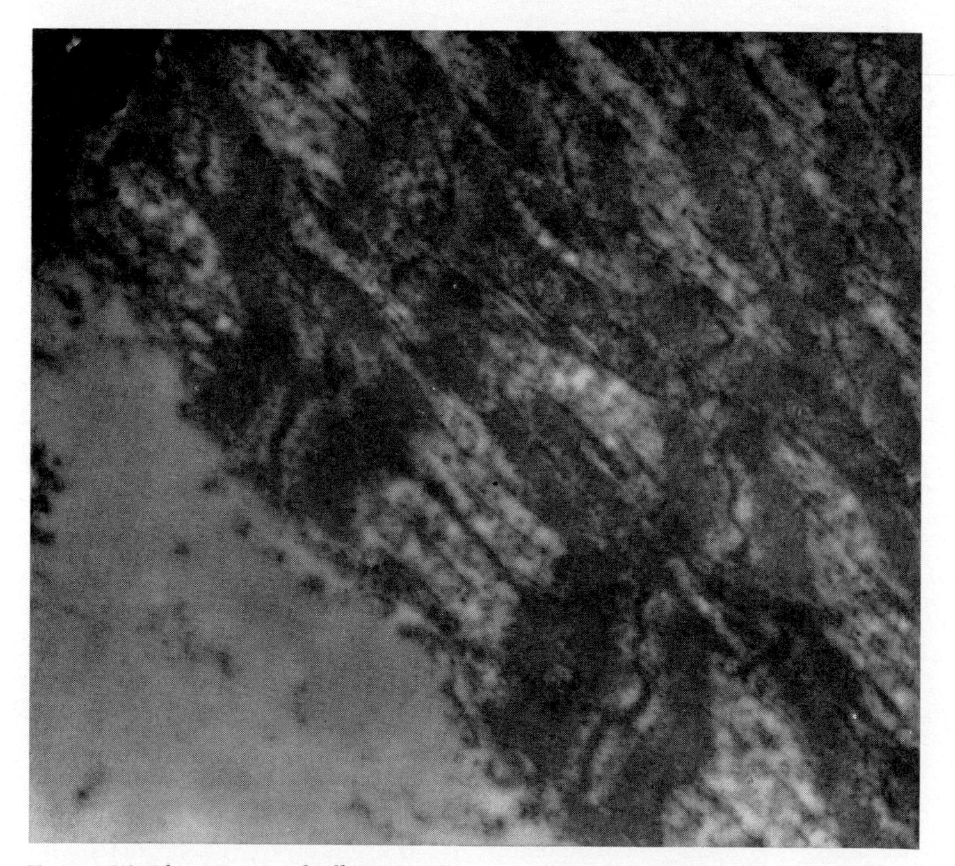

FIGURE 17. This micrograph illustrates the type of damage found in the center of an ultrasound lesion. The bands appear to be broken in the region of the H-zone.

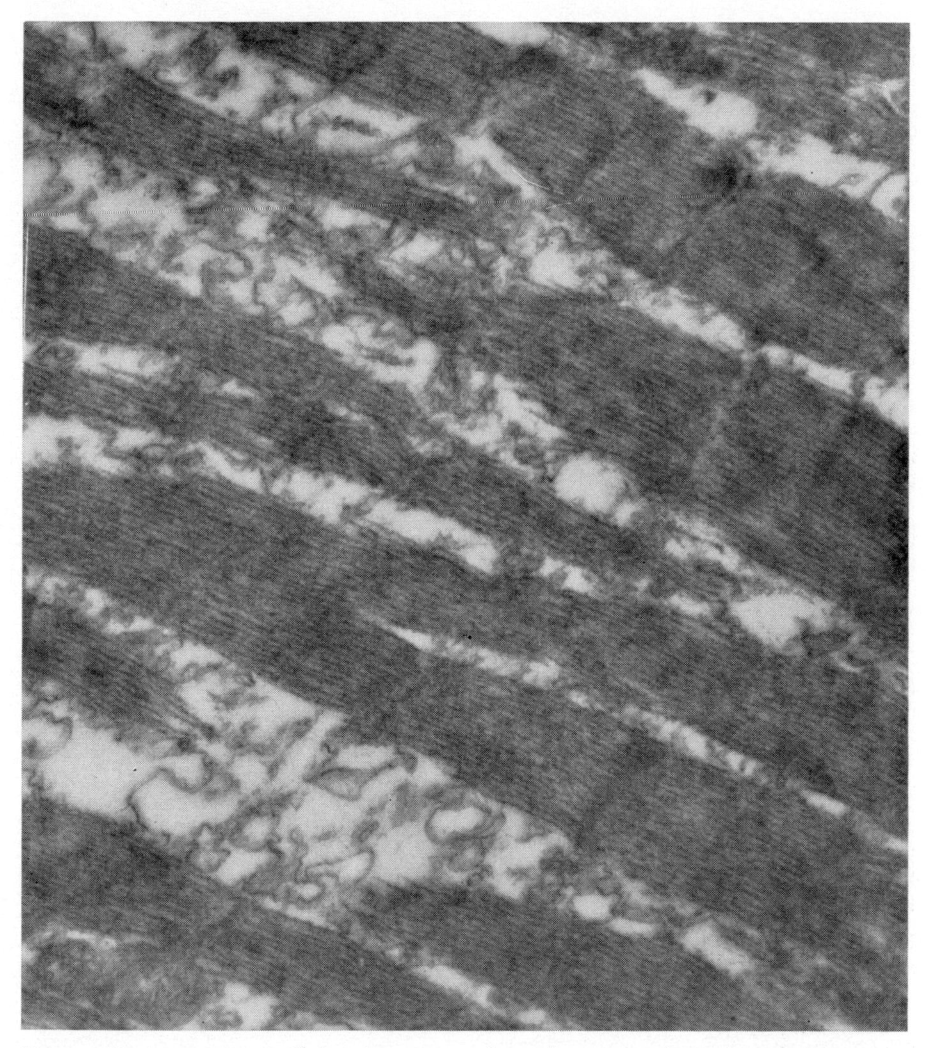

FIGURE 18. A micrograph illustrating an area from the center of an ultrasound lesion in which longitudinal filaments are present but band structure has disappeared.

ably increased, and this is explained if one assumes that the *tensile* strength of the *heated* portion of the fibers is much less than that characteristic of the unheated portion of the fibers. The muscle is held under slight tension, and as a result of this tension, the unheated portion stretches the heated portion to the point where the fibers rupture and contract away from the lesion, forming a moat. Figure 17 shows a modified band structure taken from the center of an island. If the "Z" membrane is the dark line, then each myofibril has been broken at the "M" line. Figure 18 shows an area in which the bands are not present. One of the areas of greatest damage is shown in Figure 19, but even at this level of destruction one can find evidence of mitochondria being present.

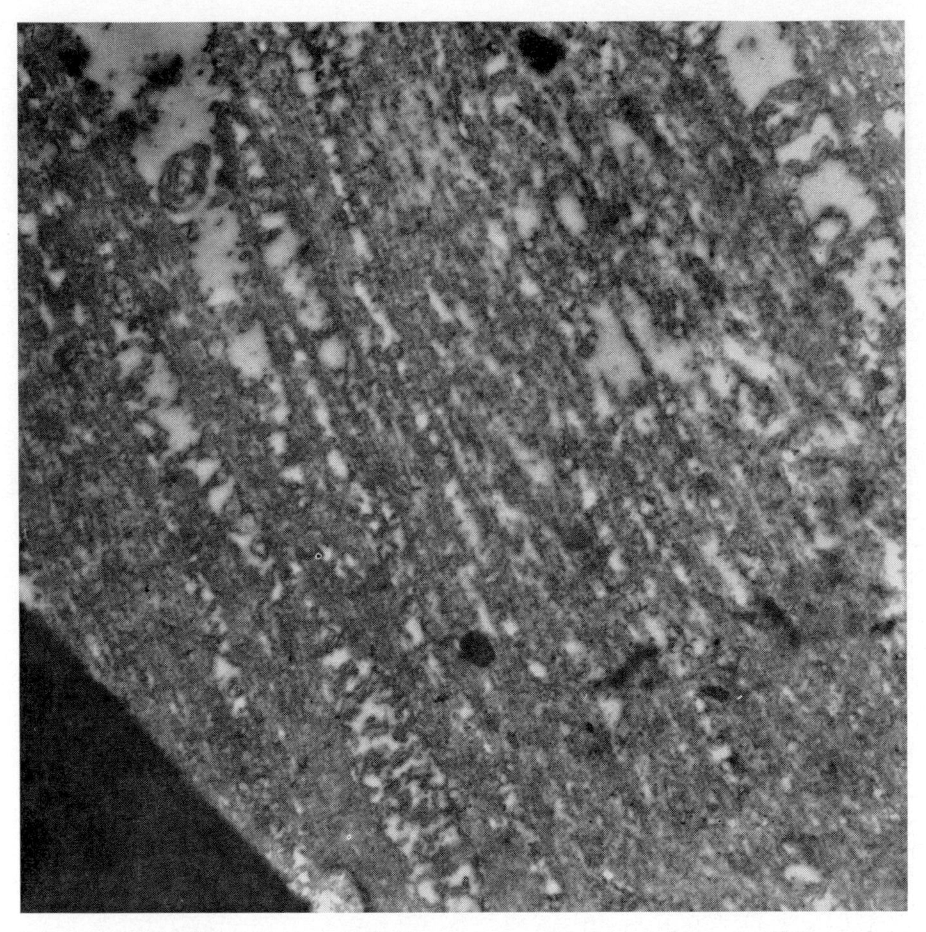

FIGURE 19. This electron micrograph illustrates an area of great damage within an ultrasound lesion. Note that mitochondria are present.

REFERENCES

1. Welkowitz, W., and W. J. Fry (1956). Effect of high intensity sound on electrical conduction in muscle. J. Cell. Comp. Physiol. *48*, 435–458.
2. Kelly, E., F. J. Fry, and W. J. Fry (1958). Effect of high intensity ultrasound on the mechanical response of excised biceps muscle of the frog. Abstract, Biophysical Society Meeting, Feb., 1958.
3. Huxley, H. E. (1957). The double array of filaments in cross-striated muscle. J. Biophys. Biochem. Cytol. *3*, 631–648.
4. Ramery, R., and J. Hampton (1959). Microscopic and submicroscopic observations on skeletal muscle from vitamin E deficient rats. Anat. Rec. *133*, 1–7.
5. Jensen, P. (1914). Weitere Untersuchungen über thermische Muskelreizung. Pflügers Arch. ges. Physiol. *160*, 333–406.
6. Mirsky, A. E. (1937). Contraction of muscle and denaturation of myosin. Exp. Biol. & Med. *37*, 157–159.
7. Buchthal, F., and E. Kaiser (1951). The rheology of the cross striated muscle fibre. Dan. Biol. Medd. *21*, 7, 1–318.

DISCUSSION

DR. CURTIS: I wonder if you would make a general statement about the range of doses that you used in terms of intensities or exposure. I wasn't clear on this point.

DR. EGGLETON: The intensities that we have used are in the range of 40 to 60 atm of sound pressure amplitude. The length of time of exposure was of the order of 1 sec.

DR. CURTIS: All single pulses?

DR. EGGLETON: Yes. In order to get more lesions per muscle, we spaced the lesions 1 mm apart. The lesion diameters were small compared to 1 mm.

DR. CURTIS: I have a question concerning the fixation. Were these 25-μ sections that you cut fixed in osmium?

DR. EGGLETON: The whole muscle was fixed in osmium, imbedded in methacrylate, sectioned on a conventional microtome, and then mounted on a microscope slide with a water base medium. We store most of our specimens in this manner. In this way we are able to scan large volumes of tissue and select portions of interest without spending a great deal of time searching with the electron microscope.

DR. CURTIS: I realize that this is a basic problem in using the electron microscope, but you are also confronted with the problem of fixation. How do you fix large pieces of muscle in osmium?

DR. EGGLETON: Fortunately, frog sartorius muscle is quite thin (not more than 1 mm in thickness); therefore it is easily possible to study fixation as a function of depth in the muscle. For example, the first section shows the fixation at a depth of 25 μ, the second at 50 μ, etc. We find that the muscle is quite well fixed throughout.

DR. FORREST: I would like to ask what, if anything, ultrasound has shown in relation to the Huxley model, and if you would like to make any comment about other models and possible future applications.

DR. EGGLETON: One of the more interesting phenomena present in some of these micrographs of muscle in which there is a loss of band structure is that the longitudinal filaments which remain after the disappearance of band structure are continuous for more than the sarcomere length. The Huxley model indicates that these fibers would be discontinuous. The model proposes that the 100-A myosin filaments extend the length of the "A" band and the 50-A actin filaments extend the length of the "I" band into the "A" band, producing a zone of overlap. These filaments are not connected and cannot account for the continuous filaments observed. In seeking an explanation for this, one can speculate that either the filaments are formed de nova or that they are continuous in normal muscle. The center-to-center distance between adjacent "A" and "I" filaments in normal muscle is the same as the spacing between filaments in muscle in which bands have been destroyed. However, it is difficult to understand how a contractual mechanism can be constructed from this data.

DR. FORREST: What prompted you to use 4 Mc instead of some other frequency?

DR. EGGLETON: Principally because the 4-Mc equipment was available to us and ready to use. It has the advantage of producing a small lesion appropriate to the size of the specimen we were using.

DR. HUGHES: May I make a suggestion? Since you have the material, it might be worthwhile to make frozen sections and estimate the water and dry weight in these by means of its appearance. Then you could relate this to changes certain of us have found in working with heated proteins. You might do this quite easily and see what, in fact, is happening to the protein in the muscle.

DR. EGGLETON: That's a good idea. Thank you for the suggestion.

DR. NYBORG: I get the impression from looking at some of the micrographs that some of the strands might be twisted.

DR. EGGLETON: Twisted around each other?

DR. NYBORG: Just out of shape.

DR. EGGLETON: Yes, as the muscle is heated to higher temperatures, there is an increasing amount of disorder in the specimen.

DR. NYBORG: I was thinking primarily of the ultrasonically treated muscles. They appear different to me than the heat-treated ones.

DR. EGGLETON: Regions can be found in the ultrasonically treated muscles that are quite similar to the heat-treated ones.

DR. GERSTEN: Did I understand you to suggest the possibility that some substance might be diffused and that this would account for this process? What evidence do you have for this?

DR. EGGLETON: We have no evidence for it, but suggested this as a possible hypothesis.

DR. WEISSLER: Did you do any experiments on cooled muscles? If the muscles were at a temperature of 2 or 5°C, presumably 0.8-sec exposure might not be enough to raise the temperature to 46°C. It would be interesting to see then whether any damage resulted. This might be one way of distinguishing thermal from other kinds of damage.

DR. EGGLETON: The temperature rise for the sound intensities we used was calculated to be about 46°C. Even an ambient temperature of 0°C would be sufficient to take it into the region of destruction.

DR. CURTIS: It would be interesting to know what changes take place at the structural level when one irradiates along the axis of the muscle fiber. It would be interesting to correlate. Have you done this?

DR. EGGLETON: No, we haven't. I agree that it would be an interesting study.

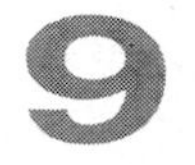

The Effect of Ultrasound in the Treatment of Cancer

KARLHEINZ WOEBER, M.D.
Luisen Hospital, Aachen, Germany, and Universitäts-Klinik für Hautkrankheiten, Bonn, Germany

Introduction by Dr. Herrick

The next paper is concerned with a very controversial subject, namely, the application of ultrasound to the treatment of cancer. This subject is of great interest to me because we initiated our ultrasound research program at Mayo Foundation on the basis of the results reported by German scientists during the period of World War II on the effect of ultrasound on tissue.

As the chairman of this session pointed out, ultrasound was introduced into Germany at the beginning of World War II principally by the work of Dr. Pohlman (1, 2). Following this, Dr. Horvath published a report concerning several patients suffering from tissue cancer, who were treated and apparently healed by ultrasonic irradiation (3–9). This report was received with great interest, but medical experts objected to the continued treatment of tissue cancer by this method without thorough investigation of the physiological bases of the results obtained by Dr. Horvath. It was for this purpose that our research team began its experimental and clinical investigations 15 years ago.

I will now briefly outline a number of conclusions resulting from our research program: (1) Carcinomatous tissue can be irreversibly modified by ultrasound of medium intensity, that is, up to approximately 1.5 w/cm^2. The effect of ultrasound is not homogeneous but corresponds to the sound field distribution. (2) The effect of ultrasound is greatly intensified by the use of a thin metallic foil, instead of a metal plate, over the quartz crystal. (3) The effect of ultrasound includes both thermal and mechanical elements, depending on the energy supply and on the means of heat reduction in the tissue. (4) The effect of ultrasound can easily be differentiated from the effect of various methods of heat production – for example, ultra-shortwaves, microwaves, or thermal bath. (5) The effect of ultrasound on carcinomatous tissue is most intense on the less mature (that is, less differentiated) cancerous tissue. (6) Low ultrasound intensities bring about biopositive effects on cancer tissue (that is, stimulating, increasing metabolic effects), which can lead to growth stimulation. The type and strength of such biopositive effects depend on the type of tissue and its degree of differentiation.

We determined that treatment of tumors by ultrasound alone is ineffective for therapy. When foil is used as the sound-transferring medium, warming of the surrounding tissue occurs and leads to heat coagulation of the cancer. This latter phenomena might explain Dr. Horvath's early successes in cancer treatment by ultrasound since foil was employed in his early equipment. Treatment of superficial tumors exclusively with ultrasound can even lead to an increase in activity of the cancer when lower intensities are used.

I should like now to present a more detailed description of our work in this field of cancer treatment. Since the beginning of radio-therapy, the use of x rays and radium has occupied an important place in the treatment of malignant tumors. Early results were poor because the destructive side effects of ionizing rays were not recognized. In studying the early techniques and utilizing the equipment that was then available, we learned how to protect the surrounding healthy tissue without diminishing the radiological dosage necessary to discourage the tumor. Thus we were able to discover new indications for x-ray and radium therapy. Nevertheless, a portion of the normal tissue surrounding the tumor was still undergoing exposure to radiation. When a radiation dosage which is lethal to healthy tissue does not differ greatly from that required by the tumor, it is always possible that healthy tissue surrounding the cancer may be destroyed. The late lesions of chronic radiodermatitis are an unfortunate complication of radiological treatment. Improvement of radiological equipment has by now reached the point where it would be difficult to accomplish greater protection of the healthy tissue surrounding the tumor (at least for superficial tumors) without running the risk of sacrificing the therapeutic effects of x ray by a further reduction of efficient dosage. For this latter reason, we have attempted to reduce the necessary radiological dosage by simultaneously applying another form of physical energy which would be capable of exerting a lethal effect on certain types of cancerous cells but would be harmless to normal tissue.

Soon after ultrasonic energy came into use for general therapy, it appeared that this agent might offer advantages over other physical agents for the treatment of neoplastic tissue, if used in combination with x rays. Our initial task, then, was to examine the action of various hyperthermic methods, particularly that of shortwave and ultrasonic energy. In our proposed animal research, we determined that all experimental specimens of cancerous tissue must have the same morphological and structural properties and that the studies must concentrate on the primary alterations of the morphological structure of the cancer cells, in order that the specific mode of action of each of the physical energies utilized might be identified. In order to compare from a biophysical viewpoint the primary modes of action of two or more forms of physical energy, it is necessary to place in evidence the specific alterations produced by each. Identical results for each agent might simply demonstrate that a certain tissue can have only a single reaction to different physical agents. Also, it must be kept in mind that the primary biological reaction of a cell can be affected by thermal processes as well as by those of a mechanical or physico-chemical nature. The reactions which follow desired therapeutic results, such as, for example, neural effects or humoral effects, are always considered to be a secondary biological reaction to a primary biophysical effect. In our first studies, Walker 256 carcinoma was transplanted to white rats, and investigations were conducted in situ and in vivo. The animals were divided into three groups, and each group was hyperthermized in a different manner. The first group was totally hyperthermized in a hot bath. The second group was exposed to electromagnetic shortwaves (diathermy), and the third group was irradiated with ultrasound of varying intensities and for various lengths of time. In order to differentiate early histological alterations from later ones, we found it necessary to fix the tissue immediately after treatment. Sixty sec after exposure of the animals, the subcutaneous tumor was excised and fixed in a special solution. Staining of the nucleotides was by the Feulgen method.

In comparatively early histological studies of mitoses of the Walker carcinoma, it was found that the hyperthermia produced by a warm water bath, in vivo and in situ, causes alterations of the mitoses, if the rectal temperature is maintained above 40°C for 60 min. Coagulation of the chromosomes increases as the temperature and time factors are increased. Finally, chromatin coagulated and tore when the temperature was maintained at 42°C for 60 min. Figures 1 and 2 show normal mitotic division (anaphase) for an untreated

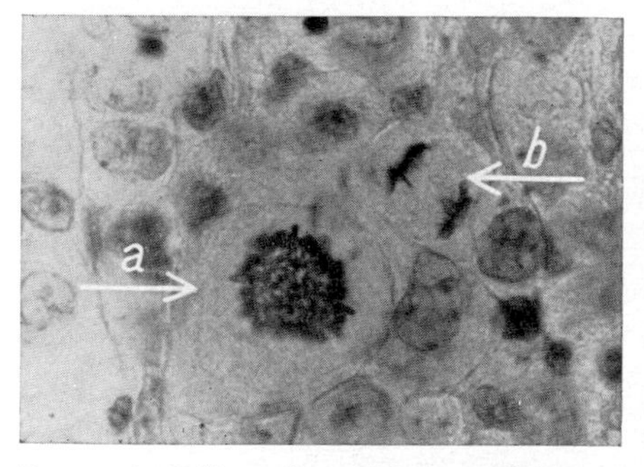

FIGURE 1. Cells, indicated by a and b, in normal anaphase stage, untreated.

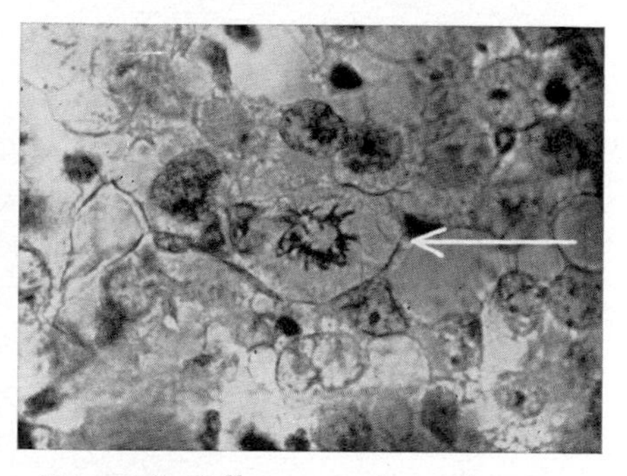

FIGURE 2. Cell in normal anaphase stage (diaster), untreated.

tissue sample. The coagulation effects of the 40°C temperature on the chromosomes are shown in Figures 3 through 6 (anaphase). These figures should be compared to Figure 7 which illustrates not only coagulation, but breaking of the chromosomes as a result of exposure of the tissue to temperatures of 42°C. The number of normal mitoses diminishes with increased temperature. For tissues subjected to temperatures above 41°C for 60 min, only pathological mitoses are found. The alterations of the mitoses are a consequence

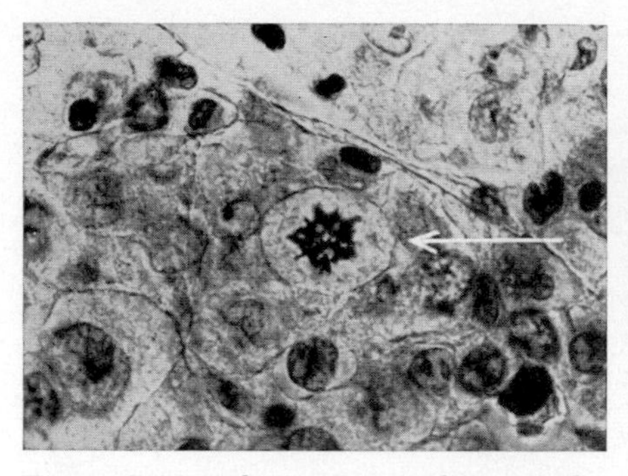

FIGURE 3. Anaphase stage with initiated coagulation of chromatin following exposure of the tissue to hyperthermia (40°C).

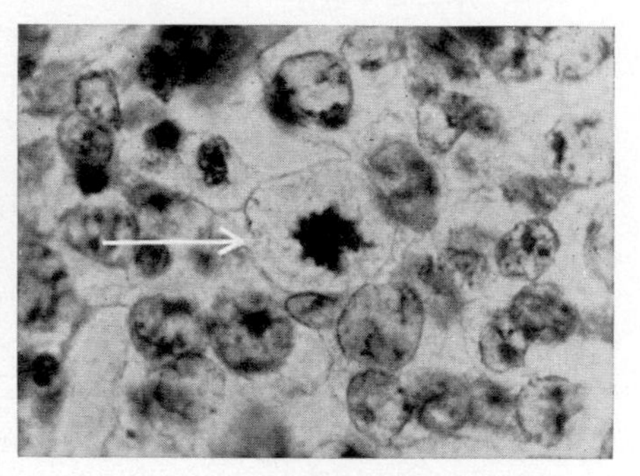

FIGURE 4. Anaphase stage in mitotic division showing coagulated chromosomes after exposure of tissue to hyperthermia (40°C).

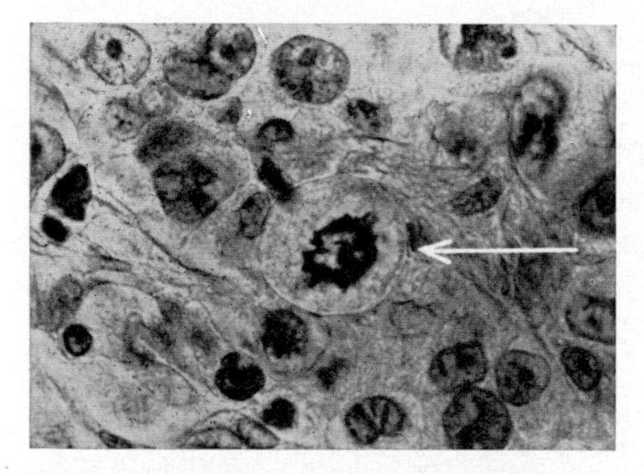

FIGURE 5. Anaphase stage in mitotic division showing coagulated chromosomes after exposure of tissue to hyperthermia (40°C).

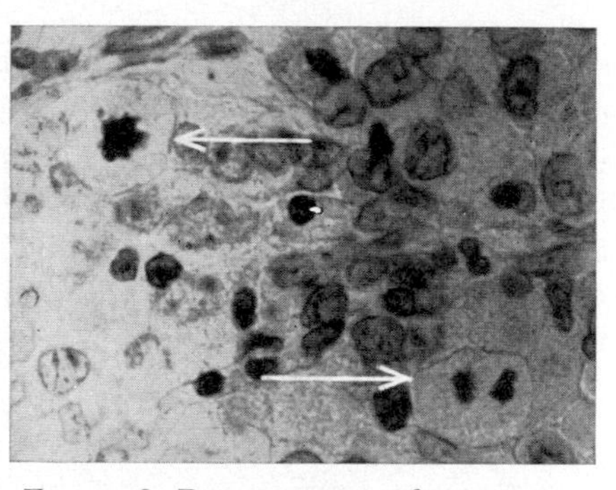

FIGURE 6. Demonstration of two mitotic divisions (anaphase) of cells from tissue exposed to temperature of 40°C.

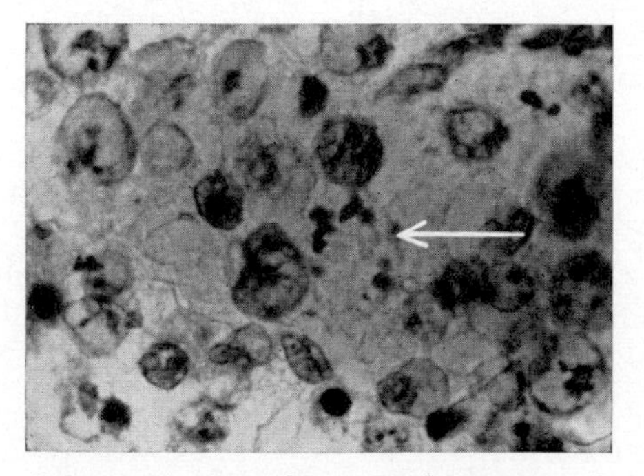

FIGURE 7. Coagulation and tearing of chromosomes after exposure of tissue to 42°C temperature for 60 min.

of a hyperthermia in the cancerous cells. They are produced according to the temperature and the time of exposure by way of the coagulation of chromatin. Since the alterations are homogeneous throughout the tissue, we concluded that the physical energy reached the tumor tissue homogeneously. We were unable to evaluate the inactive cells and the phases of mitoses which were not in the metaphasic or anaphasic stage. Tumors treated with shortwave diathermy showed the same effects as hyperthermia, if the applied energy was sufficiently intense. With the application of low energy, the alterations of mitoses were too small to be noted with the histological techniques applied. Because instrumentation for precise calibration of the shortwave energy was not available, it was not possible to establish an exact dosage which would be effective in the treatment of tumors.

Some tumors irradiated with ultrasound showed the same thermal alterations in mitoses as those treated with shortwave, but alterations were also found which were not present after hyperthermia induced by shortwave energy. Chromosomes were scattered, broken, and torn apart. This effect is known as mechanical aberrations, and its nature is not completely known. To some degree there may exist simultaneously alterations of mechanical *and* thermal nature in the same mitotic division stage. Figures 8 and 9 both show the anaphase stage, with dislocation of chromosomes after ultrasound irradiation. The coagulation and dislocation of chromatin in Figure 10 illustrate both the thermal and mechanical effects of the ultrasound. Figures 11, 12, and 13 illustrate various aberrations of chromatin after ultrasound treatment.

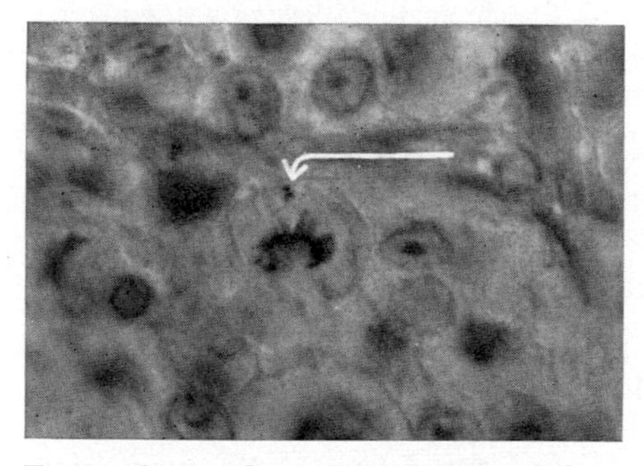

FIGURE 8. Anaphase stage showing dislocation of chromosomes following ultrasonic irradiation of the tissue.

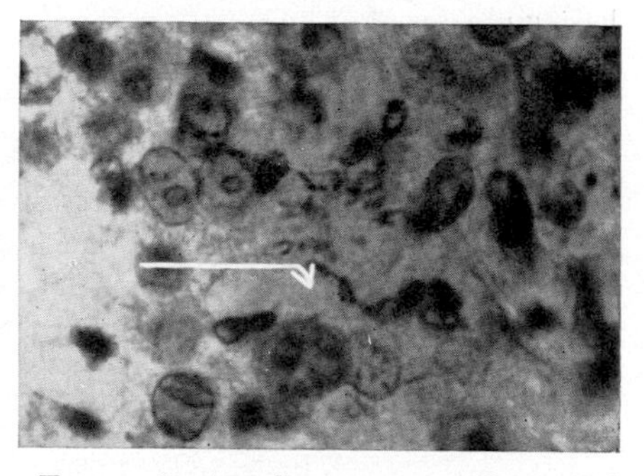

FIGURE 9. Anaphase stage with several dislocated and turned chromosomes following treatment of the tissue with ultrasound.

The sound absorption occurring at an interface between tissues of different acoustic impedance results in an increase in temperature which causes typical thermal effects such as coagulation of the chromatin. However, mechanical effects produced by ultrasonic pulsations of high magnitude are responsible for the chromosome aberrations described above, and such effects can be explained as a result of the physical properties of ultrasonic energy. The

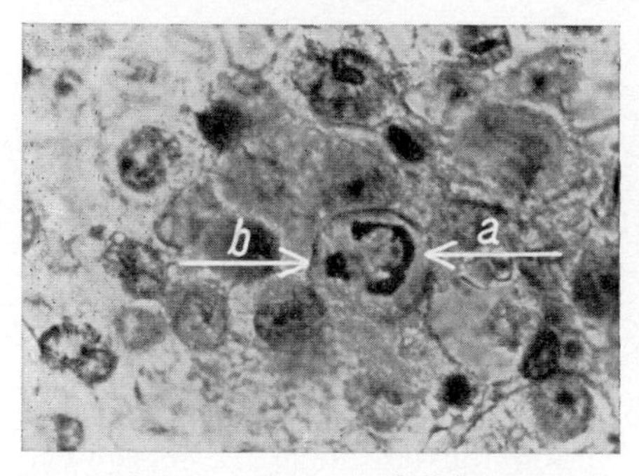

FIGURE 10. Coagulation and dislocation of chromatin following ultrasonic irradiation of the tissue, illustrating both the thermal and mechanical effects of ultrasound.

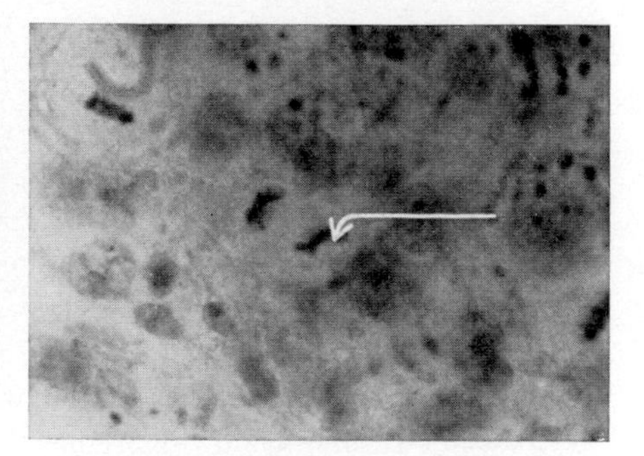

FIGURE 11. Illustration of chromatin torn apart following ultrasonic irradiation of the tissue.

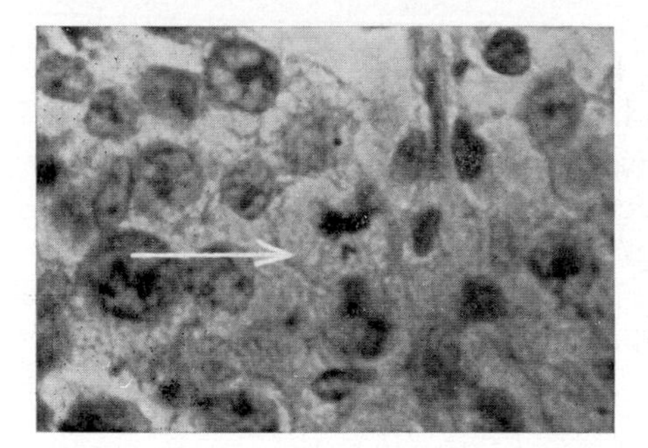

FIGURE 12. Aberration of chromatin following ultrasound treatment of the tissue.

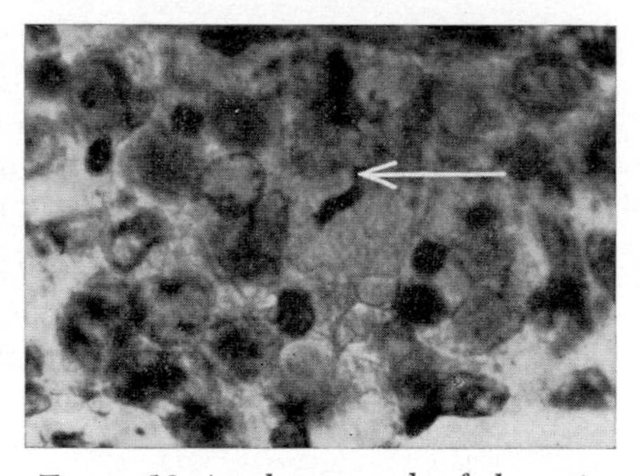

FIGURE 13. Another example of aberration of the chromatin following ultrasonic irradiation of the tissue.

above theory can be verified by reducing the thermal effect of ultrasound either by cooling the tissue or by the use of pulsed ultrasonic energy. While the coagulation of chromosomes shows a great reduction under such conditions, the mechanical aberrations can still be seen. The quality and quantity of thermal and mechanical effects are dependent upon the following conditions: (1) the magnitude of the ultrasonic intensity, (2) the quality of the ultrasonic energy (continuous or pulsed ultrasound), (3) the cooling medium between the transducer and the skin, and (4) the design of the transducer (the sound head). For each of the samples prepared, 100 mitoses were counted and it was found that more pronounced and more numerous alterations of the chromosomes were observed for the tissues irradiated with the higher doses of ultrasound.

Since we succeeded in clarifying the effects of these three types of energy on tumors by means of the histological research described above, we concluded our experiments in this field. They were, however, the foundation for further animal research. After therapeutic studies on animals, using the three methods of producing hyperthermia (shortwave electromagnetic energy, warm water baths, and ultrasonic irradiation), we concluded that it was not possible to cure tumors permanently by these means alone. A decision was made to attempt treatment of tissue cancer by combining hyperthermia *and* x rays. Experiments of Westermark (10) and Langendorff (11) on the effect of diathermy and shortwaves on transplanted tumors proved that temperature elevation increases the sensitivity of tumors to x rays. Attempts were made by various physicians to treat tumors of human patients with shortwave radiation followed immediately by x-ray irradiation. Although the medical schools at Vienna (12) and Erlangen (13) and others (14) had obtained good results with this technique in the treatment of bronchiogenic and mammary carcinoma, this method did not become generally recognized for cancer therapy because the instrumentation available was technically inadequate. Our first objective was simply to reduce the x-ray dosage normally required in treatment of cancer. We hoped to develop a combination method which would sensitize tumors which had previously proven resistant to x-ray irradiation, in order that the healthy tissue surrounding the malignant growth (which may have been irradiated several times previously) might not be further damaged by continued treatment. In order to achieve the desired therapeutic conditions, we recognized that a technique which combined two sources of energy must meet the following three requirements: (1) The control of the hyperthermia-producing energy, both in regard to magnitude and direction, must be accurate and reproducible. (2) The time necessary to produce the hyperthermia should be brief in order that it be comparable to x-ray irradiation time. (3) The technical rules which apply to x-ray apparatus must not be changed because of the addition of the apparatus required to produce the hyperthermia. The choice of ultrasonic energy as the additive to x rays was made on the basis of the three above stated requirements, as well as our previous histological studies on the effect of ultrasound, which indicated that the thermal and mechanical effects of ultrasound destroy cancerous cells. From a biological viewpoint, this method seemed feasible because the temperature increase produced by ultrasound is attained within 20 to 40 sec of application, and if the circulation is good, the temperature level should be maintained, provided that the intensity of the ultrasonic energy is properly controlled. The first equipment used consisted of two machines built by Dr. W. Lehfeldt and Co., Heppenheim, Germany, incorporating the radiation method of Chaoul (Siemens-Reiniger-Werke, Erlangen, Germany), which could be used in both animal and human work.

Our first subjects were 120 rats inoculated subcutaneously with Walker carcinoma approximately 2 cm in diameter. Thirty of these tumors were irradiated with x ray only, using 350 r at 60 kv and with 5.5-cm distance between focus and skin. Thirty tumors were irradiated with ultrasound only at 1.0 w/cm^2 for 5 min with the transducer in motion. Thirty tumors were treated with both x ray and ultrasound with the same dosages described above. Thirty tumors remained untreated as controls. The results are graphically illustrated in Figure 14. The untreated rats died after 9 days and their tumors had grown 550%. The animals treated only with x rays died after 10 days and the average growth of their tumors was 420%. The animals treated only with ultrasound died after 8 days and their tumors had grown 430%. The tumors treated with the combined therapy increased in size for the first 5 days, then receded and after 11 days all the tumors were completely absorbed. The animals remained healthy for an observation period of 90 days following the combined x-ray and ultrasonic application. In a later series, we irradiated tumors in twenty white rats with x rays only and with the same general conditions prevailing as in the first group. Our purpose was to establish the minimal dosage of x rays necessary for complete resorption of the Walker carcinoma of the same size previously treated. We found that administration of 600 r at 60 kv was necessary to obtain the same results and cause a complete resorption. This was an increase of 250 r over that required in the combination treatment. Hence, we were able to reduce the x-ray dosage by approximately 40% by using the combination of x rays and ultrasound.

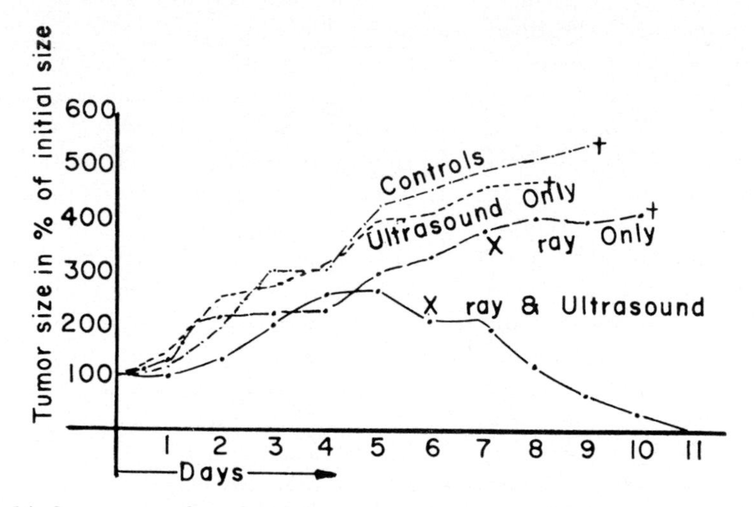

FIGURE 14. Comparison of results of three types of treatment (with one untreated control group) on 120 rats inoculated subcutaneously with Walker carcinoma. The animals were divided into four groups of thirty animals each.

We subsequently applied this combined technique of ultrasound and x rays to humans suffering from skin cancer, using equipment specifically designed for the treatment of humans. In our first experiments, we did not specialize in any particular type of cancer, for we judged it most important to observe the biological effects of our combined method on different types of cancer patients. In the course of the past 8 years, we have treated fifty patients, male and female, between forty-two and ninety-six years of age. In the majority of these cases, only one specific cancerous condition of the skin was identified; a few cases, however, showed two or more tumors of the same structure. In these cases, the two tumors were treated differently if circumstances allowed, that is, one tumor was treated with x rays alone and the other received the combined treatment. The advantage of this procedure is obvious, since the radiological reaction of similar cancerous tissue in the same part of the body to both the classical and the combined methods could be compared simultaneously on the same patient.

In the initial phase of our human work, the total roentgen dosage applied to our patients varied considerably. The optimum dosage was based on the experimental animal results according to which a 40% decrease in x-ray dosage was feasible if administered in conjunction with ultrasound. However, in order to be conservative, we adopted a 33% reduction from the customary roentgen dosages. X-ray dosages of from 3000 to 4000 r were finally used after it was recognized that this dosage level, in combination with ultrasound, gave results comparable to those achieved from simple x-ray contact therapy with dosage levels of 4000 to 6000 r. Thus, 3000 to 3500 r were used in cases of obvious basaloma and 4000 r for squamous cell carcinomas. The total roentgen dosage depended upon the ultrasonic intensity — larger doses of ultrasound entail smaller doses of x ray, and vice versa. This level of x-ray dosage combined with ultrasonic dosage of 0.2 to 0.3 w/cm^2 will lead to satisfactory results. Total dosage may be divided into fractions for daily treatments in the usual way — 400 to 600 r for daily sessions, with one series terminating after seven or eight sessions. Reactions to the classical dosage and the dosage of the combination method, as judged by erythema, epitheliolysis, and subsequent granulation and epithelization, appear to be identical.

The therapeutic results of our human program fulfilled expectations based on our experimental animal work (15, 16, 16a). We treated 35 histologically established tumors and 15 carcinomas whose manifestations made a histological confirmation of diagnosis unnecessary. The patients treated included 26 with basal cell cancer, 20 with squamous cell carcinoma, 2 with m. Bowen, and 2 with malignant melanoma. During the follow-up observation period of 6 years, one marginal relapse of a squamous cell cancer in the nose-eye angle occurred. It had evidently not been completely attacked. Regional lymph nodes appeared after 5 years in another patient who had a carcinoma of the lower lip. This carcinoma had been unsuccessfully irradiated prior to our treatment.

I would like to make a few comments now regarding the practical details of the combination technique. The contact between the transducer and the tumor tissue to be treated is produced by means of liquid paraffin, a comparatively thin film of which is applied to both the transducer and the tumor. The diameter of the irradiating surface may be chosen at random, within broad limits, and depends on the diameter of the quartz crystal of the sound transducer. The combined technique of x rays and ultrasound cannot be applied to parts of the body having considerable unevenness, such as the nose-cheek, nose-eye region, etc. In order to guarantee the very best adjustment, it has proven helpful to delineate the area of the skin which is to be treated with ultrasonic energy by means of a dermograph before applying the transducer. The ultrasonic intensity used is generally between 0.2 and 0.3 w/cm^2 which corresponds to a medium therapeutic intensity for continuous irradiation. Prior to the irradiation, the patient should be told that he should inform the physician immediately if a burning pain in the affected region appears anytime during the treatment. This periosteal pain, which occurs occasionally in cases where bone lies closely underneath the cancerous tissue, is harmless but requires a particularly small ultrasonic intensity to avoid subjective discomfort.

The research discussed in this presentation is concerned with superficial tumors or skin cancers but, as you know, attempts have been made by a number of different investigators to find a deterrent to the growth of deep malignant tumors which would act by damaging the metabolism of the malignant growth by means of increased temperature. It is not possible to discuss the results of these investigations in this presentation, but it is of interest to observe that in reviewing the literature, Selawry observed that among the so-called spontaneously healed, histologically controlled tumors, about one-third of 400 cases described showed involvement of intermittent febrile diseases such as malaria, typhus, erysipelas, etc. (17, 18). Furthermore, it seems reasonably well established that the growth-inhibiting effect of ionizing radiation can be increased by elevated temperatures (19). Selawry's investigations with human neoplastic cultured cell strains showed varying reactions of the cells in the temperature ranges studied. At 38°C an increased rate of growth occurred, at 39 to 40°C a temporary interruption of the mitotic cycle in metaphase took place, and for temperatures of 42 to 46°C irreversible heat injury occurred (20). Practical application of this knowledge to human cancer patients has not been possible because insufficient research has been accomplished. At the present time, any attempts by the physician to apply heat in combination with other agents may result in acceleration of the tumor rather than regression. It appears obvious, however, that what can be done with ultrasound and x rays for superficial tissues can be successfully applied to deeper tissues. The urgent problem is to discover whether ultrasound can be applied in a controlled manner deep within the body in combination with the agents now applied for cancer therapy, including the various types of ionizing radiation and chemotherapy. It is relatively simple to successfully treat superficial tumors with ultrasonic energy combined with some other therapeutic agent, but the question of particular interest for the scientists attending this meeting is whether ultrasonic instrumentation can be developed which would allow the successful treatment of deep tumors.

REFERENCES

1. Pohlman, R. (1939). Physik. Z. *40*, 149.
2. Pohlman, R. (1951). Die Ultraschalltherapie (G. Thieme, Stuttgart).
3. Dyroff, R., and J. Horvath (1944). Strahlentherapie 75, 126.
4. Horvath, J. (1944). Strahlentherapie 75, 119.
5. Pätzold, J., and J. Horvath (1948). Dtsch. Med. Wschr., 139.
6. Horvath, J. (1946). Klin. u. Prax. 7, 1.
7. Horvath, J. (1946). Klin. u. Prax. 7, 1.
8. Horvath, J. (1948). Strahlentherapie 77, 279.
9. Horvath, J. (1949). Ärtzl. Fortschr., 11.
10. Westermark, N. (1927). Skand. Arch. Physiol. 52, 257.

11. Langendorff, H. M. (1939). Strahlentherapie *64*, 512–519.
12. Fuchs, G. (1958). Internat. Z. Physik. Med. *11*, 134–138.
13. Birkner, R., and F. Wachsmann (1949). Strahlentherapie *79*, 93.
14. Arons, J., and B. Sokoloff (1937). Am. J. Surg. *36*, 593.
15. Selawry, O. S., and Kh. Woeber (1958). Die Bedeutung der Wärme bei kombinierter Krebstherapie, *in* "Ergebnisse der physikalisch-diätetischen Therapie (Verlag von T. Steinkopff, Dresden and Leipzig), Vol. VI, pp. 51–71.
16. Woeber, Kh. (1959). Internat. J. Phys. Med. *4*, 10–19.
16a. Woeber, Kh., and G. Stein (1963). Strahlentherapie *122*, 285–289.
17. Woeber, Kh. (1960). Arch. Phys. Ther. *4*, 351–354.
18. Selawry, O. S. (1957). Internat. Rev. Phys. Med. *2*, 78–79.
19. Selawry, O. S., J. C. Carlson, and G. E. Moore (1958). Am. J. Roent., Rad. Ther. and Nuc. Med. *80*, 833–839.
20. Selawry, O. S., M. N. Goldstein, and T. McCormick (1957). Can. Res. *17*, 785–791.

DISCUSSION

DR. MACKAY: You said that in the presence of ultrasound the difference in sensitivity between normal and cancerous tissue was increased. This seems to me to be the crux of the whole matter. Approximately what percentage was that, and how statistically reliable do you think that evaluation is?

DR. WOEBER: I think that this depends on the ultrasound intensity. If we can use a higher intensity, for example, 0.4 to 0.5 w/cm^2, we have more specific alterations than with lower intensities.

DR. KELLY: Is there a difference in thermal denaturation between cancer cells and normal cells?

DR. WOEBER: You cannot state any one temperature. Of course, as is well known, there are different kinds of tumor cells. You can only say that the more embryonic the cancer tissue, or, the less differentiated the tissue, the more easily it can be destroyed and, of course, the more easily you can have a bionegative effect. It is necessary, therefore, to know what type of cancer is involved before answering questions on what temperature or what intensity of ultrasound will affect the tissue. For example, as I indicated, the melanoma can be destroyed by heat more easily than the basaloma, which is a very differentiated tissue. This is the theoretical view in this field.

DR. KOSSOFF: When you say you irradiated the melanoma, do you mean only the primary site of the cancer was irradiated? You did not irradiate the lymph node?

DR. WOEBER: This is a so-called preblastomatotic melanoma, and we have to treat only the specific area, because we are sure in this case that there are no lymphatic metastases.

DR. KOSSOFF: And how long has your follow-up time been on the melanoma?

DR. WOEBER: Six years.

DR. MACKAY: You suggested that there are not only thermal effects of ultrasound but also mechanical effects, which enhance the susceptibility of these cells to x-ray treatment. Do you have some evidence along this line that the ultrasound acts in several ways to enhance the sensitivity of the tissues to x-ray treatment?

DR. WOEBER: I attempted to explain this in my paper. With medium sound intensity, one cannot see a mechanical effect without a thermal effect. Depending upon the intensity of the ultrasound, one generally has about 80% thermal effect and 20% mechanical effect.

DR. MACKAY: Is this what you observed or is this a hypothetical analysis?

DR. WOEBER: This is based on histological examination.

DR. MACKAY: Did you try the combination of simple direct heating and x rays?

DR. WOEBER: Several medical groups use combined heat with x rays with beneficial results. You may find a report of this in "Strahlentherapie," 29 (1954), 333–366.

DR. HUGHES: The chromosomes may be very much more resistant than other structures in the cells to these mechanical effects. I wanted to ask you whether you had done other kinds of histological examinations on this material.

DR. WOEBER: No, we did not.

DR. WEISSLER: Why did you limit your intensity in patients to 0.2 and 0.3 w/cm^2?

DR. WOEBER: This intensity corresponds to a medium therapeutic intensity for humans in the case of static treatment resulting in no periosteal pain.

DR. WEISSLER: I'm still a little concerned about this concept. This appears analogous to saying that if you have a pinprick and a sledge hammer injury, that the pinprick can alter the dosage required by the sledge hammer. You are dealing with thermal energy in comparison with x-ray energy and the orders of magnitude of these two are quite different, if you postulate a minimum mechanical effect. And yet you say that the thresholds are in some way altered by application of such relatively small amounts of energy. How can you explain that small amounts of energy applied in the thermal range will essentially alter thresholds for dosages in the x-ray range?

DR. WOEBER: There is a fundamental biological law that biochemical or biophysical effects are heightened by elevated temperatures and vice versa. The question remains whether this energy of 0.2 to 0.3 w/cm^2 applied statically to the body may be considered low.

DR. WEISSLER: It might be possible that hydrogen bonds or the tertiary or secondary structure of the complex DNA molecule are being loosened. Perhaps such a loosening-up process might contribute to the greater sensitivity of the molecules to x rays. Of course, if you had cavitation (presumably one does not), then you would get a tremendous amount of energy concentration.

DR. DYER: Dr. Woeber, you mentioned in one of your slides evidence for twisting or rotation; was this in reference to the mitotic spindle? What evidence was apparent in the slide that this was really the case?

DR. WOEBER: If you have the experience of examining 100 or more such histological pictures, especially as threc-dimensional views, and you are making counts of such cells, after a certain time you recognize the effects of simple heating such as that produced by ultra-shortwave, that is, microwave diathermy. Such coagulation effects are well known. If small doses of ultrasound are given, one begins to see these previously mentioned effects in the cells. Perhaps the cells of fast growing tissue, such as tumor, may be less resistant to the effects of ultrasound.

DR. WEISSLER: I wonder whether you had any evidence that there was shearing within the mitotic spindle? We have done this sort of thing and find that we can dislocate the whole mitotic spindle to an entirely different part of the cell and have it proceed to the vital part of the cell at the expected time and in the expected way so that in the cells we have been using, at any rate, the mitotic apparatus appears to be a pretty rigid mechanism which is highly resistant to shear. Possibly our result indicates a difference between these plant cells and your animal cells. We may be dealing with species factor. We were using 85, 94, 25 kc, etc.

DR. WOEBER: We generally used an ultrasound frequency of 1 Mc.

DR. KELLY: In your paper you mentioned the use of a foil. Could you give an explanation of the exact purpose of this foil and its location in the system?

DR. WOEBER: A thin metallic foil lying over the quartz crystal produces a thermal effect since such an arrangement results in a higher temperature in the tissue compared to the usual arrangement.

10

Biological Effects of Ultrasound on Neuromuscular Skeletal Systems

JEROME W. GERSTEN, M.D.
University of Colorado Medical Center, Denver, Colorado

Introduction by Dr. Libber

Dr. Jerome Gersten of the University of Colorado Medical Center is our next speaker. It is of interest to note that Dr. Gersten has done considerable work not only in using low intensity ultrasound as a therapeutic tool but also in applying this tool to study basic biological mechanisms.

More than 10 years have passed since research with ultrasound was first undertaken in our laboratory. Early reports of the value of ultrasonic energy had been highly enthusiastic. Yet, with the memory of exaggerated expectations in other areas of medicine fresh in our minds, we approached this area cautiously and began by probing into the physiological effects of ultrasound. Initially, we applied this form of energy for therapeutic purposes only infrequently. With the passage of time, however, we have accumulated enough clinical experience to warrant utilization of ultrasound for two general purposes, one related to connective tissue and scarring, the other concerned with membrane effects, as related to pain and muscle spasm. In addition, we have obtained some experimental data pertinent to the possible mechanisms involved. When limitation in range of motion at a joint is the result of pathology in the articular capsule or adjacent tendons, we feel that ultrasound is the treatment of choice. When pain and muscle spasm are prominent features clinically, ultrasound may be of value, though not always the best form of treatment available. I will review some of our experiences which provide some understanding of how these conclusions were obtained.

Our interest in the effect of ultrasound on water content of tendon was first aroused by observations of Hintzelmann (1), relating to changes in water content of intervertebral discs following the applications of ultrasound in rheumatoid spondylitis, and by Rollhäuser's (2) work concerning changes in extensibility of tendon following changes in the degree of hydration. Furthermore, from our own earlier work, in which a decrease in total P was noted during sounding (3), it was suggested that there might be changes in water content of muscle during application of ultrasound. Except when specifically stated all the following studies were carried out at frequencies of 1 Mc/sec with a slightly divergent ultrasonic beam. Intensities were measured with radiation pressure techniques, and indicated values always refer to the peak energy even when the ultrasound was pulsed. The intensities utilized were low, always less than 3 w/cm^2.

When frog Achilles tendon was sounded at 3 w/cm^2 (pulsed with 1 msec on, 2 msec off), under circumstances in which cavitation could not occur (degassed and in vacuo), with temperatures ranging from 5 to 25°C and with the long axis of the tendon at right angles to the ultrasound field, there was a reversible decrease in water content of this tissue (4). Maximum values were reached within 1 to 2 min after onset of sounding, with complete recovery within 1 min after cessation of sounding. When extensibility was studied under the same experimental conditions with the tendon at right angles to the ultrasound field, it was found that no change was produced by sounding provided that the temperature of the system was kept below approximately 30°C. When the situation was altered so that the temperature of the tendon was allowed to rise, extensibility increased and the amount of increase was greater as the ultrasound intensity increased from 1 to 3 w/cm^2. This relationship to temperature rise was further substantiated by comparing the effect of ultrasound to that achieved by raising the temperature of the tendon to the same level with warm water (40.9°C). The effect on extensibility was identical in the two situations (5). When the elastic limit (the point on the length-tension curve at which the slope suddenly decreases, and at which point the process changes from reversible to irreversible) was related to temperature, it was noted that no change was apparent until a temperature of approximately 30°C had been reached. Beyond this point there was a progressive decline in the tension at which the elastic limit occurred (5). From the therapeutic standpoint the elastic limit might be an extremely important point for this might be related to the ability to stretch contractures.

In general, then, when tendon was sounded at right angles to the ultrasound field, there was a decrease in hydration and no change in extensibility provided that there was no temperature increase. An increase in extensibility occurred when the temperature increased to above 30°C and seemed to be related to thermal denaturation of tendon proteins. Although marked shortening due to denaturation of collagen occurs in rat tendon at temperatures of approximately 55 to 60°C (6), some change is apparent at lower temperatures, and in the frog measurable increases in extensibility occur at 35°C. This result is pertinent to human treatment for it indicates one may obtain an increase in extensibility at a reasonably safe temperature.

The different response of muscle and tendon to sounding, as far as water content was concerned, intrigued us. Whereas tendon decreased in water content, muscle showed an increase in water content on sounding (4). It was considered that one possible explanation for this difference might be the orientation of the tendon in the ultrasound field. Since the normal direction of fluid passage along connective tissue fibrils is in the longitudinal direction (7), it is possible that the application of ultrasound at right angles to the axis of the tendon might force water out of the tissue. It has been shown that mechanical forces may squeeze fluid along the connective tissue fibrils (7). Studies of hydration and extensibility were therefore carried out with tendon sounded while in a position parallel to the ultrasound field (8). Under these circumstances it was noted that a reversible increase in water content of approximately 6% was produced under circumstances in which no recordable rise in temperature occurred. This increase in water content, completely reversible, was no longer present within 1 min after cessation of sounding. Furthermore, extensibility was markedly and irreversibly increased even though the temperature was apparently unchanged.

In order to throw more light on this extensibility increase during irradiation, in the absence of temperature rise (as measured with very fine thermocouple probes), small segments of tendon were studied. When this was done, it was noted that the effect on extensibility decreased with depth from the surface. At a depth of 6 mm there was no change of extensibility from the normal. In view of the fact that there was no demonstrable temperature rise and that the relationship between extensibility increase and depth was not exponential, one may feel a bit more secure in suggesting that this phenomenon is pressure dependent rather than temperature dependent.

Although temperature increase and nonthermal effects both played a role in increasing extensibility under in vitro circumstances, there was no evidence as to which of these two mechanisms played the greater role in in vivo situations. Despite this, it was felt that trial in the human situation was now warranted. It was likely that the shoulder and hip would prove to be two areas which might be approached frequently in order to try to gain an increase in range of motion. The hip is a region in which large metallic implants of many types might be present under therapeutic circumstances in which sounding would be indicated. Although one could predict that the temperature rise would not be excessive with metal present in the ultrasound field, this was put to specific experimental test. In fresh horse meat, with no circulatory mechanism for heat removal, the temperature rise in the irradiated area with bone present was greater than with metal at the same depth. With smaller pieces of metal, the temperature rise initiated by the ultrasound was of even lesser degree. On comparing microwaves with ultrasound, it was noted that during the application of microwaves heating of the irradiated area was consistently greater in the presence of metal as opposed to the presence of bone, while in the ultrasound field the situation was reversed (9). Studies were then extended to the anesthetized dog with a vitallium plate placed over the lateral aspect of the femur. When the vitallium plate was present, the temperature rise during ultrasonic irradiation at the surface of the plate was 25% less than at the surface of the bone under comparable irradiation conditions; in bone cortex the temperature rise was 36% smaller, while in bone medulla the temperature rise was 35% smaller. Thus, the presence of a vitallium plate in the anesthetized dog resulted in smaller temperature rises in all situations tested (9).

Since in the above experiments the thickness of the high-density medium was changed by the addition of metal, further experiments were carried out in frog with a section of the femur replaced by a steel tube of the same diameter and wall thickness. Under these circumstances it was found that temperature rise over the metal was 31% lower than over bone, while temperature rise within the metallic tube was 37% lower than temperature rise within bone after sounding at the same level of intensity. Finally, temperature recordings were made in the human under situations comparable to those which might be used therapeutically, and it was determined that the presence of metal, per se, would be no contraindication to the use of ultrasound (9).

Our second area of focus has been, in the broad sense, related to membrane effects of ultrasound, either on nerve or muscle. From the earliest days of research with ultrasound such membrane effects were suggested by observation of an increase in irritability in frog heart muscle on exposure to ultrasound (10). More recently Busnel and co-workers found that chronaxie in the rat was decreased not only by local sounding, but also by sounding at a distance (11).

In studies of isometric tension developed by frog muscle during sounding, it was noted that many of the changes were dependent upon temperature increase in the medium. In one situation, however, tension changes were not identical even though measurable temperature changes were comparable. At low levels of ultrasound (0.75 w/cm^2) there were always increases of tension after short periods of sounding. With prolongation of sounding a decrease below normal levels always resulted. This phenomenon could be duplicated entirely and exactly by any other technique of raising the tissue temperature. However, with larger doses (3 w/cm^2) there was no such initial increase in isometric tension (12).

Injury potentials were then studied, with silver-silver chloride electrodes, after 1 min of pulsed sounding at 3 w/cm^2 and after 1 min of infrared radiation. No measurable difference in temperature rise could be demonstrated with the two techniques, and the highest temperatures recorded were 34 to 35°C. Yet with infrared radiation, membrane potential remained essentially constant, while with ultrasound a marked decrease in membrane potential, consistent with a change in irritability, was noted. Following sounding there was a decrease in injury potential from approximately 46 mv to approximately 28 mv with partial recovery on cessation of sounding (12).

Since in another study carried out in our laboratory (unrelated to ultrasound) decreases in isometric tension and in phosphocreatine were parallel (13), and since Ling and Gerard had demonstrated a parallelism between phosphocreatine and the so-called A fraction of the membrane potential (14), the effect of ultrasound on creatine phosphate was investigated (3). These studies were carried out at 5°C under conditions in which cavitation was prevented (degassing and vacuo). No temperature rise was recorded (intensity of 3 w/cm^2, pulsed ultrasound). A reversible decrease in phosphocreatine of approximately 27% was produced, with an equivalent increase in inorganic phosphate, but no change in ATP. One min after the cessation of sounding there was complete restoration of phosphocreatine toward normal levels.

This change, combined with the change in injury potential, suggested that we were dealing primarily with a membrane phenomenon. The relationship to membrane changes was noted in two ways. First, the muscle was exposed to 0.5 M KCl – treatment which depolarizes the membrane. The decrease in creatine phosphate was quantitatively similar to that produced by sounding, and the process was reversible, though slower. This alone is, however, not conclusive, and the parallelism of effect does not, of course, prove that this particular phenomenon is necessarily a membrane phenomenon. To provide more evidence, the effect of cocaine was studied. Cocaine is a membrane stabilizer, blocking conduction, enhancing polarization, and reducing the depolarizing effect of KCl. It probably acts on Na transport, at the outside of the membrane. Muscle treated with a 0.1% cocaine solution did not demonstrate any decrease in creatine phosphate following exposure to ultrasound. It was suggested, as a working hypothesis, that the membrane could have some effect on the equilibrium between creatine phosphate and inorganic phosphate and that ultrasound altered this equilibrium through its effect on the membrane.

The phenomenon of contracture was studied, not only because it represented one manifestation of membrane activity, but also because, from studies in other laboratories, it was suggested indirectly that some shortening might be produced by ultrasound (15). Contracture is a prolonged reversible shortening of striated muscle, not accompanied by a propagated action potential but associated with a local partial depolarization. Temperature change and shortening were studied in frog sartorius on exposure to both infrared radiation and to ultrasound of low-intensity levels (0.08 to 1.2 w/cm^2) (27). Shortening during sounding was slow in onset, occurred without measurable temperature rise, decreased while sounding was continued, and was completely reversible – resembling contracture in all respects. The average muscle shortening with ultrasound was 300 μ, and resting lengths were reached 10 min after sounding was stopped. With infrared radiation, however, shortening began only after temperatures reached levels of 34°C and higher and was still marked 20 min after heating was stopped – a process undoubtedly the result of thermal denaturation. With application of infrared energy the shortening process does not begin until the temperature rise is quite marked, while with application of ultrasound energy, shortening begins before the temperature rise is evident. Furthermore, shortening with ultrasound is not marked and is reversible. When the membrane was destroyed by glycerolization, or blocked by cocaine, ultrasound no longer produced the shortening previously noted. Such muscle was, however, still maximally responsive to ATP.

Among the factors which should be explored in order to explain the membrane effects described is movement of ions and water across the muscle membrane. Studies of ionic flow carried out by Lota (16) and Lehmann (17) had already shown that such movement could take place. In our laboratories this possibility was explored specifically with relation to frog striated muscle (4). All experiments were carried out at 5°C, in degassed medium, in vacuo. Increase in hydration occurred following exposure to ultrasound. The process resembled a steady state, with complete reversibility within 1 min after completion of sounding. Within the temperature range of 5 to 25°C there were no differences in effect. Furthermore, interference with phosphorylation mechanisms with 2, 4 dinitrophenol (DNP) had no effect on the amount of increase in water content. The process of hydration of muscle in the ultrasound field seemed to be purely physical. When muscle was treated with 0.5 M KCl, there was a 6% increase in solids. The increase in hydration on sounding muscle treated with KCl was initially slightly greater than the increase on sounding normal muscle. This may be expected from the initially lesser degree of hydration. The subsequent return toward normal on continued sounding is very likely due to membrane depolarization with increase in permeability. If the KCl-treated muscle is sounded in distilled water, the subsequent return toward normal is not seen.

Thus, there was considerable evidence that ultrasound could affect amphibian striated muscle in vitro and that shifts in water and ions might be one mechanism whereby such effects were achieved. Studies of membrane effects were then extended to nerve, in which situation excitability might be analyzed without superimposition of the prominent function of contractility. The first experiments were carried out on frogs that had been sectioned above the midbrain level (18). Under no circumstances was an action potential found to result from sounding of either the lumbar cord or the sciatic nerve. In a second series of experiments, using the same experimental animals, thresholds were evaluated using a variable intensity, 1 msec square wave stimulus. Three situations were examined: (1) electrical stimulation of the midbrain and recording of muscle action potentials from the upper extremity, (2) electrical stimulation of the midbrain and recording of muscle action potentials from the lower extremity, and (3) electrical stimulation of the sciatic nerve and recording of muscle action potentials from the lower extremity. In all three situations the region of the lumbar cord was sounded. Temperatures were recorded in the cervical cord, lumbar cord, and sciatic nerve, using animals which were not studied from the excitability standpoint. In control situations with room temperature fluctuations between 23.6 and 24.2°C, thresholds were fairly constant over a 60-min period.

On recording from the upper extremity and from the gastrocnemius after sciatic nerve stimulation, decreases in threshold were found to be small though significant and occurred only after temperature rises had been recorded in the cervical cord and the sciatic nerve. This is in accord with previous studies on increased excitability following temperature rise within this range, provided that a short duration stimulus was used (19, 20).

When action potentials in the gastrocnemius were studied following electrical stimulation of the midbrain the picture was completely different.

Marked decreases in threshold were noted at a time when the temperature rise recorded was approximately 0.1°C. Maximal decreases in threshold occurred quickly and were maintained until the cord temperature reached 27°C. Within this range, the threshold change was a reversible process. If sounding were stopped, there was a restoration of threshold toward normal, and when sounding was again begun, there was an immediate drop in threshold. These changes were noted with extremely small doses of ultrasound and often after only a few pulses. As the temperature increased beyond this point, the threshold rose progressively until irreversible block occurred at approximately 38°C.

Experiments were subsequently carried out on the human, with sounding of nerve roots in the hemiparetic and measurement of the degree of spasticity in the elbow flexors (21). Short duration effects were demonstrable. When the sound head was moved over the spinal cord without any energy emission, there was no significant change in spasticity. With a relatively low dose of 0.75 w/cm^2 there was a significant increase in spasticity. A greater amount of force was required to passively move the extremity. If the dose was increased to 1.90 w/cm^2, there was a decrease in spasticity. Unfortunately, from the therapeutic standpoint, all of these results were reversible.

The mechanism for the above effects was not clear. It was not certain, for example, whether temperature rise could be produced within the cord itself, To test this possibility, experiments were carried out on the anesthetized dog, at frequencies of 490 kc/sec, 1 Mc/sec, and 3 Mc/sec (22). Intensities ranged between 1 and 1.5 w/cm^2. In one series, temperatures were recorded at the surface of the spinal cord at a depth of approximately 2.8 cm, in a region protected by bone (under the lamina). Under these circumstances, a significant temperature rise could be recorded within the spinal canal at the two lower frequencies. As a matter of fact, at a frequency of 490 kc the temperature increase at the spinal cord was higher than over the periosteum or the subcutaneous tissue. It is to be noted that in recent studies carried out by Shealy and Henneman reversible reflex changes were produced in the mammal on sounding of the spinal cord (23).

Our final series of observations was directed toward studies on peripheral nerve. Since there have been many pertinent studies by others in this area, I will present only the few observations that seem most difficult to interpret. When the posterior aspect of the thigh was sounded in the anesthetized dog, using a stationary technique and three different frequencies of ultrasound (490 kc, 1 Mc, 3 Mc), it was found that so-called selective heating of nerve was most marked and significant at the lowest frequency utilized (22). Repeatedly, in previous studies, interface heating has been more marked at high frequencies than at lower ones (24), and one would have predicted a smaller selective effect on nerve at 490 kc than at the higher frequencies. Cavitation is enhanced at lower frequencies, however, and one may suggest, hesitantly, that we may be witnessing a cavitation-type phenomenon in myelin sheath, even at these relatively low intensities.

Studies of conduction velocity and temperature were carried out in the human, using techniques which might be used therapeutically (25). When the sound head was moved over the skin (covering an area of approximately 75 cm^2), without energy emission, there was a decrease in conduction velocity and in temperature of subcutaneous tissue. A decrease in conduction velocity was observed until the ultrasound energy level reached 1.92 w/cm^2. When the area covered by the sound head was decreased, the temperature rise and the increase in conduction velocity observed during irradiation were greater than that observed during irradiation of larger areas. Since large areas are often covered in therapeutic use of ultrasound, we attempted to achieve further increase in temperature and conduction velocity by progressively increasing the intensity. It was noted, unexpectedly, that as the ultrasound intensity was raised above approximately 2 w/cm^2, the temperature rise was not as great as at the lower intensities. It is likely that one is dealing with vasoconstriction produced by ultrasound, but the precise mechanism is unclear (26).

In summary our studies have indicated that the major effects of ultrasound, insofar as therapeutic effects are concerned, can be demonstrated in two areas. In connective tissue one is able to demonstrate both thermal and non-thermal effects on extensibility. It is not possible, at the present time, to indicate which of these mechanisms is the more important in terms of the human therapeutic situation. Membrane effects were demonstrated during in vitro situations, under circumstances in which there was no recordable rise in temperature and often with extremely small doses of ultrasound. Unfortunately, we do not know how important these membrane effects are in human therapy, in instances of pain and spasm.

REFERENCES

1. Hintzelmann, U. (1949). Ultraschall-Therapie rheumatischer Erkrankungen, besonders des Morbus Bechterew. Strahlentherapie *79*, 607.
2. Rollhäuser, H. (1954). Experimentelle Beeinflüssung der Dehnbarkeit des Bindegewebes am lebenden Organismus. Klin. Wchnschr. *26*, 126.
3. Gersten, J. W., and E. Kawashima (1954). Changes in phosphocreatine produced in striated muscle by ultrasound. Am. J. Phys. Med. *33*, 207.
4. Gersten, J. W. (1955). Changes in hydration of muscle and tendon following the application of ultrasonic energy. Arch. Phys. Med. & Rehab. *36*, 140.
5. Gersten, J. W. (1955). Effect of ultrasound on tendon extensibility. Am. J. Phys. Med. *34*, 362.
6. Chapman, G. (1953). Studies on the mesogloea of coelenterates. II. Physical properties. J. Exp. Biol. *30*, 440.
7. McMaster, P. D., and R. J. Parsons (1950). The movement of substances and the state of the fluid in the intradermal tissue. Ann. N.Y. Acad. Sciences *52*, 992.
8. Gersten, J. W. (1956). Relation of ultrasound effects to the orientation of tendon in the ultrasound field. Arch. Phys. Med. & Rehab. *37*, 201.
9. Gersten, J. W. (1958). Effect of metallic objects on temperature rises produced in tissue by ultrasound. Am. J. Phys. Med. *37*, 75.
10. Harvey, E. Newton (1929). The effect of high frequency sound waves on heart muscle and other irritable tissues. Am. J. Physiol. *91*, 284.
11. Busnel, R-G., J. Gligorijevic, P. Chauchard, and H. Mazoué (1952). Action des

ultrasons de haute fréquence sur le système nerveux. C.R. Acad. Sci. Paris *235*, 1535.
12. Gersten, J. W. (1953). Thermal and non-thermal changes in isometric tension, contractile protein, and injury potential, produced in frog muscle by ultrasonic energy. Arch. Phys. Med. & Rehab. *34*, 675.
13. Gersten, J. W. (1952). Effect of subthreshold currents on isometric tension and phosphocreatine content of the frog gastrocnemius. Am. J. Physiol. *168*, 458.
14. Ling, G., and R. W. Gerard (1949). The membrane potential and metabolism of muscle fibers. J. Cell. Comp. Physiol. *34*, 413.
15. Fischer, E., E. A. White, S. L. Hendricks, B. A. Chevalier, and R. B. Chevalier (1954). Effect of moderate and of weak ultrasonic exposures upon normal and denervated mammalian muscles. Am. J. Phys. Med. *33*, 284.
16. Lota, M. J., and R. C. Darling (1955). Changes in permeability of the red blood cell membrane in a homogeneous ultrasonic field. Arch. Phys. Med. & Rehab. *36*, 282.
17. Lehmann, J. (1951). Die Spezifität der biologischen und therapeutischen Ultraschallwirkung. Arch. Physik. Ther. *3*, 57.
18. Gersten, J. W. (1955). Changes in spinal cord thresholds following the application of ultrasound. Proc. 4th Ann. Conf. on Ultrasonic Ther., 31–40.
19. Lapicque, M. and Mme. (1907). Influence d'une variation locale de température sur l'excitabilité du nerf moteur. C.R. Soc. de Biol. *62*, 39.
20. Schoepfle, G. M., and J. Erlanger (1941). The action of temperature on the excitability, spike height and configuration, and the refractory period observed in the responses of single medullated nerve fibers. Am. J. Physiol. *134*, 694.
21. Stillwell, D. M., and J. W. Gersten (1955). The effect of ultrasound on spasticity. Proc. 4th Ann. Conf. on Ultrasonic Ther., 124–131.
22. Gersten, J. W. (1959). Temperature rise of various tissues in the dog on exposure to ultrasound at different frequencies. Arch. Phys. Med. *40*, 187.
23. Shealy, C. N., and E. Henneman (1962). Reversible effects of ultrasound on spinal reflexes. Arch. Neurol. *6*, 374.
24. Lehmann, J., and W. Nitsch (1951). Über die Frequenzabhängigkeit biologischer Ultraschall-Reaktionen mit besonderer Berücksichtigung der spezifischen Temperaturverteilung im Organismus. Strahlentherapie *85*, 606.
25. Madsen, P. W., Jr., and J. W. Gersten (1961). The effect of ultrasound on conduction velocity of peripheral nerve. Arch. Phys. Med. *42*, 645.
26. Stuhlfauth, K. (1952). Neural effects of ultrasonic waves. Brit. J. Phys. Med. *15*, 10.
27. Gersten, J. W. (1957). Muscle shortening produced by ultrasound. Arch. Phys. Med. & Rehab. *38*, 83–87.

DISCUSSION

DR. HUGHES: Could you elaborate on what happened in the ion concentration studies?

DR. GERSTEN: These were not done in our laboratory, but elsewhere. Lota (16) showed that when red blood cells were exposed to ultrasound there was, apparently, an increase in permeability of the erythrocyte to K, with K appearing in the plasma in increased amounts. Lehmann (17) demonstrated increased passage of Cl through frog skin following sounding. Heating did not seem to be a primary factor in either instance.

DR. KELLY: What were the stimulus pulse durations in your studies of isometric tension?

DR. GERSTEN: The stimuli were square waves of 0.1 msec duration and were several times maximal. I don't recall the repetition rate in the isometric tetanic responses. The increase in isometric tension produced by the low-dosage ultrasound (0.75 w/cm^2) could be duplicated by infrared radiation and warm water.

DR. NYBORG: Would you mind explaining the hydration change brought about by the sounding?

DR. GERSTEN: Our hypothesis, and I must emphasize that at this stage it is only that, is that we are dealing with radiation pressure when the tendon is sounded at right angles to the ultrasound field. McMaster and Parsons have shown that dyes, such as pontamine sky blue, may be squeezed along the surface of connective tissue fibrils by mechanical forces. Our suggestion is that ultrasound provides such a "squeezing force" although of small magnitude. With muscle I have no suggestions and feel that one should probe more deeply with radioisotope techniques.

DR. KELLY: How were temperatures measured?

DR. GERSTEN. In our early experiments we used either thermistors or relatively large copper-constantan thermocouples. With these, temperature recordings could not be made until 5 to 10 sec after sounding was stopped. Subsequent to this, and in most of our experiments, we used 0.5-mil thermocouples and were able to record during the sounding.

DR. KELLY: Did you put a hole in the bone for insertion?

DR. GERSTEN: If necessary, yes. Let me make one final comment with respect to temperature recordings. When we were studying isometric tension and injury potentials, we did not record temperatures simultaneously because of the possibility of damage by the thermocouple, even when small. We did one series of experiments on tension or injury potential and another on temperature. We didn't try to study all of these phenomena at one time.

11

Action of Ultrasound on the Internal Ear

MICHELE ARSLAN, M.D., and O. SALA, M.D.
The Department of Otolaryngology, University of Padova, Italy

Introduction by Dr. Libber

Dr. Michele Arslan of the University of Padova was scheduled to be our next speaker, but unfortunately Dr. Arslan was not able to attend the meeting. As many of you know, Dr. Arslan did the early work on the application of ultrasound for the treatment of Ménière's disease. This disease is considered to be due to a vasomotor disorder with secondary development of edema of the labyrinth. Outward manifestations of the disorder are a type of dizziness and postural imbalance. Dr. Douglas Gordon, our medical colleague from England, has visited Dr. Arslan's laboratory in Italy and is quite familiar with his work. Dr. Gordon has consented to read Dr. Arslan's paper.

Patients suffering from severe Ménière's disease have been systematically treated by direct ultrasonic irradiation of the posterior labyrinth. This technique has been used by Arslan since 1952. Numerous publications have reported favorable results from the application of this method (1–6, 10, 12, 13, 15–17, 20, 22, 23).

It is well known that ultrasonic irradiation is accompanied by a heating effect that takes place in the irradiated tissue. This effect is due to two factors: (a) the electrical energy of the ultrasonic generator not transformed into ultrasonic energy, which becomes thermic energy at the level of the treatment head (Fig. 1),[1] and (b) the effect due to absorption when passing through tissue, particularly bone tissue which has the highest ultrasound absorption coefficient (14). As soon as the treatment head is placed in direct contact with the bone labyrinth – without any interposition of structures that may slow down or impede the propagation of the ultrasonic beam (for example, cavities containing air, such as mastoid cells of the bony bulla in animals) – and the ultrasonic beam has reached the vestibular receptors,

[1] The technical characteristics of the Arslan-Federici apparatus are briefly summarized in the first publication on the subject by M. Arslan (Minerva Otolaringol. *3* [1953], 4).

there occurs a nystagmus of the eye with the fast component directed ipsilaterally to the irradiated labyrinth (so-called "irritative" nystagmus). The jerks of the nystagmus follow the plane of the irradiated semicircular canal, though a functional preeminence of the horizontal nystagmus may be observed in man and in the animal even when the vertical canals are being irradiated. When the ultrasonic irradiation is continued, after a certain period, varying according to the animal species, the intensity of irradiation, etc., the nystagmus grows progressively fainter (the jerks become less marked and less frequent) and is replaced after about 20 to 30 min by a nystagmus in the opposite direction, that is, with the fast component directed toward the labyrinth which was not irradiated (so-called "paralytic" nystagmus) and by the typical syndrome of unilateral labyrinthine destruction (tonic deviation toward the irradiated side, etc.).

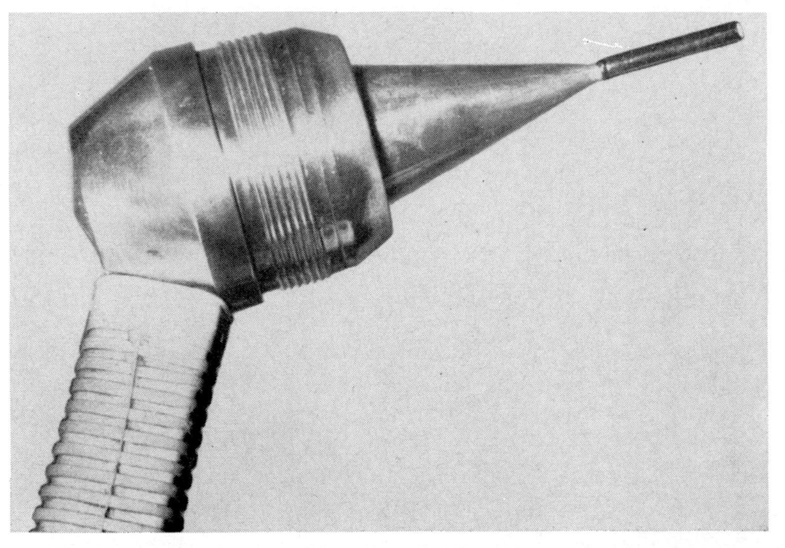

FIGURE 1. Arslan-Federici ultrasound treatment head, with transducer and applicator rod. Ultrasound waves are irradiated only from the tip of the rod. A sleeve around the applicator prevents lateral diffusion of ultrasound beam.

These complex phenomena, which we have briefly summarized, have led to the discussion of interesting problems of labyrinthine physiology. While carrying out our experimental research work on the rabbit, our aim was to study some of these problems, namely, to establish the following points:

I. Whether the eye nystagmus (of the "irritative" type) which appears during ultrasonic irradiation is due to the histofunctional modifications induced into the ampullar receptors by the ultrasonic beam, or whether it is due only to the endolymph currents which are generated by the heating effect attending the ultrasonic irradiation (that is, by a thermal stimulus, with the same mechanism which lies at the base of nystagmus).

II. Whether during ultrasonic irradiation, it is possible to demonstrate a modified activity of the otoliths by a difference of those ocular compensatory positions which arise in the animal by varying the position of its head in space.

III. Whether during the ultrasonic irradiation, there are any variations in those modifications of nystagmus by caloric stimulus which, as is well known, always occur by varying the position of the head during the appearance of the nystagmus by thermal stimulus.

IV. Whether the nystagmus phenomena which appear at the end of the irradiation, or after it, are due to the ultrasonic effect upon this epithelium, and not to that heating effect which developed in the treatment head and which is the cause of nystagmus during irradiation. In the interpretation of these phenomena, consideration must be taken into account of the histological findings of destructive lesions of the ampullar neurosensorial epithelium (which arise after ultrasonic irradiation as per Arslan's method [8, 9, 11, 17]).

In our experimental work we made use of the rabbit for various reasons: (a) It lacks any active eye movement. (b) In the rabbit, one can clearly separate the ocular phenomena of ampullary origin from those of otolithic origin. (c) When the appropriate procedures described by Bötner and Sala (7) are carried out, it is very easy to uncover the periotic bone which is particularly compact and does not have interpositions of any pneumatic bone containing air cells. In addition, it is possible, by ultrasonic irradiation, to obtain a clear nystagmus, as the lateral semicircular canal runs remarkably near to the external mastoid cortex. On a preliminary group of animals (twenty rabbits) the following experimental program was carried out:

(1) Observation of the well-known ocular compensatory positions of otolithic origin (Magnus phenomena) in the following positions of the head in space: (a) *normal position, namely, with a 30° anterior flexion of the head*; (b) *at 90° rotation of the head and body to the left*; (c) *at 90° rotation of the head and body to the right*; (d) *with head up*; (e) *with head down* (in the last two positions the animal's body must be kept perfectly vertical); (f) *in a supine position.* After being firmly fixed on a special retaining table (Fig. 2) the body of the animal was rotated in toto so as to avoid any interference of cervical reflexes upon the eye muscles (Magnus' reflexes). An asymmetric cross, drawn on the anesthetized cornea of the animal by means of a heated needle and made conspicuous by white China ink, allowed us to evaluate all the space modifications of the eyeballs both in the transversal plane and in the front-parallel plane.

(2) Direct ultrasonic irradiation of the left posterior labyrinth was carried out by placing the applicator rod into direct contact with the mastoid surface and by employing other technical devices described by Bötner and Sala (7) for the same experimental animal. During the experiment the intensity of ultrasonic irradiation was always kept at a value of 13 w/cm^2 measured by the Federici dosimeter. The timing of the transducer was constantly checked by means of an appropriate frequency meter. We noted that if the irradiation is made while the head of this animal is in its customary posture, there appears a nystagmus, caused by ultrasonic irradiation, with jerks along the

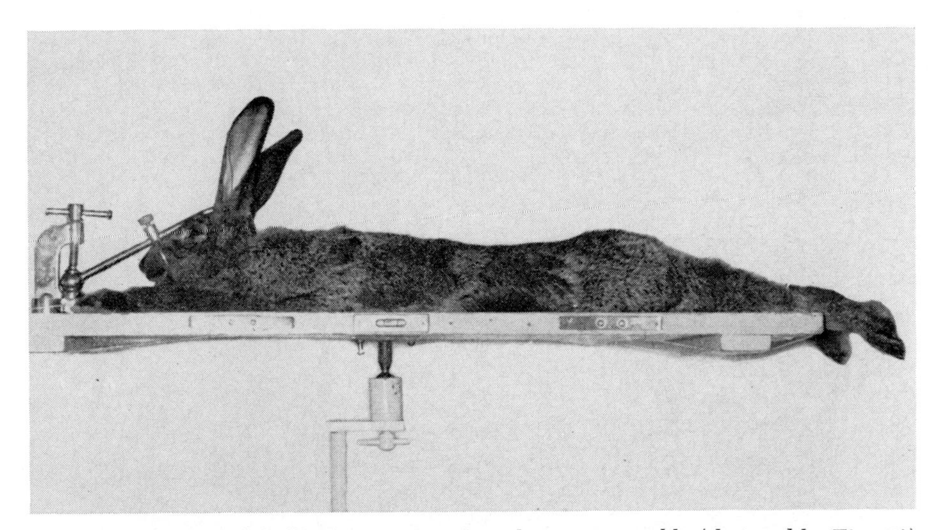

FIGURE 2. The animal (rabbit) is positioned on the retaining table (designed by Fioretti) with the head fixed in the customary position both as to space (position [a], head bent 30° forward) and to the body (to avoid any interference of Magnus' cervical reflexes upon the eye muscles).

transverse plane of the orbit, which, when the left labyrinth is being irradiated, is caudally directed in the left eye and rostrally directed in the right eye (21). While the irradiation was continued, the animal was slowly rotated so as to make it reach the positions in space we described under 1 (a), (b), (c), (d), (e), (f) above and in which we had formerly observed the appearance of the well-known compensatory modifications of the eyeballs. For each test, we varied the position from which the experiment started, the order of succession of the various positions, and the period of time the animal was left in the different positions. The results observed in this first group of animals can be summarized as follows:

In position (a), that is, in the customary posture of the animal's head and body, a left ultrasonic irradiation is constantly followed by the appearance of a nystagmus along the transverse plane of the orbit, caudally directed in the left eye and rostrally in the right one (Fig. 3), which lasts for about 40 to 50 min irradiation time, thereafter growing fainter. If the irradiation is continued in this position, after 40 to 50 min we observed a reversal of nystagmus ("paralytic" nystagmus) and the appearance of a clear spontaneous unilateral labyrinthine destruction syndrome (rolling phenomena, cephalic nystagmus, etc.) which grows fainter and disappears in the days following.[2]

In position (b), which is reached during irradiation by a slow 90° rotation

[2] The difference in ultrasonic irradiation time and intensity necessary to produce unilateral labyrinthine destruction in the rabbit and in man (values are clearly lower in man, in whom a less intense and shorter ultrasonic irradiation is sufficient to provoke a "paralytic" nystagmus) is explained by the fact that the ultrasonic beam has to pass through a thicker layer of bony tissue in the rabbit than in man.

Figures 3 through 8 show: (1) the compensatory ocular positions (left eye) with asymmetric cross on the cornea, (2) the direction and intensity of nystagmus (the length of the arrow indicating the direction of nystagmus is proportional to its intensity), (3) a sketch of the animal's skull as seen from the left side, and (4) the left posterior labyrinth with the ampulla of the lateral semicircular canal (l.s.c.) in black ("x" represents the most external portion of l.s.c. where the ultrasonic heating effect is highest). The length of the arrow indicating the direction of the endolymphatic flow is proportional to the flow intensity.

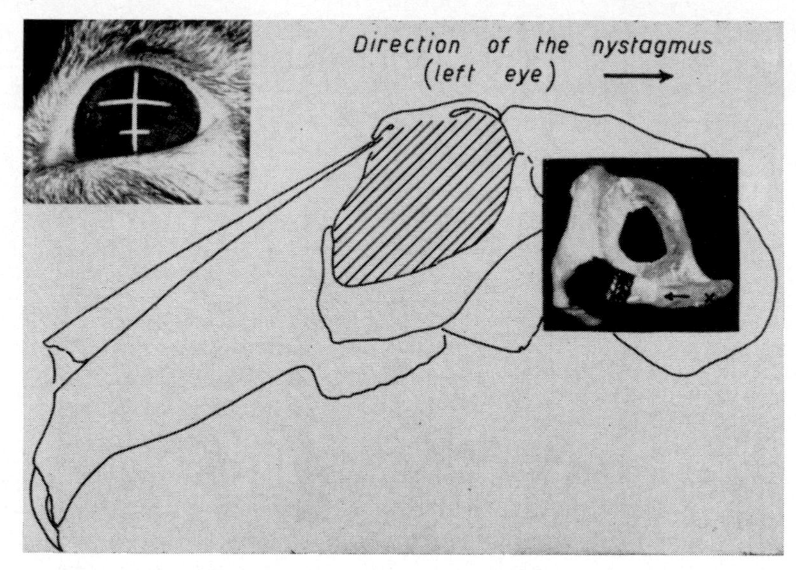

FIGURE 3. Position (a). The animal's head is in the customary posture. The eyes are in the customary position, symmetrically to the eyelid rima. The nystagmus from ultrasonic irradiation is of moderate intensity and in the direction of the irradiated side. The heating effect of ultrasonic irradiation, which is at its highest in the most external portion of the l.s.c. ("x"), causes a utriculopetal ascending endolymphatic flow, because the l.s.c. ampulla is located on a higher position with respect to point "x."

of the animal to the left, after a few seconds we observe a reversal of the nystagmus which has been observed in position (a), namely, the nystagmus jerks, though still moving along the transverse plane of the orbit, are rostrally directed in the left eye and caudally directed in the right eye (Fig. 4). On the other hand, the compensatory ocular deviations persist unchanged. By once more placing the animal's head in position (a), after a few minutes the nystagmus again assumes the characteristics described above and the eyeballs go back to their customary symmetrical position.

In position (c), obtained by a slow 90° rotation of the head (and body) to the right, the nystagmus, which moves along the transverse plane of the orbit in this case also, grows less frequent and to a smaller extent. When some small movements about this position are imparted to the animal's head, the nystagmus obtains the same extent and speed, both in the slow and in the fast phases (so-called "undulatory" or "pendular" nystagmus), and sometimes ceases to exist (Fig. 5).

In position (d), that is, with the animal's head up and its body kept per-

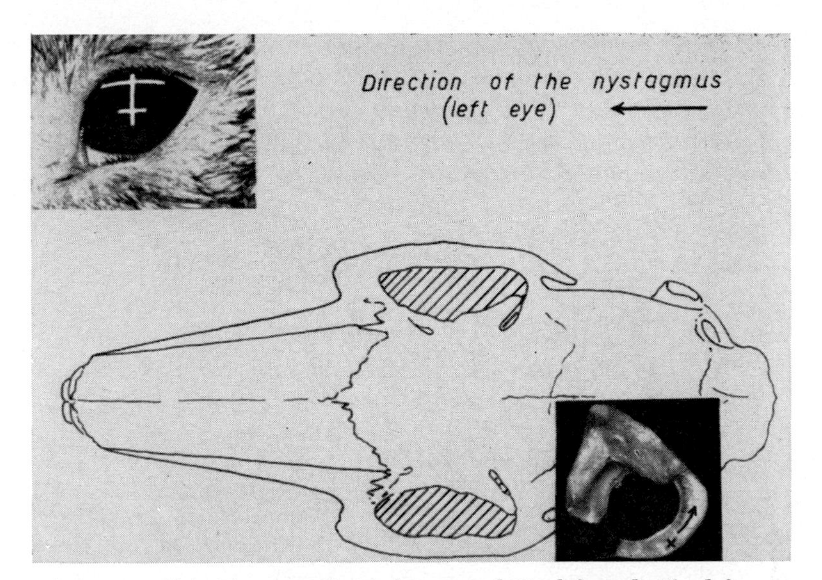

FIGURE 4. Position (b). The animal's head is rotated 90° leftward. The left eye, owing to the compensatory positions, is displaced upward. The nystagmus from ultrasonic irradiation is very intense and directed toward the nonirradiated side, namely, in direction opposite to (a). The ultrasonic irradiation heating effect, which is highest in the most external portion of the l.s.c. ("x"), causes an utriculofugal ascending endolymphatic flow, because the l.s.c. ampulla lies on a lower position with respect to point "x."

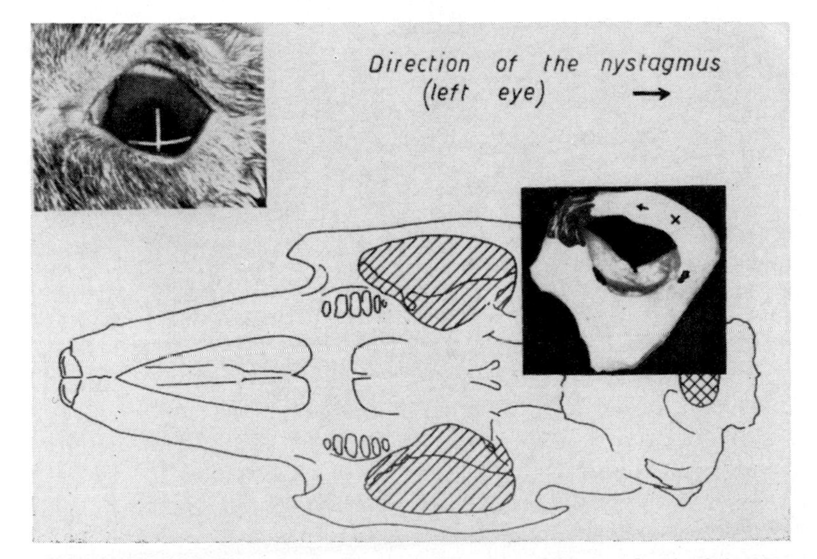

FIGURE 5. Position (c). The animal's head is rotated 90° rightward. The left eye, owing to the compensatory positions, is displaced downward. The nystagmus from ultrasonic irradiation is negligible and directed toward the irradiated side. The ultrasonic irradiation heating effect, which is highest in the most external position of the l.s.c. ("x"), causes an utriculopetal ascending endolymphatic flow of fairly low intensity because the l.s.c. ampulla is located on the same or on a slightly higher position with respect to point "x."

fectly vertical, it may be observed that the jerks of the nystagmus present in position (a) above become more frequent and of a greater breadth, and, though remaining along the transverse plane of the orbit, this nystagmus also acquires an oblique component directed upward in the left eye and downward in the right one (Fig. 6).

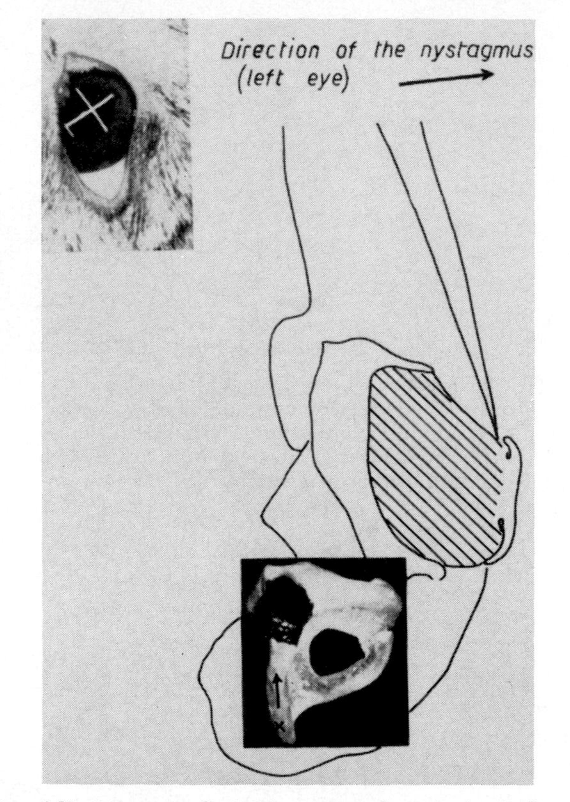

FIGURE 6. Position (d). The animal's head is upward, with the body perfectly vertical. The left eye, owing to the compensatory positions, is slightly displaced forward and slightly rotated counterclockwise. The nystagmus from ultrasonic irradiation is very intense and directed toward the irradiated side, with a slight oblique component upward. The heating effect of ultrasonic irradiation, which is highest in the most external portion of the l.s.c. ("x"), causes an utriculopetal ascending endolymphatic flow because the l.s.c. ampulla is located on a higher position with respect to point "x."

In position (e), that is, head down and body perfectly vertical, after a few seconds' interval, the nystagmus is reversed and, though still moving along the transverse plane of the orbit, it acquires an oblique component directed downward in the left eye and directed upward in the right eye (Fig. 7).

In position (f), in which the animal is lying down with its body perfectly horizontal and its head bent forward at about 30° from the horizontal plane the nystagmus moving along the horizontal plane disappears and there appears a vertical nystagmus directed upward and backward in the left eye and downward and forward in the right eye (Fig. 8).

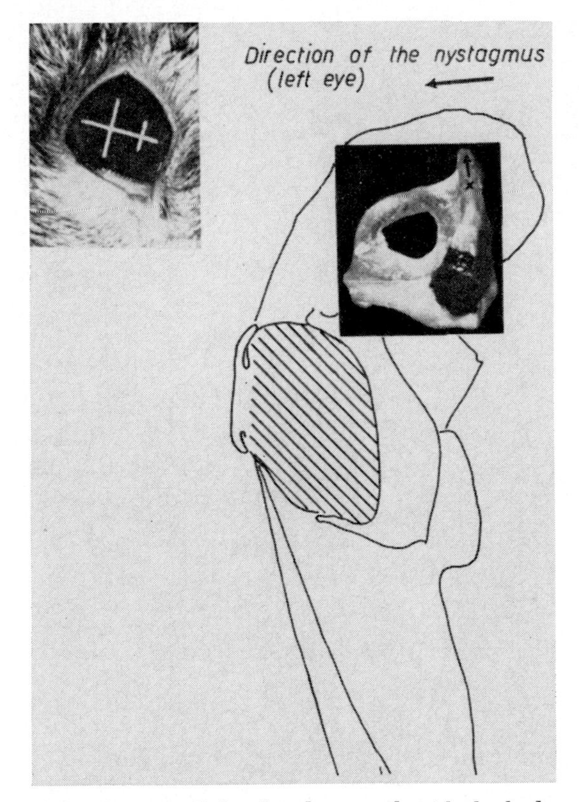

FIGURE 7. Position (e). The animal's head is downward, with the body perfectly vertical. The left eye, owing to the compensatory positions, is slightly displaced backward and slightly rotated clockwise. The nystagmus from ultrasonic irradiation is of a moderate intensity, with a slight oblique component downward. The heating effect of ultrasonic irradiation, which is highest in the most external portion of l.s.c. ("x"), causes an utriculofugal ascending endolymphatic flow, because the l.s.c. ampulla is located in a lower position with respect to point "x."

As previously mentioned, the aim of the present investigation is to provide information on four problems (I to IV) associated with ultrasound irradiation of the internal ear. The results of the research outlined above indicate the following:

I. The nystagmus which appears *during* ultrasonic irradiation does not seem to be related to a *direct* stimulation of the sensorial neuroepithelium. In fact, in some particular positions of the head in space, it is possible to invert its direction, though the direction of the ultrasonic beam is kept unmodified. Hence, this "irritative" nystagmus is, no doubt, provoked by the heating effect which accompanies the ultrasonic irradiation, that is, by the endolymph currents which heat induces in the lateral semicircular canal (s.c.) which, in the rabbit, has a major functional importance over the other canals and which is more easily reached by ultrasonic irradiation owing to its particular location. When the ampulla of the lateral s.c. happens to be at a higher level than the outermost tract of the lateral s.c. (where the heat-

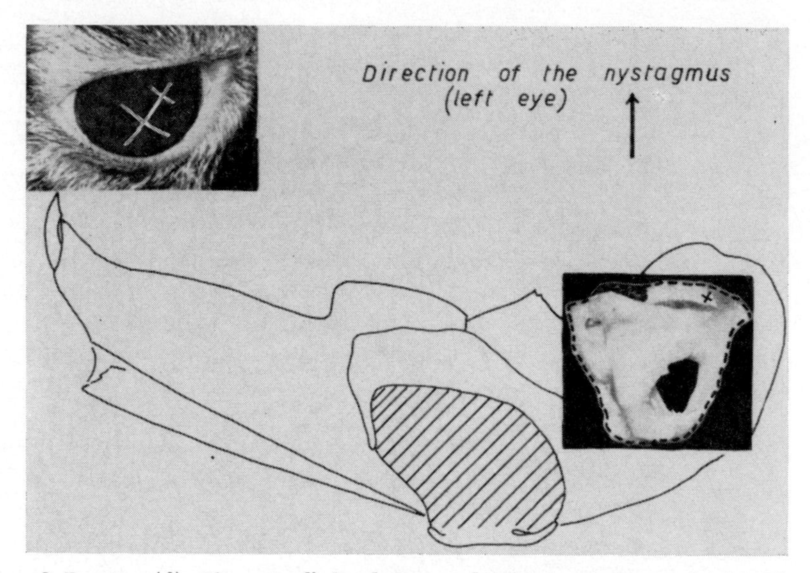

FIGURE 8. Position (f). The animal's head is rotated 180° (animal on its back). The eyes are in a symmetrical central position with slight clockwise rotation in the left eye. The nystagmus from ultrasonic irradiation is of moderate intensity and directed in the vertical plane, because the lateral semicircular canals are in the "indifferent position."

ing effect is greater), the endolymph currents directed toward the utricle are of an intensity which increases the more the lateral s.c. approaches the vertical (positions [c], [a], and [d], respectively). On the other hand, it is well known that the intensity[3] of the eye nystagmus (in our case, along the transverse plane of the orbit) is proportional to the intensity of the endolymph currents which originate in the lateral s.c. The endolymph currents have, however, a utriculofugal direction when the cupola is below the outermost tract of the lateral s.c., where, as we mentioned above, the heating effect is greater. Hence, in this case, the direction of the eye nystagmus is reversed, though still remaining in the transverse plane of the orbit. Here too the intensity of nystagmus is proportional to the intensity of the endolymph currents which, because of the above mentioned reasons, are more evident in position (e) than in position (b).

In the supine position (f), with the body of the rabbit horizontal and its head bent 30° forward, the lateral s.c. is practically on a horizontal plane, namely, in the least favorable condition ("indifferent" position) for the creation of endolymph currents. On the other hand, the vertical semicircular canals are in the most favorable position and, therefore, during ultrasonic irradiation, there arise endolymph currents which provoke a nystagmus which moves along the vertical plane. Also, the space position of the cupola of the lateral s.c. may have some importance as it happens to be in a direction which is just the opposite (downward directed) to its normal position (up-

[3] By nystagmus "intensity," we mean the ratio between frequency of the jerks in a given time and the breadth of the jerks.

ward directed). In fact, in position (a) also the lateral s.c. is in a position which is very near the "indifferent" one, and yet in that case we succeed in inducing an eye nystagmus along the transverse plane of the orbit, as we have described. These results and their interpretation have been confirmed by some control research work carried out in the rabbit by means of prolonged irrigation (15 to 20 min) with water at a temperature of 10°C (such as to induce endolymph currents of a direction contrary to those obtained by ultrasonic irradiation). In this case, the identical modifications of the position of the head in space (positions [a], [b], [c], [d], [e], [f]) are followed by nystagmuses which are absolutely equal but in the opposite direction.

II. With regard to the question whether, during ultrasonic irradiation, we can prove a modified activity of the otolith, the results make it possible to conclude that ultrasonic irradiation cannot modify the compensatory ocular positions caused by the otoliths.

III. With regard to the question whether ultrasonic irradiation causes any variations in those modifications of the nystagmus provoked by thermal stimulus, which appear when the position of the head in space is changed, the experimental results indicate that ultrasonic irradiation does not change the development of these phenomena.

Question IV is concerned with the biological importance of the heating effect which accompanies ultrasonic irradiation, which is caused by factors (a) and (b) described in the introduction of this paper. It must, however, be added that other elements also have a bearing on the matter, namely, the intensity of irradiation, the length of the ultrasonic wave, the conversion power of the electric energy into ultrasonic energy at the level of the transducer, the thermic characteristics of the treatment head, etc. With regard to this point, the research work done by J. Angell James and co-workers (2) is worthy of particular attention. These researchers studied the physical characteristics of ultrasonic irradiation at the level of the temporal bone, determining the mode of penetration of the ultrasonic beam into the bone, and the importance of the heating effect both upon the irradiation surface and in the temporal bone, particularly when, during irradiation, the mastoid cavity was undergoing a continuous irrigation of 39°C water (50 cc/min). Among the important results they obtained was the destruction of the neurosensorial epithelium, which they ascribed to vibration and cavitation caused by ultrasonic irradiation. Even though the question we have postulated is strictly limited to the biological point of view of the problem, it is nevertheless very complex. We define here just a few of its aspects, namely, (A) study of the nystagmus phenomena which appear when we apply on the bony labyrinth a pure caloric source (without ultrasound) whose intensity corresponds exactly to the thermal curve obtained by the foregoing measurement, (B) study of the phenomena which appear during and after an ultrasonic irradiation carried out with the same physical characteristics mentioned in (A) above, but during which the temperature of the treatment head is maintained by means of a cooling system at 38°C (the rectal temperature of the rabbit – 12 animals).

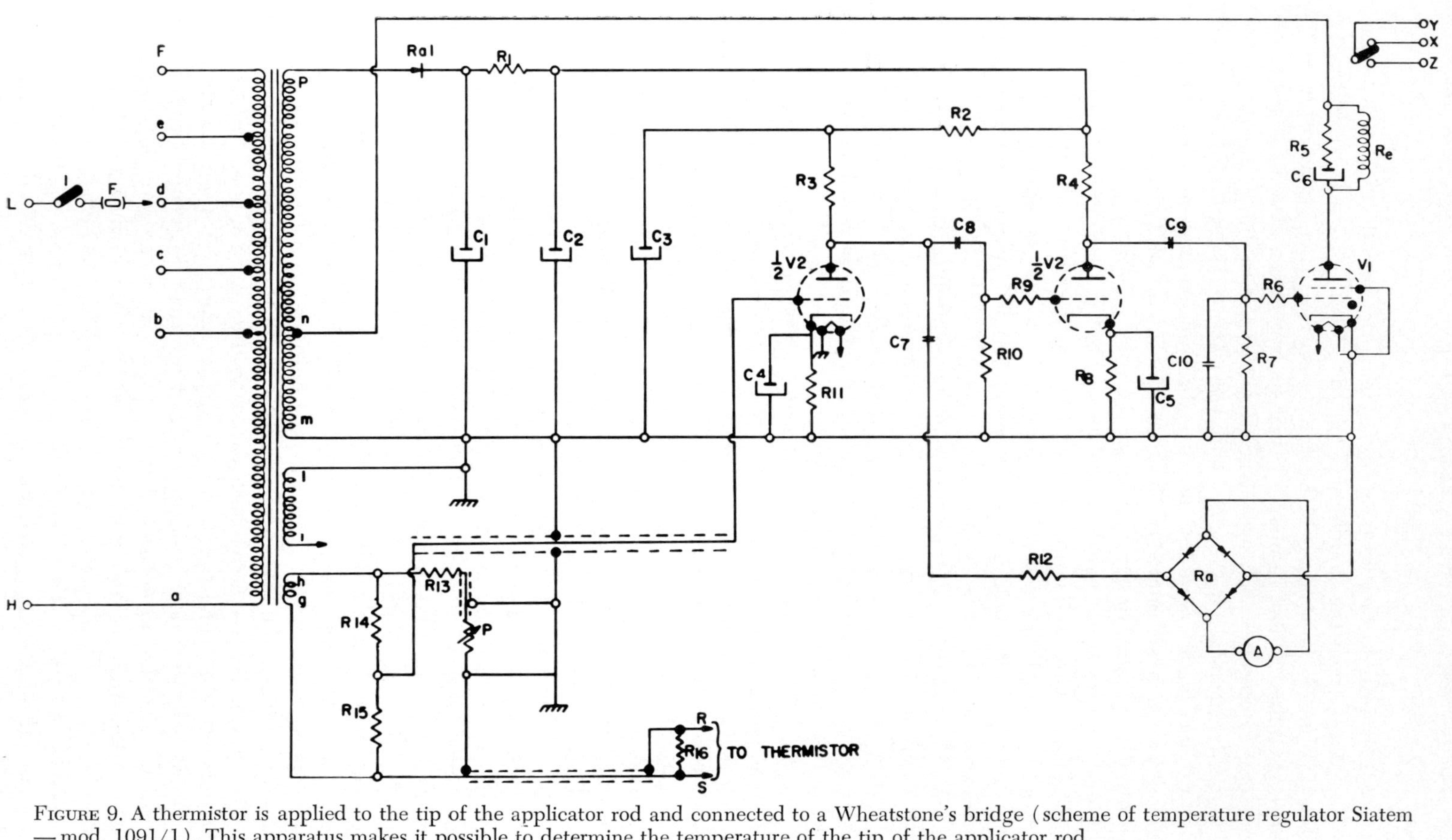

FIGURE 9. A thermistor is applied to the tip of the applicator rod and connected to a Wheatstone's bridge (scheme of temperature regulator Siatem — mod. 1091/1). This apparatus makes it possible to determine the temperature of the tip of the applicator rod.

For study (A), we arranged a source of heat to repeat the same thermic curve obtained at the tip of the treatment head during ultrasonic irradiations of various intensities (Figs. 9, 10). Thus, we had a copper rod (Fig. 11) made of the same dimensions as the ultrasonic applicator rod and equipped at the tip with an electrical resistance whose temperature was adjusted by a thermistor connected to the circuit shown in Figure 9. Once the copper rod had reached a temperature of 80°C, it was applied directly upon the same left semicircular canal — following the method we mentioned above — and there, under these conditions, it was kept for a period of time ranging from 45 to 120 min. As soon as the copper rod was applied to the temporal bone, there appeared an "irritative" nystagmus in the transversal plane of the orbit which

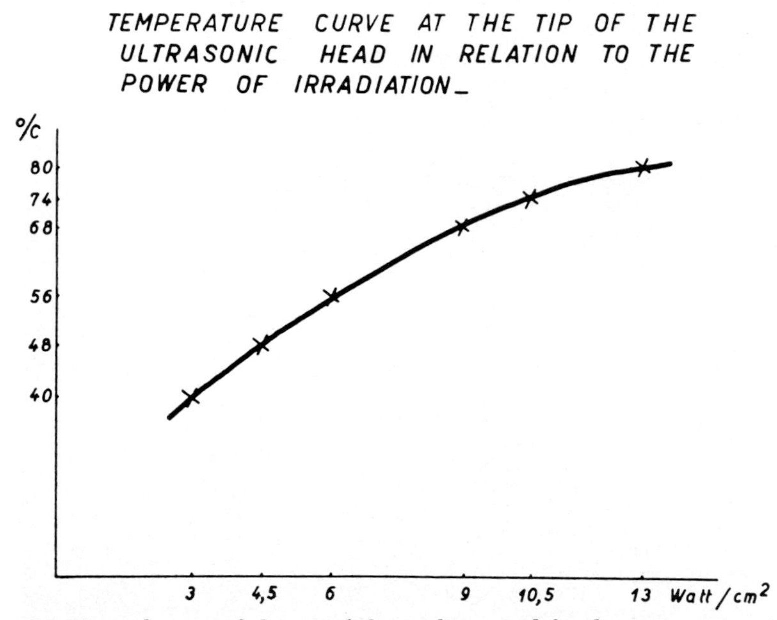

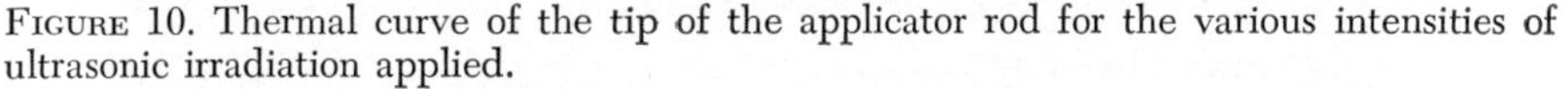

FIGURE 10. Thermal curve of the tip of the applicator rod for the various intensities of ultrasonic irradiation applied.

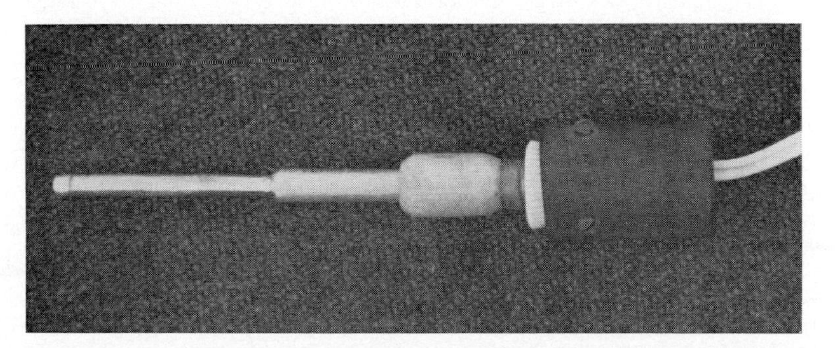

FIGURE 11. Copper rod, with an electrical resistance and a thermistor, of the same dimensions as the ultrasonic applicator rod (see Fig. 1). Connecting the electrical resistance and the thermistor according to the scheme explained in Figure 9, the temperature of this copper rod can be controlled and kept at a preestablished value.

disappeared after about 10 min; the eye nystagmus appeared again, though always for a short time (2 to 3 min), either when the animal was set in position (d) (animal vertical with its head up) or when the copper rod was again applied on the temporal bone, after suspension of the caloric irradiation for a few minutes. Under these conditions we never observed the appearance of a "paralytic" nystagmus, either at the end of the application of the copper rod or during the above mentioned intervals, between one period of heating and the following one, even if it had gone on uninterruptedly for a period of 2 hr. To obtain a "paralytic" nystagmus, that is, the syndrome of unilateral labyrinthine destruction, we were compelled to raise the temperature of the copper rod considerably (over 110 to 120°C) and to apply the rod uninterruptedly for a period of time which we discovered had to be not shorter than 2 hr. Histological research work is now being carried out to determine what lesions appear in the labyrinth of animals which underwent such heating effects and how these lesions differ from those induced by ultrasound as described by G. B. De Stefani (9) and others.

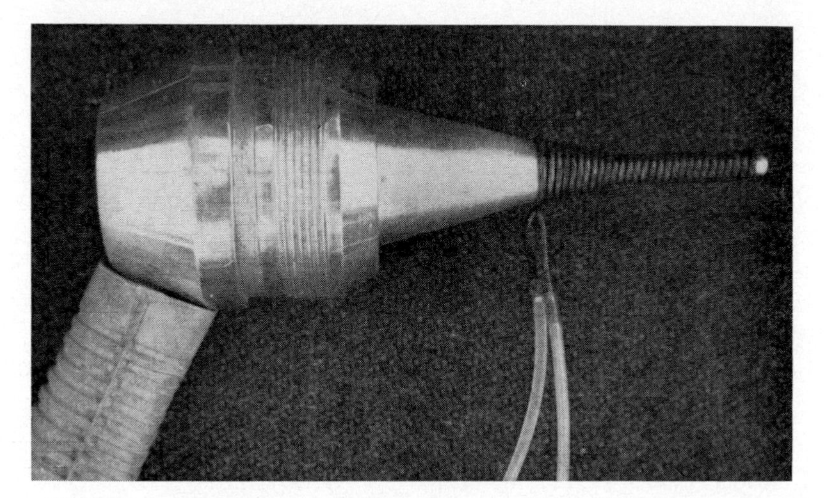

FIGURE 12. Ultrasonic applicator rod (see Fig. 1), with coiled thin copper pipe in which water circulates at variable temperature and speed in order to maintain the temperature of 38 to 38.5°C (rectal temperature of the rabbit). The temperature of the applicator rod was also checked by a thermistor.

For study (B), ultrasonic irradiation was carried out in the manner described above (upon the left labyrinth, at an intensity of 13 w/cm^2, irradiation time 40 to 50 min). The ultrasonic applicator rod, however, was constantly maintained at a temperature of 38°C by means of a cooling system consisting of a thin copper pipe coiled around the applicator rod (Fig. 12), in which water circulated at variable temperature and speed. In this case also the temperature of the applicator rod was checked by a thermistor, as described above. This cooling system differs from the method of continuous irrigation in the whole operation cavity by means of a coolant, as first used by J. Angell James and co-workers. In our research work we proved that a "cold" ultrasonic irradiation is not followed, during irradiation, by any nystagmus even though the animal's position in space was changed (positions [a], [b], [c], [d], [e], [f]). A few groups of slight jerks appeared only when some very slight and transitory variations at the tip of the applicator rod occurred.[4]

After the irradiation no "paralytic" nystagmus appeared but if the animals were prodded so as to make rapid movements, they walked unsteadily and there appeared groups of twitches of a sometimes paralytic and sometimes irritative nystagmus. This condition of latent lack of balance increased after 36 to 72 hr and then disappeared slowly. Acceleratory stimulation, made 20 to 30 days later, proved the presence of hyporeflexia of the irradiated labyrinth (18). A group of six animals was therefore subjected to a continuous "cold" ultrasonic irradiation for 2 to 2.5 hr always at the same intensity (13 w/cm^2). At the end of the irradiation we observed the appearance of an "irritative" nystagmus which continued for several hours and was not reversed when the position of the animal's head in space was modified according to the usual method described above (positions [a], [b], [c], [d], [e], [f]). We could thus exclude the possibility that nystagmus obtained in this way was caused by endolymph currents provoked by a heating effect of any kind whatever. This "irritative" nystagmus grew fainter and, after 8 to 12 hr there appeared a "paralytic" nystagmus, attended with the well-known unilateral labyrinthine destruction syndrome, which, though growing fainter, persisted during the days that followed. This "paralytic" nystagmus was not reversed, of course, when the position of the head in space was changed. These phenomena did not seem to be any less conspicuous than those obtained by ultrasonic irradiation performed without a cooling system.

As a result of our research work we can view the phenomena which appear in the posterior labyrinth in consequence of direct ultrasonic irradiation using the Arslan technique in the following way:

(1) The heating effect developed by the transducer and by the applicator rod during ultrasonic irradiation causes the appearance of endolymph currents and of consequent "irritative" nystagmus of the eye. The heating effect generated by the transducer, therefore, precedes the heating action developed

[4] During the "cold" ultrasonic irradiation the temperature of the applicator rod was sometimes caused to vary below and above 38°C. In the former case (temperature below 38°C) a "paralytic" nystagmus appeared in the transversal plane of the orbit, that is, rostral directed in the left eye (the ultrasonic irradiation affected the left labyrinth) and caudal in the right eye. In the latter case (temperature above 38°C) there appeared an "irritative" nystagmus, that is, caudal directed in the left eye and rostral in the right one.

These phenomena were observed when the animal was kept with its body and head in its customary posture (position [a]). When we modified the position of its head in space (positions [b], [c], [d], [e], [f]), the eye nystagmus obtained in the above mentioned manner, namely, by making the applicator rod temperature vary above and below 38°C, showed some modifications absolutely identical to those described in the first part of this note (Figs. 3 through 8).

by the ultrasonic beam itself upon the irradiated tissue and, modifying its state of molecular aggregation, aids the diffusion of the ultrasonic beam (19). These endolymph currents in the semicircular canals last all through irradiation, which in this research work was of the intensity of 13 w/cm^2, and become more intense as the plane of the canal approaches the vertical.

(2) The nystagmus, following the endolymph currents which originate during ultrasonic irradiation, shows a breadth of twitches and an intensity which progressively grow fainter owing to the progressive formation of endocellular lesions due to the action of ultrasound (vibratory, heating, and cavitational action) at the level of the neurosensorial epithelium. At a certain moment the lesions of this epithelium grow so extensive that they induce a functional paralysis of the vestibular receptor which manifests itself by the appearance of "paralytic" nystagmus. The preliminary heating effect generated by the transducer, therefore, does not interfere with the effects produced by the ultrasound energy on the labyrinth.

(3) The selective destruction of the neuroepithelia of the cristae ampullaris is due to the directionality of the ultrasonic beam, that is, to its property of propagating only in the direction in which it is emitted. This destruction, proved by histological research, takes place only when ultrasonic irradiation is continued for a certain period of time and is connected with the intensity of the ultrasonic beam, its wavelength, and other factors. The appearance of a "paralytic" nystagmus at the end of irradiation is the functional manifestation of this destruction. It causes a functional deficit when reaching a certain degree, both because of the number of neurosensorial cells affected and because of the severity of the endocellular lesion. Arslan and others have shown that the destruction is never completed at once, because even after the irradiation there still remain certain reflex phenomena which, in most cases, are replaced by areflexia within 2 to 3 months.

(4) If the effect of the ultrasonic irradiation is less intense (because of lower intensity or shorter time of application), there is no destruction of the receptor at the end of the irradiation, as an "irritative" nystagmus appears only at a later time (that is, after the irradiation has been discontinued). This nystagmus, however, is not reversed by causing changes in the position of the head in space, and it is, therefore, due to the presence of some mild histological modifications induced into the neurosensorial epithelium by ultrasonic irradiation, and not to the presence of endolymph currents. Most probably these endocellular histological modifications, the formal aspect of which is still unknown, cause an "irritative" condition in the neurosensorial epithelium (that is, not in the cupola). Only during the days following ultrasonic irradiation, and only if it has been intense enough, does there appear a "paralytic" nystagmus which, however, is never accompanied by a clear unilateral labyrinthine destruction syndrome.

(5) The phenomena observed in the animal and their interpretation make it possible to explain many of the phenomena observed in man during direct ultrasonic irradiation of the posterior labyrinth using Arslan's method, as it is carried out in severe cases of Ménière's disease.

REFERENCES

1. Altmann, F., and J. G. Waltner (1959). The treatment of Ménière's disease with ultrasonic waves. Arch. Otolaryngol. *69*, 1.
2. Angell James, J., G. A. Dalton, M. A. Bullen, H. F. Freundlich, and J. C. Hopkins (1960). The ultrasonic treatment of Ménière's disease. J. Laryngol. & Otolaryngol. *74*, 730.
3. Ariagno, R. P. (1960). Treatment of Ménière's disease with ultrasound. Arch. Otolaryngol. *71*, 573.
4. Arslan, M. (1953). L'applicazione diretta degli ultrasuoni sul labirinto osseo nella cura delle labirintosi. Minerva Otolaringol. *3*, 4.
5. Arslan, M. (1958). Ultrasonic surgery of the labyrinth in patients with Ménière's syndrome. Scientia Medica Ital. 7, 301.
6. Beck, C. (1958). Ultraschallwirkung am menschlichen Bogengan. Arch. Or. Heilk. u. Hals *172*, 513.
7. Bötner, V., and O. Sala (1960). L'irradiazione ultrasonica diretta del labirinto posteriore secondo Arslan nell'animale: rilievi tecnici e sperimentali. Boll. Soc. Ital. Biol. Sper. *36*, 914.
8. Brain, D. J., B. H. Colman, R. B. Lumsden, and R. F. Ogilvie (1960). The effects of ultrasound on the internal ear: a histological investigation. J. Laryngol. & Otolaryngol. *74*, 628.
9. De Stefani, G. B. (1956). Gli ultrasuoni nell'otosclerosi. Ricerche cliniche e sperimentali. Arch. Ital. Otolaringol. Rinol. Laringol. Suppl. 27.
10. Dubs, R. (1957). Über die Ultraschallbehandlung des Morbus Ménière nach der Methode von Arslan. Practica Otolaryngol.-Rhinol.-Laryngol. *19*, 401.
11. Fischetto, A. (1959–60). Rilievi istologici sulle modificazioni indotte dall'irradiazione ultrasonica diretta del labirinto posteriore secondo Arslan nel coniglio. Tesi di Specializzazione in Clinica O.R.L. (Padova).
12. Fortunato, V. (1955). Ultrasons et labyrinthe antérieur. C.R. Congr. Soc. Franç. d'Otolaryngol.-Rhinol.-Laryngol. (Paris).
13. Grandis, G. (1958). La cura delle vertigini e degli acufeni nella malattia di Ménière con la distruzione ultrasonica dell'apparato vestibolare. Valsalva *34*, 138.
14. Güttner, W. von (1954). Die Energieverteilung im menschlichen Körper bei Ultraschall-einstrahlung. Acustica *4*, 547.
15. Ironside, M. S., and J. R. Lindsay (1959). Ultrasonic therapy for relief of vertigo due to Ménière's disease. Laryngoscope *69*, 899.
16. Lumsden, R. B. (1958). Treatment of Ménière's disease with ultrasound. Proc. Roy. Soc. Med. *51*, 617.
17. McLay, K., M. Flin, and F. C. Ormerod (1961). Histological changes in the inner ear resulting from the application of ultrasonic energy. J. Laryngol. & Otolaryngol. *75*, 345.
18. Molinari, G. A. (1960). Il comportamento del nistagmo post-rotatorio, nel coniglio, dopo irradiazione ultrasonica diretta del labirinto di diversa intensità. Boll. Soc. Ital. Biol. Sper. *36*, 924.
19. Muzzioli, L. A. (1961). Los ultrasonidos. Ed. by Univers. de Concepción (Chile).
20. Sala, O., and G. B. De Stefani (1955). Applicazione bilaterale diretta di ultrasuoni sul labirinto osseo in un caso di gravissima labirintosi bilaterale. Arch. Ital. Otolaringol. Rinol. Laringol. *66*, 208.
21. Sala, O., and G. A. Molinari (1960). Il comportamento del nistagmo vestibolare da stimolazione ultrasonica diretta del labirinto secondo Arslan a seguito di cambiamenti della posizione della testa nello spazio (ricerche sperimentali nel coniglio). Boll. Soc. Ital. Biol. Sper. *36*, 927.
22. Tato, J. M. (1961). Trattamento chirurgico della sindrome di Ménière con la

distruzione ultrasonica dell'apparato vestibolare. Ann. Laringol. Otolaringol. Rinol. Faringol. *60*, 143.
23. Wolfson, R. J. (1961). Ultrasonic therapy for vertigo with chronic suppurative mastoiditis. Arch. Otolaryngol. *74*, 387.

DISCUSSION

DR. LIBBER: Thank you very much, Dr. Gordon. Would you be willing to discuss Dr. Arslan's paper?

DR. GORDON: I would be honored.

DR. WEISSLER: With reference to the discussion of the neurosensory membrane and the canal I have two questions: Could you say something concerning the elementary histology of the connections of the nerve fibers to the neurosensory epithelium; and is it your feeling that the disruption of the neurosensory epithelium is related to fluid streaming or to cavitation? It is my understanding that this is not simply a temperature effect.

DR. GORDON: No, that is the point. You see, the nystagmus is apparently an effect of temperature from convection currents produced in this field. Now it is being rather hard on a radiologist to ask him to talk about neurohistology, but I shall do my best. Enlargements of the actual nerve cells with light microscopy indicate that nothing has happened to these nerve cells. There is no doubt that some damage is being done to the fine structure in the cells of the cresta, but the ganglion cells are in the wall, and since the nerve fibers and the cells on the irradiated and nonirradiated side look quite similar, one has great difficulty in believing that there can be any direct physical action on anything more than the very superficial part of the nerve cells.

DR. HUGHES: In Ménière's syndrome, the space on the left side, the one filled with endolymph, becomes distended and there is pressure throughout the whole of the endolymphatic system which results in the pushing of that membrane (Reisner's membrane) to the left, into the perilymphatic space. The necrosis is probably due to the disfunction of that tissue toward the top of the triangle (Stria vascularis). It appears that this tissue throughout the vestibular apparatus serves the main endolymph, and it seems to be a disfunction of that which produces Ménière's syndrome. This is why it is surprising that investigators look for the destruction of the nervous element rather than for the destruction of the epithelium. We have measured the metabolism of these various tissues and found that this tissue is the most active of any in the body in terms of respiration. It is this tissue, I think, that one wants to affect. Do you agree?

DR. GORDON: No, I do not, and in this regard I would like to point out that, under certain conditions, the vestibular functions of a patient can improve. Once the pressure inside has been diminished, one gets a better reaction within the cochlea.

DR. HUGHES: I should add that the endolymph and perilymph are quite different in composition. The endolymph has high potassium and no sodium, and the perilymph has high sodium and no potassium.

DR. VON GIERKE: Do you destroy hearing?

DR. GORDON: No, you improve it. You are taking advantage of the fact that the sound is coming off almost at right angles to the direction of the semicircular canal, so the acoustic coupling of waves that are going around that part is very poor. There is a temporary falling off on the audiogram for about 24 hr in all cases, but, in the long term, the improvement is substantial in a fair proportion of the cases.

DR. KOSSOFF: I understand that you have a new type of ultrasonic instrument for application to Ménière's. How many clinical operations have you performed on patients?

DR. GORDON: Five so far. I'm sorry to say we have run out of patients with Ménière's disease in London. Not that I wish anyone any harm. It seems that Ménière's disease has a very strange geographical distribution. It appears to be very prevalent in the Po Valley, fairly prevalent in New York, and quite rare in Britain.

DR. KOSSOFF: We have the same problem. Concerning nystagmus, what sort of observation of nystagmus did you get using the new type of equipment?

DR. GORDON: The nystagmus reaction is sometimes very slight and rather unconvincing. We had to do our best largely by dead reckoning. We felt that when we had given 10 min at about 8 w/cm^2, it was time we stopped. We were generating very little heat with the ultrasound. There was no heat, hence there were no convection currents.

DR. KOSSOFF: We have done operations at 3 Mc and basically had no pain.

DR. NYBORG: To understand the mechanical action involved in this technique it seems necessary to know the coefficient of absorption for bone. Dr. Dunn quoted a value of about 8 to 9 db/cm for this coefficient. This seems considerably less than the values which, I believe, have been reported by British workers.

DR. GORDON: The work on the parietal bone using the echo technique, which I completed 2 or 3 years ago, showed 4.5 db/mm. This was at 1.25 Mc. This is fairly close to the figure observed in machined slices of petrous bone by the Bristol workers, namely, values of the order of 4 to 6 db/mm. Bone is not like, shall we say, fat or muscle. The variations in the physical structure of bone are much greater than those of most other tissues, so one can have wide variations in the results of different workers. These variations are a reflection of the different pieces of bone they have been using rather than of their technique.

DR. VON GIERKE: Is this always continuous irradiation or are there interruptions?

DR. GORDON: The interruptions are all entirely unintentional. I would say they were interrupted because of the instability of the machine. J. Angell James interrupted every 5 min in order to recheck his doses. We do not interrupt unless we begin to have trouble with an air lock in the water circulation; that is, we try to make it as continuous as possible and as steady in level as possible.

Dr. von Gierke: Why is pulsed energy not used since the heating effect is not desirable?

Dr. Gordon: We were trying to get a fairly long total period of treatment to be able to observe the nystagmus. When giving a long period of treatment, there is nothing to be gained by giving short pulses, unless there is danger of overloading your crystal, and at the levels at which we are working that doesn't arise.

Dr. von Gierke: Yes, but if I understand you correctly, the nystagmus is really not necessary, and even undesirable. It somehow clouds the picture. You could use higher intensities.

Dr. Gordon: No, if higher intensities are used there is greater risk of generating heat by absorption in bone, and this is conducted to the facial nerve. There is no doubt that in Arslan's apparatus the heat conducted from the metal affected the facial nerve much more than the ultrasound. The faster it is done, the bigger the temperature gradient. It is more manageable when you are working at low intensities. It is a bit tiring if you must irradiate for 40 min, but 10 min is perfectly acceptable.

12

Destruction of Transplantable Ascites Tumors by Means of Intense Ultrasound

TOSHIO WAGAI, M.D.
Department of Surgery, School of Medicine, Juntendo University, Tokyo, Japan

YOSHIMITSU KIKUCHI
Research Institute of Electrical Communication, Tohoku University, Sendai, Japan

Introduction by Dr. Libber

Next, we are to hear from Dr. Wagai, another of our colleagues from Japan. The work discussed in this paper is the result of a collaborative effort between Dr. Kikuchi, who spoke to us earlier on ultrasonic cavitation, and Dr. Wagai, who is a physician. It gives us great pleasure to have the opportunity to hear Dr. Wagai present this paper.

A number of reports concerning the effects of intense ultrasound on biological tissues have been published by many investigators. We have been studying the problem of whether intense ultrasound can selectively destroy tumor cells while leaving the normal cells intact. In this research we used various kinds of transplantable ascites hepatoma cells, that is, AH 130, AH 13, AH 7974, and Yoshida sarcoma in rat. The intensity of ultrasound was 1 to 2 w/cm^2 and the frequency was 1 Mc.

Figure 1 shows the ultrasonic generator used in these experiments. This apparatus produces frequencies of 0.4, 1, 2, or 4 Mc, but in this paper we will report only the results obtained with a frequency of 1 Mc. By using a barium titanate transducer of 1 Mc with a pair of reflectors, as shown in Figure 2, we were able to achieve a wide ultrasonic field above the transducer. Figure 3 shows the ultrasonic field above the reflector, with many cavitation bubbles.

In the first experiments, we irradiated 1 ml of the ascites cells in vitro at an ultrasonic intensity of 2 w/cm^2 and at a frequency of 1 Mc. Control AH 130 tumor cells are shown in Figure 4; Figures 5 and 6 show the AH 130 cells after 3- and 10-min periods of irradiation, respectively. We observed a slight destruction of the tumor cells after about 1-min irradiation, and complete de-

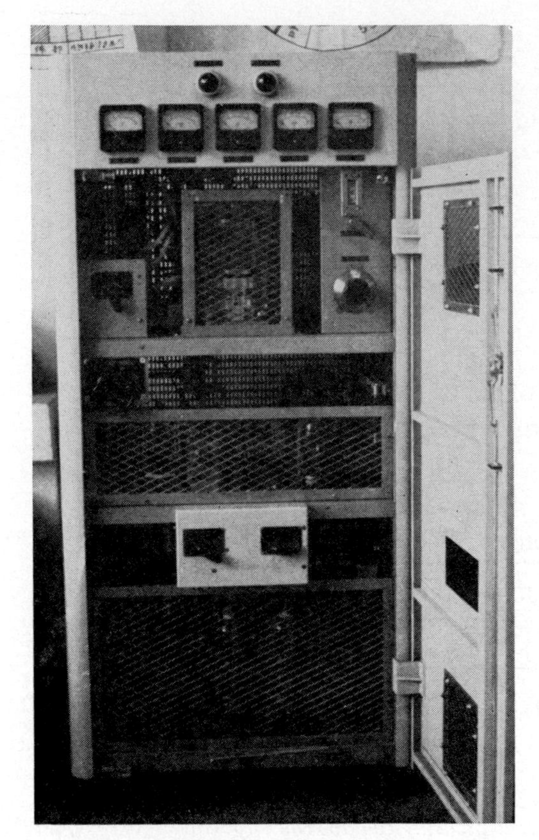

FIGURE 1. Five-hundred-watt high-frequency generator.

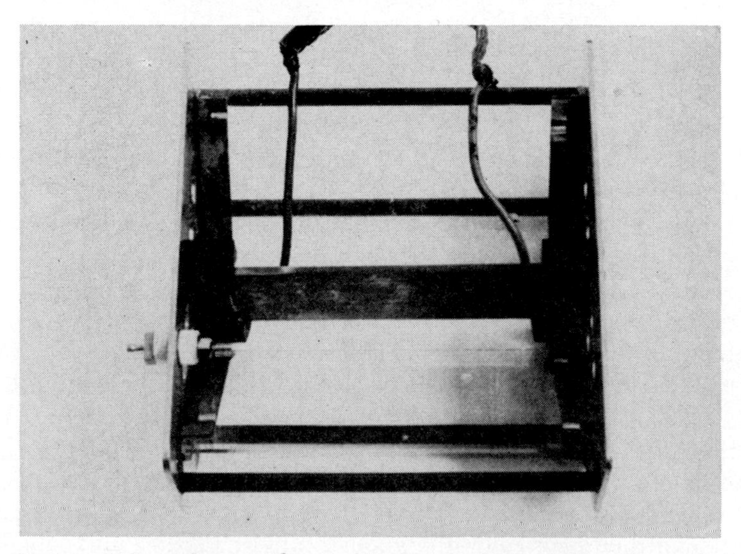

FIGURE 2. Transducer with pair of reflectors (viewed from the top).

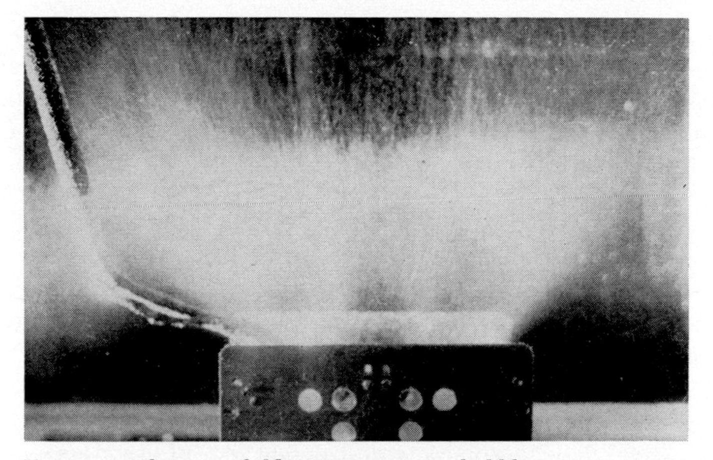

FIGURE 3. Ultrasonic field. Note cavitation bubbles.

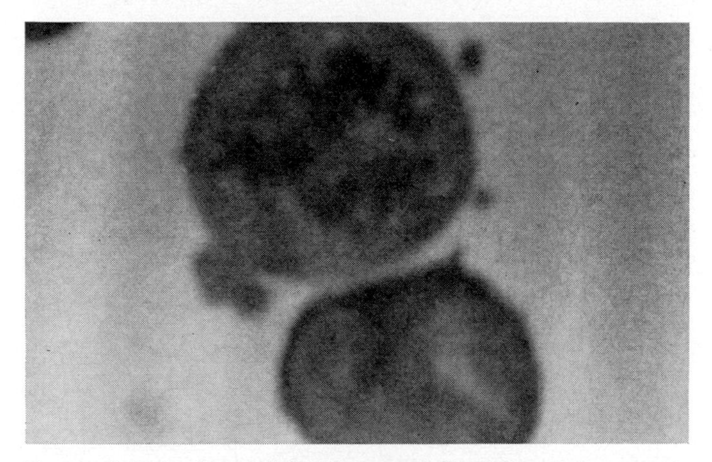

FIGURE 4. Unirradiated AH 130 tumor cells x900.

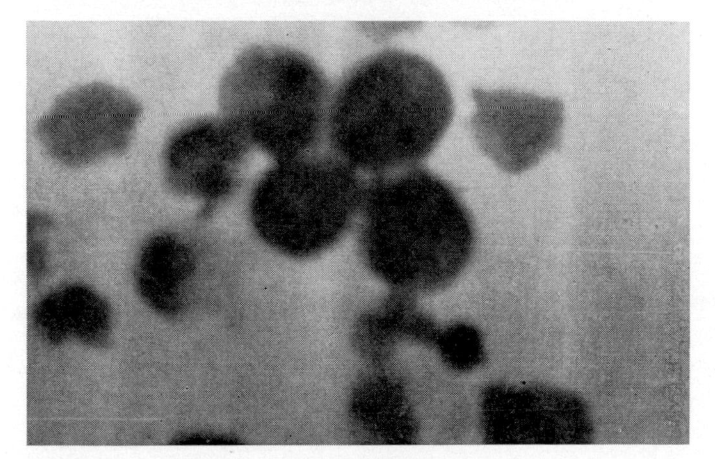

FIGURE 5. AH 130 tumor cells irradiated 3 min.

struction of the cells was evident after 10-min irradiation. Only slight changes were observed after 10-min irradiation of AH 13 cells. Control cells of AH 7974 in Figure 7 show a characteristic island structure. However, it can be seen in Figure 8 that AH 7974 tumor cells were not destroyed by a 10-min exposure to ultrasound and the characteristic island structures were not isolated. A comparison of Figures 9 and 10 shows a slight change in Yoshida sarcoma cells after a 10-min exposure to ultrasound, but human blood cells were not affected.

The comparison chart (Fig. 11) shows that AH 130 cells were destroyed completely within 10 min by an ultrasonic exposure of 2 w/cm^2, while the other tumor cells were not destroyed. The important finding in this series of experiments was that there is a remarkable difference in the destructive effect of ultrasound depending upon the variety of tumor cells.

We discovered that the complete destruction of all these tumor cells took

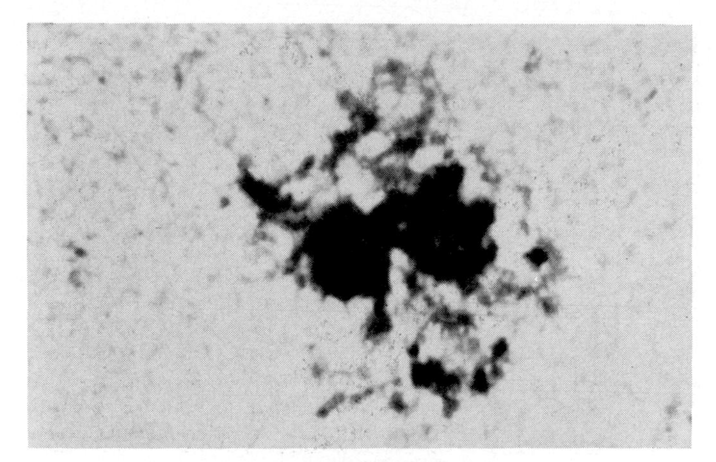

FIGURE 6. AH 130 tumor cells irradiated 10 min.

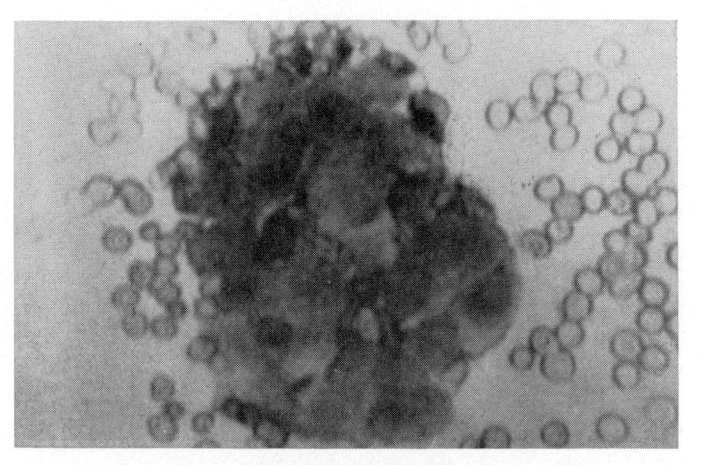

FIGURE 7. Unirradiated AH 7974 tumor cells.

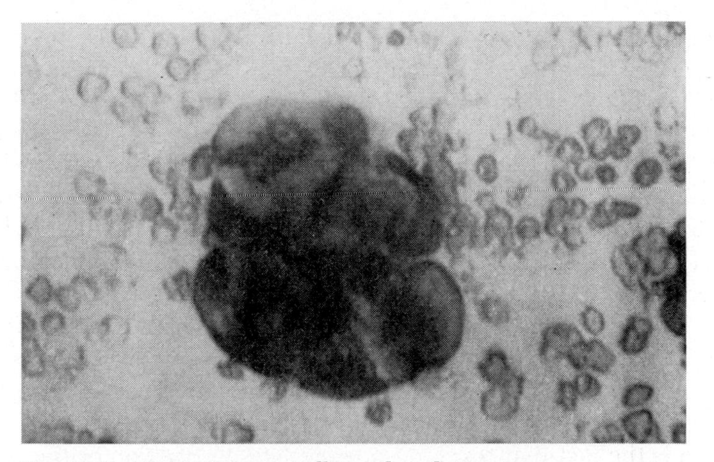

FIGURE 8. AH 7974 tumor cells irradiated 10 min.

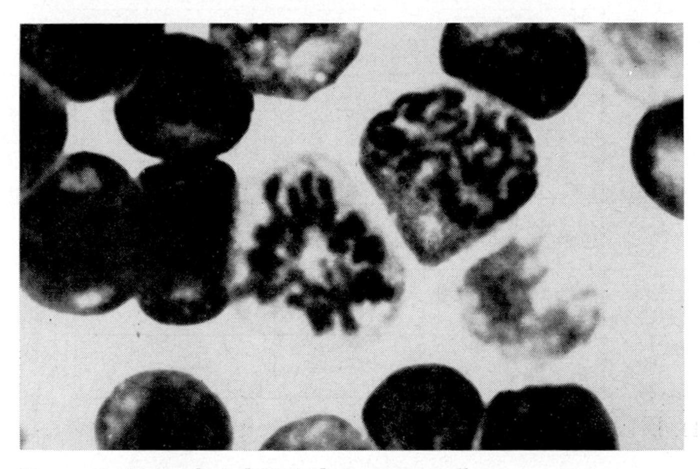

FIGURE 9. Unirradiated Yoshida sarcoma cells.

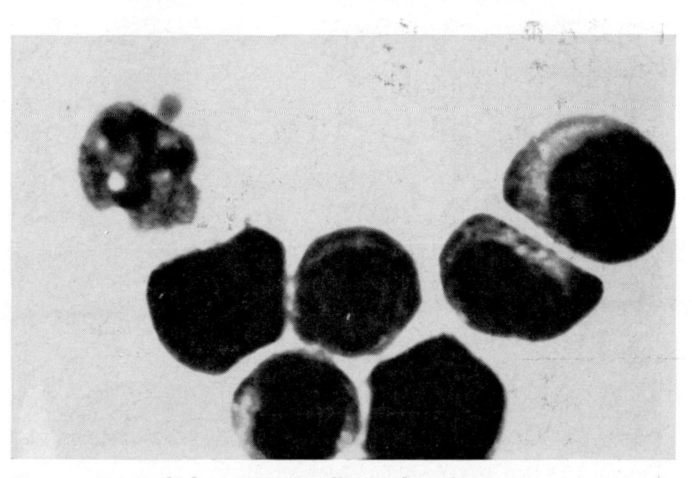

FIGURE 10. Yoshida sarcoma cells irradiated 10 min.

place when a small amount of metal colloid was added to ascites cells which were to undergo ultrasonic irradiation. Figure 12A indicates the appearance of the control Yoshida sarcoma cells while Figure 12B shows Yoshida sarcoma cells irradiated by ultrasound with 0.01 mg of gold colloid added to 1 ml of ascites. The complete destruction of tumor cells was observed within 5-min exposure. The AH 7974 tumor cells in Figure 13 were completely destroyed within 5 min by the same method. These phenomena are observed not only with gold colloid, but also with mercury or silver colloid. Human blood cells, however, with gold colloid added were not destroyed by exposure to ultrasound. The mechanism of this phenomenon may be based on the fact that the metal particles in a colloidal state collide with the tumor cells, since both of them are accelerated by ultrasound to a high relative velocity, and thus immediate destruction of the tumor cells may take place. In support of this assumption is the fact that this kind of complete destruction of the tumor cells

INTENSITY / TUMOR CELLS	2 W/cm²	ADDING GOLD COLLOID US 2 W/cm²
AH 130	+++	+++
AH 13	±	+++
AH 7974	—	+++
YOSHIDA SARCOMA	—	+++
HUMAN BLOOD CELL	—	—

FIGURE 11. Destructive effect of 1 Mc ultrasound on tumor cells and human blood cells in vitro.

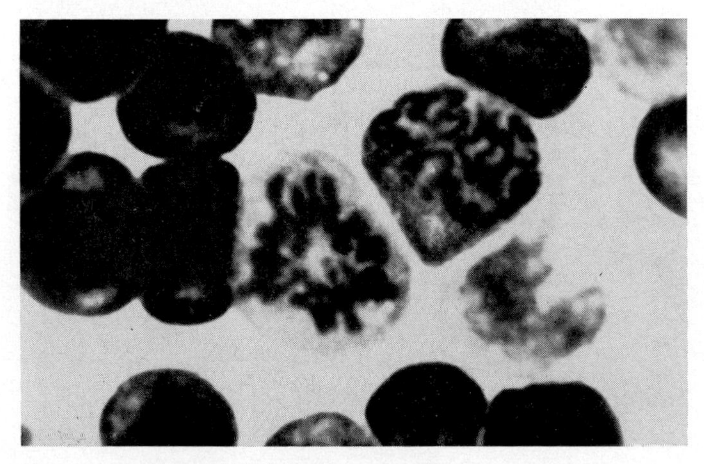

FIGURE 12A. Control Yoshida sarcoma cells.

by ultrasound is not observed when various chemical agents, such as anticancerous alkylating agents, are added instead of a metal colloid to ascites.

As a screening test we used 100 rats transplanted with Yoshida sarcoma. We injected 0.2 mg of gold colloid into the abdominal cavity of the rats after which the whole body of the rat was irradiated with ultrasound for 10 min. The intensity of ultrasound was 2 w/cm^2 and the frequency was 1 Mc. Figure 14 illustrates the method of whole body irradiation. As a control, we irradiated a group of intact rats with the same ultrasonic dosage and found no histological changes in the various tissues of the liver, heart, small intestine, lung, and kidney 30 days after irradiation. Figure 15 shows graphically the results of tests on the destructive effect of ultrasound on the tumor cells. Curve 1 is the survival curve of untreated Yoshida sarcoma and Curve 2 represents the cases which received only one shot of ultrasonic irradiation on the third day after transplantation. Curve 3 shows results for one shot of ultrasound on the first day after transplantation. A comparison of Curve 2 with Curve 3 indicates

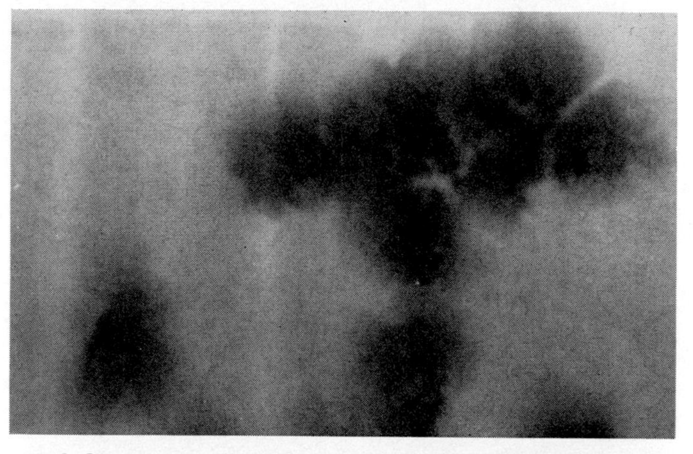

FIGURE 12B. Yoshida sarcoma cells with gold colloid added, irradiated 5 min.

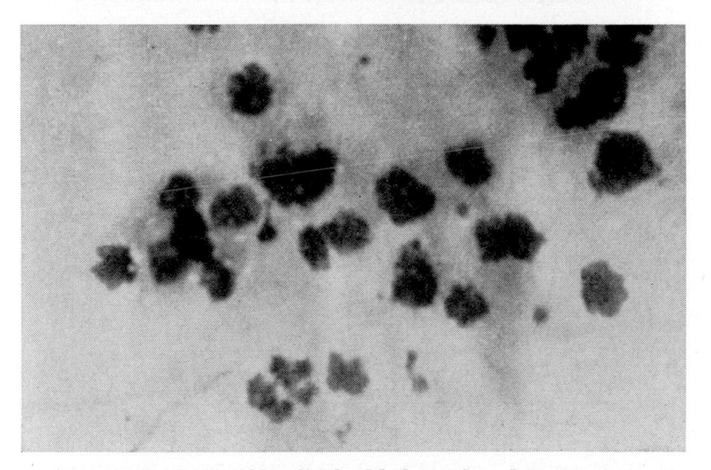

FIGURE 13. AH 7974 cells, with gold colloid added, irradiated 5 min.

that survival was highest when irradiation took place on the first day after transplantation. Many problems remain to be solved in regard to the ultrasonic dosages and the amounts and kinds of colloids to be injected into the rats before this method will result in complete success in obtaining survival of rats transplanted with ascites tumor.

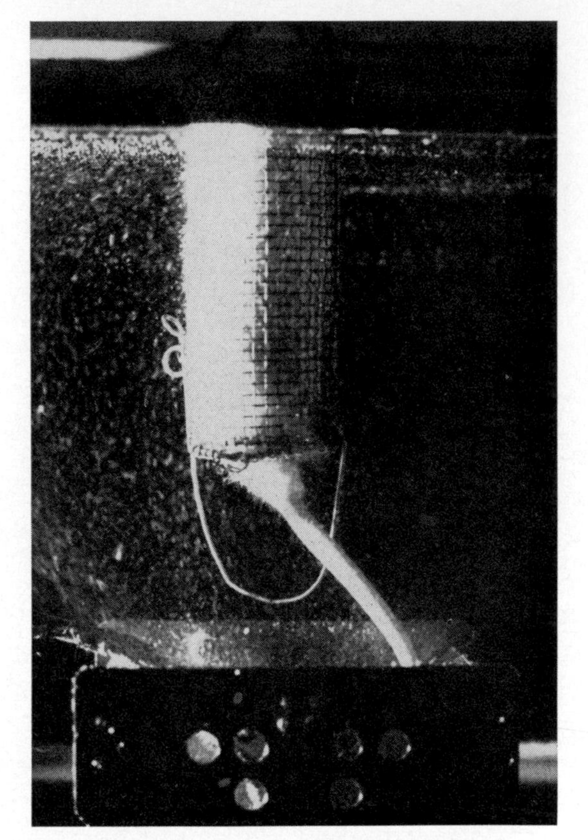

FIGURE 14. Irradiation of whole body of rat.

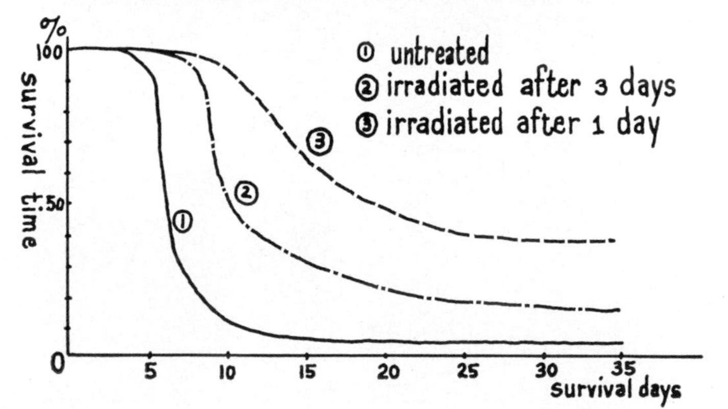

FIGURE 15. Screening tests of Yoshida sarcoma. 0.2 mg gold colloid injected into abdominal cavity of rats. Irradiated once with ultrasound at 1 Mc, 2 w/cm^2 for 10 min.

DISCUSSION

DR. CURTIS: In this experiment with animals did you do any type of controls in which you exposed the whole body to irradiation? Did you find out how long they would live after this treatment was administered? If I understand correctly, untreated means they were not irradiated. It would be interesting to know whether or not these animals would survive just the ultrasonic treatment.

DR. KIKUCHI: Figure 15 shows the results for rats with Yoshida sarcoma, plotted as Curve 3, in comparison to the untreated which were not irradiated until after 3 days of Yoshida sarcoma transplantation. Dr. Wagai states that normal rats irradiated with the same intensity and the same frequency of ultrasound have shown no change.

DR. CURTIS: Do the animals without any tumor cells survive this treatment indefinitely?

DR. KIKUCHI: Yes, Dr. Wagai has shown that for the controls, the irradiation has no effect on survival. Histological studies of liver, lung, heart, small bowel, and kidney tissue of the intact rat, irradiated with the same intensity ultrasound, indicate no effect of the irradiation.

DR. CURTIS: How much of the sound is actually getting into these animals? It looked as if no hair had been removed from them. It is my understanding that a great proportion of the energy would be absorbed by the hair. Were any measurements made to determine how much energy was getting into the animal?

DR. KIKUCHI: The abdomen was shaved prior to irradiation.

DR. WOEBER: Even though I don't think it will be possible to cure cancer in any animal by using ultrasound, I should like to have more information on this in vitro investigation. We have undertaken many investigations on the biological application of ultrasound in which we found the problem is mainly one of biological dosage. You are able to destroy cells in vitro by using metal in colloidal suspension, a method we have not used. We have been interested in destroying bacteria with antigens. Previously we mixed the antigens by different techniques, as for example, chemically. Today, however, we tend to do it by mechanical means, that is, by ultrasound. At the University of Bonn, a colleague and I prepare antigens for prevention of tuberculosis. We are able to make a diagnosis, sensitize, immunize, and so on. Now, if one used ultrasound for a similar application on carcinoma cells and destroyed such cells, perhaps an antigen for the treatment of cancer could be found. This was what I was looking for in your report. If you have the opportunity to work in the bacteriological field, I suggest that you go on and make the same tests on the melanoma. I hope I have stimulated your interest in discovering an antigen which can destroy carcinomatous cells in the same way that we can destroy bacteria.

DR. KIKUCHI: Did you irradiate cells with ultrasound?

DR. WOEBER: Yes, we irradiated tumor cells until just a few weeks ago, and we have used ultrasound on bacteria. We succeeded in discovering an antigen for tuberculosis. Therefore, I think that you could discover an antigen, inject it into animals, and then reinoculate the tumor and see what results. This is a very necessary study in the field of oncology. I presume the colloid is injected for more effective heating of the cells, since this gives more interfaces?

DR. KIKUCHI: We cannot precisely explain the mechanism at this time but it seems that gold colloid is the most effective. In this method the ultrasound intensity is low enough to allow the animal to survive, but the injection of gold, silver, or other mercury colloid is the distinguishing factor. We have had some success in survival studies with the normal rat irradiated with low-intensity ultrasound, but we are searching for complete success in survival for irradiated rats with tumors.

DR. WOEBER: I don't consider the intensity you use as low, because 2 w/cm^2 is quite high for rats or mice. A higher level is not possible.

DR. KIKUCHI: We have shown that the rats can survive this irradiation without any histological effect on the tissues. Dr. Wagai has stated that the rat can live its normal life span.

DR. NYBORG: This effect of the colloid is very interesting as well as puzzling. Can you tell us whether or not the colloid is ingested into the cells? Does it eventually find its way into the interior of the cells?

DR. KIKUCHI: Such information must be gained by examination with the electron microscope, and we are planning to discover whether the gold colloid has been absorbed into the cells or is suspended very close to the cells.

DR. NYBORG: Was the colloid which you used put in in a dry state, so that it had some gas on its surface? Dr. Hughes introduced various kinds of small particles into suspensions which enhanced the ultrasonic action apparently by virtue of air, which goes into the solution with the particles.

DR. KIKUCHI: The gold colloid was wet. The colloid is prepared in a liquid state of suspension and then injected into the abdominal cavity. No investigation has been made as to whether very small microbubbles adhere to the colloid, but usually that kind of bubble cannot last for several hours, or even several minutes.

DR. WEISSLER: With respect to the action of the gold colloid on the cells, you said that you think it may be that the gold colloid hits the cell because of the differential acceleration. Is it possible that cavitation is easier because there are more interfaces between the gold and the liquid around it so that you get more cavitation, more shock wave production because of cavitation, and it's the shock wave produced in the liquid by cavitation that gives the disruption of the sarcoma cell?

DR. KIKUCHI: We made the assumption that both the gold colloid and the cells may collide with a great difference of relative velocity.

DR. NYBORG: I know from experience that it's not particularly easy to get rid of small, very thin surface layers of air on small particles. For example, in some work where we wanted to have particles whose density was very nearly equal to that of the liquid in which they were suspended so that they could indicate motions in the liquid, we had some difficulty with particles whose density was supposed to be equal. They were, instead, floating. The reason they floated apparently was because of air which was occluded on the surface. In order to get rid of this, we had to boil the water, evacuate the system, and so on.

DR. KIKUCHI: Yes, I agree that care must be taken, but it is unlikely that an air film is in contact with the gold colloid that we use because this colloid is prepared by precipitation in a solution.

13

Technical Developments of Focused Ultrasound and Its Biological and Surgical Applications in Japan

KATUYA YOSHIOKA
Osaka University, Institute of Scientific and Industrial Research, Osaka, Japan

MASUHISA OKA
Osaka University Hospital, The First Department of Surgery, Osaka, Japan

Introduction by Dr. Weissler

Two papers to be presented this morning indicate the present diversity in applications of ultrasound to biological and medical problems. The first paper will be presented by Dr. Katuya Yoshioka of Osaka University, Japan. Since Dr. Yoshioka is primarily associated with the physics and engineering aspects of the research program, his talk will emphasize the instrumentation developments required in the application of ultrasound as a surgical tool. Following Dr. Yoshioka's presentation, Professor Francis Fry will review the work at the Biophysical Research Laboratory on the use of ultrasound as a tool for investigating basic biological mechanisms.

It is a great pleasure to welcome Dr. Katuya Yoshioka.

Since 1957, research on biological and medical applications of focused ultrasound has been underway in our country, primarily at Osaka University; recently, investigators at Niigata Medical College and Juntendo University have also undertaken work in this field. The following aspects of this research will be discussed in this paper:

I. Working characteristics of the lens-type focusing transducer.
II. Direct calibration of transducers by thermoelectric probes.
III. Lesion size obtained.
IV. Relative resistivities of the nervous system and blood vessels.
V. Effect of irradiation on the hypophysis.
VI. Ultrasonic operations performed.

I. WORKING CHARACTERISTICS OF THE LENS-TYPE FOCUSING TRANSDUCER

We have recently constructed a focusing ultrasonic generator for use in surgical work. When the target is deeply seated in tissues, a focusing transducer with high energy output is required to overcome the attenuation of ultrasound. The irradiation heads are of a single-beam type consisting of multiple quartz crystals, a half-wavelength duraluminum plate, and a polystyrene plano-concave lens. The triple crystal head was used for 1.46 Mc and the quintuple head for 944 kc. Figure 1 shows the triple-type transducer. The X-cut quartz crystals (60 mm in diameter) are cemented together, the piezo-

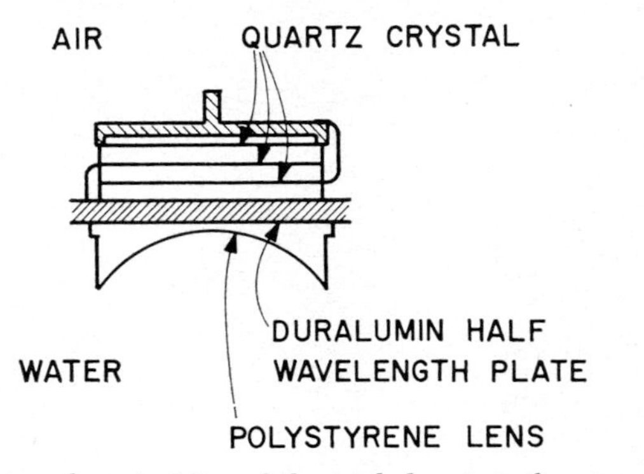

FIGURE 1. The working characteristics of the triple-lens-type focusing transducer.

electric polarity of each element being in the same direction. They are connected electrically as shown in the figure. When this transducer is driven at the resonance frequency of the thickness vibration of each element, the amplitude of the sound radiated will be, for a given electrode voltage, n times as large as that of a single-crystal system. Hence the sonic output is, for a given electrode voltage, n^2 times as large as that of a single-crystal system. This situation is confirmed by the measurement of the equivalent shunt resistance of the multiple-type transducer, which shows a decrease to $1/n^2$ of that of a single-crystal system. Since the sonic energy output of the quartz crystal is limited by the spark discharge over the electrodes, the maximum obtainable power output of the multiple system is also n^2 times as large as that of the single-crystal system. The sonic output of a focusing transducer of this type may be written at the resonance as follows:

$$I = I_0 \cdot \sigma \tag{1}$$

where

I_0: sound energy output into the lens,

σ: energy transmission coefficient of the lens.

The effect of the reflected wave from the spherical surface to the crystals was found experimentally to be small. In this case, the transducer works as if the material of the lens extends to infinity and we have:

$$I_0 \doteqdot n^2 \frac{4S}{\rho_{11} C_l} \left(\frac{\epsilon_{11}}{d}\right)^2 \cdot V^2 \tag{2}$$

where

S: area of the quartz crystal,

ϵ_{11}: piezoelectric constant,

d: thickness of the crystal,
V: electrode voltage,
ρ_{11}: density of the lens material,
C_l: propagation velocity of longitudinal wave in the lens.

Assuming that the reflected wave from the spherical surface contributes nothing to the main beam, the energy transmission coefficient, σ, is given in Equation (3) as follows:

$$\sigma = \sigma_o \cdot e^{-2at} \quad (3)$$

where $\sigma_o = I/\pi a^2 W_i$ and σ_o is the energy transmission coefficient of the lens for $t = 0$. In these expressions, I is the sonic output into water and

$$I = \int_o^{\theta_2} 2\pi r^2 \cdot \sin\theta_2 \cdot \cos\theta_1 \cdot \left(\frac{2}{L+K}\right)^2 \cdot \frac{\rho_1 C_1}{\rho_{11} C_l} \cdot e^{-2al} \cdot W_i \cdot d\theta_2$$

where

$$L = \frac{C_l}{C_1} \cdot \frac{\cos\theta_1}{\cos\theta_2} \cdot \cos 2\psi_2, \quad K = \frac{\frac{\rho_1}{\rho_{11}} + \frac{C_t^2}{C_1^2} \sin 2\theta_1 \cdot \sin 2\psi_2}{1 - 2\frac{C_1^2}{C_l^1} \sin^2\theta_2}$$

and (see Fig. 2) W_i: intensity of the incident wave at position A,

r: radius of curvature of the lens,
a: radius of the circular boundary,
θ_1: angle of refraction,
θ_2: angle of incidence,
ρ_1: density of water,
c_1: sound velocity in water,
c_l: propagation velocity of longitudinal wave in lens,
c_t: propagation velocity of shear wave in lens,
a: amplitude absorption coefficient in lens,

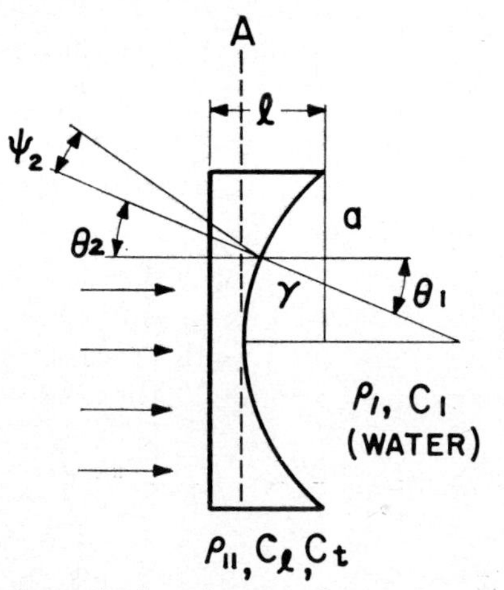

FIGURE 2. Parameters used to calculate the rate of energy transmission of the lens $t = 0$ (Equation [3]).

l: thickness of lens at the boundary,
ψ_2: angle of reflection of shear wave in lens,
t: thickness of lens at the center,
ρ_{11}: density of the lens material.

The graph in Figure 3 shows the coefficient, σ_o, of energy transmission of lenses of polystyrene and polymethyl methacrylate as functions of the diameter. The calculated value of energy transmission of the lens was equal, within the accuracy of experiment, to the measured value of the electroacoustic conversion efficiency of the focusing transducer. This shows that most of the energy loss in a focusing transducer of this type is the loss through the lens and that the lens loss is actually of the magnitude calculated here.

Figure 4 shows the temperature dependence of the sound energy output of one of the focusing transducers when unit voltage is applied to the electrode. This is deduced from the measured values of the equivalent resistance and

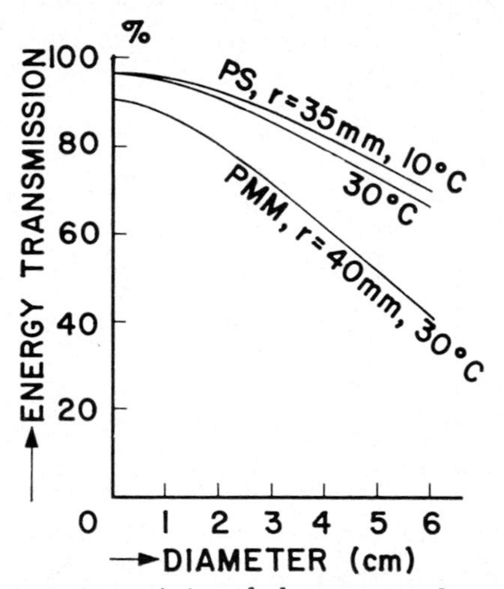

FIGURE 3. The rate of energy transmission of plano-concave lens t = 0. PS, polystyrene; PMM, polymethyl methacrylate.

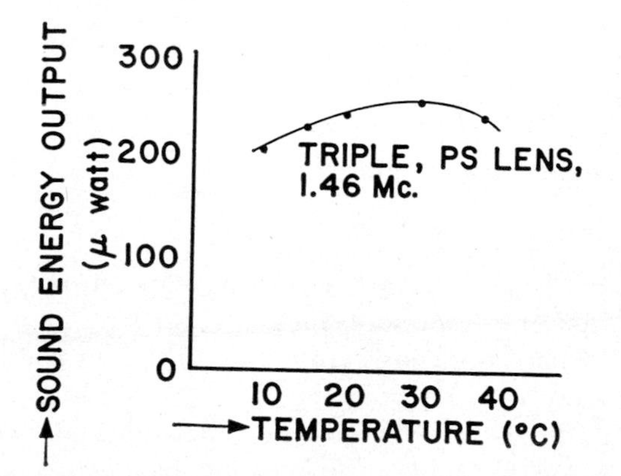

FIGURE 4. Temperature dependence of the sound energy output of a focusing transducer. PS, polystyrene.

the calculated rate of transmission of energy of the lens. The multiple-crystal-type transducers mentioned above were found by frequent calibration to be sufficiently stable. They are driven by a tube generator of 1.4 kw electric output, and the frequencies are controlled by quartz crystals at 1.46 Mc and 944 kc. The transducer is mounted on a stereotaxic irradiation device which gives it five degrees of motion: vertical translation, horizontal translation in two directions, rotation in a vertical plane, and translation along the transducer axis. The headholder for humans or animals is connected to this device by an adjustable coupler.

II. DIRECT CALIBRATION OF TRANSDUCERS BY THERMOELECTRIC PROBES

The focal intensity and the intensity distribution in the focal region were measured in the measuring tank by varying the electrode voltage of the transducer. The measuring tank was filled with degassed water which is separated from the air above by plates of polyethylene floating on the water surface. The intensity measurement was made by a thermoelectric probe method developed by Professor Fry (1, 2).

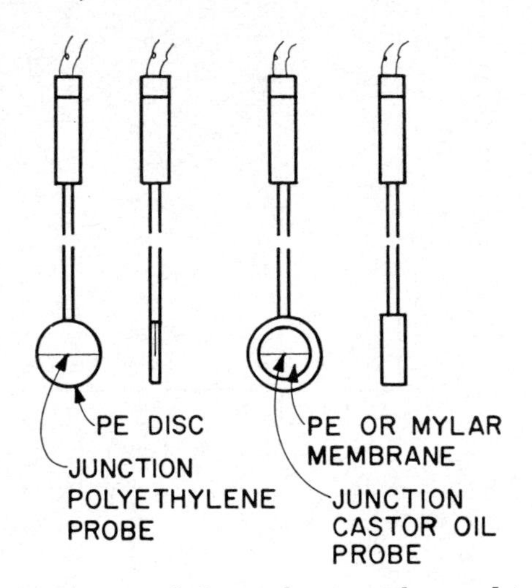

FIGURE 5. Structure of two types of thermoelectric probes used in direct calibration of the transducer.

We constructed two types of thermoelectric probes, one using polyethylene and the other, castor oil as absorbing media. Figure 5 shows the structure of these probes. The probe is placed in water normal to the direction of sound propagation. The change in the thermocouple temperature is photographically recorded after exposure to the sound wave of constant amplitude for a short period. The ρ c of polyethylene is very close to that of water, and we found the polyethylene probe to be more sensitive, especially in frequency ranges below 1 Mc, than the castor oil probe. For intensities of over 100 w/cm^2 the indication of the polyethylene probe became erroneous. It is compact, however, and may be useful for intensity measurements in living tissues.

The temperature change recorded with the castor oil probe was obtained directly (not by extrapolation) with the following procedure for absolute intensities as high as 1000 w/cm^2 and above: For the thermocouple junction parameters shown in Figure 6, extrapolate the interval $b - c$ to $t = 0$, t being the time of exposure, and obtain T_v, the initial rise of temperature. Subtracting T_v from the rise in the junction temperature, one obtains $\triangle T$. Since $\triangle T$ is determined solely by the sound absorption in the absorbing medium distant from the junction, $\triangle T$ is introduced into the equation as follows:

$$\frac{dT}{dt} = \frac{\mu}{\rho \cdot C_p \cdot K} \cdot e^{-\mu d/2} \cdot I = f\ (T) \cdot I, \qquad (4)$$

where T: temperature of the absorbing medium,
t: time of irradiation,
μ: intensity absorption coefficient per cm,
ρ: density of the medium,
C_p: specific heat of the medium for constant pressure,
K: mechanical equivalent of heat,
d: thickness of the absorber disc,
I: sound intensity at the junction (in the absence of the probe).

When the intensity multiplied by the time of exposure is small, $b - c$ is linear and one obtains the sound intensity from the equation directly, considering μ, ρ, C_p, and T_v to be constant. If the intensity, I, multiplied by the time of exposure, t, is increased, the rise in the junction temperature will show departure from a linear function of $I \times t$. In this case, the equation for Figure 6 is integrated at different base temperatures, the results being shown in Figure 7. Data regarding the temperature dependence of the absorption coefficient and the specific heat were supplemented by our experiments. Taking time, t, in the interval $b - c$, one gets the corresponding rise $\triangle T_1$ in the junction temperature. For the first approximation, one obtains from this value $\triangle T_1$ and t_1 the sound intensity, I, on the curve given in Figure 7. For the second approximation, the decrease in T_v during the irradiation is taken into account, which is caused by the decrease in the shear viscosity with the rising temperature.

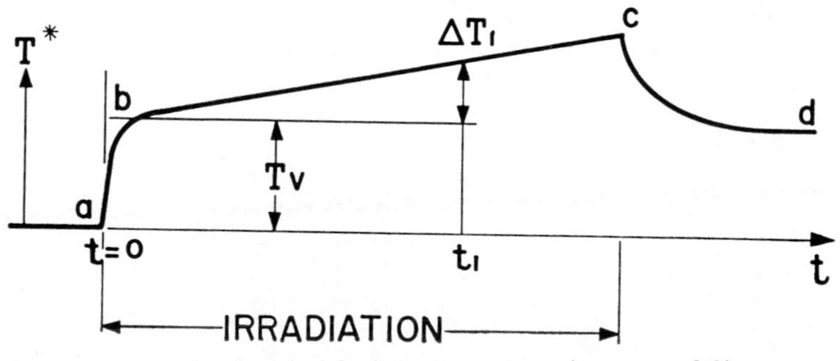

FIGURE 6. Temperature record of thermojunction (Equation [4]).

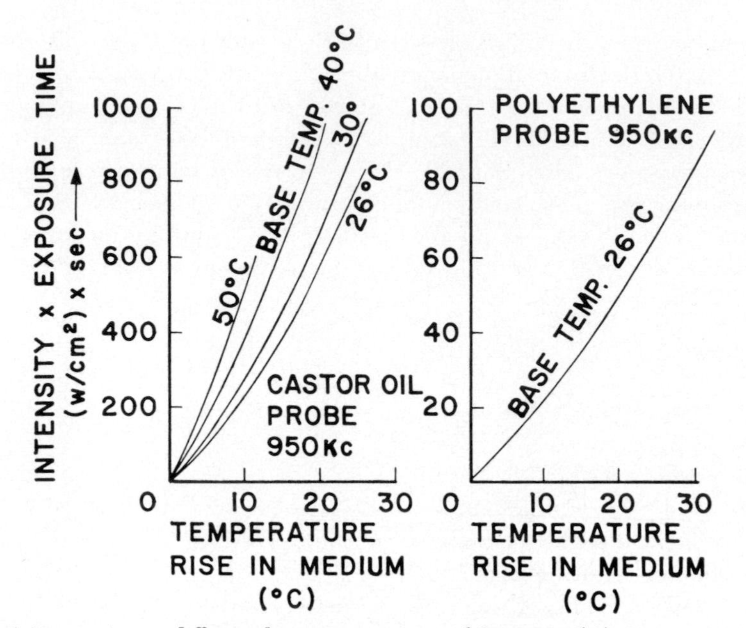

FIGURE 7. Integration at different base temperatures of Equation (4). I, intensity; t, time of exposure; T, temperature rise in the medium.

In order to determine the correction concerning the decrease in T_v, measurements were made for different base temperatures and different sound intensities. Figure 8A shows the results of these measurements. The abscissa gives the intensity which is derived in the first approximation and to which the correction is to be added. Figure 8B shows the required correction which is obtained directly from the curves in Figure 8A.

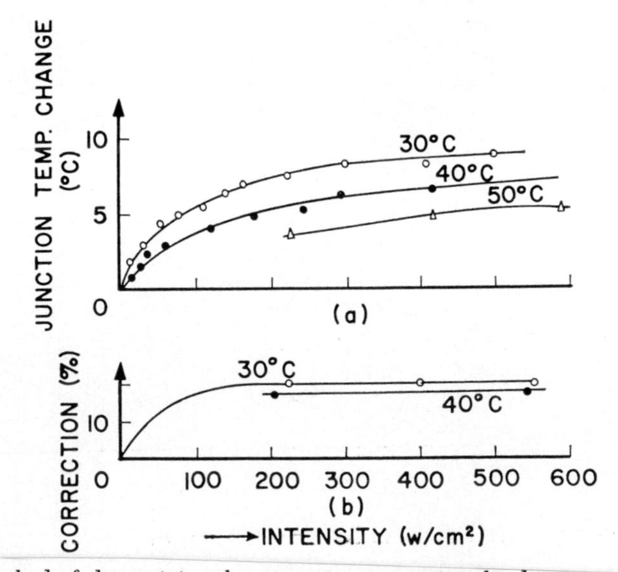

FIGURE 8. Method of determining the correction concerning the decrease in T_v.

Figure 9 shows an example of the results obtained with the polyethylene and castor oil probes. The probe was placed at the focal point of the sound beam from the transducer in a measuring tank filled with degassed water. All the measurements were made in the cavitationless state. The intensity values from the two types of probes were in good agreement. The intensity obtained was accurately proportional to the square of the driving voltage up to about 1.5 kw/cm^2. Further increase of the sonic output of the transducer frequently induced cavitation in castor oil.

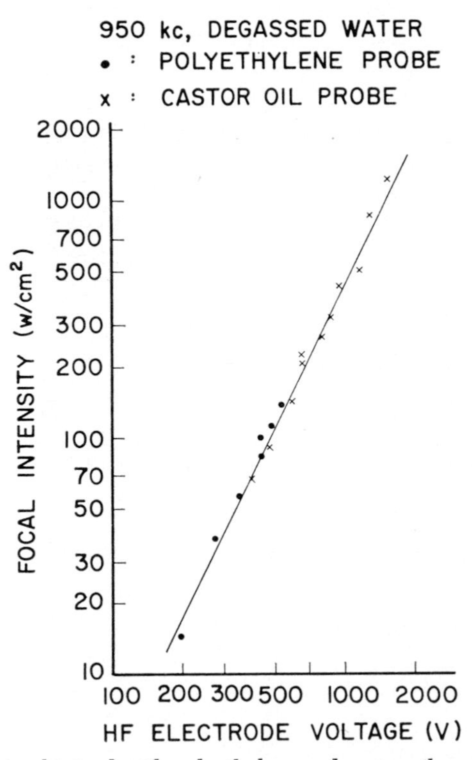

FIGURE 9. Intensity data obtained with polyethylene and castor oil probes.

III. LESION SIZE OBTAINED

In order to gain useful knowledge for surgical work, the lateral diameters and the axial diameters of the ultrasonic lesions produced in cat brain were measured. Frequencies were 1.46 Mc and 973 kc. For irradiations of 3 sec or less, one pulse of irradiation was given. For irradiation times between 3 and 6 sec, an initial pulse of 3 sec was given and the remaining time was given in a second shot. The rest interval between shots was 4 sec. For longer irradiations, the irradiation times were divided similarly.

Figure 10 charts the size of lesion obtained. The lateral diameters of the lesions were of the same order as the half-power focal diameter, while the axial diameters of the lesions were approximately half the length of the half-power axial diameter. The axial diameter is far smaller than is expected, taking

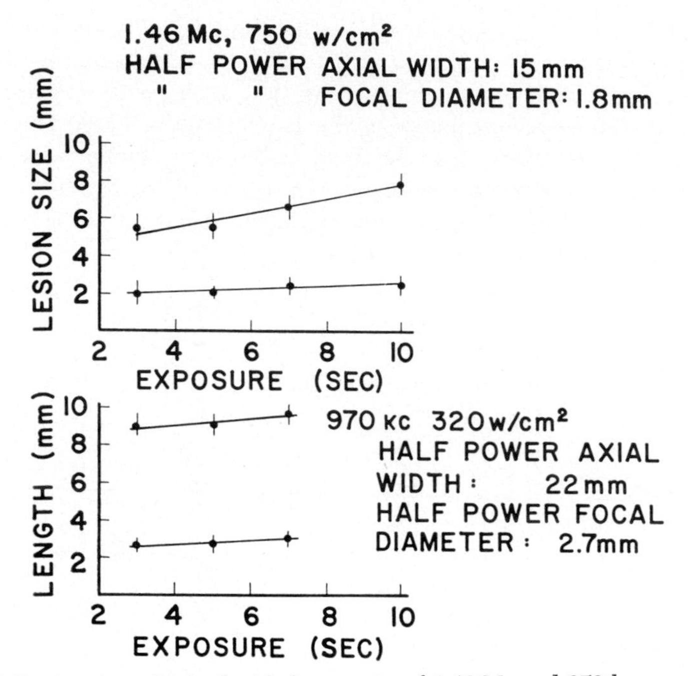

FIGURE 10. Lesion sizes obtained with frequencies of 1.46 Mc and 973 kc.

into account the attenuation coefficient. These results were used as one of the bases of our ultrasonic operations.

IV. RELATIVE RESISTIVITIES OF THE NERVOUS SYSTEM AND BLOOD VESSELS

With paralysis observed on the evoked electromyogram as a physiological endpoint, structures in cat brain and spinal cord and the sciatic nerve were irradiated. The irradiation times, above which activity disappeared in all animals used, are listed in Table I.

TABLE I. IRRADIATION TIMES ABOVE WHICH ACTIVITY DISAPPEARED IN ALL ANIMALS IRRADIATED. FOCAL INTENSITY 750 W/CM², 1.46 MC-FREQUENCY.

Site irradiated	*Irradiation time (sec)*
Motor area of cerebral cortex, nerve cells	3
Anterior horn cells in the spinal cord (lumbar segment)	2.5
Internal capsule and pyramid decussation	3.5
Nerve fibers in the spinal cord (lumbar segment)	4
Sciatic nerve	8

The nerve cells in the motor area of the cerebral cortex lost their activity after ultrasonic irradiation of 3 sec; the anterior horn cells in the spinal cord which innervate the gastrocnemial muscles became inactive after ultrasonic irradiation of 2.5-sec duration. The motor nerve fibers in the internal capsule lost their conductivity after irradiation of 3.5 sec, the motor nerve fibers in the spinal cord after irradiation of 4-sec duration. The nerve fibers in the brain and the spinal cord did not seem to be so vulnerable to ultrasonic irradiation as the motor nerve cells. The peripheral nerves seemed to show greater resistance to ultrasonic irradiation than those in the brain and spinal cord.

The irradiation studies were further extended to the hypophysis, liver, kidney, blood vessels, and mammary glands. Blood vessel and the hypophysis studies will be reported on here.

The blood vessels in the white and gray matter were irradiated with focused ultrasound, and the changes induced were observed. The frequency was 1.46 Mc and the focal intensity was 750 w/cm^2. When the irradiation time was of 3 sec or less, no morphological changes were observed. When the irradiation time ranged from 4 to 9 sec, no trace of bleeding was found but morphological changes were induced, such as edematous swelling of endothelial cells and decreased staining of the nucleus. Such changes disappeared within 3 weeks following ultrasonic irradiation. With irradiation of 10 sec or more, capillary vessels were destroyed and bleeding took place. Small veins were destroyed with irradiation of 15-sec duration or more, and when the irradiation time exceeded 20 sec, destruction of arterioles occurred.

V. EFFECT OF IRRADIATION ON THE HYPOPHYSIS

The hypophysis of a cat was irradiated for 3 sec through a skull opening with focused ultrasound of 1.46-Mc frequency, and 750-w/cm^2 intensity. The ultrasonic lesion was made at the stem of the hypophysis. Histological changes in the lesion area took place, and the number of β-cells seemed to decrease. To investigate the endocrinological change in the function of the irradiated hypophysis, ACTH tests were made before the irradiation and 3 months after irradiation. After the administration of eight units of ACTH, 17 OHCS was measured in the urine. The results of ACTH tests are shown in Table II. Tests

TABLE II. FUNCTIONAL CHANGE OF ADRENAL CORTEX OF CAT FOLLOWING IRRADIATION OF HYPOPHYSIS BY FOCUSED ULTRASOUND. CHANGES IN 17 OHCS CONTENT OF URINE AFTER ADMINISTERING BU OF ACTH ARE SHOWN.

	17 OHCS content (mg/day)					
	Before irradiation			*3 months after irradiation*		
Animal	*Control level*	*After administering ACTH*	*Reactivity of adrenal cortex*	*Control level*	*After administering ACTH*	*Reactivity of adrenal cortex*
1	0.1	1.8	1.7	0.4	0.4	0
2	0.1	1.1	1.0	0.3	0.5	0.2
3	0.1	1.9	1.8	0.8	0.7	—0.1
4	0.2	1.8	1.6	0	0.7	0.7
5	0.6	1.6	1.0	2.3	0.8	—1.5
6	0.8	1.6	0.8	1.0	0	—1.0
7	0.6	1.6	1.0	1.0	0.4	—0.6
8	0.8	1.8	1.0	1.0	0.7	—0.3

made 3 months after irradiation distinctly showed lowered reactivity of the adrenal cortex.

VI. ULTRASONIC OPERATIONS PERFORMED

Since the first stereotaxic ultrasonic operation in 1957 to destroy spike foci which were deeply seated in the forebrain and detected on electroencephalograms, six successful ultrasonic operations have been performed in place of lobectomy, stereotaxic partial thalamic destruction and hemispherectomy. The ultrasonic operations were further extended to mammary tumor, as a substitute for mastectomy. The destruction of the glandular tissue and the extension of the proliferated fibrous tissue to the former were observed.

REFERENCES

1. Fry, W. J., and R. B. Fry (1954). Determination of absolute sound levels and acoustic absorption coefficients by thermocouple probes – theory. J. Acoust. Soc. Am. *26*, 294–310.
2. Fry, W. J., and R. B. Fry (1954). Determination of absolute sound levels and acoustic absorption coefficients by thermocouple probes – experiment. J. Acoust. Soc. Am. *26*, 311–317.

DISCUSSION

DR. WEISSLER: Thank you very much, Dr. Yoshioka, for giving us this broad view of the large amount of work that you and your colleagues have been doing. How are the three quartz crystals connected to each other?

DR. YOSHIOKA: They are cemented together with aryldite cement.

DR. WEISSLER: I would like to ask whether the University of Illinois group made the same type of corrections in using the castor oil probe at very high intensities?

DR. DUNN: We avoid having to make such corrections by employing the thermocouple probe at acoustic intensities for which the second phase of the response can be assumed linear and then extrapolate to higher intensities, that is, the actual operating intensities, by assuming the transducer output to be a linear function of the applied voltage. Our actual calibration intensities are of the order of 10 w/cm^2, at which the temperature rise in the probe is less than a degree centigrade, whereas the operating intensity may be of the order of 10^3 w/cm^2.

DR. NYBORG: Some years ago Dr. Heuter made some investigations of the action of the thermocouple probe at higher sound levels, and he observed acoustic streaming around the thermocouple. I wondered if you had confirmed this or found it not to have occurred, or if it is in any way important.

DR. DUNN: As the acoustic intensity level, at which the probe is exposed, is increased, many of the nonlinear acoustic phenomena become apparent. Streaming is a very likely phenomena to appear due to the rather high absorption of the fluid in the probe and it is, of course, very difficult, if not impossible at present, to correct for it.

DR. CURTIS: I was interested in the slide relating lesion size to the time of exposure (Fig. 10). It appears that you have a very shallow slope in relation to the exposure time. I would expect stronger dependence of the lesion size on the duration of exposure.

DR. KIKUCHI: I am not an investigator in this research, but I am only acting as an interpreter. Dr. Yoshioka says the lesion produced by ultrasonic irradiation is almost constant regardless of the duration of exposure. However, the length is shorter than the half-intensity length of the beam in a free field as measured by the thermocouple probe.

DR. CURTIS: The only point that I make is that you are continually putting energy into this system which affects the temperature of the system, and I should think you would create larger and larger volumes in which the temperature would be producing irreversible changes.

DR. BELL: In Dr. Ballantine's group at Massachusetts General Hospital we found that very minute changes in exposure time result in very large changes in lesion size. During irradiation of the brain of a cat at an intensity of 1700 w/cm^2, a change in exposure time of 0.05 sec would possibly more than double the size of the lesion. The exposure times used in this series were, as I remember, 0.20, 0.25, 0.30, 0.35, and 0.40 sec at a frequency of 2.7 Mc. We found that going from 0.2 to 0.3 sec we actually went through a threshold region. So the change of time was exceedingly important, even though the duration was very short.

DR. VON GIERKE: I believe the lesions Dr. Bell refers to were much smaller than these.

DR. BELL: Oh, yes.

DR. VON GIERKE: I think that is the point. The lesions increase in size as a function of irradiation time.

DR. F. J. FRY: At 1 Mc, and for acoustic intensities in the range from 10^2 to 10^3 w/cm^2, the range of exposure times, from those necessary to produce a light lesion in white matter to those required to produce a gray matter lesion, is quite appreciable; that is, there is a time interval of the order of seconds during which selectivity of the production of white matter lesions in preference to gray matter lesions can be accomplished. However, at higher frequencies, at 4 Mc, for example, an equivalent time interval is of the order of 10^{-1} sec.

DR. WEISSLER: Thank you very much, Dr. Yoshioka. We will go on now to the next paper.

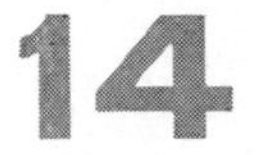

Recent Developments in Ultrasound at the Biophysical Research Laboratory and Their Application to Basic Problems in Biology and Medicine

FRANCIS J. FRY
Biophysical Research Laboratory, University of Illinois, Urbana, Illinois

Introduction by Dr. Weissler

Professor Francis Fry will now discuss the recent progress of the ultrasound research program here at the Biophysical Research Laboratory. For those of us who attended the previous symposia, it is a great pleasure to have the opportunity to learn about the current research and compare it with the status of the work at the time of the previous meetings. The progress in this field has been most stimulating.

During the past 5 years a variety of basic biological problems have been investigated and associated instrumentation developments have been pursued in the Biophysical Research Laboratory. The work of the laboratory thus falls into two major categories. First, we are primarily concerned with biological systems and the solution of problems pertaining to them. Therefore, we are involved with the methodology of attack on these problems and thus with the interaction of operating apparatus with these biological systems. Unfortunately, it is quite frequently true that the apparatus desired for a research investigation is not available commercially and a major effort must then be expended on the design of equipment. The second major category of work is, therefore, the development of apparatus, and in conjunction with this, the utilization of existing instruments as auxiliary equipment, for example, computers, to further the research activity.

The biological investigations include: (1) structure and function of the central nervous system of animals, such as monkey and cat, (2) modification of central nervous system of man for treatment of neurological disorders, (3) physical mechanism of action of ultrasound on components of central nervous systems — mouse spinal cord, (4) structure of skeletal muscle, (5) differential modification of the hypophysis, and (6) measurement of basic acoustic properties of tissue, for example, spinal cord, lung, etc. High-intensity ultrasound has been applied as an investigative tool in all of these programs. It should be noted that the specific studies are not, in general, directed at the observation of ultrasonic changes, for example, lesions, per se, but each has a broader scope as will be discussed here and in other papers presented in this symposium.

The application of high-intensity ultrasound to the treatment of human neurological disorders has been performed at the State University of Iowa Hospitals, and this work is a joint research program between the Biophysical Research Laboratory of the University of Illinois and the Division of Neurosurgery of the State University of Iowa Hospitals, of which Dr. Russell Meyers is chairman (1–6).

Under apparatus development, one can consider three general classifications: (1) mechanical, (2) electrical and electronic, and (3) electromechanical. In order to insure reproducible results in the use of high-level focused ultrasound as applied to tissue, it is necessary to control precisely the sound field parameters, as well as the parameters which determine the state of the tissue and consequently which determine the type of interaction. This applies not only in the case of irreversible changes in tissue, in which the selective action of ultrasound on various tissue components is desired, but also in the case of reversible interactions, in which tissue is not permanently affected. Control of the sound field parameters begins with the construction of reasonably stable transducers, which in turn are driven by appropriate electronic equipment. The problems associated with the design of this electronic apparatus will be discussed in another lecture at this session.

Transducers of a variety of types have been and are being used for the irradiation procedures. The frequency of the ultrasound used initially on animals was 1 Mc/sec and this frequency has continued in use on humans. Since the major fraction of the neuroanatomical investigations on experimental animals of interest to us at the present time demand small lesions, 4 Mc/sec sound has been used for most of this work. Reflecting, multi-beam, and single-beam focused transducers have all been employed in the irradiation procedures. However, for the past 5 years the majority of the animal irradiations have been performed with a single-beam, lens-focused transducer, while the human patients have been irradiated, up to the present, with a focused multi-beam irradiator.

A schematic view of a single-beam, 4-Mc irradiator is shown in Figure 1. A view of one electrode face of the quartz crystal is shown resting against the stainless steel housing, and this face is continuous with the electrical ground. The opposite electrode is in electrical contact with a thin gold foil which lies partially beneath the back-up gasket. The latter maintains the crystal in electrical and mechanical contact with the front part of the housing. The lens, in this case a plastic plano-concave unit, is held at an appropriate spacing distance, one-quarter acoustical wavelength at the operating frequency, from the crystal. Castor oil or silicone oil[1] is the coupling medium

[1] Dow-Corning Type 7d.

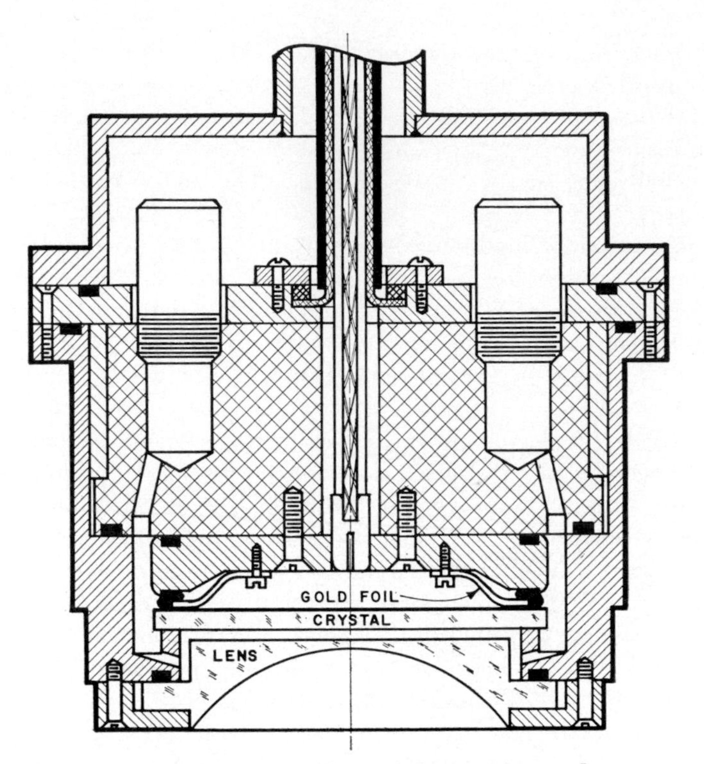

FIGURE 1. A schematic view of a single-beam, 4-Mc irradiator.

between the lens and crystal. Ports provide a free interchange for this medium to flow to the region surrounding the circumference of the crystal, to provide electrical insulation for the applied driving electric field. The lens is held in such a way that it can expand sideways relative to the housing. Thus, it does not flex in the center to produce variations in transducer output due to the differential temperature expansion between the housing and the lens. It should be noted that for calibration of the sound output of this type of transducer we use a thermocouple probe that is calibrated in absolute units by a radiation pressure procedure based on measuring the deflection of small diameter metal balls positioned in the sound field (7, 8). With a transducer of the type described it is possible, by careful assembly and subsequent storage in a constant temperature oven at, for example, 37°C (with the unit immersed in a sterilizing fluid such as benzakonium chloride), to obtain the type of transducer output data illustrated in Figure 2. The ordinate represents the r.f. voltage level on the transducer required to obtain a constant sound level at the focus. The abscissa refers to the time interval, in days, following filling of the space between the lens and crystal with oil. As one can see, the sound output exhibits a relatively slow drift pattern coupled with apparently random, day to day, variations. These random short time variations amount to $\pm 0.7\%$ and are within the limits of the overall accuracy of recording the data.

Accurate geometric placement of lesions in the brain of both humans and experimental animals requires a rigid tie between the skull and irradiator. In our earlier animal research studies, we employed modified Horsley-Clarke head holders, but for our later investigations we designed completely new types of head holders. For humans we designed a rigid head holder utilizing four stainless steel pins which fit hemispherically prepared indentations in the skull bone, two in the front and two in the rear. Each pin is supported by a post which provides three directions of motion, with a repositioning accuracy determined by micrometer readings. The accuracy of repositioning in the holder is such that, in general, ventriculography is *not* done for each irradiation procedure. Figure 3 shows a patient mounted in this type of head holder at the State University of Iowa Hospitals. Figure 4 shows the head holder in use with the apparatus for irradiation clearly visible. A local anesthetic is infiltrated into the tissue at the sites at which the pins penetrate the scalp. Although the forces along the pin axes are of the order of 50 to 75 lb, the patients do not usually complain. A sensation of compression is not a common occurrence, but some patients experience a transient compression feeling which is perhaps suggested by their visual observation of the turning of the pin tightening nuts.

Figure 5 shows a similar type of head holder which we designed and installed at the Medical Center of the University of Indiana. Dr. Robert Heimburger, Head of the Division of Neurosurgery there, is using this instrument. (Lesions are produced electrolytically.) Figure 6 shows a patient in this apparatus.

As one can readily see from an examination of these figures, both the mechanical rigidity of supporting the head of the patient and the accuracy of repositioning his head in the instrument have been prime considerations

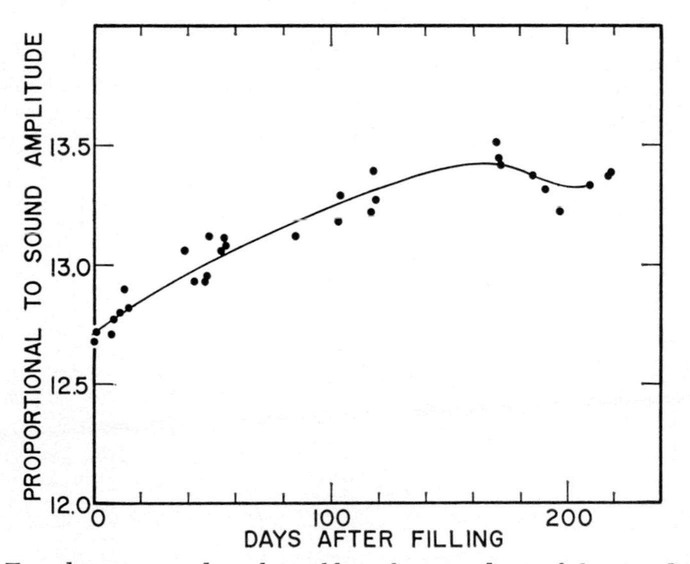

FIGURE 2. Transducer output data obtainable with a transducer of the type described.

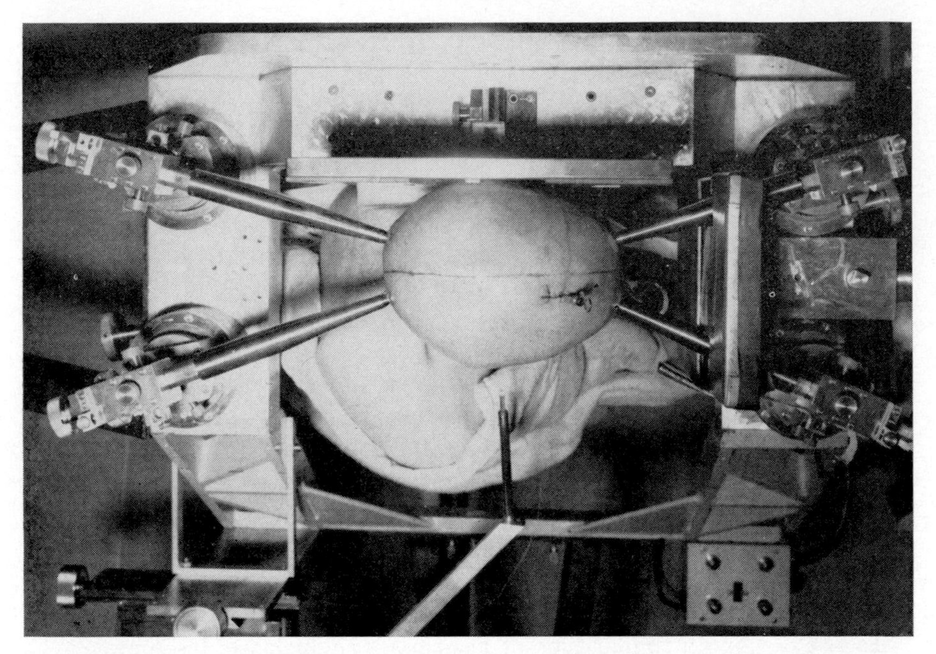

FIGURE 3. A patient at the State University of Iowa Hospitals mounted in the new type of head holder.

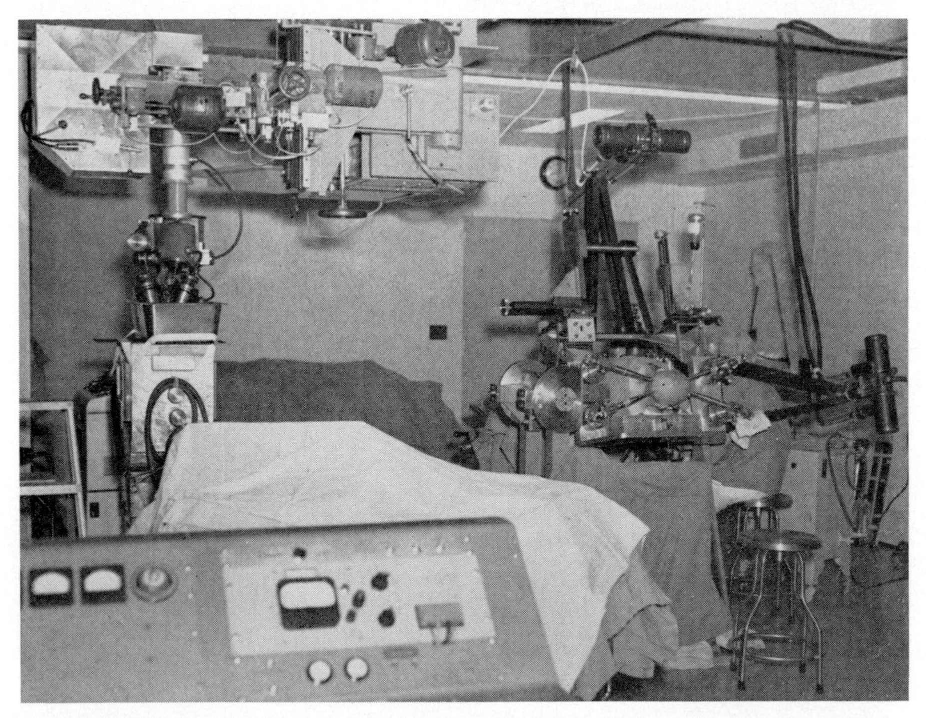

FIGURE 4. The head holder in use at the State University of Iowa Hospitals with the apparatus for irradiation clearly visible.

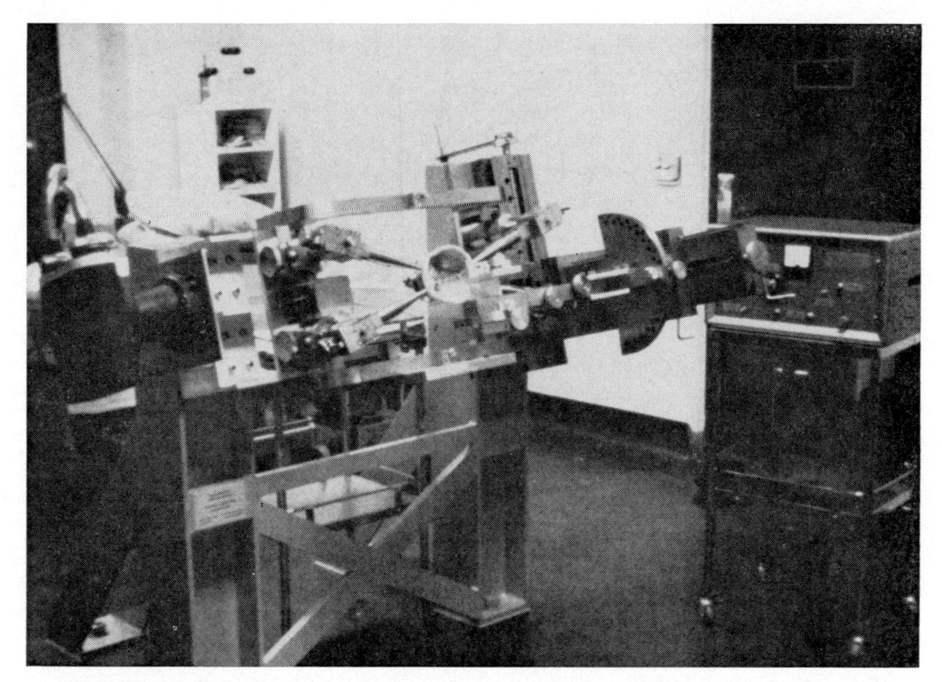

FIGURE 5. A similar type of head holder installed at the Medical Center of the University of Indiana. A piece of skull is mounted in the holder.

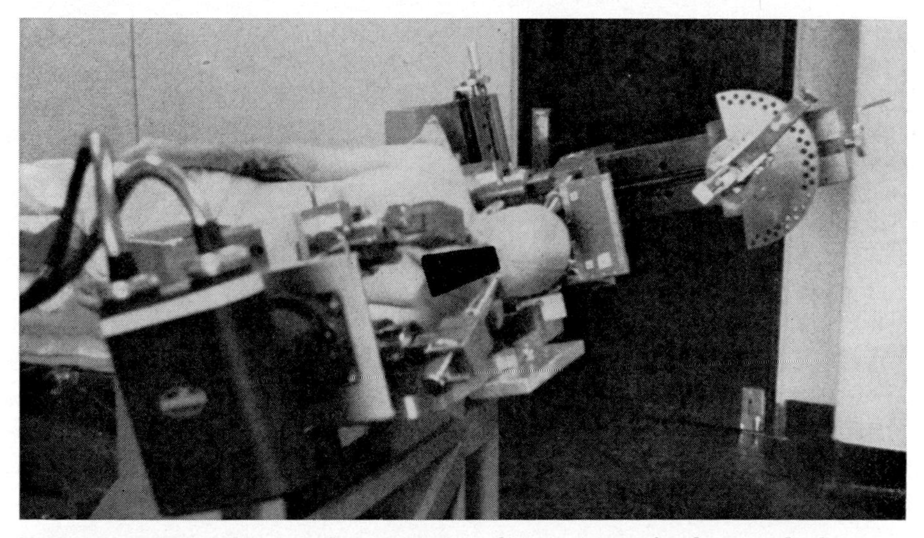

FIGURE 6. A patient shown in the apparatus at the University of Indiana Medical Center.

in the design of these head holders. In order to achieve reasonable accuracy in the determination of the coordinates of prechosen anatomic sites in the brain of the human or experimental animal, internal landmarks must be employed, except in cases where it is possible to localize a structure by reference to bony landmarks alone, for example, the pituitary gland. For the animal studies at the Biophysical Research Laboratory, the techniques have progressed from the simple ear bar zero method to an x-ray procedure employing internal bony landmarks and, finally, to the procedure involving x-ray ventriculography (9). For successful introduction of the x-ray opaque medium into the ventricles of the experimental animal, we have devised an electrical impedance measuring device which indicates by pointer deflection on a meter when the ventricle is entered by the penetrating cannula. Figure 7 shows the concentric arrangement of the cannula and the inner electrical insulated lead. In the lateral view of the cat skull shown in Figure 8, one can see that the needle, oriented vertically downward and driven by a mechanical positioning system, has just penetrated the roof of the lateral ventricle. At this point, the inner conductor is withdrawn and the x-ray opaque medium is introduced into the ventricle. One can see clearly the outlines of the lateral and third ventricles, and the anterior and posterior commissures are readily identified. A vertical view of these same structures is shown in Figure 9. A modified but similar ventricular cannula as that shown in Figure 7 has been devised for human use. Figure 10 shows a patient in a head holder with the ventricular needle held by the associated positioning system. A three-

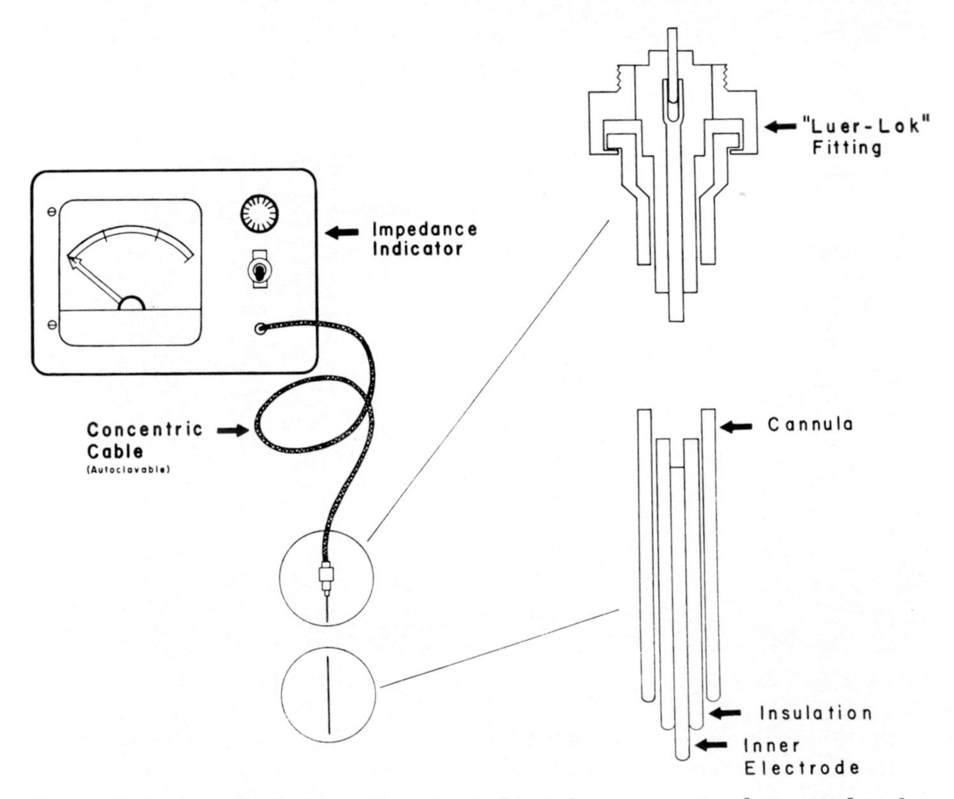

FIGURE 7. A schematic drawing of an electrical impedance measuring device used in the introduction of the x-ray opaque medium into the ventricles to indicate when the ventricle is entered by the penetrating cannula. The concentric arrangement of the cannula and the inner electrical insulated lead is shown.

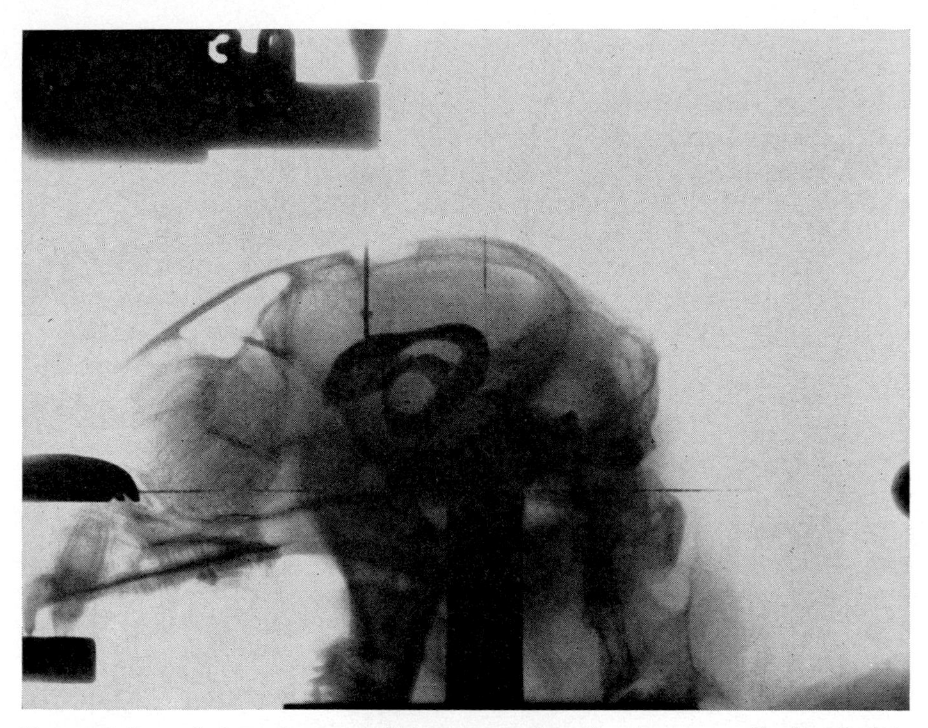

FIGURE 8. Lateral view of a cat skull showing the hypodermic-type needle described in Figure 7 penetrating the roof of the lateral ventricle. The outlines of the lateral and third ventricles are visible.

view x-ray technique is employed to localize the ventricular system of the patient in space: (A) lateral view, (B) anterior-posterior view, and (C) a view along an axis in the direction from the superior frontal sinuses to the base of the neck on its dorsal aspect.

The x-ray opaque medium we used for the earlier ventriculography on the human was Thorotrast, but this is no longer employed for this purpose. Figure 11 shows a group of three x-ray photographs taken with panopaque [2] filling. The anterior and posterior commissures are clearly visible on the lateral view (A). The length of the intercommissural line, which varies from patient to patient, is used for longitudinal scaling. The position of the midline of the third ventricle is based on the anterior-posterior information contained on the two views (B and C). After the x-ray photography is completed, most of the medium can be removed from the patient by draining it out through the cannula in the lateral ventricle.

The irradiation procedure and equipment have undergone continuous modification and evolution during the course of the work on the human. Figure 12 shows a schematic view of the configuration of some of the elements of the equipment used during the irradiation. A patient's skull is shown clamped in a head holder. In this case, a 1-Mc multi-beam transducer is used

[2] Brand of ethyl iodophenylun decylate, 30.5% iodine, distributed by Westinghouse Electric Corporation, X-ray Division, Baltimore, Md.

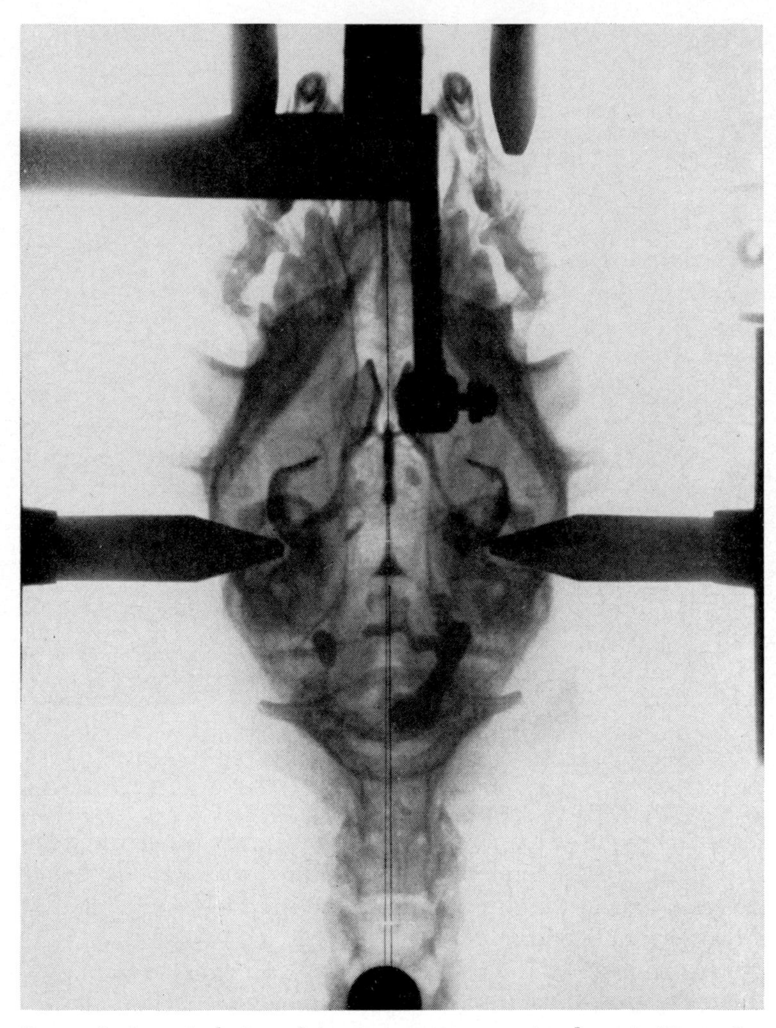

FIGURE 9. A vertical view of the same structures pointed out in Figure 8.

and the coupling pan (in which the degassed liquid is held and the transducer partially immersed) does not rest on the patient's head but is suspended from the side. In the first stage of evolution of the technique involving human patients, we employed a procedure in which the bone opening was made on the day of irradiation. The brain was irradiated transdurally, the excised bone was replaced, and the opening closed. The entire procedure was rather long and stressful. It has since been replaced with a procedure in which the bone is removed under general anesthesia during the initial preparation, the scalp is closed over the bony defect, and the irradiation procedures are carried out at a later date under nonsterile conditions, with the radiation traversing the intact skin. A variety of types of patients in the category of the hyperkinesias, for example, Parkinsonism, athetosis, dystonia, and in-

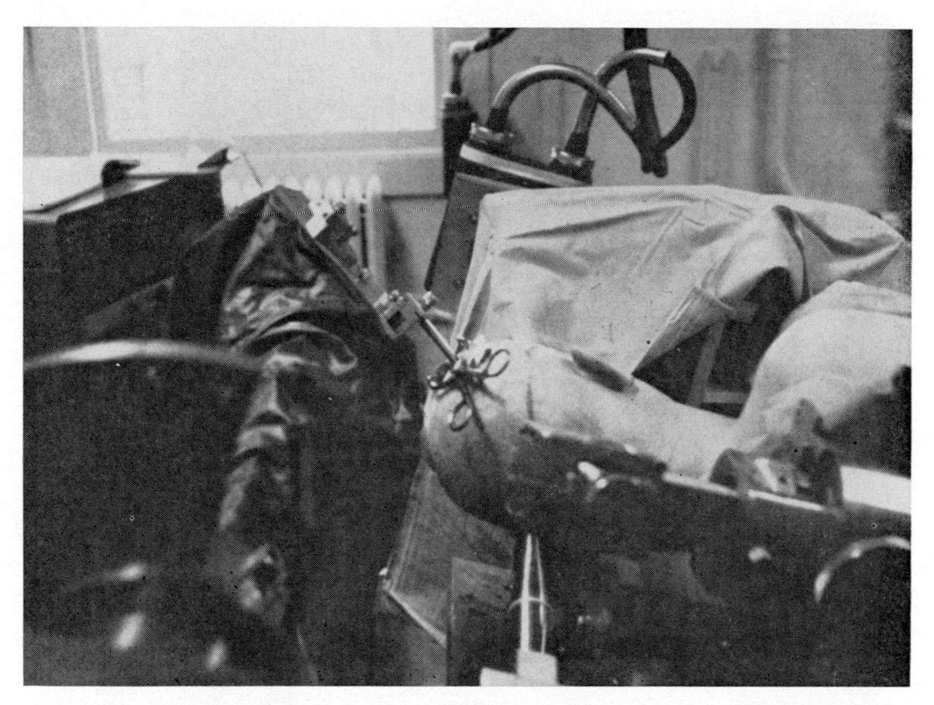

FIGURE 10. A patient in place in a head holder with the ventricular needle held by the associated positioning system.

tention tremor have been treated. Some work has also been accomplished on phantom limb and other intractable pain cases.

With regard to the effects that have been observed in the central nervous system of experimental animals on exposure to high-level ultrasound, it is abundantly clear that the white matter is more susceptible to irreversible damage than is the gray matter. This is shown by the group of pictures in Figure 13. A classic example of this differential susceptibility is shown in the illustration showing the lesion in the subcortical white matter of the cat (A). Irradiation was performed by placing a multiplicity of exposures spaced laterally at equal intervals. The overlying gray matter experienced the same dose received by the white matter. The selective destruction of the compact white matter is strikingly apparent. The figure also shows the mammillothalamic tract selectively destroyed (B), a subcallosal fornix lesion (E), and a lesion in the medial part of the medial mamillary nucleus (D). Part C of this group shows a lesion interrupting fibers of the cingulum, and part F shows a two-step sheet lesion produced in thalamic gray matter with one of the steps extending into the internal capsule. The dimension of the sheets in the anterior-posterior direction is a few tenths of a millimeter. Extensive histological studies have shown that the neural components of the tissue are, in general, more susceptible to the action of the ultrasound than are the nonneural components.

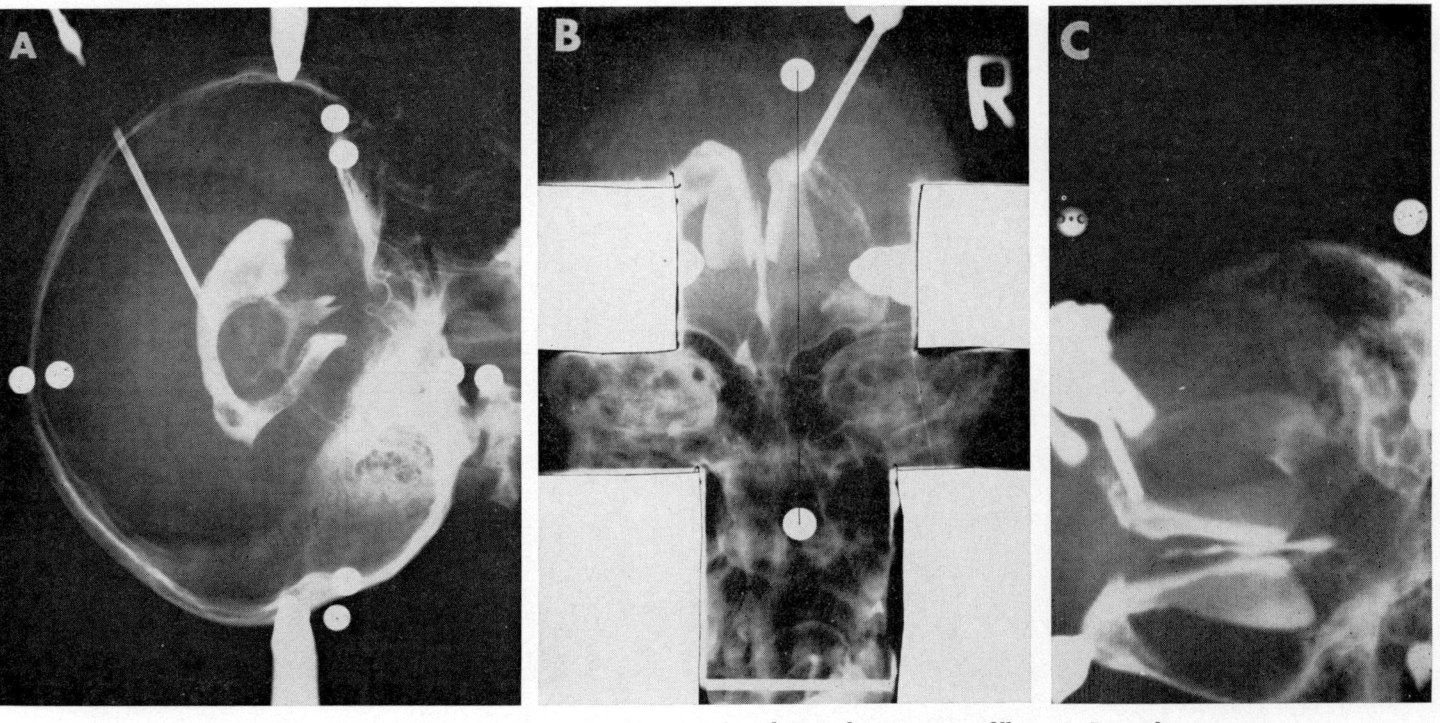

FIGURE 11. A group of three x-ray photographs taken with panopaque filling. A. Lateral view. B. Anterior-posterior view. C. View approximately in the mid-sagittal plane of the brain along an axis in the direction from the superior frontal sinus to the base of the neck on its dorsal aspect.

Unfortunately, it is not possible in the time available to discuss in any detail the many other programs underway. I will, therefore, simply mention some of the other areas in which we have worked. As you probably know, we have investigated the use of high-intensity sound to produce *reversible* effects in the central nervous system (10). In this investigation it was shown that it is possible to markedly affect the evoked potentials in the occipital cortex in response to light flashes at the eye, while focusing ultrasound at various sites in the lateral geniculate nucleus.

In the experimental animal behavioral studies, under the direction of Garth Thomas, the mammillothalamic tract of animals has been severed bilaterally, both totally and partially (11). Ultrasound is also being used to produce the refined lesions required for a comprehensive neuroanatomical study, now in progress, on the mammillary nuclei and associated complex. So far, this study has provided a considerable amount of new anatomic information (12) and the quantitative neuroanatomical studies which will be forthcoming in the future will provide much more.

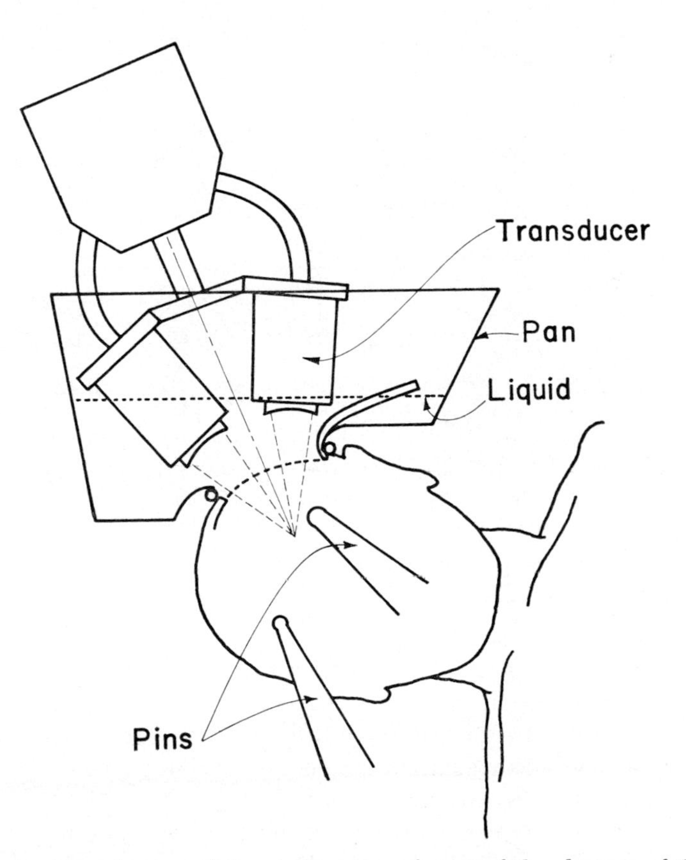

FIGURE 12. A schematic view of the configuration of some of the elements of the equipment used during human irradiation. A patient's skull is shown clamped in the head holder.

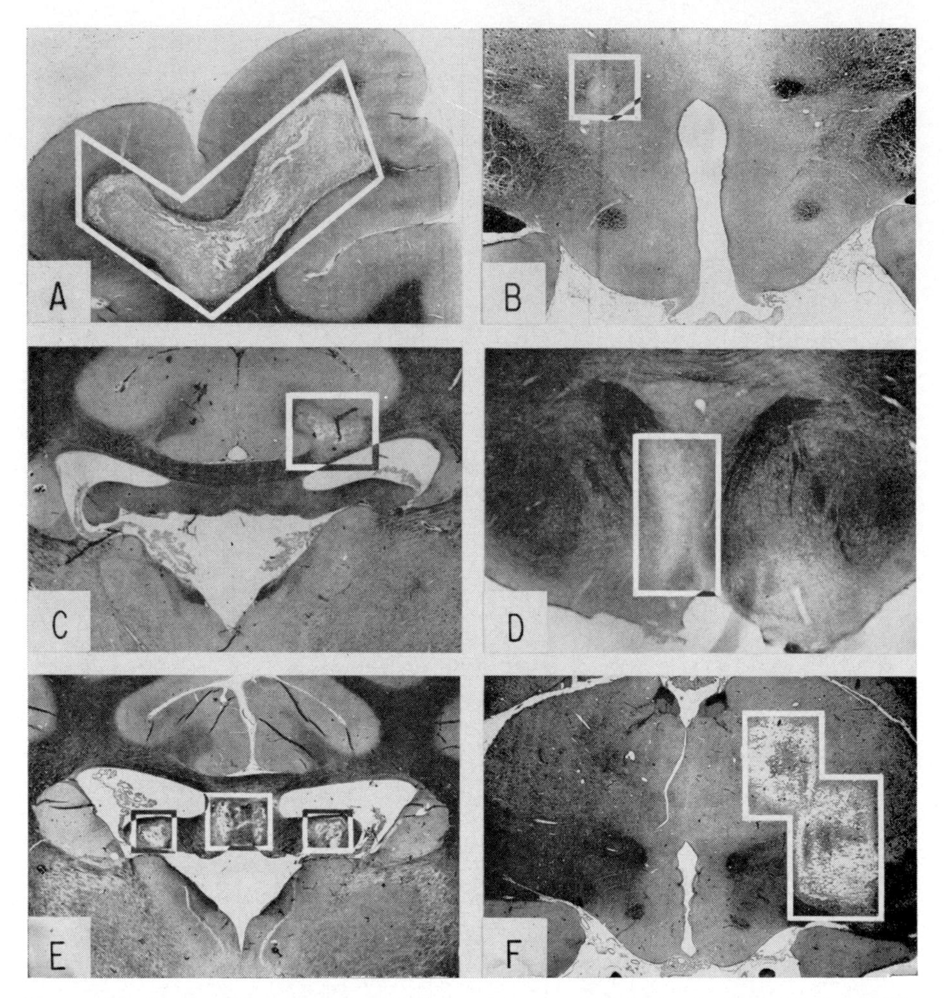

FIGURE 13. Photomicrographs of stained tissue sections of cat brain illustrating the differential susceptibility of white and gray matter to irreversible damage by high-level ultrasound. A. Selective disruption of subcortical white matter. B. Mammillothalamic tract selectively interrupted. C. Interruption of longitudinally running fibers of the cingulum. D. Destruction of the medial part of the medial mamillary nucleus. E. Three lesions in the subcallosal fornix. F. Two rectangular sheet lesions in thalamic gray and structures ventral to thalamus.

Data on man is being obtained from histological studies of the brains of patients who have succumbed, for a variety of reasons, subsequent to ultrasonic irradiation. Of the 86 patients irradiated, none have died as the immediate result of an irradiation procedure, although two deaths have occurred within 10 days after irradiation.

DR. WEISSLER: As part of his paper, Frank Fry has a film to present. Unfortunately, there is insufficient time to show it now, so the film is scheduled for the afternoon session, when Dr. Ballantine will be presiding as chairman.

REFERENCES

1. Fry, W. J., R. Meyers, F. J. Fry, D. F. Schultz, L. L. Dreyer, and R. F. Noyes (1958). Topical differentia of pathogenetic mechanisms underlying Parkinsonian tremor and rigidity as indicated by ultrasonic irradiation of the human brain. Trans. Am. Neurol. Assn., 16–24.
2. Meyers, R., W. J. Fry, F. J. Fry, L. L. Dreyer, D. F. Schultz, and R. F. Noyes (1959). Early experiences with ultrasonic irradiation of the pallidofugal and nigral complexes in hyperkinetic and hypertonic disorders. J. Neurosurg. *16*, 32–54.
3. Meyers, R., F. J. Fry, W. J. Fry, R. C. Eggleton, and D. F. Schultz (1960). Determination of topological human brain representations and modifications of signs and symptoms of some neurologic disorders by the use of high level ultrasound. Neurology *10*, 271–277.
4. Fry, W. J., and F. J. Fry (1960). Fundamental neurological research and human neurosurgery using intense ultrasound. IRE Trans. Med. Electron. *ME-7*, 166–181. Reprinted in Proc. Biomed. Eng. Symposium (San Diego, 1961).
5. Fry, W. J., F. J. Fry, R. Meyers, and R. C. Eggleton (1960). The use of ultrasound in neurosurgery. Proc. 3rd Internat. Conf. on Med. Electron., 453–458.
6. Fry, W. J., and R. Meyers (1962). Ultrasonic method of modifying brain structure(s). 1st Internat. Symposium on Stereoencephalotomy. Confinia Neurologica *22*, 315–327.
7. Fry, W. J., and R. B. Fry (1954). Determination of absolute sound levels and acoustic absorption coefficients by thermocouple probes – theory. J. Acoust. Soc. Am. *26*, 294–310.
8. Fry, W. J., and R. B. Fry (1954). Determination of absolute sound levels and acoustic absorption coefficients by thermocouple probes – experiment. J. Acoust. Soc. Am. *26*, 311–317.
9. Fry, W. J., F. J. Fry, G. H. Leichner, and R. F. Heimburger (1962). Tissue interface detector for ventriculography and other application. J. Neurosurg. *19*, 793–798.
10. Fry, F. J., H. W. Ades, and W. J. Fry (1958). Production of reversible changes in the central nervous system by ultrasound. Science *127*, 83–84.
11. Thomas, G. J., W. J. Fry, F. J. Fry, B. M. Slotnick, and E. E. Krieckhaus (1963). Behavioral effects of mammillothalamic tractotomy in cats. J. Neurophysiol. *26*, 857–876.
12. Fry, W. J., R. Krumins, F. J. Fry, G. J. Thomas, S. Borbely, and H. W. Ades (1963). Origins and distributions of several efferent pathways from the mammillary nuclei of the cat. J. Comp. Neurol. *120*, 195–257.

FILM

Dr. Ballantine: This afternoon we will hear from several members of the Biophysical Research Laboratory. Professor Francis Fry will show a film presentation which is part two of the paper he presented this morning. It was apparent from part one of Frank Fry's paper that in order to successfully apply high-intensity ultrasound as a research tool, very rigid requirements must be placed on the design of the irradiation instrumentation. Dr. Leichner will enlighten us further on this by discussing the overall electronic design approach required in order to obtain such precise control of the effect of ultrasonic energy on the biological system. For the final presentation we are privileged to hear from our host, Professor William Fry, Head of the

Biophysical Research Laboratory, who will discuss new approaches to the study of biological systems by ultrasound.

A film will now be shown on the application of ultrasound as a neurological procedure. As most of you know, the equipment used for the ultrasonic neurosurgical work was designed and built here in the Biophysical Research Laboratory. The irraditions were performed by a research team consisting of various members of the Biophysical Research Laboratory of the University of Illinois and Dr. Russell Meyers of the State University of Iowa Hospitals. The first patient shown has a Parkinson's syndrome, and the other patient is suffering from a random movement disorder. Since the film does not have a sound track, Professor Francis Fry will explain the procedure during the film.

Dr. F. J. Fry: This is a sweeping view of the operative area (Fig. 14). You see here the ultrasound transducer, calibration tank, head holder, electronic equipment, and x-ray equipment. The patient is mounted in the machine. In preparation for the irradiation procedure, a plastic drape is placed around the suture line, so that the area of the dura corresponding to the area of bone removal is not covered with the plastic. The drape is drawn up through a metallic pan which is supported off the head-pin support posts and degassed saline is introduced into a plastic bag which is supported by the metal pan. All this draping and filling is, of course, done under nonsterile conditions. A heating coil keeps the saline at body temperature. The next view shows the multi-beam transducer being lowered into the coupling pan and medium (Fig. 15). You see here the patient in the head holder just prior to irradiation. The patient is rigidly held at the skull attachment, but otherwise unrestrained. A light indicates the period of irradiation, that is, the sound is on during the interval that the light is on. The first irradiation is of the order of

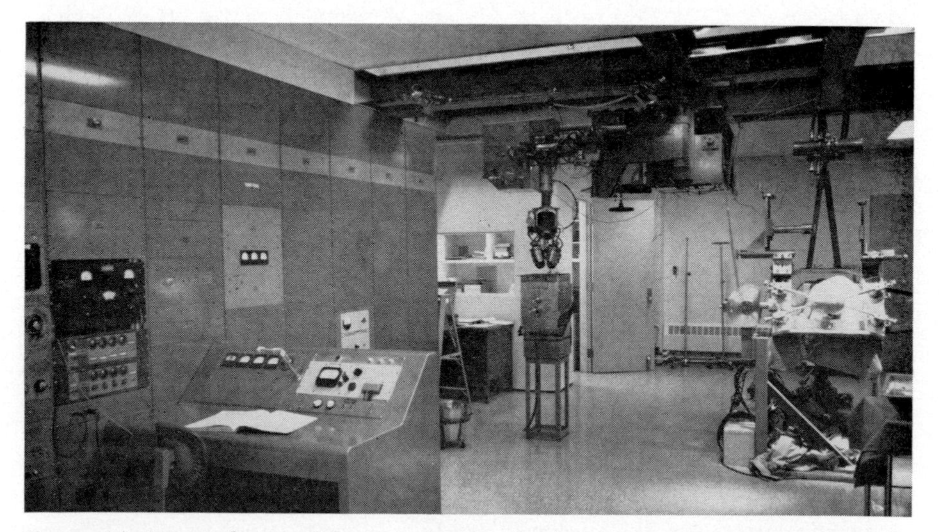

Figure 14. A general view of the operative area for the ultrasound irradiation procedure. The ultrasound transducer, calibration tank, head holder, electronic equipment, and x-ray equipment are visible. A patient is in position in the head holder.

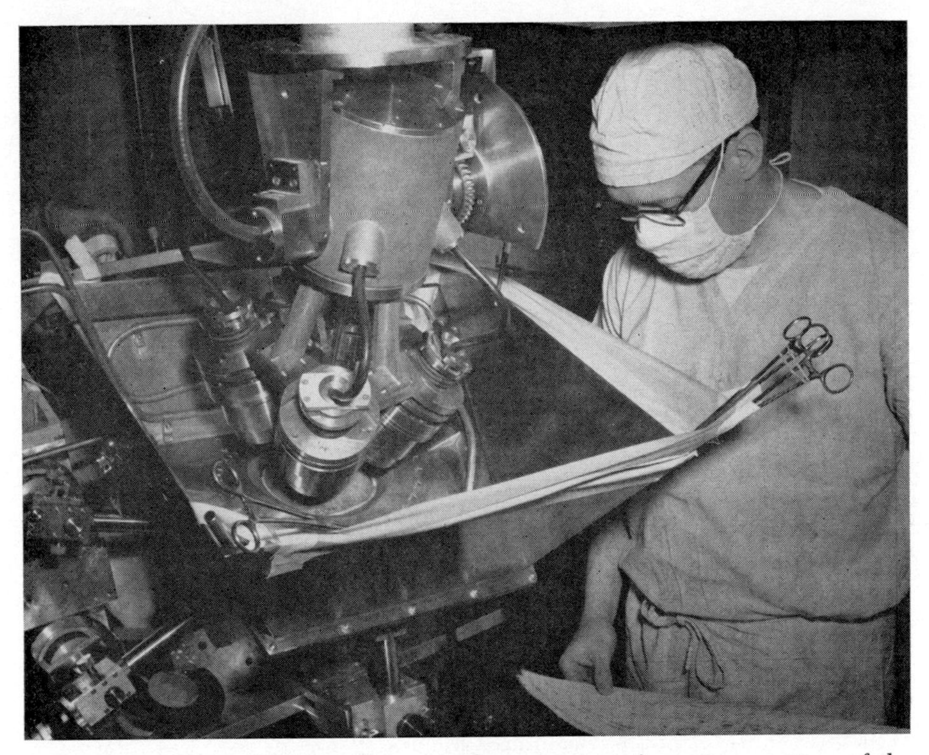

FIGURE 15. Professor W. J. Fry shown checking clearances for various positions of the transducer to be employed during the irradiation procedure.

a few seconds. A time recorder indicates the total time in minutes after the first irradiation. We usually leave a reasonable period of time between exposures for observational purposes. It is now 40 min from time of zero reference, and the sound is now on for the third exposure. In general, of course, these individual exposures have been placed in such a way as to produce some lesions at preselected areas which may or may not be adjacent to each other. The total time is now 1 hr. The total time required, of course, is dependent on the length of the time you want to observe the patient on the operating table. In some cases, the period required for the full procedure is only 1½ to 2 hr. You now see the patient after irradiation. The tremor is gone, and he is demonstrating his muscle control by successfully opening and closing a safety pin with one hand. His irradiation was unilateral with a total of three exposures.

The next patient, a thirty-two-year-old female, shows a nonpatterned intention tremor, primarily in the upper-left extremity. As you can see, she cannot accomplish the simple movement of touching hand to nose. The patient is now in the machine prior to irradiation, and the machine has been padded so she will not injure her arm and hand due to her random movements. The right side of the brain is to be irradiated, the sound is now on. Apparently the amount of tissue involved in the first sound exposure resulted in a reasonable reduction in symptoms. Each of the individual lesions encompasses a volume of tissue which is quite small (of the order of magnitude of 6 or 7 mm long and 1.5 mm in maximal diameter) and is elliptically shaped. This patient was the sort of individual who felt that nothing could ever be done to relieve her symptoms. Here, for the first time during our association with her, she manages a small smile. This view shows the patient the following day after irradiation — and as you can see, she can now perform hand to nose movement quite smoothly.

DISCUSSION

DR. GORDON: What advantage is there in using ultrasound as opposed to the accepted techniques that are being presently used in my neurological hospital, that is, the injection of Novocain and alcohol at comparable sites? I would be only too pleased to sell an ultrasonic technique to my neurosurgical colleagues but, as the hospital radiologist, I was associated with the treatment of some hundreds of cases of Parkinson's disease which have shown exactly similar cure and benefits by being treated by a small bore hole and an injection of alcohol. I would like to hear about a series of cases showing significant improvement from ultrasound treatment, as against the alcohol injection technique.

DR. BALLANTINE: The chairman will exercise his prerogative. Let us illustrate a diagrammatic cross-section of the brain, and let us say you wish to ablate a portion of the thalamus for Parkinson's disease. You place the electrode (which is bare only at its tip) down here. Previously, you put a needle through here into which you injected alcohol and Novocain. Well frankly, I don't know anybody who now injects alcohol and Novocain. Some people inject Novocain first and then alcohol, but most of the chemical techniques for ablation have more or less gone out of style in this country. The reason for this is, Dr. Gordon, that a free-flowing solution will follow planes made by nerve fibers, and so you have no way of knowing where your destructive agent is going to go. If you use an electrode, which, I would say, is one of the very common methods of ablating a certain portion of the basal ganglia, then you run into two difficulties: (1) the vast majority of the complications of this operation are secondary to the tearing of the blood vessels as you introduce your needle, and (2) control over the lesion size and shape associated with methods such as chemical destruction or heat destruction by electrocautery techniques is not as precise as that possible with ultrasound. The final point is that blood vessels are extremely susceptible to the type of heat that an electrocautery produces, and therefore there is grave danger of a hemorrhage at the site of your lesion when you are using such methods for producing lesions. So, these are the advantages of sound: (1) there is no track going down to the area that you wish to destroy, (2) control over lesion size and shape is quite precise — the destruction takes place only where your focal region is placed — and (3) as pointed out in the previous talk, the blood vessels in the lesion region are the least susceptible to the damaging effects of ultrasonic radiations.

Now, balanced against all of these advantages is the disadvantage of the necessity for removal of a large section of bone. This problem has been solved to a certain extent by Fry and Meyers since the bone flap is now removed prior to irradiation. This will strike a great many people as a handicap, however, and it is an objection that you must be prepared to meet. But there is no question, I believe, in the minds of anyone that the ultrasonic technique is the method of choice for making lesions within the central nervous system, if you can get the energy in without having to use a large craniectomy. Would you like to speak on that, Dr. Heimburger?

Dr. Heimburger: The only thing I would like to add is that the lesions that you make with electrocautery or with alcohol are roughly spherical, whereas you can make sheets of lesions with ultrasound. The anatomy of the brain is not spherical in any one area. You can interrupt tracts by sheet lesions, something that you cannot do with other methods.

Dr. Gordon: I'm well aware of these arguments, and I've done my best to put them to my colleagues and associates, but our results with these alcoholic injections are so obviously good. I want to see a long series of cases treated by ultrasonic techniques that can produce better results than the results at my hospital with other techniques.

Dr. Ballantine: If you are getting uniformly good results without complications, then I'm going to send all of my cases to England because we do not get uniformly good results without complications. We get paralysis, we get hemorrhages, and we get infection. Those are the three things that occur as complications in such a significant number of cases that we are still searching for a better way to make a lesion.

Dr. Joyner: I would like specific statistics on the exact number of patients irradiated and both the immediate and long-term results of these irradiations. Did these patients survive for 6 mo, and for those that survived, was there a return of symptoms at a later date? I am under the impression that the cases shown in the movie may be isolated cases.

Dr. W. J. Fry: In answer to your question, I would like to point out that insofar as neurological results are concerned, it is essential to distinguish between methods of making lesions and between the choice of structures in which lesions are placed. These are completely separate problems. Dr. Ballantine indicated very clearly the advantages of the ultrasonic method as the means of making changes in the brain. The neurological result is dependent upon the specific choice of structures that one modifies. If one doesn't choose a proper structure, then obviously there will not be a favorable neurological result. Now, I can comment very briefly on the latter aspect, but I wanted to clearly differentiate it from the former.

The number of irradiation procedures pertinent to the discussion are over 100. Some patients have undergone as many as four such procedures. The results obtained must be subdivided first on the basis of the various categories of disorders treated — about half a dozen different types. In addition, we modified at least half a dozen different structures in Parkinson patients alone. Therefore, because of the large number of combinations, I cannot answer your question in detail in a few minutes. But I can say that if one considers a Parkinson patient with a tremor, then irradiating or modifying the tegmental field of Forel will result in the elimination of tremor in an extremely large percentage of cases, certainly above 90%, and I suspect that we could accomplish elimination of the tremor in 95% of the cases. This result is not true of modifying, for example, the base of the ventrolateral nucleus of the thalamus. By modifying this region one can affect tremor to some extent, one reduces rigidity markedly, but one does not eliminate tremor in such a high percentage of cases. These constitute examples of the types of results that can now be achieved. One could also, of course, place a coagulating electrode into the tegmental field of Forel and if the lesion included the appropriate region, then one could also eliminate the tremor. Does that answer the question?

DR. JOYNER: I agree with your statements, but I would still like to know how many patients with Parkinson's disease have been irradiated.

DR. W. J. FRY: We have treated 86 patients – probably 60 Parkinson patients.

DR. JOYNER: And of those 60, how many are now living, and what is the extent of the improvement of their original symptoms?

DR. W. J. FRY: Of the Parkinson patients that we have irradiated during the five years since the start of the program, four died for various reasons, in addition to the two that were mentioned this morning. The complications – paresis and paralysis – that were produced in some early members of the series when we were working with the medial globus pallidus were the result of impinging on the internal capsule. In addition to Parkinson patients, we worked with a small number of intractable pain cases, seven patients in all. We started the series by modifying the ventroposterior lateral nucleus of the thalamus which receives an input from the medial lemniscus. If one irradiates the basal portion of the ventroposterior lateral nucleus, one may produce anesthesia, and this occurred in the first phantom limb case that we treated. This individual had the right-upper extremity severed midway between the wrist and elbow, and he experienced a phantom of the severed portion, pain in the phantom, as well as pain in the stump. In this case, immediately following the irradiation of the ventroposterior lateral nucleus, the patient exhibited an analgesia over a portion of the corresponding side of the body, and he later developed a thalamic syndrome. In the next patient we moved more medially and had no complications of analgesia and no delayed thalamic syndrome. However, the original discomfort returned within a couple of months postirradiation. In a third phantom limb case irradiated more medially – border zone of the centromedian nucleus – the phantom and discomfort were eliminated and did not return. This is an example of the way the program evolved in the modification of intractable pain disorders. We also worked with several patients exhibiting a thalamic syndrome, and in these we modified the ventrolateral and lateral border region of the centromedian nucleus. In two cases we were able to produce a normal neurological sensory status, but the favorable results obtained were not sustained. Within a few months the symptoms of the thalamic syndrome returned. Are there any other specific points you would like to have discussed?

DR. BALLANTINE: I think Dr. Joyner has raised an extremely important point in attempting to obtain an analysis of the results of the irradiation of patients with ultrasound. I may say that I find it a great pleasure to be on the same side of the fence as Bill Fry from time to time. In answer to Dr. Joyner's question, I would like to say that I do not believe that Bill Fry and Russell Meyers are advocating at the present time the ultrasonic method of ablation for the treatment of all cases of Parkinson's disease. I think this would be a gross exaggeration if anyone did say this, because I think there are certain fundamental disadvantages associated with the technique, which incidentally have led us in our laboratory to postpone the use of this in the central nervous system. This is a matter of opinion, but I would feel that if I were going to have "my Parkinson's disease" treated, I would still probably have it done by more conventional techniques. But this does not detract from the potential advantages of the focused ultrasound method. I think that while it would be nice to know exactly what the percentage of complications is in a particular series, or the mortality figures, which is what you were asking for in "X" number of cases, I think you will agree that with cardiac surgery, neurosurgery, and all new methods which have to be developed, the percentage of good results increases with the number of operated cases. If there were 50% complications — I don't think there are, don't misunderstand me — but suppose there were 50% complications in this series of ultrasonically irradiated cases, I would simply say that they were on that portion of the curve which represents the necessity of gaining experience in order to translate a potentially good result into an actually good result. I think that there are many problems that we must overcome in the use of focused ultrasound in the making of lesions. But (I made this statement in conversation here, and I'll make it in public) there is no question in my mind but that if anyone is interested in studying neuroanatomy or neurophysiology by ablation techniques in animals, the ultrasound method is the only method to be used and I wouldn't give a damn for any electrode or chemical introduced into the brain as opposed to the use of ultrasound. This is a proven method, and it eliminates so many of the artifacts inherent in other methods of making lesions that it represents a prime event.

DR. JOYNER: There is no doubt that the advances in localization represent a great improvement, but the point is, if you are to move into the so-called clinical sphere with an experiment of clinical design, then you must have some idea of where you are going as you go along.

DR. BALLANTINE: I think this is very important, and I agree with you on that point.

DR. W. J. FRY: I want to second the comment made that we certainly wouldn't recommend the ultrasonic method for general therapeutic use at this time. We are still in the process of improving our methods. As Frank indicated here this morning, since the start of the human work, the technique has been greatly improved in reducing the total time involved in an irradiation procedure. Formerly, 12 to 14 hr were required to accomplish the craniectomy and irradiation at a single procedure. This should be compared with the 2-hr procedure now employed for irradiation. However, we are still not anywhere near the completion of the evolution of all of the practical details so important to the recommendation of a method for routine therapy.

Dr. Gordon: I fully agree with you on the question of the production of experimental lesions, and I hope to do some work along this line myself within the next couple of months, and I also agree with you in that I feel for the time being the conventional techniques are the best bet.

Dr. Ballantine: But I don't think this removes the stigma which you have attached to your neurosurgeons by not being imaginative enough to explore new areas and new methods. They can't be content with the old as we are in Boston. You've got to move forward as they do at the University of Illinois.

Dr. Dunn: Where does the ultrasonic method presently fall as compared to the other methods for treating humans?

Dr. W. J. Fry: If we include every patient that we have done, we have had complication in certainly 20% of the cases. If we consider only the last twenty or thirty patients with Parkinson-type complications, we experienced probably no more than 5%.

Dr. Dunn: How does that compare with alcohol or other methods?

Dr. Ballantine: You have just introduced another barrier. All I can say is that I would have a hunch that there are statistically significant differences that would lead me to employ the electrode or the freezing technique, whatever method you like, because I think that the results are probably in the 70 to 80% range. If you consider the possible complications and the percentage relief of tremor and rigidity, there would be a variation from neurosurgeon to neurosurgeon, as well as from technique to technique. Just as clinicians had difficulty 5 or 10 years ago in trying to find out what the results of cardiac surgery were, so we have the problem of trying to assess the validity of certain clinical reports of all procedures. However, I still feel that we would have to call ultrasonic neurosurgery a developmental and experimental method which should be restricted to one, two, or three centers at the present time.

Dr. Howry: Where was the lesion located in the patient shown in the film with the nonpatterned intention tremor?

Dr. W. J. Fry: This can best be shown by a diagram (Fig. 0–1) which includes the red nucleus and fibers called the tegmental field of Forel. We placed the center of the first site in the area designated "lesion"; the beam was coming in at an angle of approximately 45°. You noticed that the first site completely eliminated the abnormal movement, but nonetheless, we extended the irradiation in an anterior-posterior direction, 2 mm anterior and 2 mm posterior in the tegmental field of Forel.

Dr. F. J. Fry: I would like to indicate that we plan a histological study on the brains of those patients who succumbed to some ailment or other in the course of the 5 years, roughly, since the time we initiated these irradiations. The brains have been embedded in celloidin and special apparatus has been constructed so that we can determine how accurately we have placed the lesions with respect to the landmarks we used at the time of ventriculography.

We also want to check on the accuracy of the scaling methods applied in attempting to place the lesions within a given structure.

DR. BALLANTINE: Can you tell us something about the differences in the irradiation parameters both stereotaxically and from the standpoint of the energy requirements when you irradiate through the scalp as opposed to when you irradiate transdurally?

DR. W. J. FRY: We have effectively considered the skin and muscle to be much the same as brain.

DR. F. J. FRY: We measured the muscle and skin thickness and averaged this over a number of precise craniectomies. The muscle is rather thin over the major part of the area, but we take an average value.

DR. W. J. FRY: We found the absorption coefficient of this muscle layer to be essentially the same as that in the brain, and we compensate for the additional thickness, averaging out the fact that the muscle which comes up

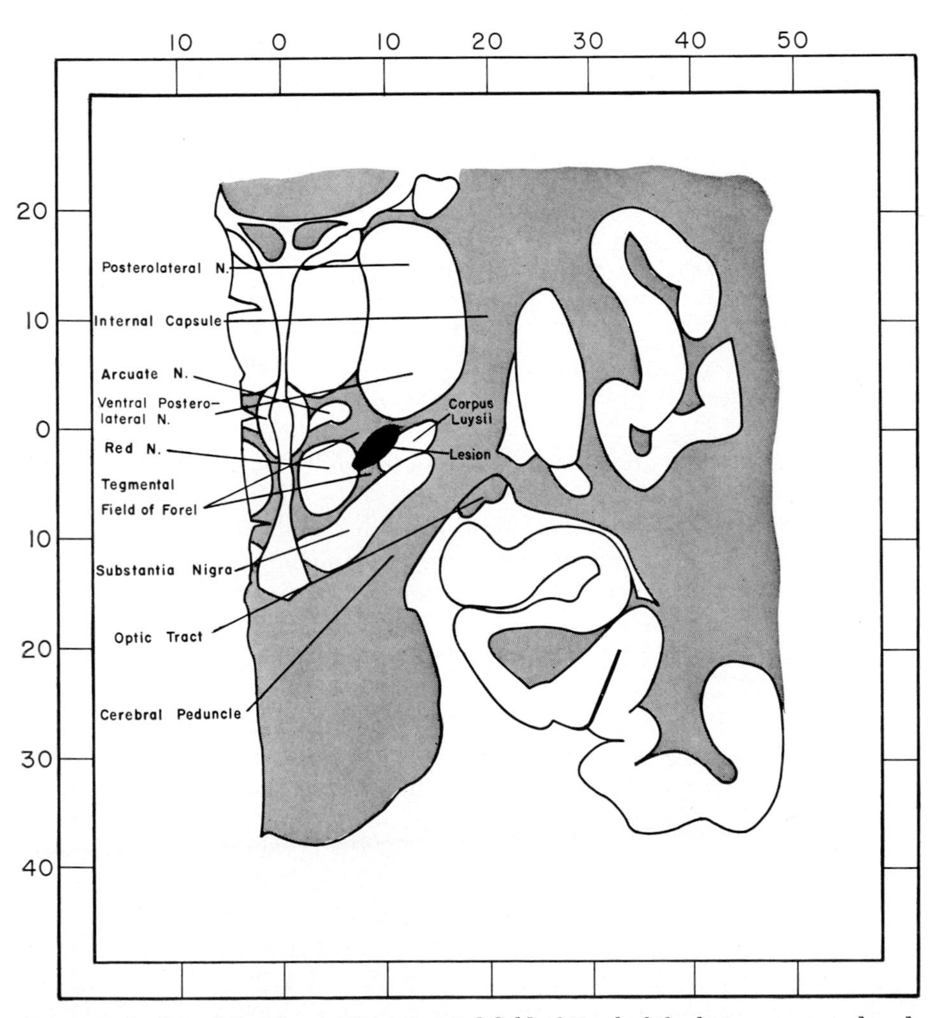

FIGURE 0–1. One of the sites in the tegmental field of Forel of the lesion array produced to relieve intention tremor.

over the temporal region is tapering off fairly quickly. We have seen no apparent difference between the effect in terms of localization, as we interpret it from the functional endpoint, in irradiating transdurally or transcutaneously.

DR. HERRICK: Do you still use a sort of hunting technique to detect the reversible effect?

DR. F. J. FRY: On the human patients, of course, our apparatus is not set up to do any sort of reversible suppression, but one could use the reversible technique as an adjunct to localization with a ventriculography procedure. We used this technique on one patient. It is not generally true that irradiation at one site, for example, in the Parkinson-type patient, would necessarily produce the cessation of the tremor or modify it sufficiently to be able to tell by looking at the endpoint whether one were actually in an appropriate region. Therefore, the reversible technique with the apparatus available at that time was not really ideally suited for this problem. However, in the case of one patient, in order to demonstrate this as a possibility, we repeated the process at one site at a sublethal dose, so to speak, approximately ten times, with intervals of 5 to 10 min between each, to show that one could, in effect, first suppress and then have complete recovery with this many cycles for irradiation at one particular site. It just happened to turn out that this patient could be suppressed at that one site. This would not necessarily be true of all types of patients.

DR. HERRICK: That process is time-consuming.

DR. F. J. FRY: Yes, it is quite time-consuming, but as I say, unless you are set up to cover more tissue or scan with the beam, so that you can suppress some function by irradiating a reasonable volume, you may not be able to utilize the method of reversible suppression very efficiently. But in this case we did demonstrate the reversible phenomena. The question of whether or not we produced a lesion can only be based on the finding that the patient had no apparent change in the tremor after approximately ten cycles of sublethal irradiation.

DR. HERRICK: I thought you did this to establish that there might be some analogous site in the brain for relief of these disfunctions and you said that this technique would insure accurate placement of your lesions.

DR. W. J. FRY: No, this we never did on human patients, primarily from the point of view of apparatus insufficiency. We relied entirely on the ventricular pictures for our localization.

DR. MACKAY: I wonder if you would care to comment, for the sake of the record, on something we noted before lunch, namely the fact that in your transducer there is a $\lambda/4$ spacing between the piezoelement and lens whereas Dr. Yoshioka this morning showed a $\lambda/2$ spacing.

DR. W. J. FRY: I can show here roughly how the output from a transducer varies as a function of this spacing dimension.

A half-wave spacing is, of course, the choice that one makes if he simply wants to achieve the effect of no spacing at all. In other words, if zero spacing is inconvenient, one can employ a half-wave. But a half-wave is not the best choice from the viewpoint of obtaining maximum power transfer for a given driving field strength across the crystal. One can obtain much more power from the transducer for a fixed driving voltage by choosing dimensions and characteristic impedances of the coupling media in other ways.

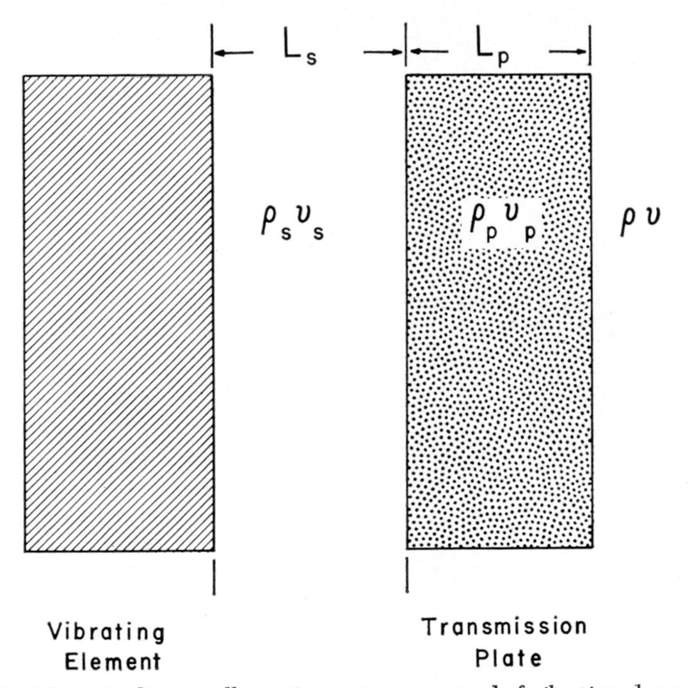

FIGURE 0–2. Schematic diagram illustrating system composed of vibrating element, spacing material with thickness L_s and characteristic impedance $\rho_s v_s$, transmission plate with thickness L_p and characteristic impedance $p_p v_p$, radiating into a medium of characteristic impedance ρv.

Consider the system shown in Figure 0–2 – a vibrating element coupled to a medium of characteristic acoustic impedance ρv by a two-layered assembly. The gain, G_p, is defined as the ratio – at equal driving voltages – of the power output of the indicated configuration divided by the power output of the vibrating element when radiating directly into the medium. Of course, the operating frequency is the same in each case. The gain obtained by this scheme arises as a result of the modification of the electrical input impedance at the terminals of the piezoelectric elements which allows the element to draw more current and more power for the same driving voltage from the electronic generator. The characteristic acoustic impedances of the transmission plate and spacing material are, respectively, $\rho_p v_p$ and $\rho_s v_s$, and the corresponding thicknesses of these two media are, respectively, L_p and L_s. For all values of the ratio $[\rho_p v_p / \rho v] > 1$ and for any fixed thickness of transmission plate, it is possible to realize values of the gain $\overline{G}_p$ greater than unity by choosing L_s equal to an odd multiple of a quarter wavelength. It is possible by appropriate choice of the acoustic parameters to realize rather high gains, for example, 10 to 100. For this case, the gain is given by

$$\overline{G}_p = (\rho v/\rho_s v_s)^2 \left[\frac{1 + \tan^2 \left(\frac{\omega L_p}{v_p} \right)}{1 + \frac{1}{(\rho_p v_p/\rho v)^2} \tan^2 \frac{\omega L_p}{v_p}} \right] \quad (1)$$

where $L_s = (\lambda_s/4)\ (2m - 1)$ and $m = 1, 2, 3, \ldots$. Large values of $\overline{G}_p$ are obtained by choosing materials such that the ratios $\rho v/\rho_s v_s$ and $\rho_p v_p/\rho v$ are large. The optimum thickness of the transmission plate, for high gain, is one-quarter wavelength. The graph of Figure 0–3 shows the bracketed factor of Equation (1) plotted as a function of L_p/λ_p (the thickness of the plate

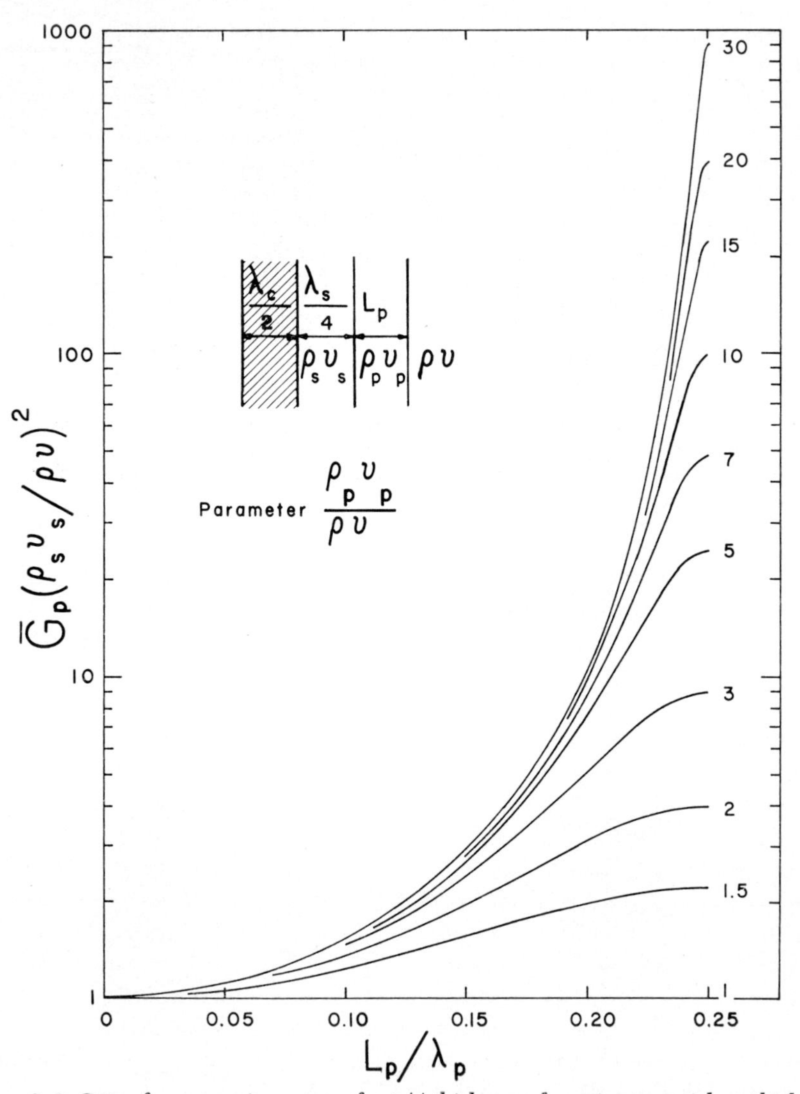

FIGURE 0–3. Gain of a composite system, for $\lambda/4$ thickness of spacing material, vs thickness of the transmission plate. Symmetrical about $L_p/\lambda_p = 0.25$ and repeats every $L_p/\lambda_p = 0.5$.

divided by the wavelength of sound in the plate). The parameter from curve to curve is $\rho_p v_p / \rho v$.

The gain, $\underline{G}_p$, is equal to or less than unity if $[\rho_p v_p / \rho v] > 1$ and if the thickness of the spacing material is zero or any multiple of a half-wavelength for all thicknesses of the transmission plate. For this case, the gain is given by:

$$\underline{G}_p = \frac{1 + \tan^2\left(\frac{\omega L_p}{v_p}\right)}{1 + (\rho_p v_p / \rho v)^2 \tan^2 \frac{\omega L_p}{v_p}} \tag{2}$$

where $L_s = (\lambda_s/2)m$; $m = 0, 1, 2, \ldots$. Figure 0–4 shows $\underline{G}_p$ plotted as a function of L_p/λ_p.

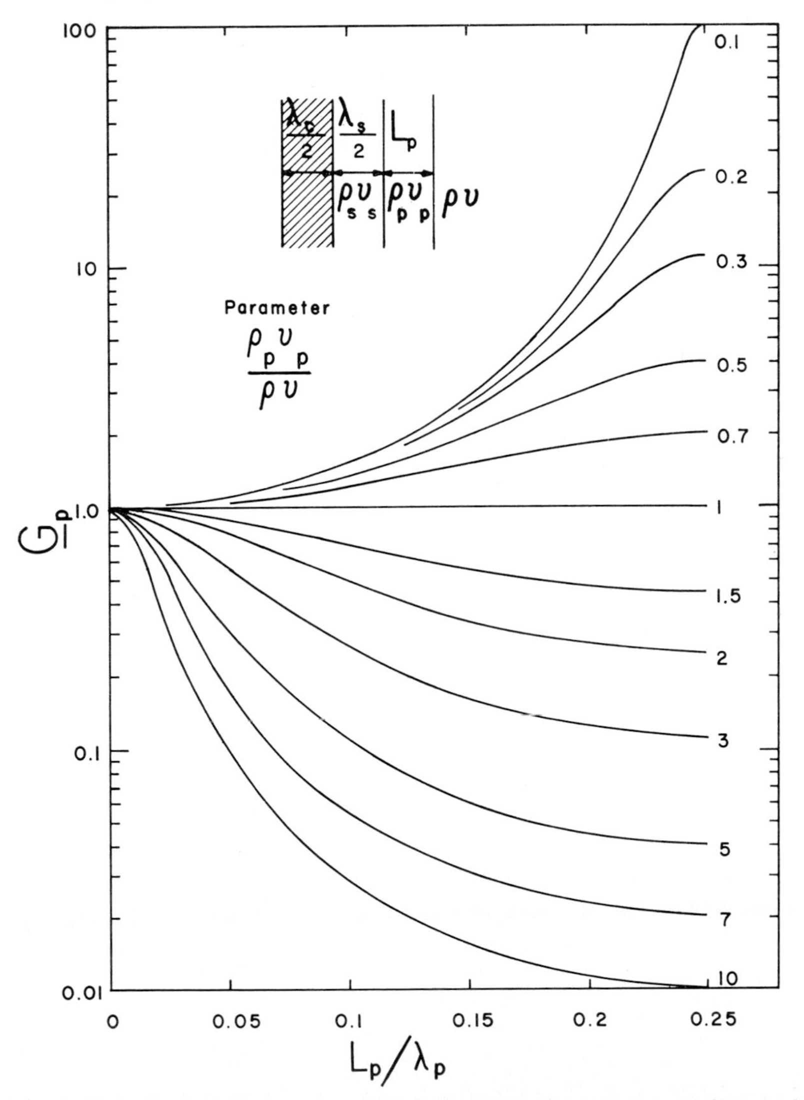

FIGURE 0–4. Gain of a composite system, for $\lambda/2$ thickness of spacing material, vs thickness of the transmission plate. Symmetrical about $L_p/\lambda_p = 0.25$ and repeats every $L_p/\lambda_p = 0.5$.

However, I should mention that the achievement of high gains by the procedure just described would result in a relatively sensitive transducer from the viewpoint of the variation of its characteristics with changing temperature.

DR. MACKAY: Would it be fair to say that this loading process changes the characteristic impedance of the transducer but doesn't help the impedance matching problem?

DR. W. J. FRY: It's probably better to say that it lowers the input impedance at the crystal face so that for a given electric field strength a higher power can be transferred.

15

Concepts of Electronic Design for Precision Ultrasonic Lesions

GENE H. LEICHNER
Biophysical Research Laboratory, University of Illinois, Urbana, Illinois

I. INTRODUCTION

In order to produce precise ultrasonic lesions of predictable size in brain tissue, an overall or complete system approach is necessary, including the establishment of accurate standards for equipment calibration. The final goal to be accomplished, namely, delivering a precise dose of ultrasonic energy to the tissue site, must be kept in mind to avoid being sidetracked onto separate secondary problems. If, for example, it is found that power line voltage variations are causing errors in lesion size, an overall system review may show that it is more desirable, either technically or economically, to redesign the irradiation equipment so that it is less sensitive to power fluctuations than to launch into a precision power supply design program.

A recent statistical study at our laboratory on the effect of ultrasound on the spinal cord of one-day-old mice illustrates the necessity of precisely controlling the ultrasound level. A possible relationship between sound level and sound duration for a given probability of producing paralysis of the hind quarters is being investigated and the approximate relation is shown in Figure 1. It was found that very slight errors in sound level caused significant errors in the time determination, and, in fact, random errors of only a few per cent in sound level would completely prevent the construction of any meaningful curve. Consequently, the obtaining of overall results with a modest accuracy of 5 to 10% required sound level control to the rather strict limits of 0.2 to 0.4%. Detailed anatomical studies of the brain, using ultrasonic techniques, also require precise control of the ultrasound level in order that only the desired structures are affected. Here again, errors of only a few per cent can completely mask the effects being sought.

A reasonable approach to the problem of precise control begins by summarizing as many sources of error as can be predicted in advance. Table I

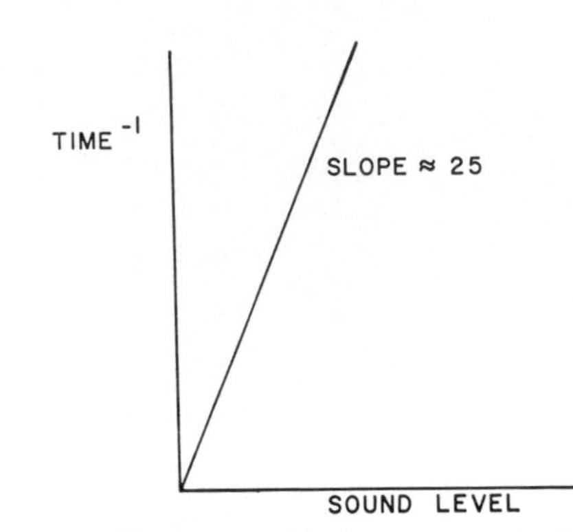

FIGURE 1. Illustration of high sensitivity to dose settings.

indicates some of the possible sources of error which have been considered in our investigations. Obviously, however, such a tabulation is compiled as a result of an attempt to obtain precise data and not after a priori contemplation. Consequently, following the initial exploratory phase in which the need for further improvement of the equipment is recognized, it is necessary to interrupt the experimental investigation and to formulate a new procedure, or system, which can eliminate the difficulties observed to date. In most instances the new system will probably not be the ideal one since compromises in design will be required for reasons of cost or lack of a technical solution to a particular phase of the problem. The theoretical ideal should be retained, however, and rechecked periodically to see whether new techniques or approaches can make the ideal more nearly attainable.

If we choose as a specific example the goal of producing a lesion of precise size in brain tissue, the ideal solution might be as follows. First, establish an approximate sound level which is certain to produce a lesion, provided the sound is applied for a sufficient time, as determined by preliminary experi-

TABLE I. SOURCES OF ERROR IN ULTRASOUND LEVEL.

Source	*Possible causes*
Driving signal changes	Frequency and amplitude changes caused by tube aging, power supply variations; temperature and aging effects on components.
Transducer changes	Resonant frequency drift caused by crystal clamping pressures and temperature effects. Crystal activity variations. Focus and field shape changes caused by changes in lens element spacings and temperature-induced distortions.
Instrumentation errors	Aging components, temperature effects, and drifts in calibration standards.
Changes in tissue	Temperature changes in the tissue and variations in the amount of, or nature of, intervening tissue, such as might be caused by slight motions with blood pressure pulsations.

mental investigations. Second, use the duration of the sound as a precise control of the size of lesion, and finally, consider measuring the lesion *as it forms*. Neglecting the practical problems involved for the moment, let us review briefly the many advantages of such a procedure. If the necessary size measurement could be made, then every one of the possible sources of error in Table I would be avoided. Each one would have an effect, to be sure, on the precise duration required, but the lesion size would be correct regardless of the time needed to produce it.[1] The sources of error would thus be reduced to a very few, namely, those associated with the lesion measurement and such questions as whether the lesion continues to grow after the sound is removed.

The general principle illustrated here is the measurement, as directly as possible, of the quantity to be controlled, in this case, lesion size, and the generation of a control signal, which is based on the comparison of desired to actual performance and which will bring these two variables into agreement.

II. A PRACTICAL SYSTEM AND ITS COMPROMISES

The example of lesion formation in brain tissue may now be further pursued, departing from the ideal approach above only as far as necessary. Unfortunately, the first compromise is a far-reaching one. It is not practical, as yet, to measure the lesion as it forms. The insertion of simple measuring devices into the irradiation site would destroy the advantages associated with the use of ultrasound and remote measurement devices are not yet available. Consequently, not only can the lesion not be measured as it is formed, but also the sound level cannot be measured where it matters most, that is, in the lesion area. Various alternatives must be considered.

From an overall feedback viewpoint it appears that the portion of the system beyond the transducer will have to remain outside the control loop (see Fig. 2). It would, of course, be preferable to bring the transducer activity

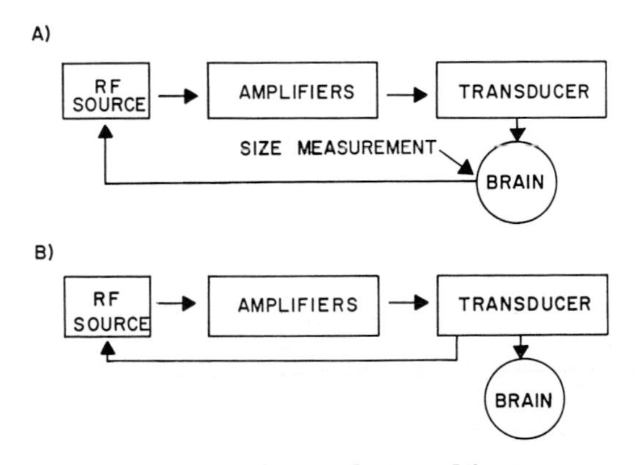

FIGURE 2. Idealized feedback control loop and its modifications as a result of the first compromise.

[1] This statement is obviously meant to apply only to errors of the order of 10 to 20% or less. Very large errors could prevent a lesion from ever forming.

and focus changes, the intervening tissue attenuation effects, and the tissue characteristics at the irradiation site inside the feedback loop as shown in Figure 2A. However, it now appears that the best available solution is to include as many as possible of the other error-producing elements in the measurements made at the transducer. The portion of the system beyond the transducer must operate in a so-called "open loop" mode. Error-producing changes there evoke no corrective or compensating signals.

The measuring procedure in present use at the University of Illinois Biophysical Research Laboratory samples the voltage applied to the transducer. Such a procedure thus introduces a second compromise – this time for a less compelling, but still practical, reason. Some of the transducer changes could be detected and included in the feedback system by sampling the sound field in the water between transducer and brain, but the necessity for developing a stable sampling device that would not unduly distort the field has delayed the implementing of this procedure. There is no denying its desirability, however. A summary of our position, therefore, shows that all sources of error beyond the applied voltage at the transducer will go uncorrected. All error sources at earlier stages will evoke automatic compensation.

Essentially all of the sources of error in Table I must now be dealt with directly and individually, as opposed to automatic correction, with the exception of those concerning the driving signal. While the frequency of the driving signal might still be bothersome, in that it must match the transducer resonant value, drifts in frequency are easily prevented by the use of crystal oscillators. These devices are sufficiently stable that they essentially remove frequency stability as a problem. The question of whether the transducer frequency is stable or not is another matter; it simply must be checked periodically.

In an effort to observe and compensate for transducer variations the transducers are calibrated periodically using the same applied voltage each time. Very small thermocouple probes are used to plot the sound field and to measure the sound output at the focus. Thus, any drifts which are occurring over a period of time can be detected and the necessary adjustments in applied voltage can be made during the experimental irradiation procedures. However, the use of "small" thermocouples (accurate plotting of the sound field requires very fine thermocouple junctions) brings with it several new problems. The probes are delicate and easily damaged. They therefore require low sound levels during the calibration procedure, which in turn results in very small output voltages. The necessity for stable low-level amplifiers is thus introduced. Small transducer driving signals now must be used for calibration in place of the large signals normally used for irradiations, which means the control circuits must be capable of accurate scaling from low to high levels. Furthermore, the manner in which the transducer output varies as a function of drive voltage must be assumed to be the same at high levels as it is at low levels. Clearly, additional tests are necessary to investigate further the above factors.

In order to check possible long-term drifts of the transducer and calibration equipment, periodic animal irradiations are performed, the animals sacrificed, and the lesions measured. This procedure also serves as a check on the methods by which the attenuation of the sound through the intervening tissue is computed, as well as the positioning procedure.

One last source of error of lesion size is the temperature of the tissue at the irradiation site. Here again it is not practical to measure directly at the site. It has been established, however, that larger lesions result from increased tissue temperature. Thus the problem becomes one of insuring that the irradiation site itself is at a standard temperature during irradiation. The Biophysical Research Laboratory has established a reasonably effective method for obtaining the desired control. Rather than measure temperature directly at the site, a measurement is made at the posterior end of the brain, where the influence of a thermistor-carrying needle on the region under study should be slight. In order that there be no excessive temperature gradient between this point and the irradiation site, the temperature of the cat's entire body is controlled by means of a heat exchanger wrapped around its midsection. Since the cat's own internal temperature control system is largely disabled under anesthesia, this control process is quite effective and usually maintains the temperature in the rear of the brain to an accuracy of $\pm 0.1°C$. Whenever the temperature exceeds these limits, the irradiation is stopped until the control system returns the temperature to the required value. Deviations of the temperature sometimes occur during the irradiation which the external controller must overcome, such as those brought about by anesthesia level changes.

A summary of the procedures for producing precise lesions indicates that a heavy price is paid for the inability to measure the lesion directly during its formation. Feedback control techniques are applied over as large a portion of the irradiation system as possible, while that portion of the system not inside the feedback loop must be separately measured and calibrated. It is clear that the latter portion of the system requires human cognizance of the possible sources of error. In contrast to this, all sources of error inside the feedback loop are automatically included by the comparison of desired to actual end results. Much of our instrumentation and calibration effort therefore stems from the single inability to measure the lesion directly as it is formed.

III. LONG-TERM ACCURACY PROBLEMS

A number of the study programs involving the use of ultrasound require the ability to reproduce a particular sound level several months or even years later. For example, in a behavior study involving irradiation of a specific brain structure, there is considerable delay between irradiation of different animals. Time is required to train the animal before irradiation and to study the effects of the irradiation on the behavior pattern, so that the interval over which it is necessary to be able to deliver exactly the same dose to a second animal may extend over a number of months. The study would be dangerously disturbed by a sound source which gradually increased or decreased in output.

Thus it is necessary to have a number of standards of comparison available for instrument calibration only — standards which are inherently stable and, if possible, self-checking. These standards must be kept in a protected environment and used only as reference devices rather than subjected to the rigors of daily use. In general, the devices should be as simple as possible to minimize the chances of their changing and to facilitate checking their operation. Our laboratory keeps several such standards. The simplest is an accurate thermometer for a temperature standard, against which all thermistor probes are checked periodically. Others are an accurate DC voltage source which uses a standard cell as a reference, and a thermocouple-type meter for r.f. voltage measurements. The latter instrument uses the transfer principle for an internal self-check on DC, and this portion is then checked periodically against the DC source as an additional safeguard against undetected drifts. Perhaps the best example of standards, however, is the one used to check the thermocouple probes, which plot the sound field and calibrate the transducer. What is required is a device which can verify whether the thermocouple probe produces the same output for a given sound field strength as it has in the past. To do this, a strictly mechanical procedure has been developed which uses the radiation pressure of the sound field as a measure of its strength. A small metal ball, usually gold, is suspended from thin nylon threads, and its horizontal deflection is measured optically during irradiation at a sound level which produces a reference level of output from the thermocouple probe. In this way an output curve can be developed for each thermocouple over a period of time. The standard itself is easily built, though some care is required, and has the additional advantage that its performance can be checked by direct calculation, providing a plane field is used for the tests (1–3). Here, then, we have an example of what must be done ultimately for all standards. They must compare to an arbitrary standard, such as the standard meter at the Bureau of Standards, or they must produce results which are calculable in terms of such standards.

IV. CONCLUSION

Attempts to produce precise lesions in brain tissue with ultrasonic techniques have led to a continuous program of upgrading of equipment. The introduction of feedback control systems has made it possible to eliminate several sources of error while periodic systems studies have pointed the way toward more ideal approaches. Finally, the problem of long-term drift has been attacked by setting up calibration standards of the secondary standard type.

REFERENCES

1. Fry, W. J., and R. B. Fry (1954). Determination of absolute sound levels and acoustic absorption coefficients by thermocouple probes – theory. J. Acoust. Soc. Am. *26*, 294–310.
2. Fry, W. J., and R. B. Fry (1954). Determination of absolute sound levels and acoustic absorption coefficients by thermocouple probes – experiment. J. Acoust. Soc. Am. *26*, 311–317.

3. Fry, W. J. (1958). Intense ultrasound investigations of the central nervous system, *in* "Advances in Biological and Medical Physics," C. A. Tobias and J. H. Lawrence, eds. (Academic Press, New York), Vol. VI, pp. 281–348.

DISCUSSION

DR. VON GIERKE: On your first diagram you chose to monitor the voltage at the transducer. Did you consider monitoring the vibration amplitude or velocity amplitude at the crystal face? Couldn't that be done relatively simply and wouldn't it include some of the factors that you have just discussed?

DR. LEICHNER: It may not be too easy, but it does sound like a good idea.

DR. CURTIS: Holding the voltage on the transducer constant when the impedance of the load is changed seems to be a dubious procedure.

DR. LEICHNER: But monitoring the current by *itself* would suffer the same difficulties; you would have to monitor both current and voltage. These measurements must be made right at the transducer, as close as one can get.

DR. KIKUCHI: I quite agree with your program of employing a feedback circuit to control the amplitude of the irradiation. I have been thinking about this problem for some time and I have used a feedback system of picking up the voltage applied directly to the transducer. It was compared to a standard DC voltage, then the difference was fed back to an amplifier of an AGC (automatic gain control) type. This technique is successful in keeping the velocity amplitude at the crystal face at a predetermined value. In regard to the final objective of this equipment, namely, control of the intensity of the ultrasound in the brain, has there been any attempt to use a brain electrical wave as a signal source? If there is a significant signal, is it possible to analyze such electrical brain waves? As you know, in a computer the analysis of a particular signal can be picked up almost immediately using correlation techniques. It may be possible, therefore, to use the electrical brain-wave signal as a source of computer control. Has any work been done in this direction, and have you investigated the significance of brain-wave patterns while you were projecting ultrasonic waves into the brain?

DR. LEICHNER: That certainly is an interesting idea, and we have given some thought to it. I might ask Bill to describe some of the things he has considered in this direction.

DR. W. J. FRY: The question arises whether one could possibly monitor some electrical activity from the brain as a whole, I presume, to determine the dosages. I would say that the chances of detecting a change on the surface (where you would necessarily place the electrodes, otherwise you would revert to the old disadvantage of inserting a number of probes into the brain), which manifested any variation in a small volume of a deep structure, would be very small. That is to say, the opportunity of producing a major change in any arbitrary structure by controlling the irradiation parameter of the sound by this method would be slight. Of course, one can produce changes in deep structures, using various cortical potentials as an indication of change in a specific region, but it is not possible to do this in all cases – for example, in the case of the mammillothalamic tract. During my talk, I shall discuss another method which I think might serve as a monitor.

DR. BALLANTINE: I should like to ask a question. What order of predictability do you wish to have with your lesions, and how do you determine whether you are in the ball park or not?

DR. LEICHNER: Well, as to whether you are in the ball park or not, you must always evaluate after the fact, that is, you evaluate the histological evidence. In the case of a human patient you might see whether it had the desired effect, but that, clearly, is not a suitable indication. Therefore, the histological evidence is the criterion for determining if the lesion has the intended dimensions. I would say that the lesion should be, certainly, within 10% of the size at which you were aiming. Bill, do you think that is a reasonable figure?

DR. W. J. FRY: I think perhaps a better way to describe the reproducibility is in terms of the dosage curves. For the preparation previously discussed, one-day-old mice, where you choose as an endpoint a paralysis of the hind legs following irradiation of the lumbar enlargement of the cord, one can determine a dosage curve, that is, a relation between time of irradiation and sound level. This can be accomplished quite accurately, and one can discuss the requirements of stability in terms of the variation of the points which define the curve. The particular result that Gene quoted a while ago, an uncertainty in the time equal to 25 times the uncertainty in sound level, that is, a 25% variation in time as a result of a 1% variation in the level, was taken from a dosage curve. Therefore, if one wishes to obtain curves accurate to, say, 5% on the time scale over the range of values of the parameters in which the situation just described obtains, then one requires a 0.2% accuracy in the sound level. So that in our case, for the dosage work in the physical mechanism studies, we attempt to reproduce sound levels to a couple of tenths of a per cent in order to achieve a 1 or 2% accuracy in the determination of the dosage curve itself. From the viewpoint of a histological evaluation of reproducibility, one can consider as a criterion, for example, interruption of the mammillothalamic tract with no interference to surrounding structure. However, this latter basis for considering reproducibility is probably not as definite as one based on the variation of points on a dosage curve.

DR. BALLANTINE: We have been using, for the past 8 years or so, a single-beam irradiator at a frequency of 2.7 Mc for our work with animals, and in a very tentative fashion, with humans. The thing that has plagued us has been this question of reproducibility of lesion size, shape and control. As Gene Leichner so beautifully expressed the problem, there are a number of parameters that can go wrong in the irradiation equipment, things that we were not aware of for a long time, such as ridiculously small variations in temperature of the coupling medium or of the brain, etc. We finally worked out what we considered to be a satisfactory piece of apparatus and a satisfactory method of calibration, which has been published in the March issue of the Journal of Physiology.[1] One thing that we have done since that time, which has been fun

[1] P. P. Lele. A simple method for production of trackless focal lesions with focused ultrasound: physical factors. J. Physiol. *160* (1962), 494–512.

to do and which has been more or less helpful, is to produce lesions in plastic.[2] Figure 0–1 (A to H) shows a series of such lesions produced in plastic. We found that there is a relationship which is fairly constant between the dosages required to make lesions in methylmethacrylate and in the brain of a cat.[3] Figure 0–1B shows a series of these so-called lesions in a stressed bar of methylmethacrylate, viewing in a cut across the length of the lesion. Figure 0–1G shows the effect on the size of the lesions in the plastic bar of decreasing the duration of the ultrasonic irradiation, these being two different views of the same lesions. With a constant intensity and irradiation time, but with pulsed energy applied, Figure 0–1H indicates the effect of decreasing the number of pulses, that is, the effect on the size of the lesions. You also see that these lesions tend to become more globular as the pulsed energy is used, rather than the CW techniques. Figure 0–2 shows the relation between pulse duration and lesion volume, on log scales for three different intensities, the bars representing the variations in four different lesions made at these points. Can you see that, except for its threshold, these bars are very small indeed, showing that we do have, I think, a reasonable control over the volumes of the lesion, at least in methylmethacrylate? Finally, Figure 0–3 shows the effect of increasing path length through the medium to be affected, the effect on lesion size. You see again the effect of absorption. It is apparent, therefore, that variation in lesion size and shape in this bar of plastic follows very closely the variations that one sees in the cat brain. We found this to be a method of quick calibration, a quick look at the geometry of our focal region.

DR. NYBORG: How do you see these assimilated lesions?

DR. BALLANTINE: You see them with polarized light.

DR. GORDON: I would like to confirm how really valuable this technique is. I've seen it in use in London.

DR. BALLANTINE: I believe that in England Dr. Warrick also has worked with the plastic bars, although I don't think he has published it. For our calibration techniques, Gene, you might be interested to know that we do use the thermocouple, but we use it primarily for locating and delineating our focal region and we do that about once a month. Then, for immediate pre-irradiation calibration we use a simple Siemen's "Sonartest" which we have adopted.

DR. MACKAY: You suggested that the bar was prestressed. Did you mean this?

DR. BALLANTINE: Yes, you have to get the stress marks out of it. Unless you anneal it, you get all sorts of breaks in the plastic (Fig. 0–1A).

DR. MACKAY: We have been taking ours right out of the stock pile, and we usually obtain good pictures.

---

[2] P. P. Lele. Irradiation of plastics with focused ultrasound: a simple method of evaluation of dosage factors for neurological applications. J. Acoust. Soc. Am. *34* (1962), 412–420.

[3] L. Basauri and P. P. Lele. A simple method for production of trackless focal lesions with focused ultrasound: statistical evaluation of the effects of irradiation on the central nervous system of the cat. J. Physiol. *160* (1962), 513–534.

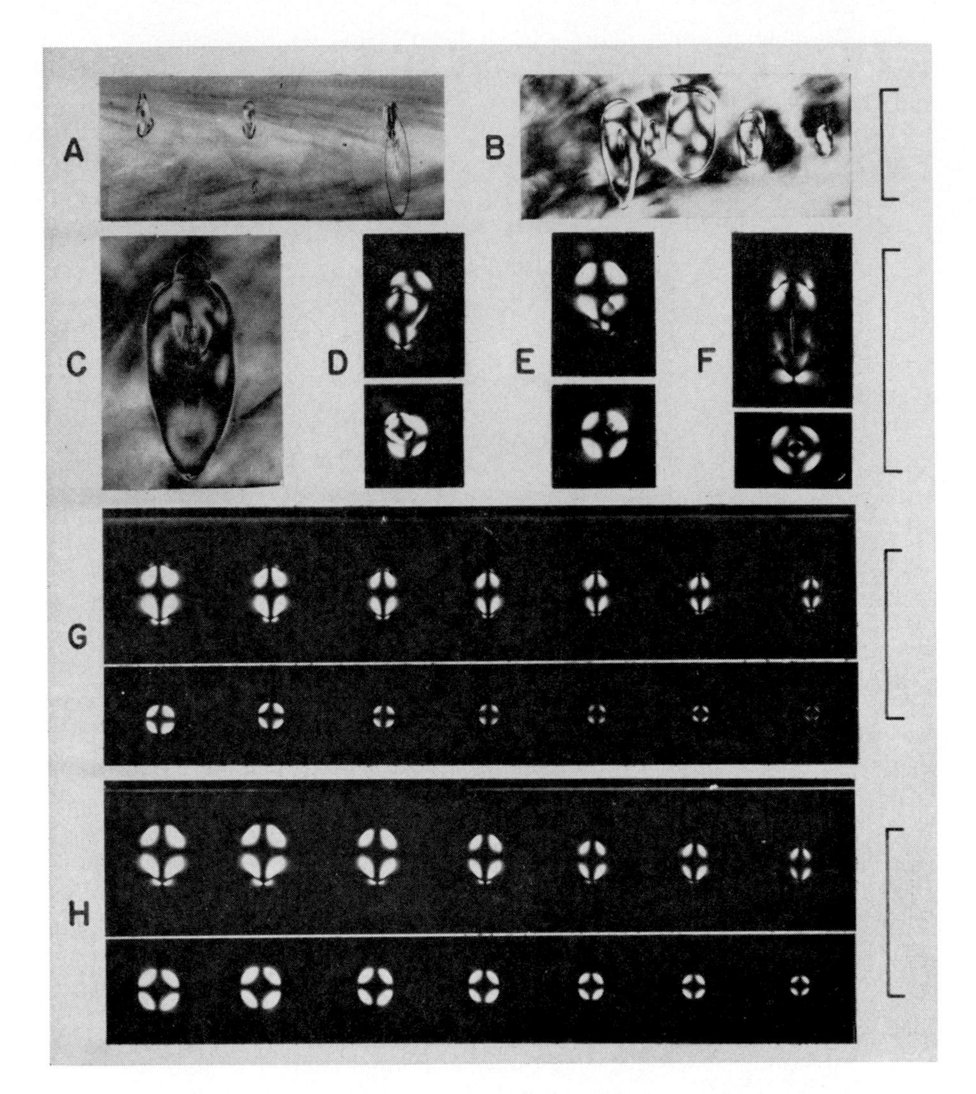

FIGURE 0–1. Photographs of "lesions" in plastics. Calibration mark = 1.0 cm. A. Polystyrene bar showing four lesions from four different dosages. Note irregular shape and a fracture plane in relation to one lesion. B. Methacrylate bar showing lesions of irregular shape. C, D, E. Each shows two overlapping lesions in methacrylate. In D and E (and all subsequent illustrations) the bar was annealed before irradiation to remove preexistent strain. Two views of lesions are shown at right angles to (top) and in the axis of irradiation, respectively (bottom). F. "Acorn"-shaped lesion with disfiguration and discoloration in the long axis resulting from a high dose. G. A series of lesions each made with a single pulse. The pulse duration was decreased in steps from left to right. The two rows show the two views of lesions as in E. H. A series of lesions each made with multiple pulses of a constant pulse duration. The number of pulses used decreases from left to right. The two rows show two views of the lesions as in G. (Reprinted with permission from J. Acoust. Soc. Am. *34* [1962], 412–420.)

DR. BALLANTINE: Well, yes, but it doesn't give you as pretty a picture. At least it doesn't give us one. Maybe you have a better plastic than we do.

DR. KIKUCHI: I would like to ask Dr. Leichner a question regarding the four-beam-focused irradiator. If the four beams travel through this presumably uniform medium, the phases of the waves coincide, but if you irradiate the sound in an oblique direction, then the beams may not be in phase if the medium is not really uniform, since the velocity is somewhat different. In that case, the four beams cannot coincide. Have you attempted to confirm this?

DR. LEICHNER: I believe the answer to your question is yes. We have made such measurements with the human irradiator containing four transducers, which I believe is what you are referring to. The small thermocouple probe allows us to plot the beam, and we find, as you would expect, one main beam, that is, one main focus, and four smaller lobes. It is a long and tedious process, but we adjust and determine this pattern until we get the ratios between the

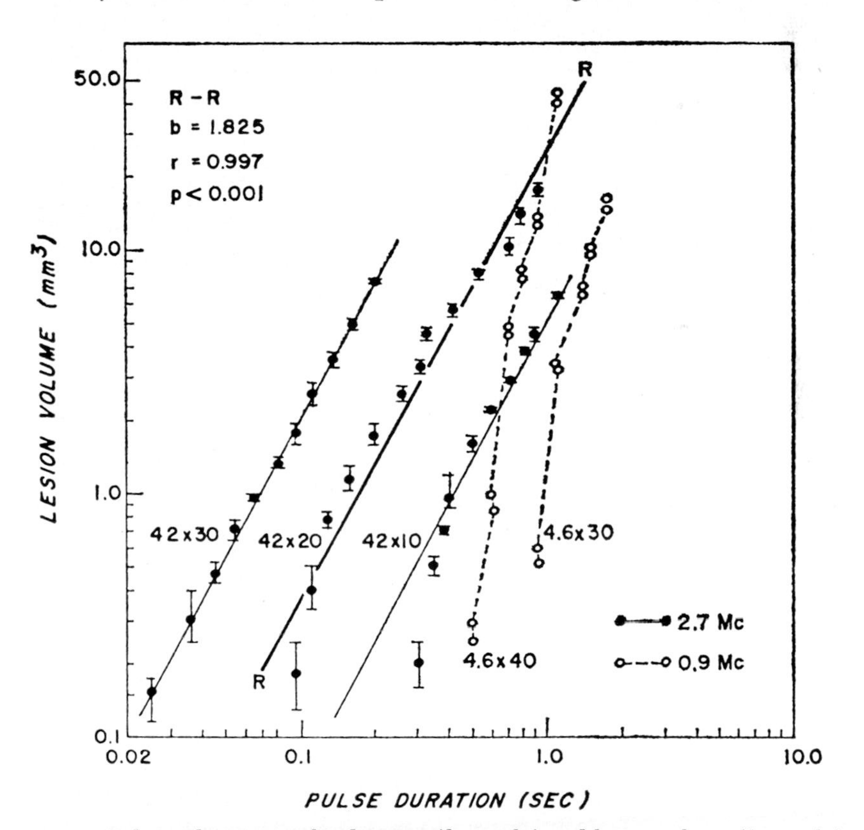

FIGURE 0-2. Relation between pulse duration (log scale) and lesion volume (log scale) at different intensities and 2.7 Mc. Each point is a mean of four different lesions. The bar represents the range of variation. Each lesion was made using a single pulse. Calculated regression line R-R is shown for 42×20 w/cm^2 average focal intensity at 2.7 Mc. Regression lines for other intensities were parallel to the one shown. For comparison, data obtained at $I_{av\,f} = 4.64 \times 40$ w/cm^2 and 0.9 Mc are also included. (Reprinted with permission from J. Acoust. Soc. Am. *34* [1962], 412–420.)

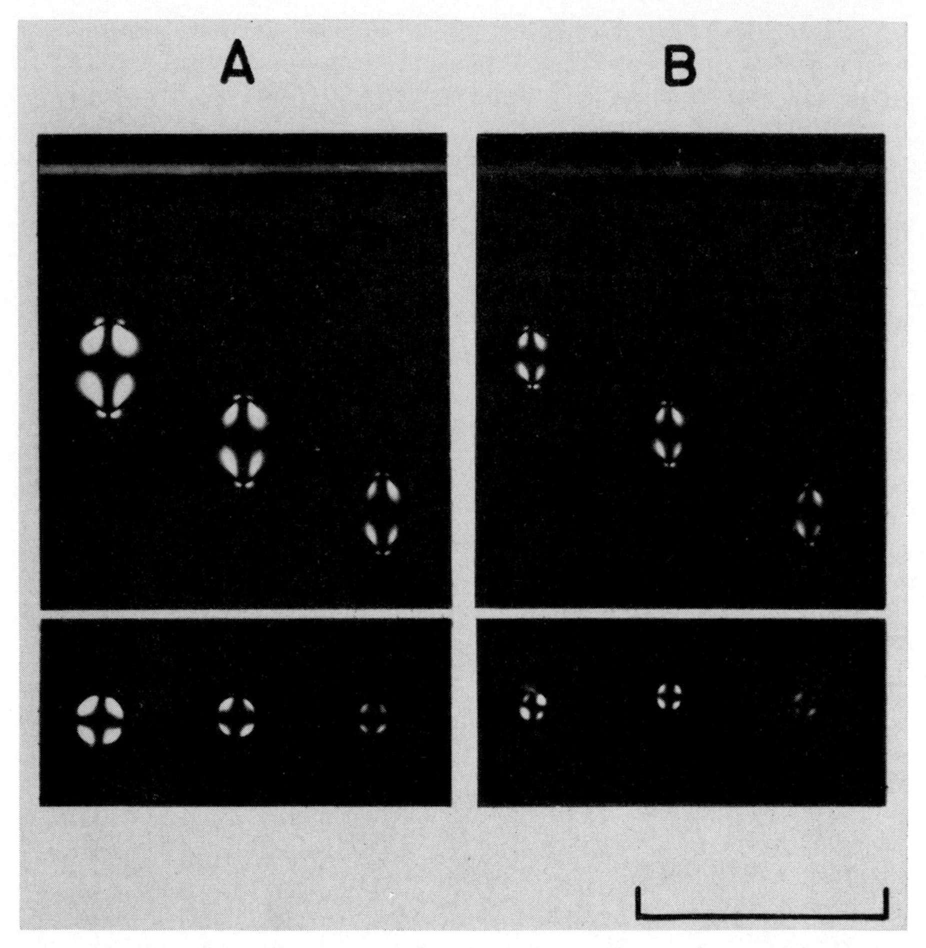

FIGURE 0-3. A. Relation between path length of ultrasound in medium and lesion size. Note progressive diminution in diameter and sphericity. B. Results obtained by compensating for attenuation at different depths by increasing duration of irradiation, thus obtaining lesions of the same size at different depths. (Reprinted with permission from J. Acoust. Soc. Am. *34* [1962], 412–420.)

main-lobe amplitude and those of the smaller side lobes as great as we can. We do this by adjusting the phasing of the transducers and by changing their angles of orientation.

DR. KIKUCHI: I know that, but I was referring to the problem that the four paths might be somewhat different lengths, that is, just slight difference in length might cause a large difference in sound level at the focus since the wavelength is so small; if one beam is retarded a little relative to the others, it is out of phase. This makes the intensity very low.

DR. LEICHNER: I agree with your statement that this can happen. I don't believe that we correct for that. One cannot detect the presence of such a condition in the brain, and we cannot, therefore, correct what we don't know. If the energy comes from some other path, then you have a different shaped field.

DR. W. J. FRY: With respect to difficulties resulting from changes in relative phasing along different paths, it wouldn't make any difference if one worked with a single beam or with many beams. The solid angle subtended is the important parameter. We check the extent of phasing shifts directly by inserting an entire excised brain, or a major portion of one, into the focused beams with the geometry arranged so that the focus lies outside the tissue. In this way the shape of the focus and the acoustic level can be directly measured after the beam traverses the entire thickness of the tissue.

16

New Approaches to the Study and Modification of Biological Systems by Ultrasound

WILLIAM J. FRY

Biophysical Research Laboratory, University of Illinois, Urbana, Illinois, and Interscience Research Institute, Champaign, Illinois

As you all know, present methods of ultrasonic visualization of soft-tissue structure depend upon the existence of differences in the characteristic acoustic impedance at tissue interfaces – that is, differences in the product of the speed of sound and the density. Therefore, it is possible to detect only those structures, that is to say, interfaces between structures, that are characterized by different values for these parameters. This means that in the normal brain no structure is discernible except the ventricles, since only at the ventricular boundaries does the value of the impedance undergo sufficient change for successful visualization. The procedures that have been used up to the present time for the placement of electrodes in the brain or for irradiating specific nuclei with various types of energy have depended on various landmark systems. The most accurate of these systems employs the ventricles as references. Obviously, a method which would enable one to view brain structures directly would be extremely valuable in the field of applied neurology, including neurosurgery, and also in basic neuroanatomic and neurophysiologic research. I would like now to describe such a method which, in principle, will enable us to see all major brain structures directly.

Figure 1 illustrates diagrammatically the basic principle involved. Two beams of pulsed, focused sound are employed. Let us consider as an example the case of concentric beams – that is, an inner conical beam with an outer or enveloping beam surrounding it. The inner beam induces transient changes in the temperature of the medium of the order of a few degrees. If this is accomplished fast enough, let us say in a time interval of the order of 1 sec, then steep temperature gradients will be produced in the tissue at anatomic sites where the value of the absorption coefficient changes as a boundary is crossed.

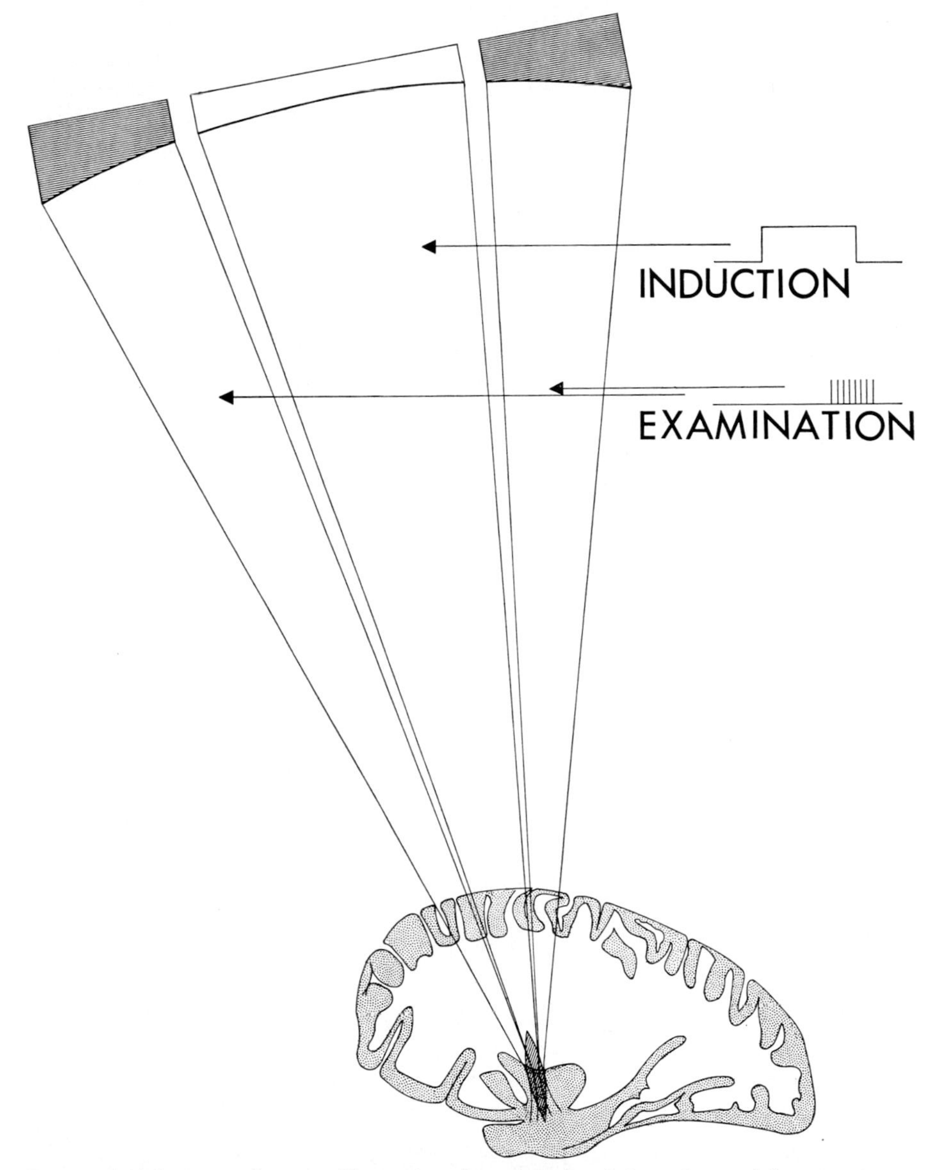

FIGURE 1. Schematic diagram illustrating the principle of detecting and locating interfaces between brain structures characterized by different values of the ultrasonic absorption coefficient. The relatively long duration pulse of the focused induction beam produces transient temperature gradients and therefore gradients in the speed of sound at interfaces between such structures. A second focused beam, consisting of a train of short duration pulses synchronized in appropriate time relation with the induction beam, locates the boundaries by echoing from the sites of the induced acoustic impedance gradients.

Measurements indicate that the value of the absorption coefficient for white matter is considerably higher than for gray matter — approximately 50% greater. Therefore, by this method one can produce at a white-gray matter boundary a transient thermal gradient with a temperature difference of at least 2°C without causing damage. Since the speed of sound is dependent upon the temperature, a corresponding gradient in its value would result. A gradient in sound speed implies a change in characteristic impedance, and since the sites of impedance differences are detected by present methods, the examining beam of Figure 1 is synchronized with the first so that a train of pulses of short duration is produced and echoes are detected as in the reflection methods used up to the present time. Thus, this new method provides the possibility of detecting any interface between two structures, if a sufficient change in the magnitude of the absorption coefficient exists. This happens to be the case for brain, since the white and gray matter exhibit such a difference in absorption coefficient. Other tissue interfaces should also be characterized by different values of the absorption coefficient, but we have not yet planned a measurements program. The indicated method would also be applicable in those cases where tissue structure is detected with difficulty by the older, presently employed method since one could expect to enhance the contrast by employing this new method.

In addition to directly visualizing major structures of the brain, the method described here will also make possible the viewing of lesions as they are produced and will thus provide a direct control of their position, shape, and size. Ultimately, present landmarking systems will probably be eliminated and lesion production would then be under the direct and automatic control provided by the visualization method itself.

Of course, one must use considerably higher acoustic energy levels for the temperature-inducing beam than those applied in present visualization methods, but the temperature gradients required to produce detectable changes in acoustic impedance would be of the order of only a few degrees.

At the present time, it is completely impossible to use the ultrasonic method in a controlled fashion for the modification of brain structure by transmitting sound through the intact skull. However, successful development of the method described here would provide the possibility of spreading the incoming ultrasonic energy over a major fraction of the area of the skull so that the ultimate objective for brain modification in the human — the complete elimination of all surgical procedures — might be achieved. The problems that will be encountered in reaching this objective are not simple, and the instrumentation that will be required will be extremely elaborate by comparison with present ultrasonic and other instrumentation used in brain-modification work.

Now, if anyone has any questions on this aspect of our proposed work I would be happy to answer them before going on to discuss other research plans.

Dr. Howry: I would simply like to comment that the concept you have just outlined is very worthwhile and has tremendous possibilities. You are to be congratulated.

DR. GREENWOOD: I would like to ask if you have any data on the strength of the echo from the lesion after it has been produced and after the thermal transient has passed and whether this might be a way of controlling dosage.

DR. W. J. FRY: No, we do not have such data, but of course one would not necessarily have to observe the lesion after it is produced. That is, it could be observed during the period corresponding to the induced temperature change accompanying lesion production. In answer to your second question, I would expect that echo strength could be used to control the dosage.

DR. GREENWOOD: Echoes from a lesion would not necessarily be reflections from the thermal region per se but could be reflections from immediately surrounding tissue.

DR. W. J. FRY: Yes, this would certainly be a possibility. And in regard to this, when ultrasound is used to produce selective lesions, we have noted that histologically one does not see any general breakdown in the tissue structure for some time after irradiation, so it may not be possible to see the lesion immediately unless a thermal gradient is used. Of course, after a time, the breakdown of structure is very apparent.

DR. CURTIS: If I understand you correctly, you would use this new technique to visualize the tissue structure before you place the lesions. The usefulness of the method would then be very dependent upon knowing what sort of injury was associated with the associated very small temperature change.

DR. W. J. FRY: No injury would accompany the use of the method. In fact, one could employ previously obtained data to deduce limitations on the radiation conditions in order to restrict the effects to reversible changes. For example, at 100 w/cm^2 one can irradiate the lateral geniculate nucleus for about 30 sec at a frequency of 1 Mc/sec and still induce only reversible changes. I would expect the maximum dosage required for implementing the new visualization method (as applied to brain) to be about an order of magnitude below this.

DR. CURTIS: Do you know what sort of temperature changes you are producing at the reversible level?

DR. W. J. FRY: We have not measured these specifically for the reversible dose levels. However, for the irreversible levels we measured temperature changes of 10°C (gray matter) to 20°C (white matter) for exposures of 1 sec at an "intensity" of 800 w/cm^2. (I will use the parameter "intensity" to indicate approximate sound levels here even though we do not feel that it should be used in any precise description of the exposure conditions.) In the visualization method now proposed it should be possible to restrict the temperature to levels that might be associated with a high fever — but, of course, for a comparatively negligible period of time.

DR. CARLIN: Have you done any calculating of pulse lengths, repetition rates, etc.?

DR. W. J. FRY: Yes. The basic feasibility of the method depends upon whether one can produce the requisite temperature change in the time available before conduction levels the thermal gradient. Computations indicate for intensities in the neighborhood of 100 w/cm^2 and time durations of the order of 1 sec, that thermal conduction would not destroy induced reflecting interfaces for practical values of range resolution.

DR. CARLIN: It seems to me you are talking about longitudinal waves almost entirely, but you may have had in mind more than this. Normally, in passing from a tissue with a low absorption coefficient value to one with a high absorption coefficient value there would be quite a temperature gradient because of the generation of heat. In addition, if one has reflection without this temperature gradient, then there is probably generation of shear waves at the boundary and an even stronger effect. That is, at a boundary that gives rise to reflection of longitudinal waves, there must be generation of shear waves which would give rise to a very localized heating effect. As you know, it is possible to see these reflections without the temperature gradient so we might consider your concept as a way of increasing contrast in tissue that you can already visualize.

DR. W. J. FRY: Yes, that is correct.

DR. VON GIERKE: What temperature gradient do you think is needed?

DR. W. J. FRY: I would say of the order of 3°C across the interface. This would probably produce a change in the magnitude of the impedance of the order of 1%.

DR. REID: In order to produce this at the interface, aren't you going to need a larger initial temperature difference?

DR. W. J. FRY: The induced temperature changes would be of the order of 6°C above the base temperature in white and 3°C in gray matter.

DR. CARLIN: If the time of travel of the ultrasound wave is of the order of, let's say, 20 to 30 μsec and the pulse length is 1 sec . . . , I wonder if you would explain your timing in greater detail?

DR. W. J. FRY: Both the temperature-inducing and the examining beams are focused into the same region. The inducing beam is pulsed on first, and the temperature increases. Then toward the end of the pulse – for example, 1-sec duration – the examining beam, which consists of a train of short pulses, is turned on and partially reflected from the region of induced impedance gradient if the focus of the induction beam is positioned in a tissue volume where the absorption coefficient is spatially nonuniform in value.

DR. REID: Perhaps I missed something in the train of logic with regard to tissue interfaces from which we now receive reflections, but it would seem to me that, since the change in impedance caused by the temperature rise is related to the attenuation coefficients, we might very easily destroy an existing impedance discontinuity – equally probable, we might enhance it. That is, I do not see that the probability is any greater than 50-50 that you would achieve an enhancement rather than a destruction of the impedance difference.

DR. W. J. FRY: I do not quite agree with your conclusion. The chances are that the tissue on both sides of an interface will have the same algebraic sign for the temperature coefficient of velocity. So, one should have at the interface an impedance difference equal to that before temperature-gradient induction plus the difference caused by the transient induced gradient.

Dr. Dawe: I would like to point out a couple of physiological facts here. The only person I know who has changed the temperature in deep areas of the brain is Hardy at Yale, and he finds some rather profound changes in the entire organism due to this temperature variation. One must remember, if he is going to affect the deep portion of the brain or to make a thermal scan of the brain, that every portion that is heated is going to require a little more oxygen because of the increased metabolic rate. From a physical standpoint your experimental approach looks very good, but you have to be careful that you do not make physiological changes in the animal.

Dr. W. J. Fry: I agree. One must make the measurements in a short period of time. In the case under discussion, the peak of the temperature rise does not last more than a few tenths of a second. In our research on the production of lesions in brain by ultrasound and on the induction of reversible effects, we have produced greater temperature changes than those necessary in the new visualization method, so we do know what sort of temperature increases the tissue can experience without damage for the periods of time required.

If there are no further questions, I should like to amplify the statement I made previously regarding the possibility of ultimately irradiating directly through the intact skull. The possibility is remote at the moment, but I would like to indicate briefly the basic difficulties that prevent irradiation through the skull at the present time and also some possible means of circumventing these difficulties. First, refraction drastically limits the area of skull through which one can pass an ordinary converging ultrasound beam to produce a focus of small volume in the brain. The skull is so nonuniform in shape on the scale of importance here and the angles of entry of different portions of a large aperture converging beam are so different that the possibility is remote that the "rays" entering from various positions will superimpose accurately after transit. A second basic difficulty is the determination of dosage because of the variations in skull thickness as a function of position. In addition to evaluating the effect of absorption, the determination of dosage must take account of differences in the value of the deflection coefficient from position to position. A third difficulty arises from the fact that the amount of energy required in a transcranial irradiation procedure for focal lesion production in depth is such that the cortex would be damaged by heat unless the incident acoustic radiation is spread over a major fraction of the area of the cranial vault.

Now, let us consider how the proposed new visualization method would aid in the solution of these three difficulties. It is apparent that, in principle, the first difficulty could be handled because it would be possible to superimpose, by direct observation, individual incident beams of small cross-section. That is, the new method would show where each beam path is located in the tissue structures and would thus provide the information to permit them to be superimposed at a desired anatomic site by individual adjustment of the positioning systems which support the separate transducers. Thus, one could in principle, solve the refraction problem. With respect to the problem of dosage, the new visualization method provides the possibility of direct determination of the dose at the common intersection by measuring the magnitude of the induced temperature gradients. The third difficulty—overheating of the tissue-neighboring bone at the port of entry of the sound—is a messy one, but since we have shown, in principle at least, how the first two difficulties might be handled, we can now consider spreading the incoming energy over a very large fraction of the skull. A computation shows that conceivably one might operate at a frequency as high as 1 Mc and still allow sufficient energy to penetrate the skull without overheating the cortex.

Therefore, in principle there exists the possibility of eliminating all three major difficulties which currently present a barrier to the direct ultrasonic irradiation of deep brain sites via the intact skull.

DR. BALLANTINE: Do you ultimately replace the bone flap in the work you are doing at Iowa?

DR. W. J. FRY: Ultimately a plastic replacement is inserted.

DR. BALLANTINE: Why don't you replace the bone flap with plastic immediately?

DR. W. J. FRY: This represents a difficulty. We hope that one of our next advances in method will be the development of a suitable replacement for the bone. Any ordinary piece of plastic cannot be used as a bone replacement since the same refraction difficulty would be present as with the original bone. We have been giving some thought to the design of a "sound transparent" replacement.

I would like now to present some other topics that are of interest to us. We reported a number of years ago on the reversible changes in function induced in the visual system of the cat by ultrasonically irradiating a lateral geniculate nucleus while flashing light in the animals' eyes. We showed at that time that one could obtain a three-dimensional "functional" mapping of this portion of the brain by using the sound focus as a probe to modify the relations between the stimulus or input and the output in the form of cortical-evoked potentials. Figure 2 shows the type of map that we published at that time. If one subjects the eye of an anesthetized cat to single flashes of light while maintaining the temperature and level of anesthesia fixed, a reproducible form of the evoked potential is elicited. Under the experimental conditions obtaining for the map and with the electrode placed at the cortical position indicated, the normal response was of the form appearing in the lower circle of the right side of the figure. Now, by focusing the sound into the lateral geniculate nucleus, we showed that one could produce drastic temporary modifications of the form of the potential, the extent of the change depending on where the focus is placed. For example, the response appearing in the upper circle of the right side of Figure 2 shows that all later components of the evoked potential can be suppressed without affecting the first. For some other electrode positions, one observes modifications of the form of the initial response. Therefore, the ultrasound focus, when employed in the manner indicated, constitutes an analyzer for modifying the relations between stimulus and response.

To indicate the potential versatility of ultrasound from the viewpoint of determining maps of brain function, I would simply like to compare its use with that of electrodes alone to obtain comparable information. If one em-

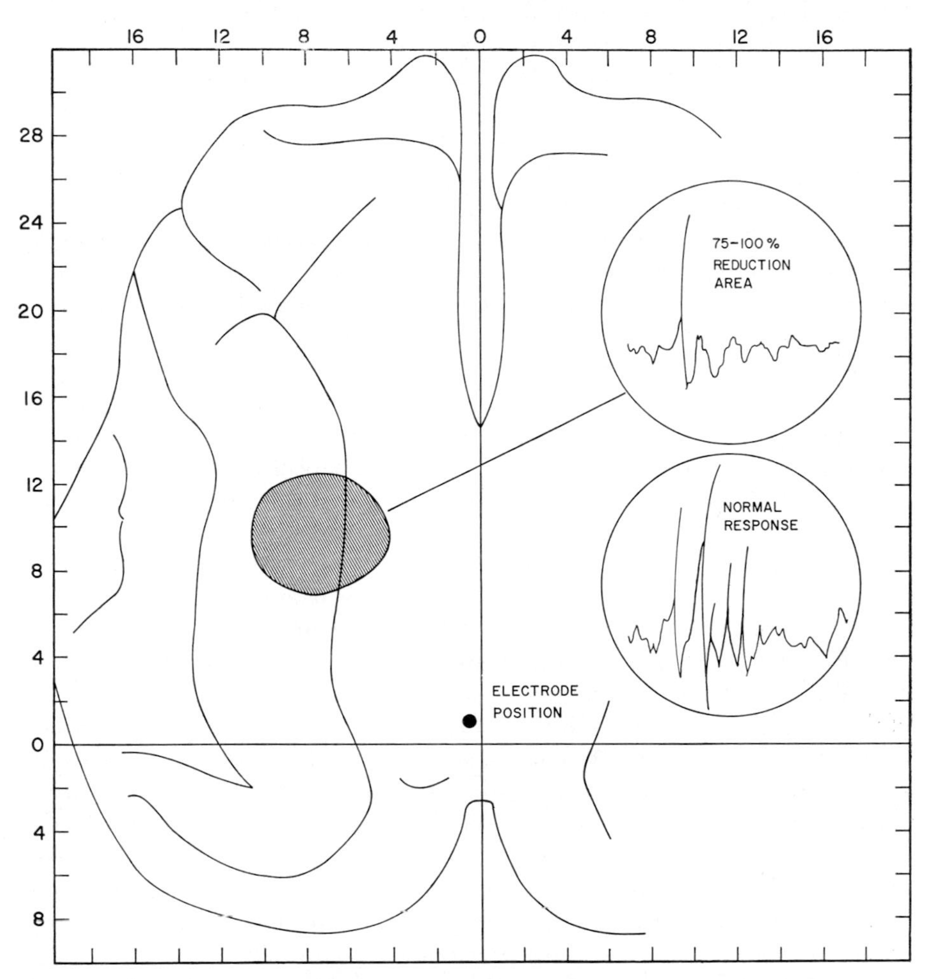

FIGURE 2. Induction of reversible changes by ultrasound in the cortical electrical response induced by subjecting the eye of an anesthetized cat to single flashes of light. The normal response for the level of anesthesia and brain temperature employed appears in the lower encircled area on the right. A number of readily distinguished components can be seen in the response pattern. When an ultrasound beam is focused into the region of the lateral geniculate nucleus and appropriate irradiation parameters are employed, the cortical evoked response pattern can be modified temporarily to assume the form illustrated in the upper circle of the diagram. The gray patch on the left side of the figure is the area, at the vertical level corresponding to the approximate middle of the lateral geniculate nucleus, in which the center of the focus can be placed to produce the result indicated. The cortical pattern of the cat brain is shown to indicate the position of the receiving electrode and also to indicate the approximate positions of the sites of irradiation in the longitudinal and lateral coordinate directions (scales are in millimeters).

ploys 4 Mc/sec ultrasound, as we do routinely for work on the cat brain, then the moving focus of the beam constitutes an analyzer of relatively small dimensions (the diameter, at a pressure amplitude $1/\sqrt{2}$ of the peak value, of the beam perpendicular to the axis of propagation is 0.6 mm). This focus can be moved anywhere in the brain consistent with the portion of the skull cap that is removed, and therefore one has an analyzer capable of modifying the mechanisms of operation in a very large number of positions. For example, it is not unreasonable to anticipate that 100,000 positions could be temporarily modified in a single brain. Obviously, it is completely impractical to consider placing anywhere near that number of electrodes in a brain. In fact, if a dozen electrodes are inserted into even a large structure, one worries whether the system has been disturbed to such an extent that observed function may not bear any resemblance to that of the normal structure. Of course, one can modify the function of neural circuits in various ways; for example, the relation between input and output events might be changed by inhibiting information transfer at specific locations or by potentiation. At the present time we are unable to specify the specific mechanism by which the sound acts on the lateral geniculate to disturb the "normal" mechanism relating the light stimuli and the evoked cortical responses. It may well be through suppression of some events, or it may be through enhancement of others. It should be noted in this regard that we do see enhancement of the amplitude of cortical evoked potentials under some experimental conditions of irradiation.

Considered in the manner described here, focused ultrasound might well provide a tool for the study of complex behavior which would permit some elucidation of the vast array of events which occur in the neural circuitry. Of course, one would require a considerable amount of instrumentation in order to initiate an effective program in this area and I will simply mention some of the types here. Data analysis for the simple experiments we have performed thus far—the measurement of latencies and amplitudes of electrical events—requires a week of one investigator's time to handle the information received at a single electrode by hand measurement and computation methods. In slightly more sophisticated experiments information would be recorded from a number of electrodes simultaneously so that data analyzers, programming equipment, and apparatus for presenting the results of the analysis would be required in order that the information could be processed and assimilated fast enough to determine the future course of the experiment. Some machine representation of the anatomy is necessary so that the investigators can "see" the present path and the history of the position of the focus in the brain. Obviously, automatic positioning and irradiation-control instruments are a prerequisite to such studies.

Some of the data pertinent to the irradiation procedure is now represented by diagrams of the type illustrated in Figure 3. The different shaded squares in the figure represent various sites in a number of nuclei on one side of the brain of a human. This particular diagram was constructed for use during the irradiation of a patient with Parkinson's disease. In this particular case,

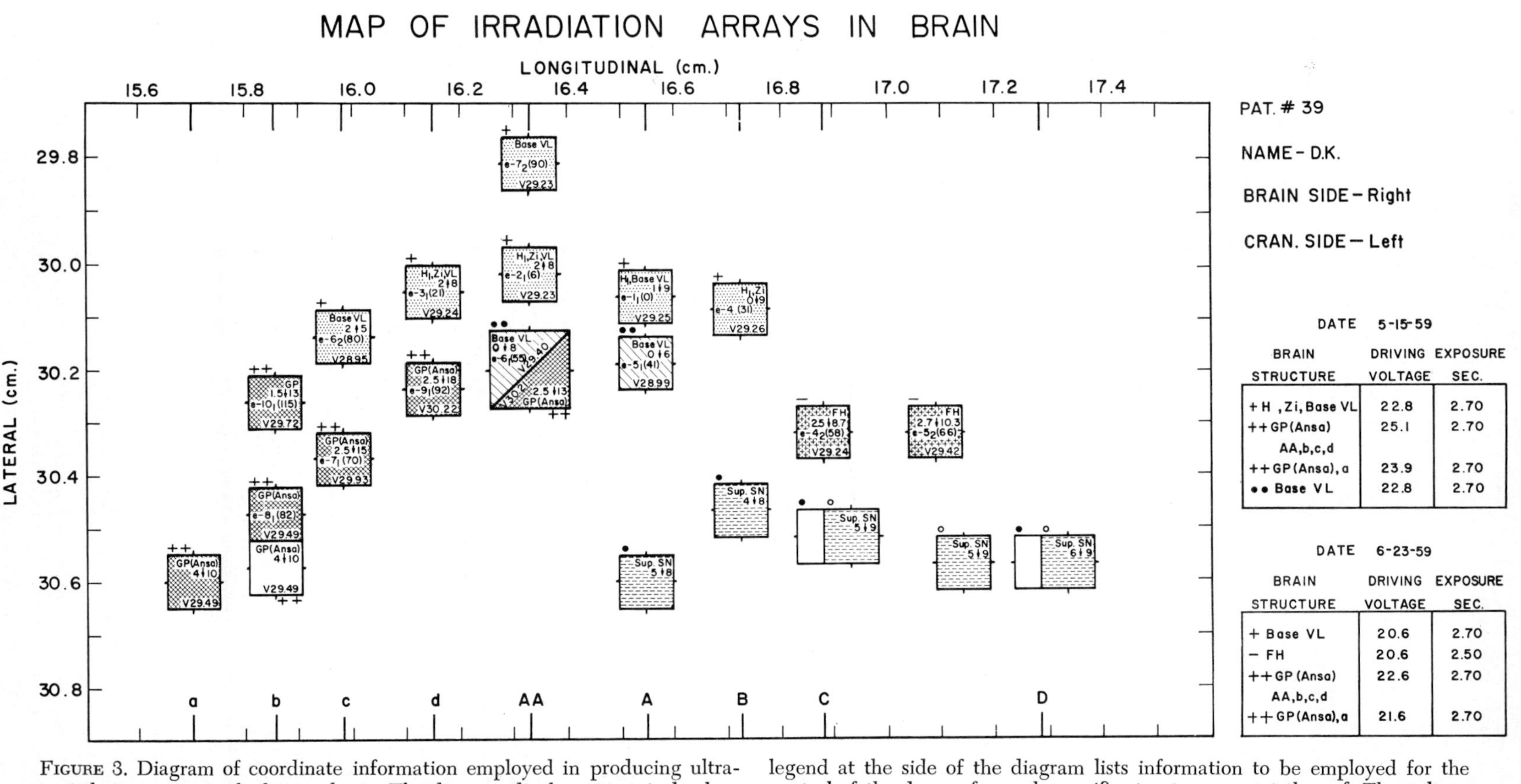

Figure 3. Diagram of coordinate information employed in producing ultrasonic lesion arrays in the human brain. The diagram displays numerical values for the coordinates of reference sites in various brain structures of interest in the modification of hyperkinetic and hypertonic symptoms. The array of reference sites lies on one side of the midsagittal plane (right side). The legend at the side of the diagram lists information to be employed for the control of the dosage for each specific structure or part thereof. The voltage listed is proportional to the driving level applied across the transducer and the column labeled "sec" indicates the duration of each exposure in seconds.

squares with cross hachure, +, represent sites in the tegmental field of Forel (FH); squares with diagonal box cross hatching designate positions in and at the base of the medial globus pallidus (GP); and squares with dotted stippling and with diagonal line cross hatching indicate positions at the base of the ventrolateral nucleus (VL) of the thalamus. Squares with horizontal line segment hachure indicate sites in the substantia nigra (SN). The specific sites indicated in the diagram constitute only a reference set and one does, in general, consider many other positions. Obviously, the representation of the diagram is a planar one, that is, only two of the three coordinate directions are designated by axes. The longitudinal direction or ordinate of the diagram corresponds to the anterior-posterior direction in the brain and the lateral direction of the diagram corresponds to a direction in the transverse plane at an angle of approximately 55° with respect to the vertical axis. The vertical[1] coordinate position is designated by a number in each of the shaded squares. It is readily apparent that it is rather difficult to "visualize" how the brain anatomy corresponds to this representation.

With further regard to information processing, we have found in work with awake human patients that the data obtained during the step-by-step production of changes in their neurologic state represent a quite complex array of information, and it has become apparent that machine aids for processing and presentation are necessary if this information is to serve its maximum utility in determining the lesion arrays to be made. The complexity of this information is illustrated by the diagram of Figure 4. This diagram shows the changing state, in a single ultrasonic irradiation procedure, of hypertonus[2] of different muscle groups all over the body in a Parkinsonian patient as a function of the positions of lesions placed in different anatomic sites. On such a diagram, one can note the changes in tone that occur in each particular muscle group by following the lines connecting lesion sites, indicated on the array of transverse sections in the diagram, with the position of the muscle group in the body. To conclude my comments on this topic, I would emphasize that one would like, during the course of an irradiation procedure on a patient with Parkinson's disease, to maintain an awareness of all of the data of the diagram and, in addition, of information pertinent to other symptoms. Clearly, data-processing and presentation instruments are necessary aids.

I would like now to mention briefly a major goal of our work on the pituitary gland. Basically, we are interested in seeing if the hypophysis can be redesigned by appropriate treatment with ultrasonic radiation — that is, we wish to determine if its hormonal output can be permanently changed to modify the endocrine state of the animal. This possibility is suggested by the histologically observed fact that the population ratios of the various glandular cell types can be affected to a marked extent by irradiation. For example, one can depopulate a region of glandular cells and the repopulation that follows need not duplicate that originally present.

---

[1] The vertical direction is perpendicular to the plane determined by the other two coordinate directions.

[2] The gradations in rigidity are represented by the hachures indicated in the legend of the diagram; the complete absence of stipple represents normal muscle tone.

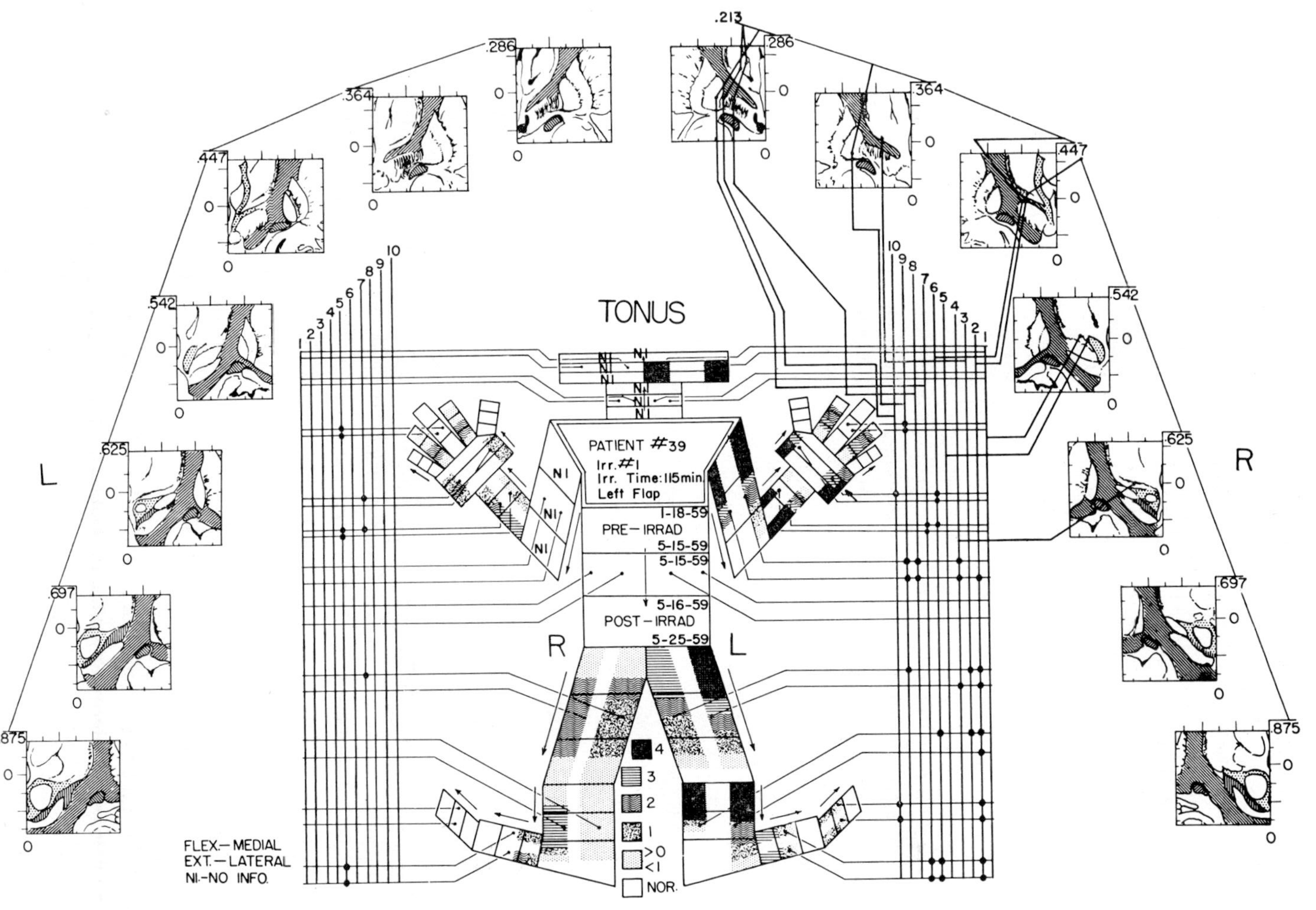

Figure 4. Diagram representing the sequence of changes in the tonus of the various muscle groups of a Parkinson patient undergoing brain modification for the relief of symptoms. The positions of the individual lesions, which result in changes in tone in each of the muscle groups, are designated by dots on the diagrams of the brain sections, and lines connect these sites with the vertical columns of lines on the right and left hand of the figure. The numbers at the top of each column refer to the lesions in the chronological sequence in which they were produced. The small black circles in the columns of lines indicate which lesions produce changes in specific muscle groups as shown by connection with the horizontal lines that terminate on the representation of the body.

It seems appropriate to comment here on our interest in ultrasonic absorption spectroscopy at very high frequencies (100 to 2000 Mc/sec). The work of Carstensen, Schwan, *et al.* on hemoglobin and other biologic materials demonstrates that absorption coefficient values for proteins depend upon the composition of the ionic environment, the degree of hydration, and other factors. It would be extremely interesting to extend such measurements to the high-frequency range indicated and thereby possibly determine the entire extent of the relaxation spectrum.

As you know, many soft tissues exhibit an almost linear relation between the frequency and the value of the absorption coefficient per unit path length. It is desirable to investigate this dependence at the higher frequencies to determine where marked deviations from the "linear" form occur. Up to the present time, although one can discuss analytically the observed absorption coefficient dependence on the frequency, it has not been possible to ascribe the absorption to specific dynamic events. That is, one can describe the data phenomenologically in terms of a distribution of relaxation frequencies. However, further work on the investigation of protein solutions might well show that different macromolecular configurations of biologic significance are distinguished by considerably different relaxation spectra. If this is the case, it might then be possible to derive information on the distribution of various macromolecular species within the cellular elements of tissues by employing ultrasonic microscope principles.

A number of years ago, I proposed a new form of ultrasonic microscope. In this regard, it should be noted that the development of an ultrasonic instrument of high resolution cannot be achieved by applying the design principles employed in light microscopy, for example, the use of lenses, because at the frequencies of operation necessary to obtain appropriate resolution (1000 Mc/sec and higher) the absorption coefficient values are too great to permit the use of the long transmission paths required. However, the type of design which I proposed would surmount this difficulty by: (1) employing plane waves that travel only a short distance to reach the specimen in which they are partially absorbed and (2) detecting the transmitted energy distribution by an array of thermocouple probes placed immediately adjacent to the specimen. The instrument would reveal structural features by localizing sites where the absorption coefficient experiences a gradient.

I will finish this outline of new approaches to the study and modification of biologic systems by ultrasound by noting that we are still pursuing the investigation of physical mechanisms. We feel that this aspect of our program is very important since results obtained will undoubtedly suggest new ways to employ acoustic energy to elucidate structure and function in such systems.

DISCUSSION

Dr. Gersten: In the investigations of the reversible effects are the changes in excitability only at the focal point?

Dr. W. J. Fry: We can discuss that on the basis of resolution, that is, how much does one have to move the focus in order to see a change occur. This is a convenient way to localize the volume of tissue responsible for the observed change. The data that I showed was taken at 1 Mc where the resolution is not as high as one would like. The amount of movement of the focus that would result in a detectable difference in the responses would probably be of the order of half a millimeter or so. Now with 4-Mc frequency, we can increase this resolution to somewhere near a tenth of a millimeter.

DR. BALLANTINE: I would like to comment briefly on some of the results and publications of our laboratory at Massachusetts General Hospital because I think they bear on this question of the localization of the areas to be destroyed, or to be studied by the investigator. First, as I previously mentioned, there are the two publications by Lele [1] and Basauri.[2] Young and Henneman [3] and Shealy and Henneman,[4] who were working both in our laboratory and in the Department of Physiology at Harvard, have published in the Archives of Neurology. It seems to me that there are two methods which should be borne in mind for such a study. One is the anatomical method for visualization of tissue through ultrasound, and the other is the physiological method. Young and Henneman showed fairly conclusively that there was an immediate effect on peripheral nerve, which was differential and reversible. The differential part of this may be open to some question in regard to its reproducibility. We don't know yet but we are repeating some of the experiments. However, the reversibility of the effect on the compound action potential of peripheral nerve is, I think, fairly well established. Accompanying this effect was an initial enhancement of the compound action potential. Similarly, Shealy and Henneman, working with the cat's spinal cord, were able to demonstrate an effect on the monosynaptic and polysynaptic reflex response. With thirty pulses of ultrasound, one a second, there was a rather large enhancement of the potential of the monosynaptic reflex discharge, and then a falling off to almost zero and then after a period of 25 min, a recovery. In yet another experiment, in which both the monosynaptic and polysynaptic reflexes were investigated, there was, following an initial enhancement, a depression of polysynaptic reflexes and a slow recovery. It seems reasonable to deduce that if you can reversibly affect peripheral nerve and monosynaptic and polysynaptic reflexes in the spinal cord, that such reversibility should be feasible in the brain, and in addition, it may be possible that the ultrasound stimulation response could be used as a physiological indication of the location of the sound beam in the brain. I'd like to ask Dr. Fry if he has seen any such stimulation in the patients who were irradiated at the University of Iowa.

[1] P. P. Lele. A simple method for production of trackless focal lesions with focused ultrasound: physical factors. J. Physiol. *160* (1962), 494–512.

[2] L. Basauri and P. P. Lele. A simple method for production of trackless focal lesions with focused ultrasound: statistical evaluation of the effects of irradiation on the central nervous system of the cat. J. Physiol. *160* (1962), 513–534.

[3] R. R. Young and E. Henneman. Reversible block of nerve conduction by ultrasound. Arch. Neurol. *4* (1961), 83–89; and R. R. Young and E. Henneman. Functional effects of focused ultrasound on mammalian nerves. Science *134* (1961), 1521–22.

[4] C. N. Shealy and E. Henneman. Reversible effects of ultrasound on spinal reflexes. Arch. Neurol. *6* (1962), 374–386.

Dr. W. J. Fry: We did not see any motor stimulation during the irradiation of structures of interest to us from the viewpoint of relieving the symptoms of the hyperkinetic disorders, but we do have some evidence for stimulation in patients who were irradiated for the relief of intractable pain. The sensations experienced by these patients indicate stimulation, but, of course, at the time we were treating these patients we were concerned with making irreversible changes, so that we can't say in these cases that the stimulation was unaccompanied by irreversible change in the neural tissue. These patients, who were conscious during treatment, experienced various sensations over the surface of the body, for example, heat waves. Some of them would describe the sensations very vaguely because they hadn't experienced them before. Some were described as very desirable sensations and others as not so desirable. So there is no doubt that one does produce stimulation but I don't believe, in the present instance, that we could use these results to support the view that reversibility would also accomplish stimulation. However, we have other data that might support the view that one can produce stimulation with reversible change, namely, the enhancement of evoked cortical potentials. In our work on the production of reversible effects by ultrasound, we noted enhancement of these potentials, so that one might consider this as evidence for stimulation during the production of reversible changes.

Dr. Ballantine: One other point which I believe needs reemphasizing is that probably a larger volume of tissue needs to be irradiated to produce a lesion, or to produce an effective lesion, than is encompassed in the single lesion produced by a single burst of sound. Wouldn't you say that was true? In the work that we have done, both with peripheral nerve, but more particularly in the spinal cord, so-called defocused ultrasound was used, that is, the focal region was slightly above the surface of the spinal cord in order to give a spraying effect to that segment of the cord to be irradiated. We have been working with various methods to focus and refocus ultrasound in order to get both a clean wave of high intensity and a narrow pencil of high intensity just near the focal region that we can use to irradiate a larger volume of tissue than we can with the ordinary focused beam.

Dr. Curtis: Would you comment on the reversible effect in the peripheral nerves, say in the C and E fibers?

Dr. Ballantine: We found that if the right parameters of irradiation time and intensity were used with pulsed ultrasound, it was possible to abolish the compound potential, and after a certain interval, to have it return. Following an attempt to analyze the compound potential and to break it down into the A and C fibers, Young and Henneman found that the A fibers were more resistant to ultrasound than the C fibers.

Dr. Curtis: How reproducible did you find this and what frequency are you using?

Dr. Ballantine: Young and Henneman felt that it was quite reproducible. We are repeating some of this work and initially found it as reproducible as they did. However, we are using slightly different parameters of irradiation, namely 1-, 1.8-, and 2.7-Mc frequency.

DR. CURTIS: I would like to ask Dr. Fry if he has tried any cortical work?

DR. W. J. FRY: Some years ago we did some work on the irradiation of the motor cortex of both the monkey and cat. Again, we were using dosages which produce irreversible effects, and we observed motor activity related to the position of the focus in the cortex. One could map the cortex in terms of ultrasonically induced muscle movement.

DR. CARSTENSEN: I would be very interested in your feeling regarding the mechanism involved in this stimulation. Is it purely thermal, do you suppose?

DR. W. J. FRY: It's probably a thermal effect; that would be my guess.

DR. CARSTENSEN: I believe that in the article by Young and Henneman, the authors indicated high-intensity ultrasound was used but they did not give precise data on the intensity values.

DR. BALLANTINE: Pulsed ultrasound was used of approximately 1300 w/cm^2. It was pulsed for very short durations. One of the problems inherent in that particular experiment, however, was that there was no adequate control of intensity, such as we have been able to achieve in later experiments; it is probable that the intensity was variable.

DR. CARSTENSEN: A scientific article which does not give ultrasound dosage is comparable to a pharmacology paper on a new drug in which no drug dosage data is presented. It is difficult to draw any conclusions from such a publication. The authors went to the trouble to give the voltage applied to the transducer, which is interesting, but fairly useless.

DR. BALLANTINE: Well, that brings me to a subject which has intrigued me for a number of years, namely, that investigators in their own laboratories use different characteristics for power measurement. Bill Fry uses acoustic amplitude and particle velocity. At our laboratory, we have used watts per square centimeter. When Lele joined our laboratory, he decided that this was a kind of arbitrary figure. Therefore, he multiplied the watts per square centimeter derived from the sonartestmeter, which I think is reasonably accurate, by the increase in gain due to the optics of the focusing system. One reads in his articles notations such as 42×15 or 42×20. I think that it is high time that we circulate a memorandum among the people working in the field and ask them for their ideas on the best measurement figure for ultrasonic power. In addition, I think it is wise to bear in mind that the choice of a unit of measurement which is familiar to the biologist and physician would be a great advantage.

DR. W. J. FRY: If one uses a radiation pressure detector for a focused beam, one has the problem of worrying about precisely what this is measuring in the focal region. The term intensity is directly applicable for plane waves or for small angle convergence lenses, but with a large angle of convergence the use of the intensity parameter alone introduces difficulties; that is, the specification of the intensity does not uniquely determine the values of the field parameters, and therefore we do not use the intensity in quantifying these wide angle converging fields. Of course, one can talk about a flow of energy, in which the pressure, particle velocity, and their relative time phase are involved, but since we use the thermocouple probe[5] for calibration and it does not yield any measure of phase, we cannot determine values for the intensity. We calibrate in a plane wave field of known values for pressure and particle velocity amplitudes and then, by analyzing the form of the response in the focused field, obtain values for pressure and particle velocity amplitudes, but no phase measurement. It is true that with this technique we have not completely specified the field, but it is probably true that insofar as the biological effects are concerned, the relative phase of pressure and particle velocity is not important.

DR. KOSSOFF: What about describing a plane wave?

DR. W. J. FRY: Well, for plane waves the specification of intensity does determine the values of the other field parameters. If the form of the field distribution is not known, I don't see any way to obtain both it and values for the particle velocity and pressure amplitudes from intensity measurements alone. Do you have some particular scheme in mind?

DR. KOSSOFF: No.

DR. W. J. FRY: Even though measurements are made with a radiation-pressure device, it is very desirable for investigators to include in their publications a complete description of the specific method of measurement so that other investigators can, at least, make some computations to translate the presented data into values of parameters of interest to them. For example, everyone does not measure pressure and particle velocity amplitudes, so one can't expect them to list values for these parameters, but if one indicates the angle of convergence of the beam and also gives some information on the field distribution at the focus, then estimates of pressure and particle velocity amplitudes can be made.

DR. HERRICK: I believe Ralph DeForrest and Ted Hueter had a standards committee in the early days, when ultrasound was being introduced into physical medicine.

DR. W. J. FRY: The ultrasonic diathermic standards are certainly very desirable but when they were set up, the use of high-power focused ultrasound was not included because of the state of development of the field. It would be very desirable now to consider this problem so that some uniformity in the method of describing irradiation conditions would be employed.

DR. BALLANTINE: I would like to second what Bill Fry has said concerning the desirability of including in publications sufficient information so that other investigators can attempt to duplicate the results. Insofar as the work at our laboratory is concerned, I believe we have finally arrived, as I said, at a satisfactory description of our equipment, of our measurements of the various parameters of dosage, and of the results obtained. If any of you read Lele's

[5] W. J. Fry and R. B. Fry. Determination of absolute sound levels and acoustic absorption coefficients by thermocouple probes – theory. J. Acoust. Soc. Am. *26* (1954), 294–310; W. J. Fry and R. B. Fry. Determination of absolute sound levels and acoustic absorption coefficients by thermocouple probes – experiment. J. Acoust. Soc. Am. *26* (1954), 311–317; W. J. Fry. Intense ultrasound in investigations of the central nervous system *in* "Advances in Biological and Medical Physics," C. A. Tobias and J. H. Lawrence, eds. (Academic Press, New York, 1958), Vol VI, pp. 281–348.

paper [6] and are in doubt as to the precise details of the experiment or feel that you can't build the equipment from the information provided in the publication, then please tell us. We like to encourage other investigators to work with the same equipment, to see whether our results will stand up under such scrutiny.

DR. DUNN: Professor Fry and I published, several months ago, a chapter in the Academic Press series, "Physical Techniques in Biological Research," in which we attempted to record principles of measurement and desirable apparatus for high-intensity ultrasound research.[7] This chapter is about 135 pages in length and discusses in considerable detail many of the problems being considered here.

DR. GERSTEN: In connection with your previous comments regarding stimulation by ultrasonic energy, have you ever recorded any propagated action potential? We never recorded such potentials, but we have been using much smaller ultrasound intensities than you have.

DR. BALLANTINE: We have not measured a propagated potential as a result of stimulation, but we have seen from time to time, particularly during the irradiation of the spinal cord, a twitch in the hind leg of the experimental animal.

---

[6] See n. 1, pp. 236, 255.

[7] W. J. Fry and F. Dunn. Ultrasound: analysis and experimental methods in biological research, in "Physical Techniques in Biological Research," W. L. Nastuk, ed. (Academic Press, New York, 1962), Vol. IV, Chap. 6, pp. 261–394.

17

Current Status of Ophthalmic Ultrasonography

GILBERT BAUM, M.D.
Veterans Administration Hospital, Bronx, New York

IVAN A. GREENWOOD
G.P.L. Division, General Precision, Inc., Pleasantville, New York

Introduction by Dr. Mackay

The first paper is concerned with the application of ultrasound for visualization of structures within the eye. This presentation is co-authored by Dr. Gilbert Baum, an opthalmologist, and Dr. Ivan Greenwood, a very clever physical scientist. Their collaboration has been very fruitful, and it is with great pleasure that I introduce Dr. Baum.

INTRODUCTION

This paper discusses the theory and lines of investigation being pursued to establish differential diagnosis between benign and malignant tissues in vivo by ultrasonography.

For many of the previous investigations in this field, ultrasonic differential diagnosis has been based primarily upon one feature, namely, gross aberration of the anatomical pattern. Differential diagnosis based on a single criterion may frequently be misleading. To broaden the base upon which differential diagnosis may rest, diagnostic criteria used in optical differential diagnosis have been considered, and the techniques for measuring the acoustic analogs developed. Differential diagnosis of tissues by optical methods is normally based upon the following tissue characteristics: gross architecture, surface and interfacial properties, internal texture, color, staining, and absorption. Table I lists these diagnostic tissue criteria and their acoustic equivalents.

ULTRASONIC MEASUREMENT TECHNIQUES

A number of methods have been developed to observe the acoustic analogs. Equipment was developed which possessed the requisite resolution and sensitivity to map ocular tissues accurately and to display the 70-db dynamic range inherent in ocular tissues (1, 2).

The following photodensitometry techniques are used to determine the average echo amplitude of ocular tissues in vivo from compound or sector scanned ultrasonograms. The apparatus compresses the 70-db dynamic acoustic range into the gray scale of the display tube and film. Upon completion of the regular serial examination, repeated undifferentiated scans are taken (at a single level of the specimen, with progressively increased attenuation, 5 db per scan) until echoes from tissue structure fall below the detectable levels.

TABLE I. OPTICAL CHARACTERISTICS OF TISSUE USED IN DIFFERENTIAL DIAGNOSIS AND THEIR ACOUSTICAL ANALOGS.

Property	*Optical characteristic*	*Acoustic analog*
Gross architecture	Gross appearance	Gross appearance
Surface and interfacial properties	Sharp Diffuse or invasive	Interfacial texture Smooth Rough Absolute amplitude of reflection at normal incidence Sharpness at transition as determined by undifferentiated vs differentiated echoes
Internal texture	Smooth Rough	Amplitude distribution of echoes Spatial distribution of echoes Absolute amplitude of reflection at normal incidence
Color	Color under white light	Examination with multiple ultrasonic frequencies
Staining	Variable affinity of tissues for various dyes	Selective alteration of the acoustic characteristics of tissues
Absorption	Optical absorption	Shadowing

Calibration is accomplished by placing special test objects (Figs. 1–4) in the path of the ultrasonic beam before and after the examination of tissues. Electrical attenuation is then introduced while the test objects are being examined. Since the tissue ultrasonograms and the standardization ultrasonograms are on the same filmstrip, both are developed under identical conditions. The data is then analyzed by an electric photodensitometer.

Preliminary observations of some of the acoustic parameters listed in Table I have been made and will be described in the remainder of this paper.

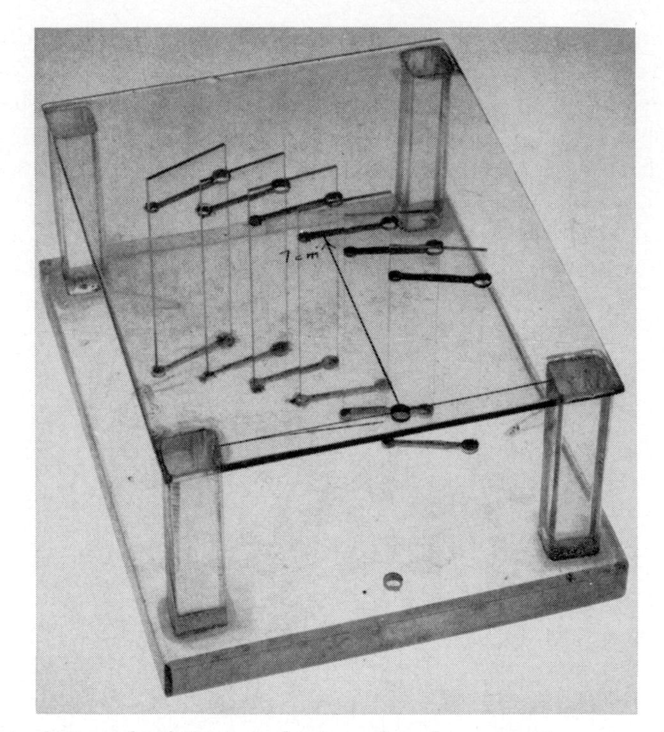

FIGURE 1. A photograph of the test object used to determine the gray scale values at various distances from the transducers, that is, film density vs attenuation in decibels. The test object consists of glass plates placed 1 cm apart. The plate marked 7.0 is placed at the focal zone and the entire test object is adjusted so that a maximum echo is produced by the 7-cm plate at normal incidence. Repeated scans are then taken with progressively greater amounts of attenuation until the reflected signal becomes undetectable. The values obtained can then be compared with the echoes obtained from tissues, thus establishing the precise strength of the tissue echoes.

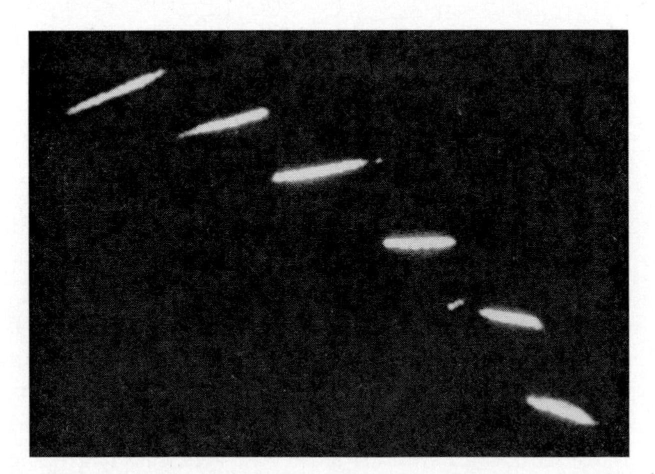

FIGURE 2. The ultrasonographic appearance of the test object with 50 db of attenuation introduced.

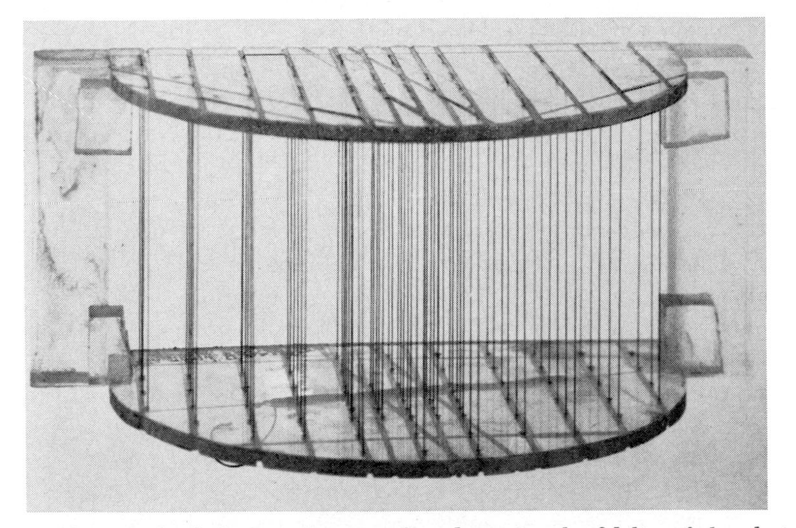

FIGURE 3. Photograph of the test object used to determine the fidelity of the electronic representation of a test pattern. The outer threads are separated by 1 cm and the threads in the inner zone by 0.5 cm.

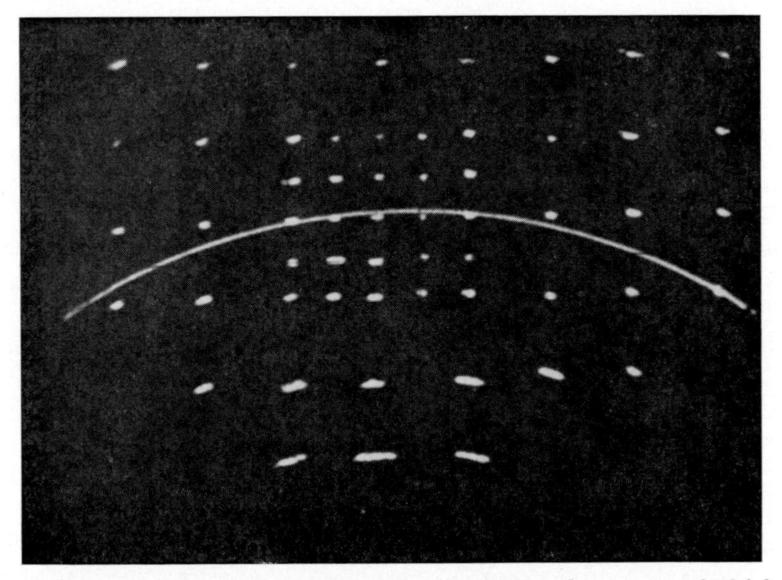

FIGURE 4. Ultrasonogram of the test object of Figure 3 which demonstrates faithful reproduction of the geometrical pattern of the test object.

ACOUSTIC DIAGNOSTIC CRITERIA

Gross Structural Alteration

The detection of gross alteration in tissue structure by ultrasonography has been reported in a number of previous papers and need not be elaborated here (3–7). (See, for example, Fig. 5.)

Acoustic Properties of Surface and Interfacial Areas

The most important property of tissue surfaces and interfaces is the magnitude of the echo at normal incidence which is a measure of the difference in acoustic impedances between the two media. Tissue surface and interfacial textures may be determined by measuring the strength of the reflection vs the angle of the sound beam with the instrumentation and techniques described. The different reflection characteristics of smooth and rough surfaces may be demonstrated on glass test blocks (Fig. 6). The sharp dip and rise in the curve for the smooth glass surface is believed to be a diffraction phenomenon. The same effect is present in the curve for the rough surface, but on a reduced scale because of the irregularity of the surface. The discovery of an improper tissue interfacial texture at an aberrant anatomical site would then be presumptive evidence of a tissue change.

Another method for evaluating interfacial and surface characteristics is to view the structures using first differentiated and then undifferentiated video signals. A differentiator in the video circuitry emphasizes the very high-frequency components of the video signals; hence it passes only the leading and trailing edges of pulses. The trailing edges are subsequently removed by clipping.

If both the differentiated and undifferentiated echoes from a tissue interface are compared with those from a glass block, it is found that a tissue interface or surface having a sharp transition in acoustic impedance will yield comparable reflections, whereas an interface having a gradual transition in acoustic impedance will yield a differentiated signal which is relatively weaker. By this means one can deduce something about the character of the interfacial transition even though its structure may not be resolved.

Confirmatory data can be demonstrated clinically. Thus, for a patient with corneal edema and conjunctival chemosis (Fig. 7), the cornea and conjunctiva of the affected eye yield a stronger corneal echo and a flatter fall-off with angle than the normal eye. In addition, both the cornea and conjunctiva are markedly thickened (Fig. 8). Thus, the disease process affects both the surface and internal textural acoustic response of the tissue. It is also valuable to measure the absolute amplitude of reflection at an interface at the normal incidence with the aforementioned method. Table II lists average values of

TABLE II. AVERAGE VALUES OF COEFFICIENTS OF REFLECTION OF HUMAN OCULAR TISSUE INTERFACES.* (Values tabulated in db relative to glass-saline interface.)

Interface	db
Cornea I vs saline	—28.3
Cornea II vs aqueous humor	—32
Lens I vs aqueous humor	—31.5
Lens II vs vitreous humor	—37
Iris vs aqueous humor	—26
Retina vs vitreous humor	—41

* The listed values have not been corrected for absorption in the intervening structure of the eye. Other measurements suggest that for these structures in normal eyes the corrections required would be less than the uncertainty associated with these values.

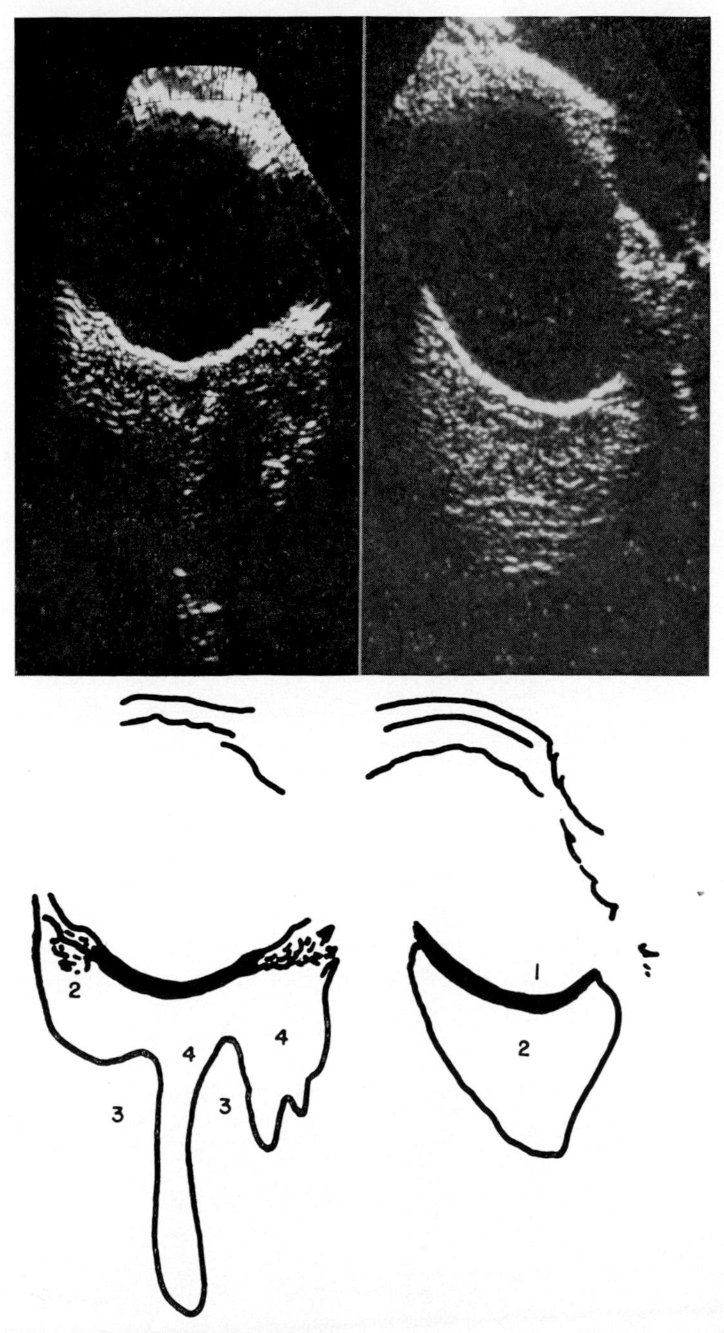

FIGURE 5. Ultrasonograms showing the difference in gross anatomical appearance between the normal orbital fat pattern (right) and the abnormal fat pattern (left) which had been produced by a tumor in this orbit. Left: abnormal eye. 1, posterior sclera; 2, fat compression characterized by more intense echoes; 3, elongation of the fat pattern; 4, echoes from the orbital fat. Right: normal eye. 1, posterior sclera; 2, orbital fat.

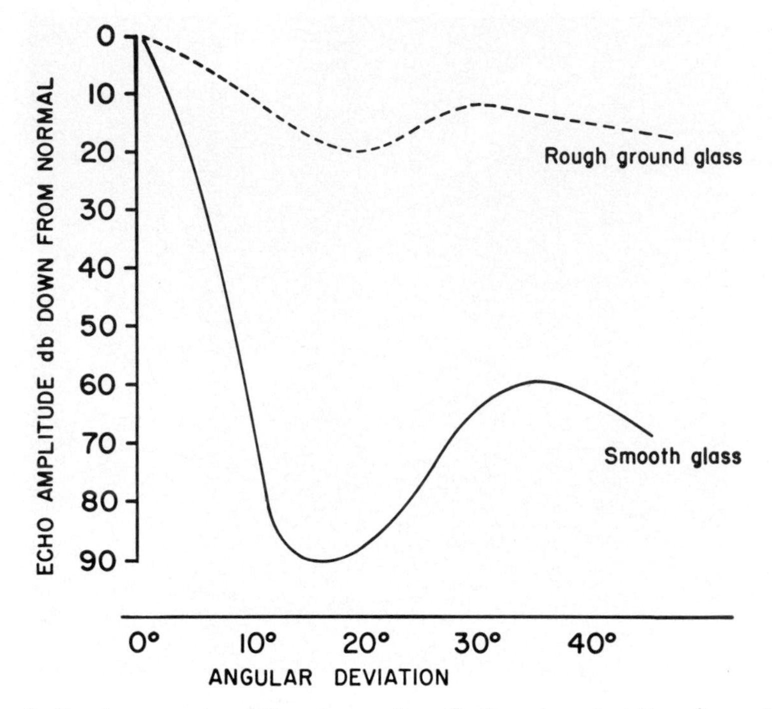

FIGURE 6. Graph comparing different acoustic reflection characteristics of smooth and rough surfaces as demonstrated on glass test blocks.

the coefficients of reflection of interfaces of the healthy eye at the normal angle of incidence.

A dense leading edge at the tumor interface has been noted in cases of proven malignant melanoma. This interface echo may be 5 to 10 db stronger than that of the adjacent surrounding structure. Melanomas produce internal echoes whose amplitudes lie between those of blood and retina. Such identification is shown in Figure 9.

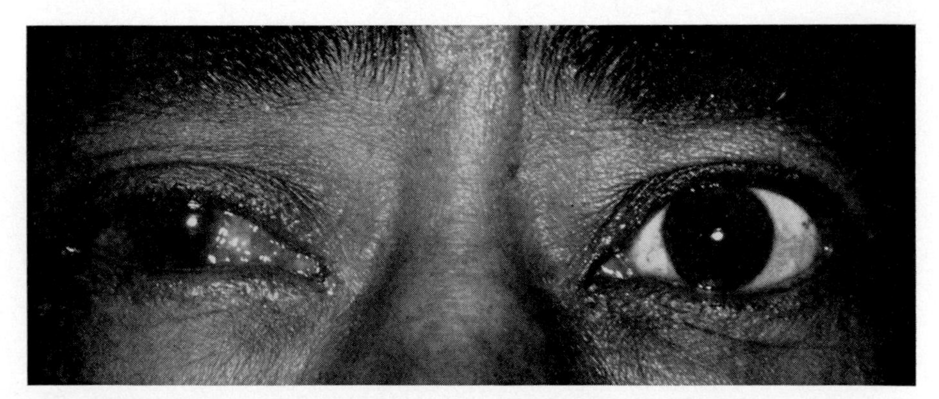

FIGURE 7. The right eye of subject has marked corneal edema, conjunctival injection, and chemosis. The left eye is normal.

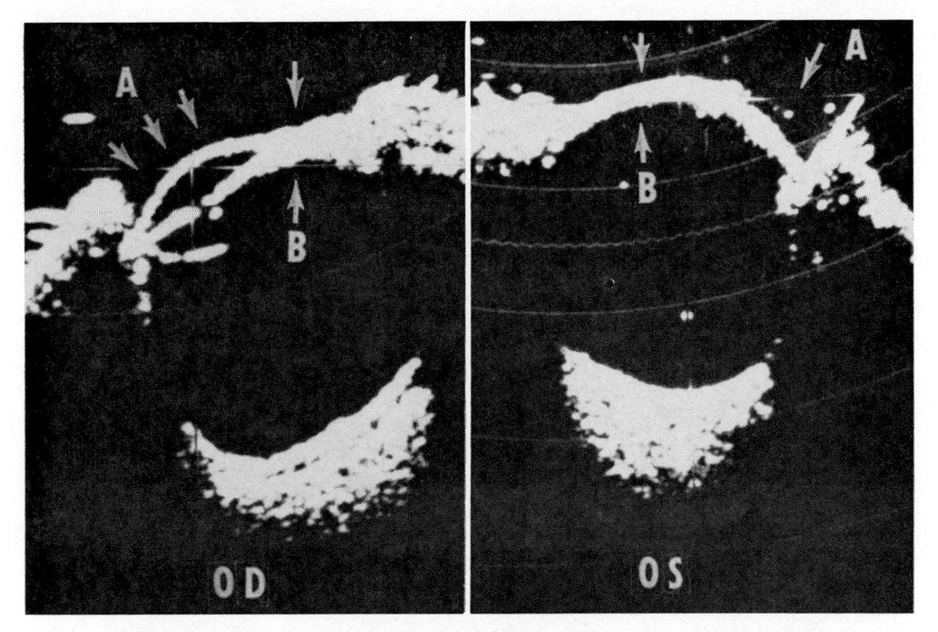

FIGURE 8. Ultrasonograms of the eyes of the subject in Figure 7 show that the edematous cornea yields a stronger and more uniform echo (arrow A). In addition, the edematous cornea and the adjacent chemotic conjunctiva are thickened (arrow B). O.S., left eye; O.D., right eye.

Internal Texture

Tissue internal texture may be classified by measuring the spatial distribution and intensity distribution of the internal tissue echoes in addition to the average intensity of reflection at normal incidence. A grid consisting of 2-mm square boxes is superimposed on the ultrasonogram and the relative size and density of the echoes contained within a 2-mm square are plotted by means of an electronic photodensitometer and ruler using the techniques previously described. At the present time, this is a long and tedious process which might be ameliorated by the use of suitable auxiliary data-analyzing devices such as frequency analyzers, flying spot scanners, and other read-out devices.

Thus, the internal texture of the normal cornea and lens are characterized by echoes from the front and back surfaces of these structures with no echo in between because of the homogenous center. The vitreous is also sonically homogenous and fails to yield echoes except when diseased. The normal sclera, choroid, and retina are solid black lines of uniform density (Fig. 10). When diseased, the opacified internal portions of the cornea (see Fig. 8 vs Fig. 10), lens (see Fig. 8), and vitreous do produce echoes. A detached retina produces multiple pinpoint echoes, and a malignant melanoma of the choroid results in choroidal thickening and internal echoes of various sizes and intensities. Note the difference in choroidal echoes exhibited

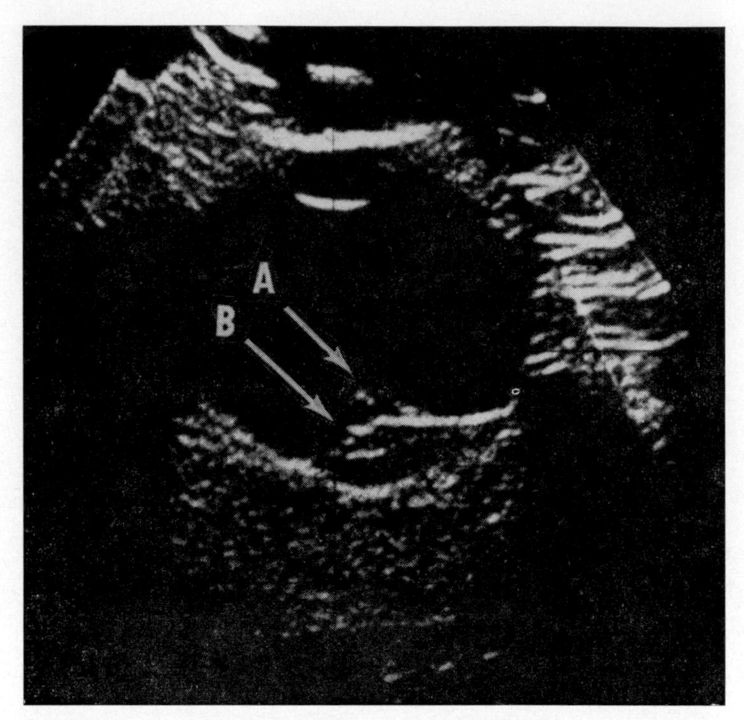

FIGURE 9. Ultrasonogram of an eye with a malignant melanoma of the choroid. Immediately anterior to the melanoma there is a small retinal detachment, which yields a very weak echo. The surface of the tumor is marked by a very intense echo (arrow A). The choroid is thickened as compared to the normal adjacent choroid and contains many echoes of variable size and variable intensity (arrow B).

in Figures 9 and 10. Hence, pathological changes within specific ocular tissues may be studied by observing their ultrasonic internal texture patterns.

Changes in the physiological state of normal tissues may also produce changes in internal echo, for example, the recti muscles produce echoes only in the contracted state (Fig. 11).

The normal characteristics of orbital fat may be determined by grid counts of the spatial and intensity distribution of the echo patterns. When orbital fat is compared with a mucocoele, the echoes of the mucocoele seem to be of lesser amplitude but greater in number. As attenuation is introduced, the internal mucocoele echoes disappear sooner than the echoes from the surrounding cyst wall and the normal tissue echoes (Fig. 12).

Color

Examination of tissues at a number of ultrasonic frequencies, or by a frequency-modulated system, is the acoustic equivalent of optical color examination. Acoustically, the number of tissue interfaces which might be visualized decreases as the operating frequency is decreased. The magnitude and type of interfacial and internal texture alterations resulting from frequency shifts may have diagnostic significance. At present, we are preparing to initiate such a study using a frequency of 10 Mc, in addition to the 15 Mc used heretofore.

Enhancement Techniques

Just as the pathologist uses staining techniques to improve the visualization of various structure in tissues, we will attempt to differentiate between tissues by altering their relative acoustic impedances. Acoustic interface reflection is analogous to optical interface reflection, that is, as sound passes from a medium of a given acoustic impedance to a medium having a different acoustic impedance, a portion of the energy is reflected at the interface. Hence, if one could differentially modify the acoustic impedances of two adjacent tissues and determine that a normal tissue interface response lay within a given range, then any change outside of that range would indicate tissue alteration. It is possible to detect 0.4% density or velocity changes at —40 db and 0.004% at —80 db by the aforementioned ultrasonic methods, so that even subtle differential responses of tissues should be detectable.

Since the acoustic impedance is the product of the density of the sub-

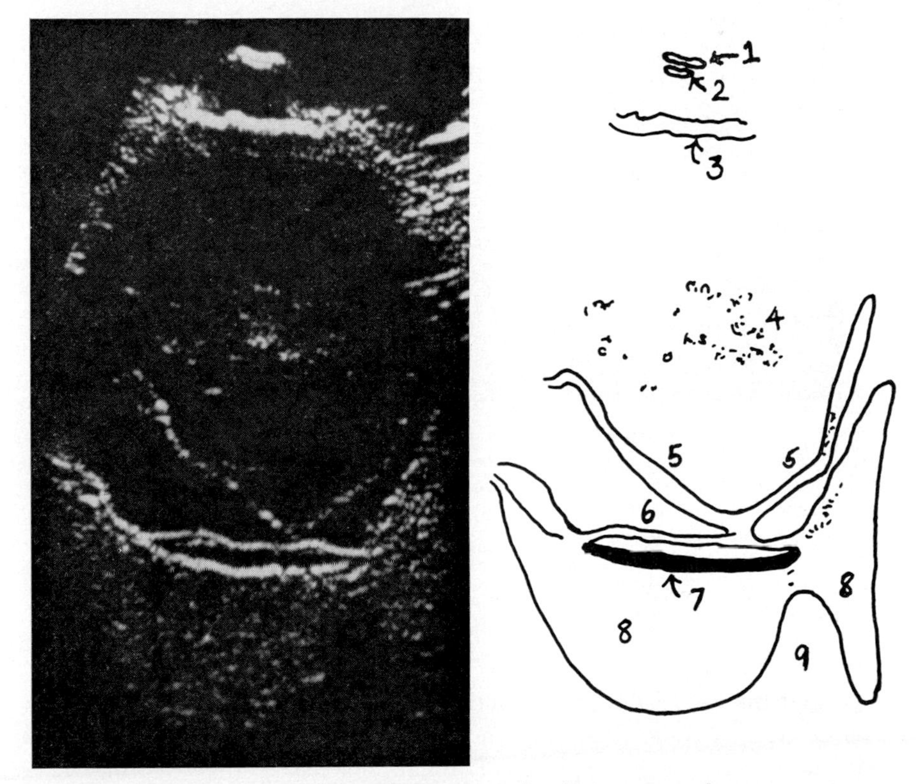

FIGURE 10. An ultrasonogram which demonstrates the characteristic ultrasonic appearance of the tissue of the eye. 1, front surface of the cornea; 2, back surface of the cornea; 3, iris; 4, vitreous opacities; 5, retina (detached); 6, choroid (detached); 7, sclera; 8, orbital fat; 9, passage in the orbital fat through which the optic nerve passes. The eye was aphakic, hence no lens echoes are present. Normal vitreous is sonically transparent.

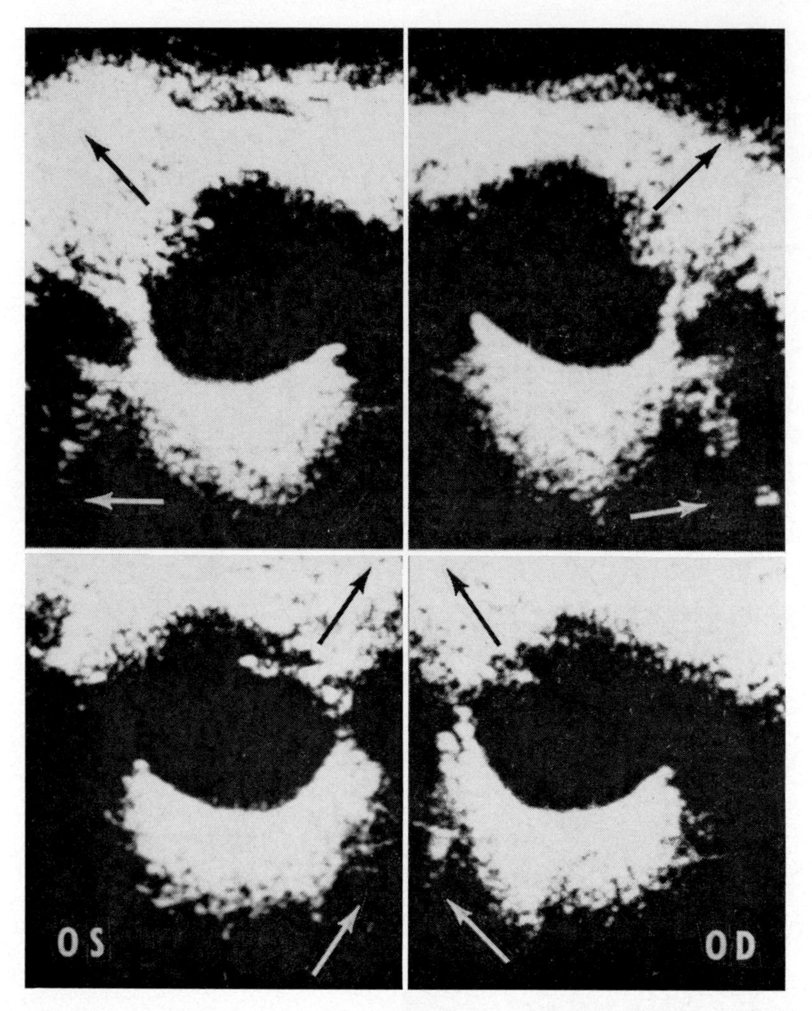

FIGURE 11. Demonstrates that the recti muscles are visualized only during contraction. Thus, when the right eye looks laterally, the lateral rectus muscle appears and the medial rectus is invisible. Further, when the eye is rotated medially, the medial rectus muscle appears and the lateral rectus muscle disappears. An identical phenomenon is noted in the left eye. The position of the cornea is indicated by the upper arrow. The lower arrow indicates the echo from the lateral recti muscles. (The ocular structures are markedly distorted because an air-backed transducer and an orbital position focus were used.) O.S., left eye; O.D., right eye.

stance and the velocity of the sound in the substance, agents which alter either or both of these tissue parameters within the physiological limits of tissue survival are to be explored. Four approaches to investigating these agents are to be used: (1) temperature changes – for their effects upon sound velocity, (2) hydration and dehydration, (3) vasodilation and vasoconstriction, and (4) ground substance modification by hyaluronidase – for its effect

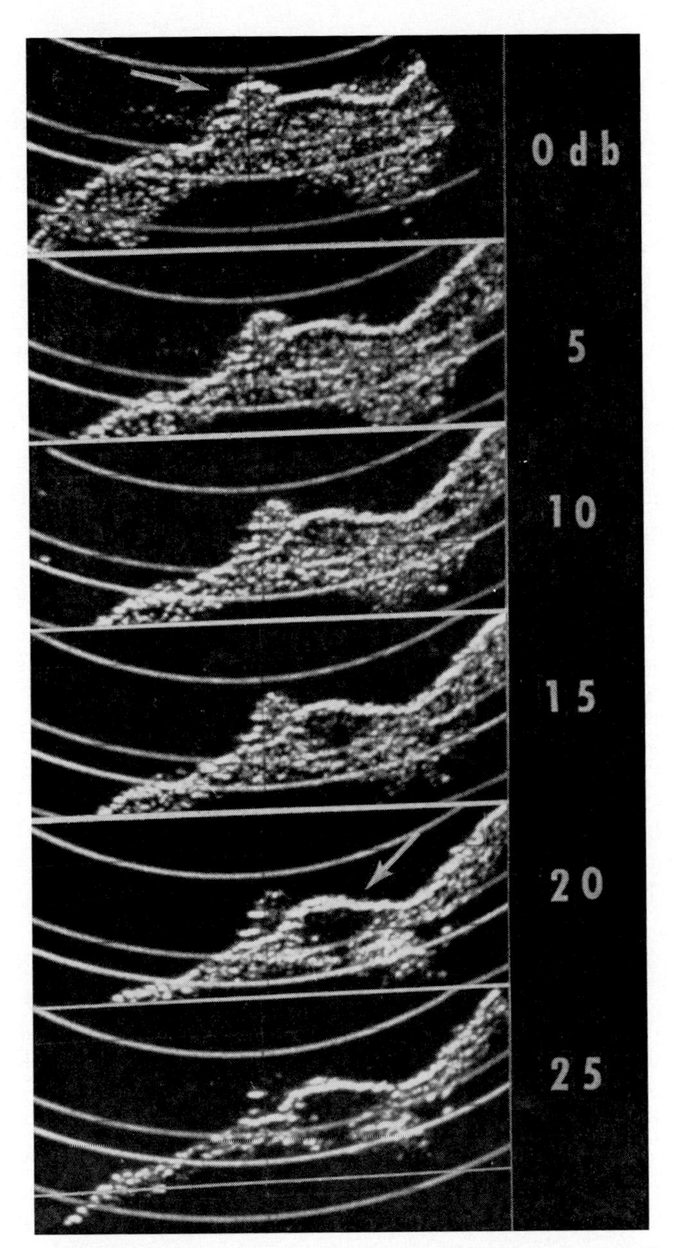

FIGURE 12. An ultrasonogram taken through the lid at the point at which the mucocoele had erupted through the surface of the skin. A bead of pus was on the surface of the skin (arrow). Without attenuation, there is a minimal difference between the echoes from the mucocoele as compared to the echoes of the normal surrounding tissues. With 10-db attenuation, the echoes from the interior of the mucocoele begin to disappear, whereas those from the orbital fat remain essentially unaltered. This effect is intensified with the introduction of 15-db attenuation. Twenty-db attenuation causes all pus echoes to disappear, only the cyst wall can be visualized, and there is total absence of the contents of the mucocoele. This change is further enhanced by the introduction of 25-db attenuation.

upon tissue density. Exposure to heat-inducing radiation such as ultrasound[1] or microwave (8) results in selective temperature rises in the component ocular tissues. Because of the selective temperature rises, differences in acoustic velocity within tissues might be achieved. As indicated by Fry (9, 10), focused ultrasound could be used to produce such localized heating in order to accomplish examination of specific areas. Hydration of tissues has been produced by the intravenous injection of 5% glucose in water and dehydration by 30% urea. The eye is unique in that a highly vascularized layer, the choroid, is sandwiched between two relatively avascular structures, the retina and sclera. Hence, vasodilators and vasoconstrictors might have a more marked effect upon the choroid than on the retina and sclera.

Absorption

Absorption measurements may be performed in vivo by comparing loss in a tissue path through a lesion with loss in a nearby tissue path. This may be done by measuring the average echo amplitude over a plane anterior to a lesion and comparing it with the average echo amplitude over a plane behind the lesion. The decrement which occurs on either side of the lesion in similar tissues represents path loss. When this figure is subtracted from the echo amplitude loss in the shadow of the lesion, the difference represents the additional absorption produced by the lesion. This measurement may be significant in differential diagnosis and is especially useful in differentiating between hemorrhage and tumor.

A marked increase in acoustic absorption has been noted immediately following tissue death. With ultrasonic techniques it is possible to demonstrate these phenomena in vivo. Thus, in a patient who has a normal lens in one eye and a hypermature cataract in the opposite eye (Fig. 13A), the marked absorption caused by the cataractous lens can be demonstrated by quantitative ultrasonic techniques. The shadowing produced by such a cataractous lens results in apparent widening of the optic nerve passageway. This phenomena is most graphically demonstrated with the introduction of approximately 20 db of attenuation. Under these circumstances, the orbital echoes from the affected eye nearly disappear, whereas those from the eye containing the normal lens still persist (Figs. 13B, 13C). Postoperatively, this shadow disappeared (Fig. 13C). Shadowing is also produced by malignant melanoma of the choroid. It would be possible in some instances to detect abnormal tissue by its absorptive properties despite the fact that such a lesion might be missed by dependency upon the other diagnostic criteria.

DISCUSSION

If differential diagnosis by ultrasonography between benign and malignant tissues is possible, we believe it will be based upon combinations of the characteristics listed above, rather than upon some single feature. Of the

[1] Unpublished data (Baum).

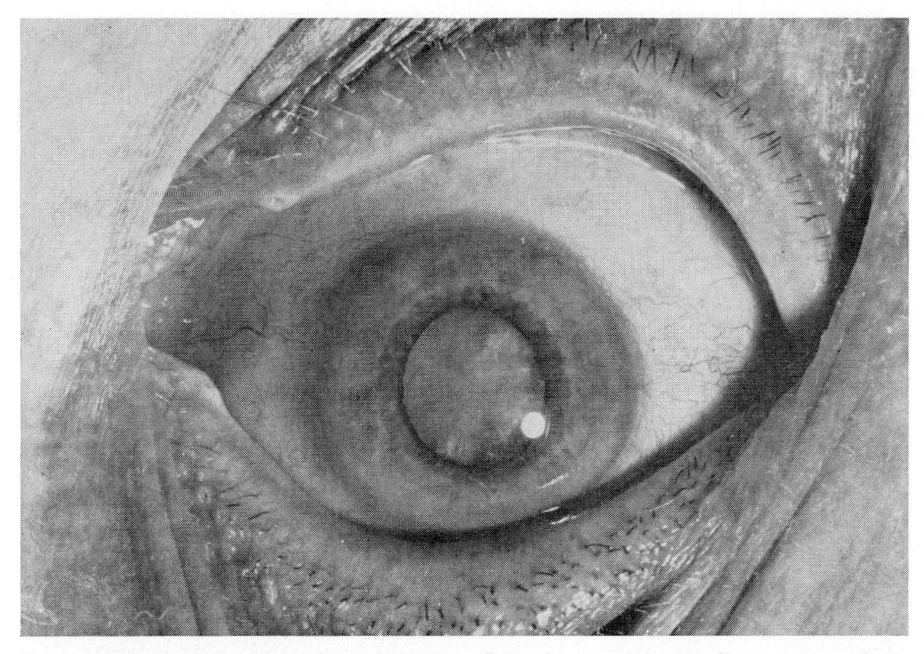

FIGURE 13A. A photograph of an eye with a dense hypermature swollen cataract of the right eye.

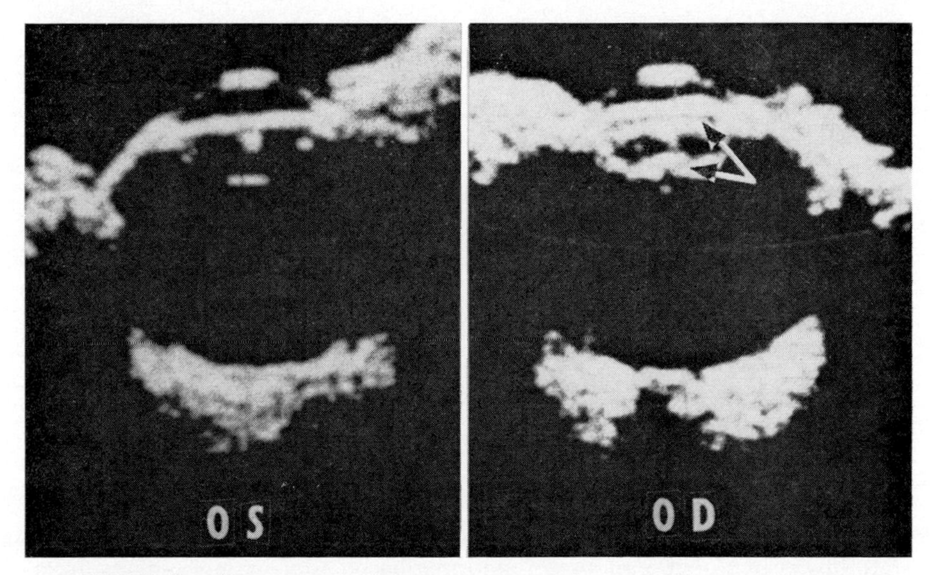

FIGURE 13B. The ultrasonogram of the cataractous right eye of Figure 13A shows considerable structure within the lens (arrow), whereas the central area of the normal lens is clear. There is marked widening of the area of the optic nerve because of the increased absorption produced by the cataract. Similar absorption is not present in the left eye. O.S., left eye; O.D., right eye.

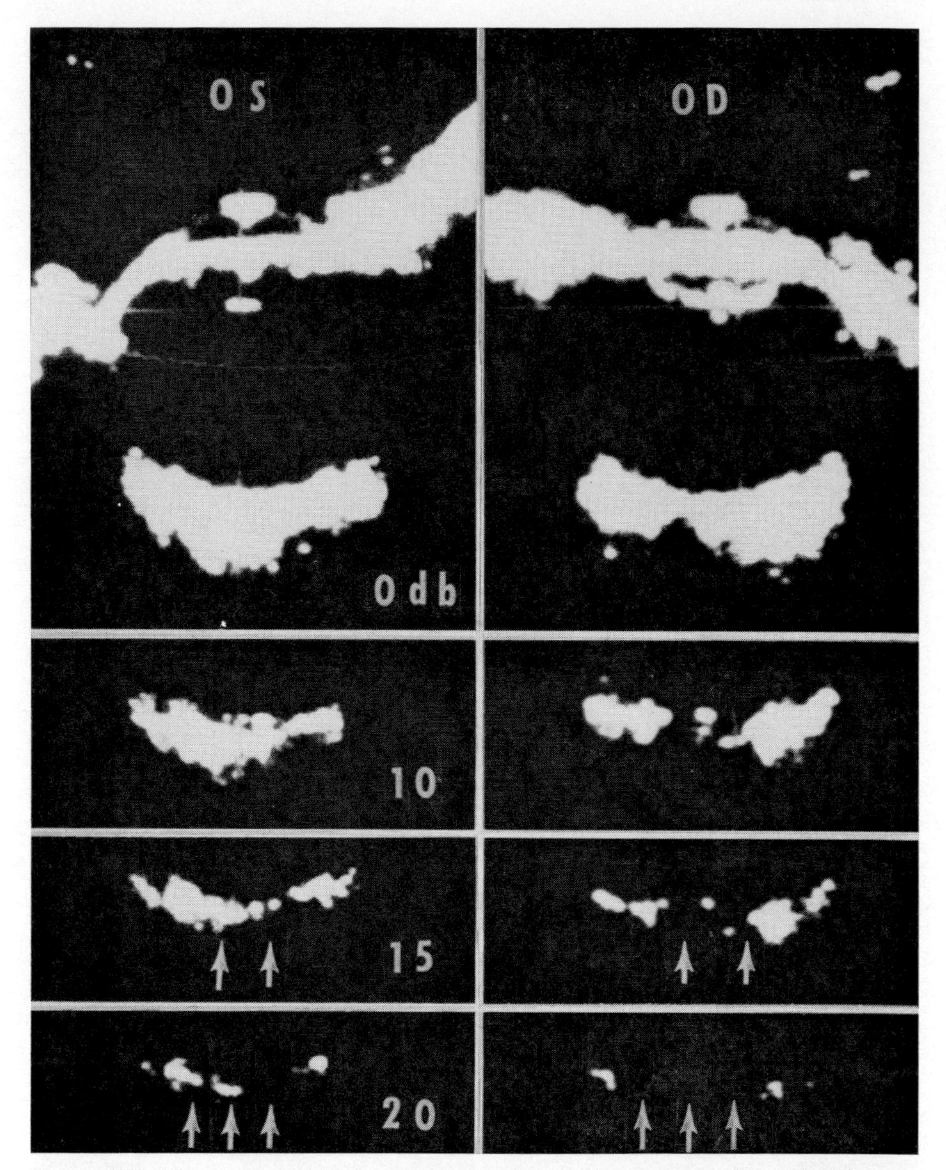

FIGURE 13C. Ultrasonograms of the same eye as that of Figures 13A and B. The difference in the appearance of the orbit is best demonstrated when viewed with increasing amounts of attenuation. Fifteen- to 20-db attenuation produce the greatest difference (arrows). O.S., left eye; O.D., right eye.

six optical differential diagnostic criteria listed, ultrasonography, in its present state of development, can supply information on four, namely, gross architecture, surface and interfacial properties, absorption, and internal texture. It should be stressed that all these data are recorded simultaneously on the ultrasonograms, so that the patient need not be subjected to numerous different examinations.

Instrumentation development, although incomplete, has progressed to the point that research, aimed at the development of the remaining two diagnostic criteria and eventual clinical application of these criteria, is possible. Other data-analyzing devices, such as spatial frequency analyzers, may be necessary to achieve these diagnostic goals. After the range of the norms has been established, it may be possible to simplify clinical equipment so as to obviate the need for the auxiliary data analyzing equipment.

SUMMARY

The major problem of diagnostic ultrasonography is the differential diagnosis of solid tumors. The six optical parameters used to achieve differential diagnosis with light-dependent instruments are listed. Techniques for measuring the equivalent acoustic parameters by quantitative ultrasonography are discussed and clinical examples are described.

REFERENCES

1. Baum, G., and I. Greenwood (1960). High-resolution ultrasonography and its application to clinical ophthalmology. Proc. 3rd Internat. Conf. on Med. Electron., Part III.
2. Baum, G., and I. Greenwood (1958). The application of ultrasonics locating techniques to ophthalmology; theoretic considerations and acoustic properties of ocular media. I. Reflective properties. Am. J. Ophthal. *46*, 319.
3. Baum, G., and I. Greenwood (1958). The application of ultrasonic locating techniques to ophthalmology. II. Ultrasonic slit lamp in the ultrasonic visualization of soft tissues. A.M.A. Arch. Ophthal. *60*, 263.
4. Baum, G., and I. Greenwood (1960). Ultrasonography—an aid in orbital tumor diagnosis. A.M.A. Arch. Ophthal. *64*, 180.
5. Baum, G., and I. Greenwood (1960). Ultrasound in ophthalmology. Am. J. Ophthal. *49*, 249.
6. Baum, G., and I. Greenwood (1961). A critique of time-amplitude ultrasonography. A.M.A. Arch. Ophthal. *65*, 353.
7. Baum, G., and I. Greenwood (1961). Orbital lesion localization by three dimensional ultrasonography. N.Y.S. J. of Med. *61*, 4149.
8. Carpenter, R. L., G. H. Hammond, D. K. Biddle, and C. A. Van Ummersen (1961). The effect on the rabbit eye of microwave radiation at X band frequency. 4th Internat. Conf. on Med. Electron. 195.
9. Fry, W. J. See pp. 242–248, above.
10. Fry, W. J., and F. J. Fry (1963). Ultrasonic visualization of soft tissue structure, based on gradients in absorption characteristics. J. Acoust. Soc. Am. 35, 1788.

DISCUSSION

DR. KOSSOFF: Have you tried any other technique besides irradiating through water, such as the application of a rubber contact as a coupling agent?

DR. BAUM: We use normal saline as a coupling medium because its acoustic impedance closely approximates that of the tissues of the eye. It is relatively inexpensive, readily available, and does not lead to irritation secondary to its use. Coupling techniques, other than saline with a face mask, all introduce troublesome problems. Because of the highly irregular configuration about the eye, it is impossible to get a precise fit between a flexible diaphragm and the eye. As a result, air bubbles are trapped between the eye and the diaphragm, leading to the production of many acoustic artifacts. Such coupling would also limit compound scanning. We have tried a contact lens but its use precludes any scanning technique whatsoever. Also, the pressure produced by a contact lens tends to deform the shape of the globe and to set up acoustic artifacts which are undesirable. Thus, although the design of a suitable face mask is difficult, this approach seems to be the best compromise. Our masks are fabricated with sufficient play between them and the side of the tank that as the patient's face moves, the mask is displaced in an accordion-like fashion relative to the rigid tank. Others have tried variations of these techniques, such as using Steridrape attached to the face to retain the liquid coupling medium.

DR. KOSSOFF: What happens if the patient closes his eyelids?

DR. BAUM: Since ultrasound can penetrate the eyelid, for purposes of ocular examination the closing of the lid does not produce any major problems. However, when the lid is closed, very weak echoes may be lost due to the added absorption. If this added absorption becomes a problem, it is then necessary to retract the lids, either manually or with a speculum. The lid may also produce marked reduplication artifacts in the orbit, so one must be on the alert for such artifacts to avoid serious interpretive errors.

DR. MACKAY: Would you indicate the physical characteristics of your device.

DR. GREENWOOD: We are using a loaded epoxy-backed X-cut quartz crystal transducer with a focusing lens, shock excited at 15 Mc. It transmits and receives pulses which are about a quarter of a microsecond long. The total dynamic range of the system is greater than 90 db, and of this range, approximately 70 db can be displayed and photographically recorded from the face of the cathode ray tube with sufficient differences in gray shades so that echo strengths can be determined by photodensitometer measurements.

Resolution both in depth and laterally is approximately 0.2 to 0.3 mm. The receiving amplifier has a bandwidth of ± 5 Mc centered at 15 Mc. The video circuits have a bandwidth of 8 Mc. The cathode ray tube is 5 in in diameter and has a double layered P-14 phosphor. The fast blue light image is photographed and the persistent yellow image is visually monitored. Photographs are recorded on 35-mm film. As many as 800 individual ultrasonograms may be taken of an especially interesting patient, although we expect that it will be possible to record a smaller number in routine clinical procedures.

DR. KOSSOFF: You made reference to a muscle contraction phenomenon. I wonder if such phenomena are being followed by anyone in this group. In studies of absorption in tissues, we started with dead tissues, then we observed the muscle of the arm and tried to get some insight into the physical mechanisms of absorption. There were those who said the proteins were mainly involved in absorption and that one could grind the tissue and get the same results; and then there were those who felt that the texture of the tissue was very important, too. Now, you have a direct clue to this phenomena. I think that may in itself be a very interesting research topic.

DR. HOWRY: Before you answer Dr. Kossoff, I would like to ask if there is anything to indicate a change in velocity with the orientation of muscle fibers?

DR. BAUM: The stronger echoes from the contracted recti muscles of the eye demonstrated in Figure 11 were caused by a change in acoustic impedance, anisotropy, a change in orientation, or a combination of these factors rather than a change in absorption since the acoustic path remained unchanged. We agree with the observations that in reflectance, velocity, and absorption measurements on muscle, factors to be considered must include condition of tissue orientation and degree of contraction. We have not attempted to isolate these factors in any of our investigations, but we concur that this would be an interesting research topic. The large increase in acoustic absorption accompanying the death of certain tissues, such as the lens of the eye, implies that in these cases, at least, absorption depends on something more than just the total protein content. Study of this phenomena would also be a very interesting research topic.

18

The Use of Ultrasound to Record the Motion of Heart Structure

JOHN M. REID
University of Pennsylvania, The Moore School of Electrical Engineering, Philadelphia, Pennsylvania

CLAUDE R. JOYNER, M.D.
Hospital of the University of Pennsylvania, Philadelphia, Pennsylvania

Introduction by Dr. Mackay

The next series of papers is concerned with the application of ultrasonic reflection techniques for recording the motion of various heart structures. We are privileged this morning to have the opportunity of hearing about the work of Dr. Edler and Dr. Hertz of Lund, Sweden, who have been in this field for a number of years. A paper will also be presented by our American colleagues, Dr. Reid and Dr. Joyner. We will postpone the discussion period until all of this morning's papers have been presented in order that all of the papers may be discussed at the same time. This is the most logical approach since all of the research work being discussed this morning is so closely related. We will hear now from Dr. Reid.

This paper will be delivered in two parts. In the introduction and the concluding remarks, I will discuss our experimental approach to the problem while Dr. Joyner will present the clinical aspects of the research program.

We have been investigating the use of ultrasound in the diagnosis of heart diseases and heart conditions. I would like to acknowledge that this work was originated by Drs. Edler and Hertz in Sweden and considerably extended by Dr. Effert in Germany. Our preliminary work was based on the information in Edler and Hertz's widely circulated publication (1). We subsequently defined our own criteria for the equipment and then constructed the required instrument. We were interested at first in determining whether or not we could transmit sound through lung tissue and obtain echoes from the heart from all directions. We did a preliminary study of lung attenuation and our conclusions were similar to those that Dr. Dunn presented here. The work with short pulses indicated considerable scattering. The pulse is stretched in time by a factor of about 10, so that the lung is completely unusable as a transmission path to obtain information about the heart with this technique.

We were primarily concerned with recording the position and velocity of the reflecting structures in the functioning heart. The distance resolution of the equipment used by previous investigators was judged to be between 2 and 5 mm, and the structure with the greatest motion has an amplitude of motion of about 2 cm. Now, if the strength of the echo changes, you will falsely record a change in the position of the echo due to the slope of the lead-

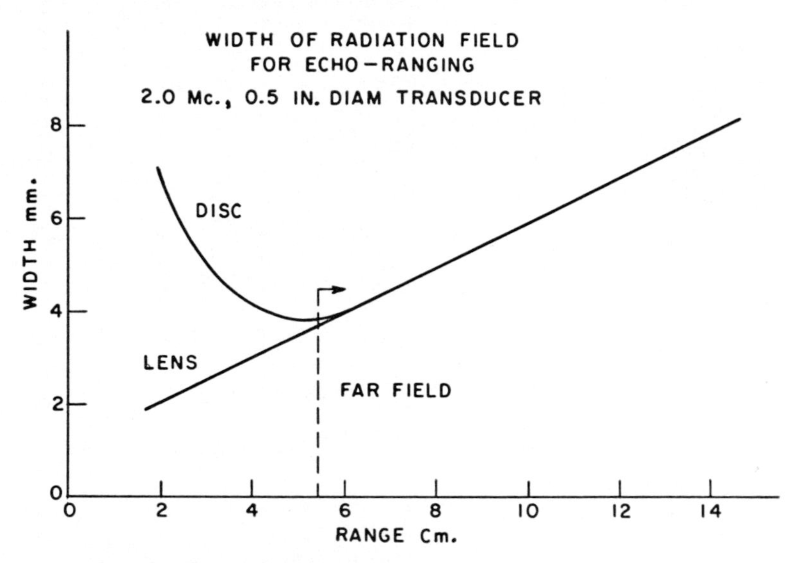

FIGURE 1. Width of radiation field between the 3-db down points. Measured in a water bath with a 2-mm diameter metal ball as a target.

ing edge. In order to hold this error to the order of 2% of the motion, our initial goal was to obtain a distance resolution of 1 to 1.5 mm. This was achieved with the use of crystals of 1-Mc frequency. With the 2-Mc crystals, there is a 3-db distance resolution of 0.75 mm, and for a change in echo amplitude of approximately 20 db, this resolution introduces a position error of a few tenths of a millimeter. The angular resolution, as measured in a water bath, is shown in Figure 1 and is much poorer than the distance resolution. The width of the field of the half-inch diameter transducers is approximately 8 mm between the 3-db down points at a range of 14 cm. This 14-cm distance is approximately the distance between the chest wall and the back wall of an enlarged heart. Therefore, in the mitral valve area the beam width is still uncomfortably large. With a plane disc, there is a near-field effect in which the field close to the transducer is wider than when it is farther from the transducer. In order to obtain better results for echoes from structures close to the chest wall and to allow preliminary work on dogs, one of the crystals was fitted with a two-element converging lens of 2.5-cm focal length.

The application of the lens did result in a contraction of the width of the near field, yielding a narrow beam for the examination of small hearts. However, the limited distance between the ribs of the patient restricted the size of the crystal to a half-inch diameter. An experiment with a larger transducer, designed to focus a narrow sound beam between the ribs, indicated that the beam width, in this case, had to be considerably smaller than the aperture between the ribs to avoid rediffraction.

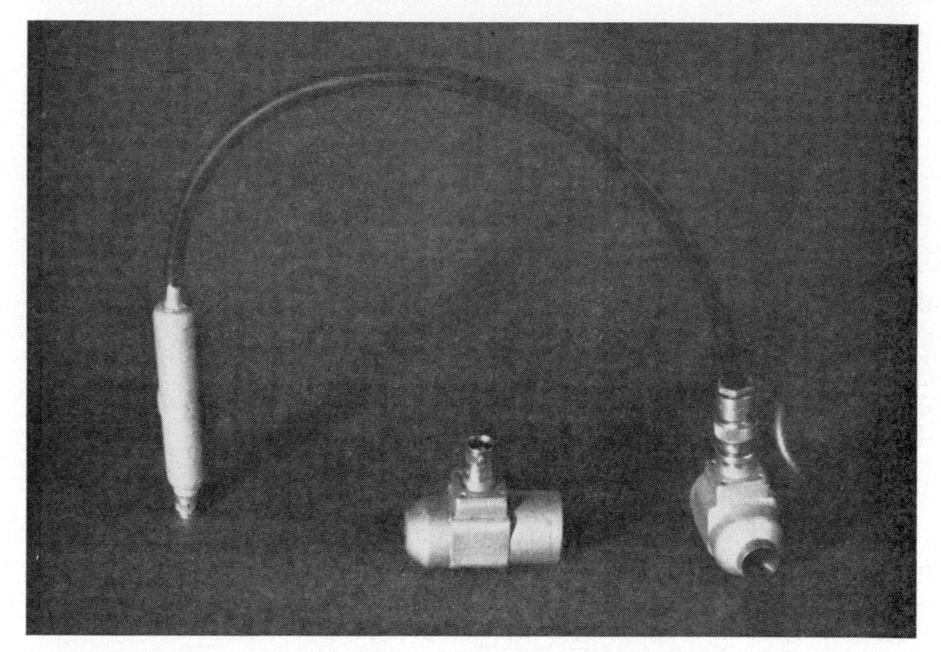

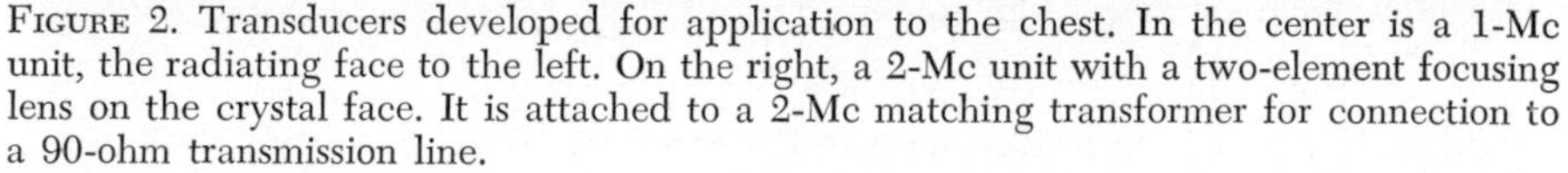

FIGURE 2. Transducers developed for application to the chest. In the center is a 1-Mc unit, the radiating face to the left. On the right, a 2-Mc unit with a two-element focusing lens on the crystal face. It is attached to a 2-Mc matching transformer for connection to a 90-ohm transmission line.

Figure 2 shows the transducers designed for application to the chest. The transducer shown in the center was designed to minimize the size of the case surrounding the crystal, which has to fit up against the interspace between the ribs. The transducer with the two-element lens is on the right; the two elements were necessary because the front face of the lens had to be flat.

The equipment in its present form is shown in Figure 3. As you can see, the recording is accomplished with a standard moving film camera and two ordinary oscilloscopes. Without the power supplies, the machine occupies a rack space of 22 in.

Figure 4 is a block diagram of the system. A half-cycle electrical pulse causes the transducer to emit an ultrasonic pulse a few cycles long. The transducer is applied directly to the patient and there is no scanning motion involved. The ultrasound beam travels into the patient, and the echoes are received by the same transducer that emitted the pulse. The resulting voltages are amplified by the receiver and displayed on an ordinary linear time base oscilloscope. The echoes also intensity modulate the beam of the second oscilloscope which simultaneously displays the electrocardiogram for comparison.

The fidelity of recording of this system is not a problem. The relative time delays of various methods of recording heart information must be known. In this application, the major time delay is due to the transmission time from the extreme range back to the receiving crystal, which amounts to some 0.2 msec. This delay is quite small when compared to the delays of other types of recording. The pulse repetition rate of 2 kc should allow one to record echo motions having frequency components extending to almost 1 kc.

The interpretation of the records can result in some confusion. You will

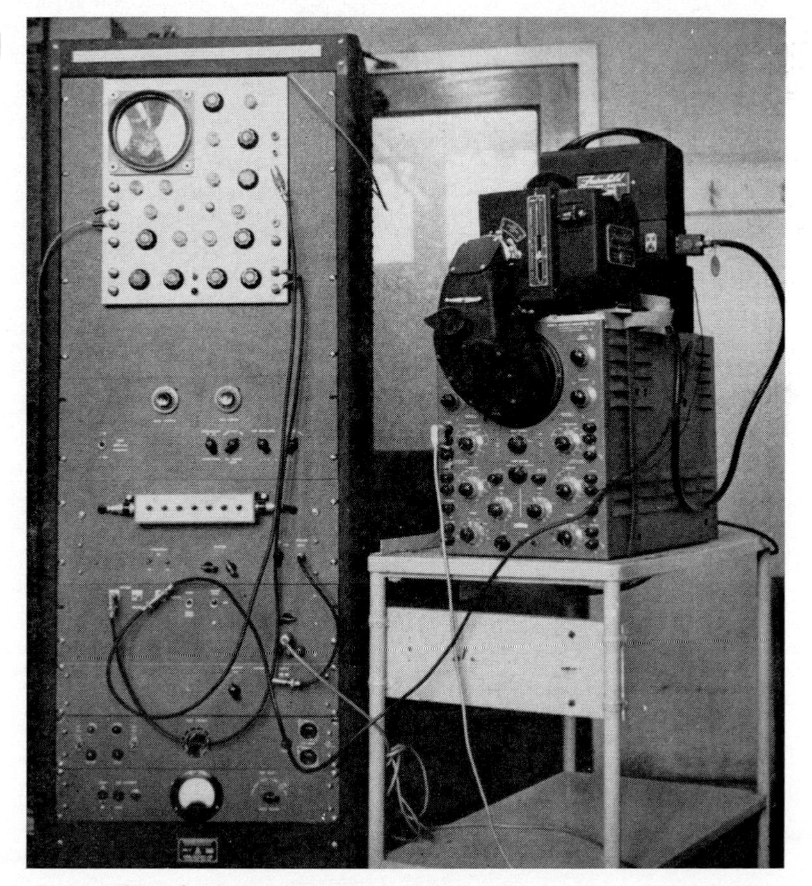

FIGURE 3. Complete ultrasonic echo-ranging and recording equipment. The basic machine at the left from the top down consists of: oscilloscope, timer and receiver control unit, receiver, video and marker mixing panel and electrocardiograph amplifier, transmitter, power distribution panel, regulated power supply and monitor, and at the bottom, two commercial power supplies. On the table are the two-beam oscilloscope and moving film recording camera.

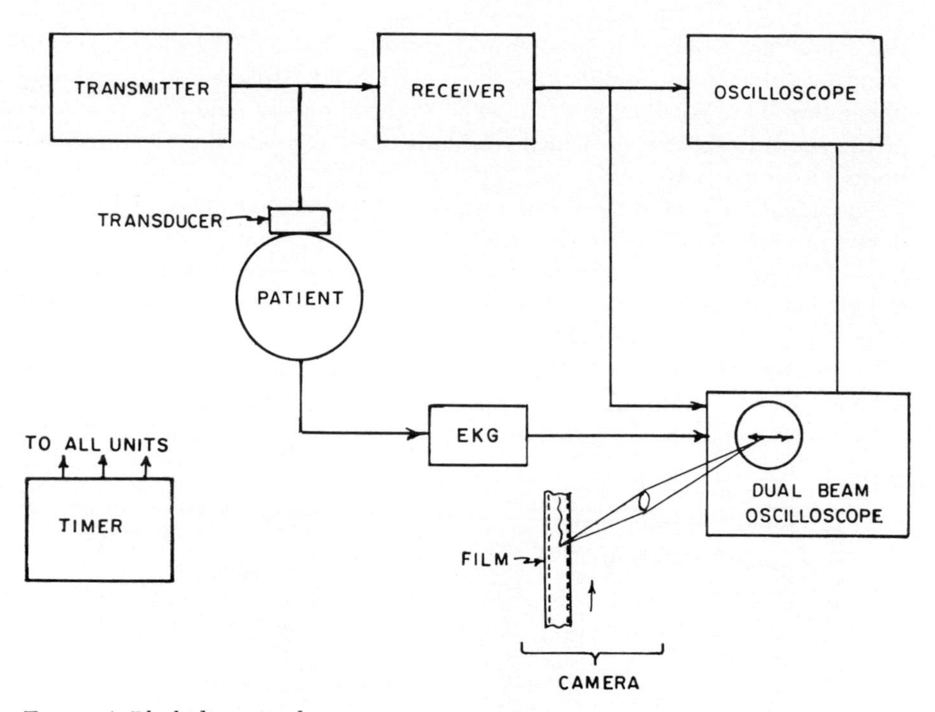

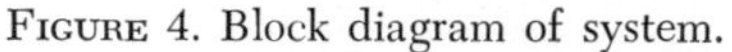
FIGURE 4. Block diagram of system.

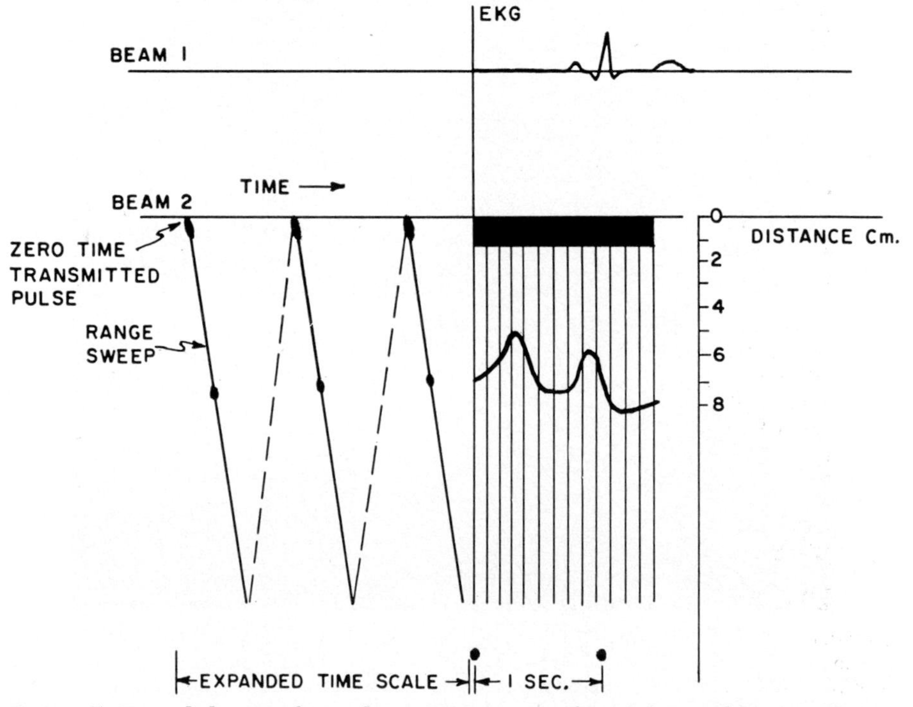

FIGURE 5. Expanded view of recordings. The time axis from left to right is provided by moving the photographic film. Beam 1 records the electrocardiogram. Beam 2 is deflected downward by a linear time-base sweep and is intensified by the echo voltages.

note that the measure of the distance to an echo is the time delay from the transmitted pulse to the receipt of that echo. Since we also wish to follow the motion of these echoes as a function of time, both coordinates of the records represent time. We move the film to provide a slow-speed time base from left to right as indicated in Figure 5. Beam 1 simply records the electrocardiograph; beam 2 is deflected by the linear time base sweep, which starts at the time that the transmitter becomes active. It is brightened when the received echo comes back. At the end of its sweep, beam 2 retraces to wait for the next transmitter pulse. Therefore, in this type of plot, distance from the chest wall is downward. Figure 5 is a rather expanded view; in the actual recording there are 2000 lines per second, so that the echoes received from a structure form a line which follows the motion of the structure. Since the velocity of sound in most soft tissues is almost constant and since its value is known, we calibrate the fast time base in distance in centimeters into the tissue. We record 1-sec time marks on the film to give us the time during the cardiac cycle.

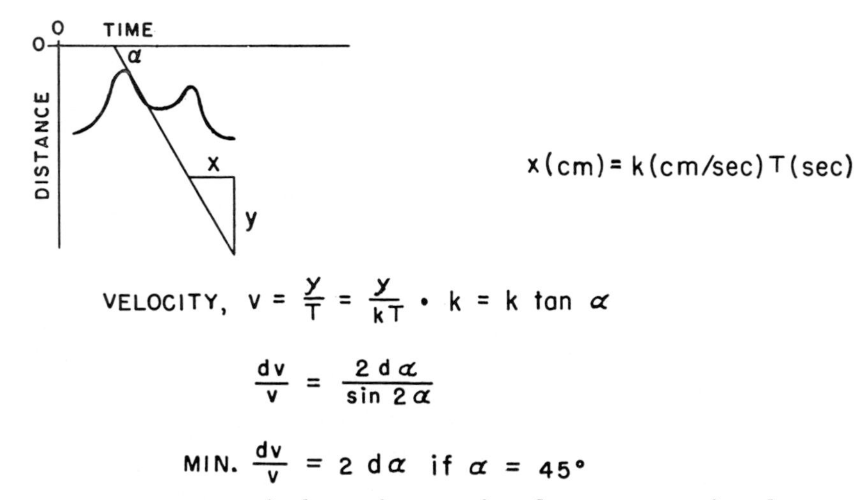

FIGURE 6. Determination of velocity of motion of a reflecting structure from distance and time scales.

Figure 6 indicates the method used to extract information from the record. Recorded here is the distance vs time graph of an echo, which is executing some complicated motion. It was originally reported by Edler (2) that the velocity of such a curve in one part of its cycle is highly significant. However, we found that various investigators have reported their results in terms of angles, rather than velocity, and this figure indicates a method for translating data from one system to the other. Alpha is the angle between a uniform velocity portion of the curve and the horizontal axis. The slope of this segment of the curve is shown measured in x and y components, using the distance calibration as reference. The length, x, corresponds to a time interval, t, with k designating the transformation factor. The velocity of a segment of the curve is equal to y/t which can be expressed as k times the tangent of the angle α. Specifications of the angle alone are not useful unless the factor, k, can somehow be deduced from the author's figures or from a knowledge of his instrument. The fractional error in velocity, caused by inaccuracy in measuring the angle, can be found by differentiating the logarithm of the velocity expression with respect to α. The error has a minimum, where $\sin 2\alpha$ equals 1, which occurs at an angle of 45°. The velocity corresponding to an angle of 45° can be adjusted by choice of the constant k. This velocity is approximately 75 mm/sec for our instrument.

Dr. Joyner will now discuss the clinical aspects of the work. I would like to emphasize that all the records he will present were taken essentially blind. The monitor oscilloscope indicated when a particular echo with both large amplitude of motion and rapid motion was present but it was not possible to judge from the monitor screen the shape of the curve of motion vs time. The records were not available for examination until 2 days to 2 weeks later. This, in effect, was a single blind experiment. Dr. Joyner knew the condition of the patient, but he did not know what was being recorded.

DR. JOYNER: I can only repeat what Dr. Reid has emphasized, namely, that the clinical aspects of this study certainly followed the work of Drs. Hertz, Edler, and Effert. We precede them in no manner, other than in the order of progression of today's business. The curves which we have recorded are from persons with cardiac disease and other persons without apparent disease. Today, we wish to present our findings in 260 patients. The procedure applied is quite simple, that is, records are obtained by applying the transducer at the fourth, or occasionally third or fifth, left interspace adjacent to the sternum. We are particularly concerned in this study with the fast-moving component of the reflected echoes. The entire procedure requires only about 2 or 3 min for each patient.

Figure 7 is the typical, characteristic curve which is obtained from normal individuals. The EKG is at the top of the record. As you can see, echoes (A) are recorded from the various surfaces such as skin, immediate subcutaneous tissue, and intercostal muscle. The wavy line designated by B apparently represents the anterior portion of the heart or the intraventricular septum, since the trajectory being employed would ordinarily pass through the heart, just to the right of the intraventricular septum, through the intraventricular septum, and into the lumen of the left ventricle. The curve of interest from the clinical viewpoint is curve C which has a range of anterior-posterior motion much greater than that of any other structure in the chest. The excursion is usually between 2 and 3 cm in the anterior-posterior direction. The horizontal lines on the record are for distance quantitation, each one representing 1 cm. The round marks at the bottom of the record are 1-sec marks. As you know, one of the serious problems is defining the origin of the echoes. As far as we are able to determine, curve C originates from the anterior leaflet of the mitral valve. The typical normal curve C shown here demonstrates motion anteriorly, or into the lumen of the left ventricle shortly after atrial contraction. At this time, the atrium empties remaining blood into the ventricle and one would expect the flow of blood to push the mitral valve anteriorly into the ventricular cavity. It is seen here that anterior motion to peak 1 is closely related to the P-wave of the EKG. This particular peak of the ultrasound curve is not seen except when the atria contract effectively. It is, therefore, not visible in patients with atrial fibrillation. The other prominent wave of anterior motion occurs in early diastole. One would expect the mitral valve to open at this time. This maximum point of anterior motion is designated as peak 4. The curve then begins to recede posteriorly as the left ventricle fills. The portion of the curve which has been subjected to quantitative analysis is the movement of this part of the curve posteriorly from its most anterior position (peak 4), since this is the portion of the curve which is distorted in mitral stenosis. The quantitation with which we have been concerned is, therefore, the measurement of the speed of motion from the most anterior position in early diastole.

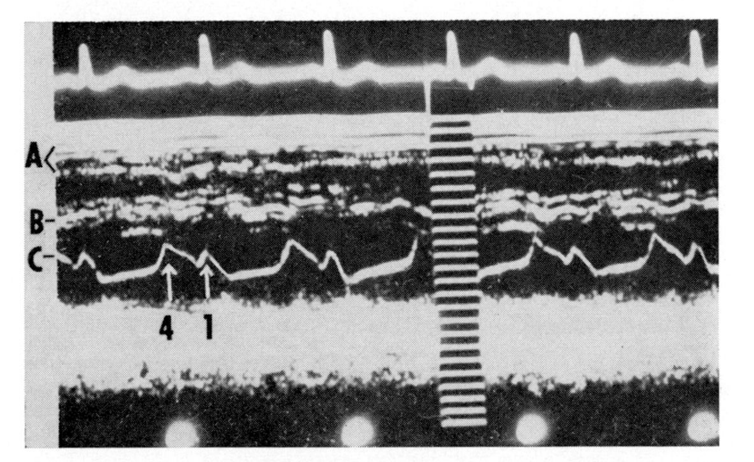

FIGURE 7. Recording of normal ultrasound pattern. The electrocardiogram is displayed at the top of the record. Echoes immediately beneath the transducer which represent the anterior chest wall are recorded in area A. B apparently represents the anterior heart or intraventricular septum. Curve C is the apparent reflection from the anterior leaflet of the mitral valve. Peak 4 in early diastole and peak 1 in late diastole form the normal curve. The horizontal lines on the record are for distance quantitation, each one representing 1 cm. The round marks at the bottom of the record are 1-sec marks.

In contrast to the typical normal pattern, Figure 8 demonstrates the pattern one obtains from patients with mitral stenosis. Address your attention to the portion of the curve which follows peak 4. In the normal, there is a very rapid posterior motion during left ventricular filling. In contrast to this normal fast slope, you see that there is a plateau configuration of the pattern in the patient with mitral stenosis. The rate of movement posteriorly from the horizontal level corresponding to peak 4 is measured in mm/sec by reference to the appropriate time and distance mark. Please note that, in spite of the restricted posterior motion in the presence of mitral stenosis, there is still a slight forward impetus following atrial contraction in this patient with normal sinus rhythm. The plateau, or limited movement of the mitral valve, is quite characteristic of the patient with mitral stenosis. This, we feel, represents a delay in motion of the mitral valve from its most open position because ventricular filling is delayed by the obstruction at the mitral valve. There continues to be an elevated left atrial pressure during ventricular diastole, maintaining the open position of the valve as long as possible. In spite of the high pressure in the atrium and incomplete ventricular filling, the mitral valve must close when the ventricle contracts. The anterior leaflet moves posteriorly, co-adapts with the posterior leaflet, and the valve is closed. This posterior motion follows closely after the QRS complex of the EKG.

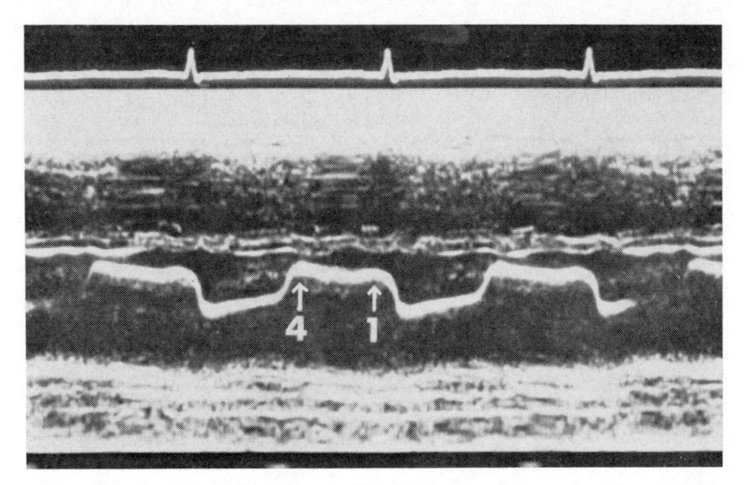

FIGURE 8. Ultrasound pattern from a patient with mitral stenosis. The posterior descent from peak 4 is delayed. Peak 1 is small.

Figure 9 shows the record of a patient with mitral stenosis who had atrial fibrillation rather than normal sinus rhythm. Again, the typical plateau of the mitral stenosis curve is seen. Since this patient had atrial fibrillation, the forward movement to peak 1 is not seen. In this individual, the speed of motion posteriorly from peak 4 was 14 mm/sec. Figure 10 is a record obtained from this same patient after the valve was successfully opened by surgery. This record demonstrates the change from the nearly horizontal line to a faster slope with a velocity of posterior motion of 37 mm/sec from peak 4.

As indicated previously, this method is no different from other echo techniques and one of the great problems is to define with accuracy the origin of the reflected echoes. It is significant that with procedures such as angiocardiography, the only structure delineated in the area from which this fast-moving curve is obtained, which has a range of motion equal to that demonstrated in this curve, is the mitral valve. However, the mitral valve leaflets do not move from a stationary base. There is associated movement of the annulus, the ring of attachment of the leaflets.

Figure 11 is the preoperative record of an individual who, as you can see, has the pattern typical for mitral stenosis. A caged ball valve mitral prosthesis was inserted at the time of open heart surgery. This is the Starr-Edwards type of valve which has been used in a number of patients for replacement of the mitral valve. The patient whose ultrasound record is seen in Figure 11 had very dense, heavily scarred mitral valve leaflets which were excised and an

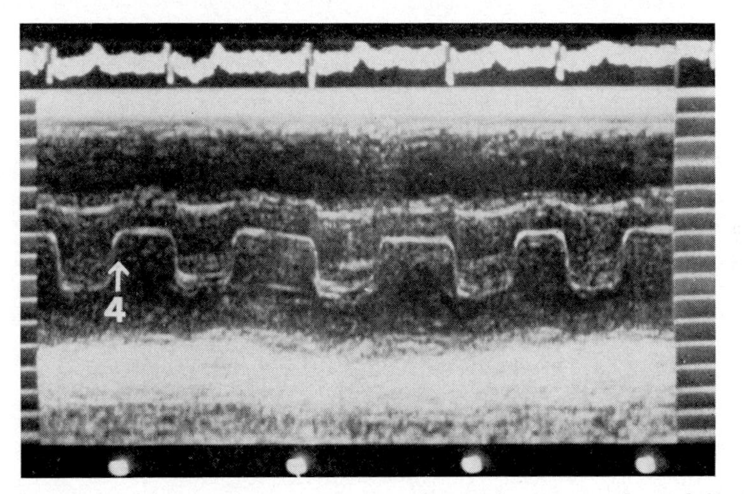

FIGURE 9. Ultrasound pattern from a patient with mitral stenosis and atrial fibrillation. The delayed slope from peak 4 is seen as in Figure 8. Peak 1 is not seen, since there is no effective atrial contraction. The horizontal lines on the record are for distance quantitation, each one representing 1 cm. The round marks at the bottom of the record are 1-sec marks.

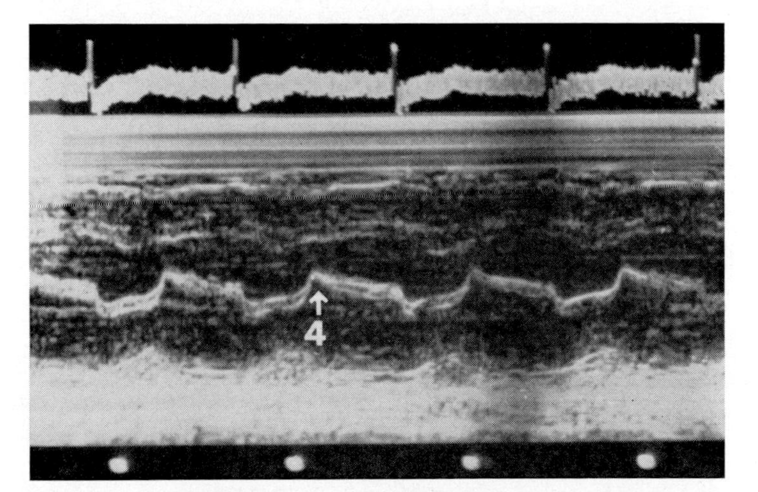

FIGURE 10. Postoperative record from same patient whose preoperative record is shown in Figure 9. The rate of descent from peak 4 was 14 mm/sec in the preoperative record (Fig. 9). The rate of descent has increased to 37 mm/sec in Figure 10.

artificial ball valve inserted in the annulus. Figure 12 is the postoperative record from the same patient as that recorded in Figure 11. You can see the multiple parallel echoes in Figure 12, recorded after the artificial valve was inserted. A similar pattern of multiple reflections is recorded if one places the ball in a jug of water or oil and jiggles the ball up and down. This adds further support to the belief that the echo originates from the mitral valve.

The extent of the correlation of the curves with the degrees of mitral stenosis are represented in the following two slides. Figure 13 illustrates the velocity of motion from peak 4 for 20 normal subjects and for 56 patients with mitral stenosis. All normal individuals had a speed of motion of 85 mm/sec or greater. The measured velocity obtained from the record of each of the 56

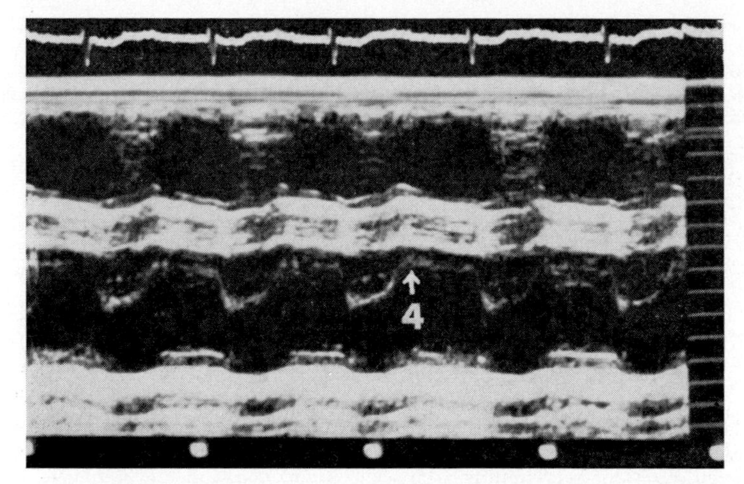

FIGURE 11. Preoperative record of a patient with mitral stenosis and a heavily calcified valve. The horizontal lines on the record are for distance quantitation, each one representing 1 cm. The round marks at the bottom of the record are 1-sec marks.

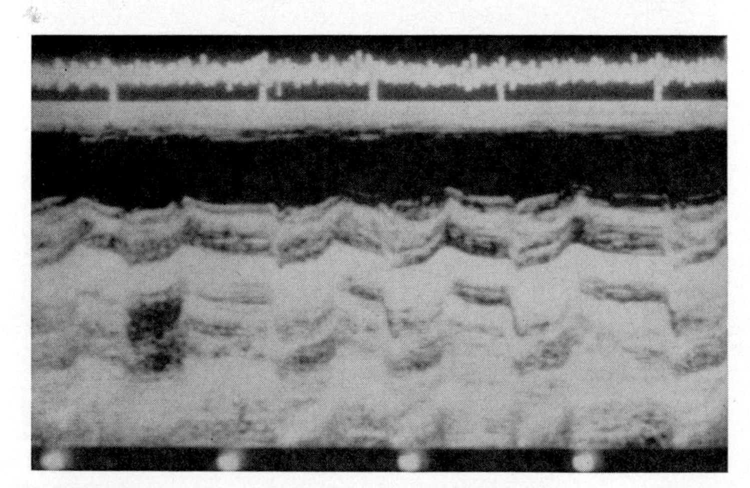

FIGURE 12. Multiple parallel echoes from a ball valve inserted in the mitral annulus in the patient whose preoperative record was shown in Figure 11.

patients with mitral stenosis is plotted with reference to the estimated valve size found at subsequent surgery or necropsy. The valve size of patients later dying was estimated by me at the autopsy; the estimation of the valve at surgery was done by our cardiac surgeon, Dr. Julian Johnson. There are obvious limitations to the accuracy of estimating the effective valve opening due to anatomical differences in the type of stenosis. However, this form of estimation which assumes a normal valve to have an orifice of "three fingers or more" has proved clinically useful. Figure 13 indicates that there is no overlap between the values obtained in the mitral stenosis patients and the values recorded from the control group.

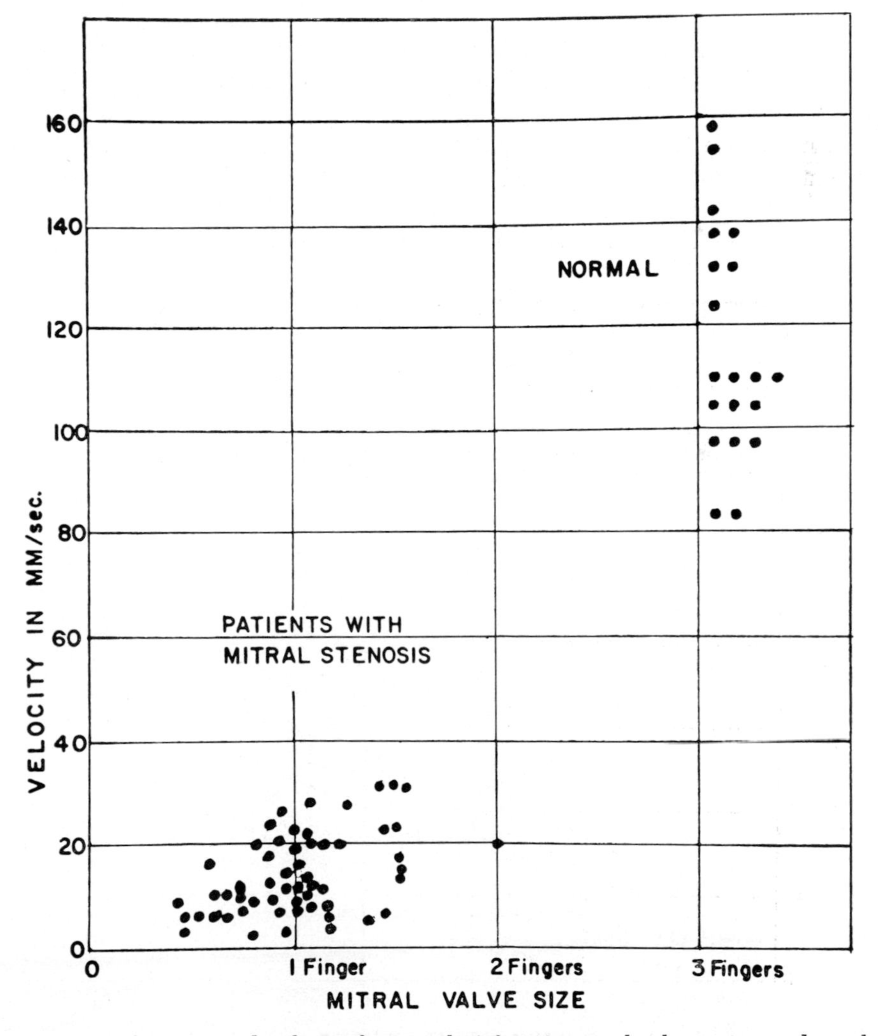

FIGURE 13. The measured velocity from peak 4 for 20 normal subjects is noted on the right of the chart. The velocity of 56 patients with mitral stenosis is noted on the left of the chart where the values are plotted in reference to the size of the mitral valve determined at subsequent operation or necropsy.

Figure 14 is a representation of 26 of the 39 patients whom we have studied before and after successful mitral valve surgery. It is apparent that all individuals had an increase in the velocity recorded after surgery, but none of the patients have had an entirely normal pattern after operation. As you can see, we did not record a velocity lower than 85 mm/sec for normal individuals nor a velocity exceeding 70 mm/sec for a postoperative patient. More study is required before it can be determined whether the velocity may increase as a longer period intervenes following operation. In addition, as yet we have not had adequate experience to determine whether the method will prove clinically useful in determining restenosis.

Other than the normal individuals and those with mitral valve disease, we have studied persons with a variety of other conditions such as hypertension, myocardial infarction, and pericardial effusion. Suffice it to say that we have not obtained a pattern of the type seen in mitral stenosis, except in patients proved subsequently to have mitral stenosis. In other words, we have not had a "false-positive" pattern for mitral stenosis to date. Also, for patients with mitral stenosis we have not failed to record the typical pattern,

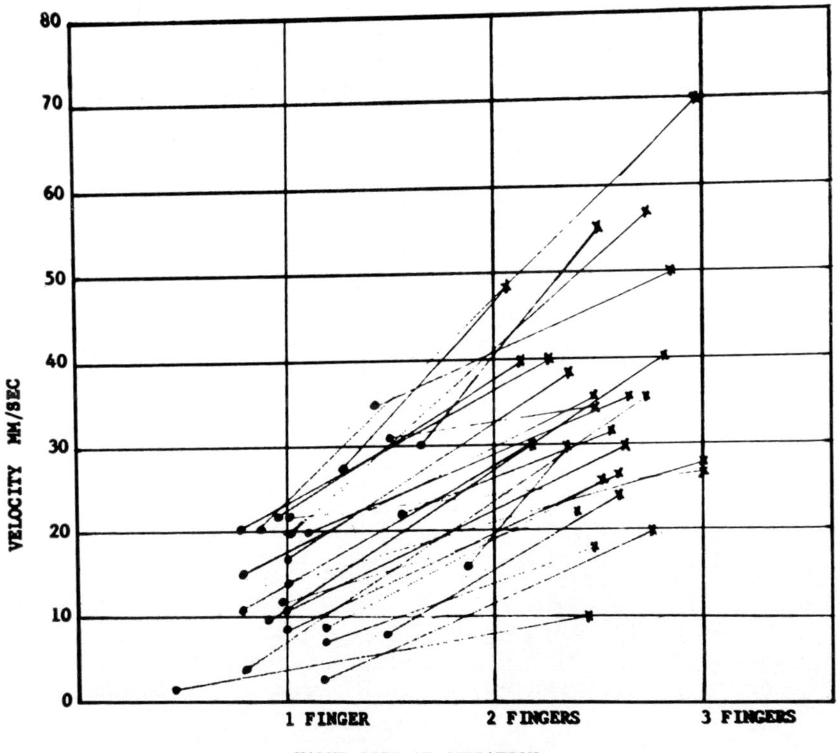

FIGURE 14. Pre- and postoperative velocities from peak 4 recorded in 26 patients having ultrasound records obtained before and after operation. The velocities are plotted against the valve size estimated before and after surgery.

unless they were one of those rare individuals in whom a satisfactory record could not be obtained. Patients from whom we were unable to obtain a record have been persons with some unusual bony configuration of the chest or those with marked emphysema.

The final curve (Fig. 15) is from an individual with pure mitral insufficiency. Peak 1 is not seen since this patient had atrial fibrillation. A prominent peak 4 is seen with a very rapid motion posteriorly from this peak. To date, twelve patients with mitral insufficiency have been studied and evaluated at subsequent surgery. They have all had a velocity of motion which was normal or exceeded our normal range. Note that the speed of motion in this individual is very rapid. In fact, it is about 300 mm/sec. A fast rate of motion has been found in three types of individuals. These have been patients with either mitral insufficiency, myocarditis with a gallop, or aortic insufficiency of a major degree. All of these are situations in which the ventricle fills quite rapidly in contrast to the extremely slow filling associated with mitral stenosis.

Dr. Reid will now continue with his portion of the discussion.

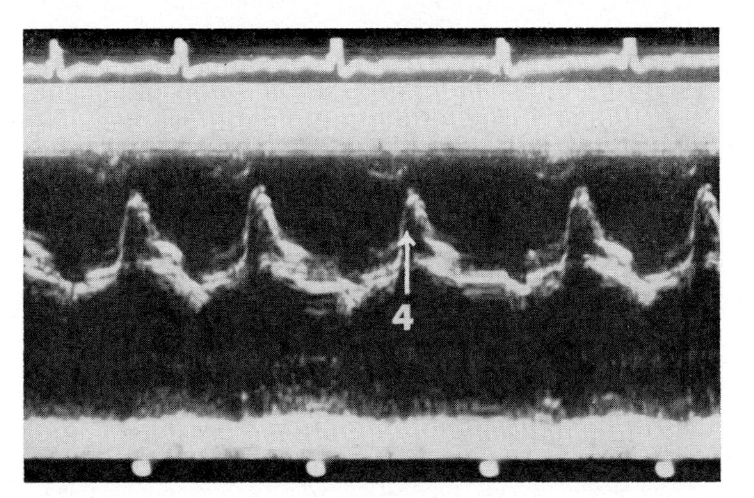

FIGURE 15. Ultrasound pattern from a patient with predominant mitral regurgitation. The velocity of posterior movement from peak 4 is 300 mm/sec.

DR. REID: One of the primary concerns in any clinical technique is the safety of the procedure. In this regard it is essential to know both the average and peak powers of the ultrasonic energy. In the present application, the average power was quite low, but the peak power was reasonably large. Since the pulses were of short duration, it was difficult to measure the peak power directly. The average power was determined by measuring the radiation pressure. A special pan of sound-absorbing rubber was fitted to an analytical balance, with the pan immersed in a container of saline solution. The transducer was dipped into the saline, adjusted, and clamped to the outside of the container. This general arrangement, often used for measuring surface tension, should measure forces as small as a fraction of a dyne. However, the damping introduced by the pan in the water reduced the sensitivity of the balance. It is possible to raise the center of gravity of the balance so that the balance becomes more sensitive. There always remains a restoring force, due to the change in the submerged volume of wire as the pan moves up and down, dependent on the wire size. Surface tension phenomena on the suspension wires required a rather lengthy series of determinations, since the zero point continuously shifted. With an automatic or chain-weighted balance, this method would be quite rapid and convenient. We measured a force of approximately 1 mg, representing a total average output of 14.3 mw. Dividing this power by the area of the transducer the average intensity in the liquid in front of the transducer is found to be 12 mw/cm^2. The heating induced by the average power is negligible. The peak intensity, calculated from the observed 3-db pulse length of 1 μsec, and the interpulse interval of 500 μsec, was 5.7 w/cm^2. Intensities this high have been used continuously in clinical therapy. Since neither heat nor cavitation occurs with the short duration pulses applied, and the only reported effects on patients at intensity levels of this order are ascribed to these mechanisms, no deleterious effect on the patient would be expected from the applied ultrasonic energy. Similar apparatus has been used on experimental animals, upon the investigators themselves, and on thousands of clinical cases. For this particular application, we feel that no danger is involved. As indicated by the work on rabbit eyes (3) and by Fry's (4) investigations of the central nervous system with high-intensity ultrasound, greater peak power can be used if the time of application of the energy is reduced. However, these results show that you cannot determine the allowable intensity by simply dividing the energy density by the time. The peak allowable intensity does not rise as fast as the reciprocal of the time, as a constant energy relation would indicate.

Figure 16 shows a cross-section of the transducers, which use a stock barium titanite disc. The bandwidth of the vibrating crystal is increased by attaching it to a backing material of high acoustic impedance. The backing is made by adding tungsten powder to an epoxy resin and centrifuging it so that the powder is packed. The highest impedance obtained by this means was approximately half that of the crystal. This backing is just adequate to give a distance resolution of 1.5 mm for a frequency of 1 Mc. The characteristic impedance of the backing is closer to that of the piezoelectric element than is the characteristic impedance of the tissue of the patient. Under these conditions the power delivered to the backing was almost ten times the power delivered to the patient, and these transducers were very sensitive detectors of energy reflected from the end of the backing material. After experimenting with several shapes, we found that coarse notches hand filed in one direction on the end of the backing gave a 20-db suppression of the back echo, but the echo remained. We added a reactive polysulfide rubber modifier to soften the epoxy resin. This increased the loss of the backing to the point where we could not see any back reflection. We could then see echoes from pulses that were getting into the metal case and traveling through it back to the crystal. The cases are now cast from epoxy resin mixture, with the addition of small air-filled bakelite spheres. This is not a final design, but such transducers can be made in any chemical laboratory containing a balance, a small oven, and a centrifuge.

In summary, the major contribution we have made is an independent confirmation, as far as the patients to date allow, of the work of Edler, Hertz, and Effert. Since this general type of investigation suffers from having too few investigators, we hope that interest in this field will be greatly expanded.

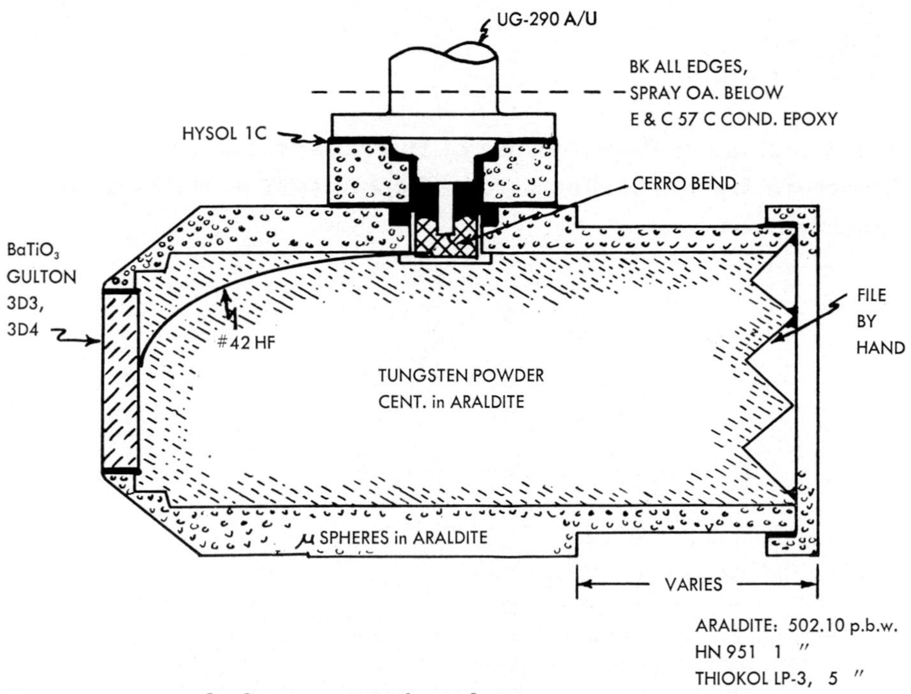

FIGURE 16. Longitudinal cross-section of transducers.

REFERENCES

1. Hertz, C. H., and I. Edler (1956). Die Registrierung von Herzwandbewegungen mit Hilfe des Ultraschall-Impulsverfahrens. Acustica *6*, 361.
2. Edler, I., and A. Gustafson (1957). Ultrasonic cardiogram in mitral stenosis. Acta Med. Scand. *159*, 85.
3. Baum, G., and I. Greenwood (1960). Ultrasound in ophthalmology. Am. J. Ophthal. *49*, 249.
4. Fry, W. J., and F. J. Fry (1960). Fundamental neurological research and human neurosurgery using intense ultrasound. IRE Trans. Med. Electron. *ME-7*, 166–181.

19

The Continuous Registration of the Movement of Heart Structure by the Reflectoscope Techniques — Methods of Registration

CARL HELLMUTH HERTZ
University of Lund, Lund, Sweden

Since certain heart diseases have become operable, the demands on the accuracy of the diagnosis preceding the operation have increased tremendously. As a result of this, several new diagnostic methods have been developed, such as the measurement of the pressure in the heart chamber by heart catheterization and the various methods of angiocardiography. Nearly all of these new methods are complicated and require a relatively large medical staff. They are uncomfortable for the patient, and therefore cannot be repeated frequently for control purposes.

In 1954 the authors showed that heart structures reflect ultrasound and that echoes could be obtained from the heart by placing a 2.5 Mc/sec transducer of a commercial reflectoscope, designed for material testing, externally on the thorax of the patient (Edler and Hertz, 1954; Edler, 1961). The typical pattern on a reflectoscope oscilloscope screen as a result of such an application is shown in Figure 1, where the echoes, R, directly following the zero marker, O, are due to reflections from the chest wall while the echoes, E, are due to reflections from heart structures. The latter can easily be verified because these echoes pulsate in position and size synchronously with the heart beat of the patient. Since the lung tissue surrounding the heart has a very high absorption coefficient for ultrasound, with a frequency of about 2 Mc/sec, no echoes from other body structures are obtained. On the other hand, the heart can be located by this method only from a relatively small area on the thorax of the patient, where no lung tissue lies between the heart and the chest wall.

Since the movement of these echoes represents the movement of heart structures, it was clear that this method could eventually be used for diagnostic purposes, since in the diseased heart we would expect that these typical movements would be greatly altered. Two methods for the recording of these movements were therefore developed.

In the photographic method of recording heart movements, the screen of the CRT of the reflectoscope is projected by a lens, O, on a 0.3-mm slit, S, in such a way that the horizontal zero line on the CRT lies just under the slit (Fig. 2). In this way the 24-mm film, F, which moves smoothly across the slit at a speed of 12 mm/sec, is exposed only to the echo signals projected on the slit. Thus, if the echo is constant (for example, the zero marker, O) a straight line will be marked on the film, while a pulsating echo will generate a curve as shown in Figure 3S. These curves which are generated by pulsating echoes from the heart are called ultrasound cardiographs (UCG). For more accurate inspection of these curves the X-axis of the reflectoscope was expanded electronically approximately three times, resulting in a magnified curve showing more detail (Fig. 3M). These magnified curves were frequently used in the diagnosis of heart valve diseases. In the diagnostic application of this instrument it is very important to record the UCG-curve and at least one ECG-curve simultaneously (Hertz and Edler, 1956). This can be achieved by reflecting a light beam with the small mirror, M, of an ECG-sling-oscillograph onto the screen of the CRT in such a way that a thin vertical line is formed on the screen (Fig. 2). If the current from the ECG amplifier is applied to the oscillograph, this line vibrates along the direction of the X-axis, thereby creating an ECG-curve on the film simultaneously with the UCG (Fig. 3M).

The advantages of the photographic recording method are that an un-

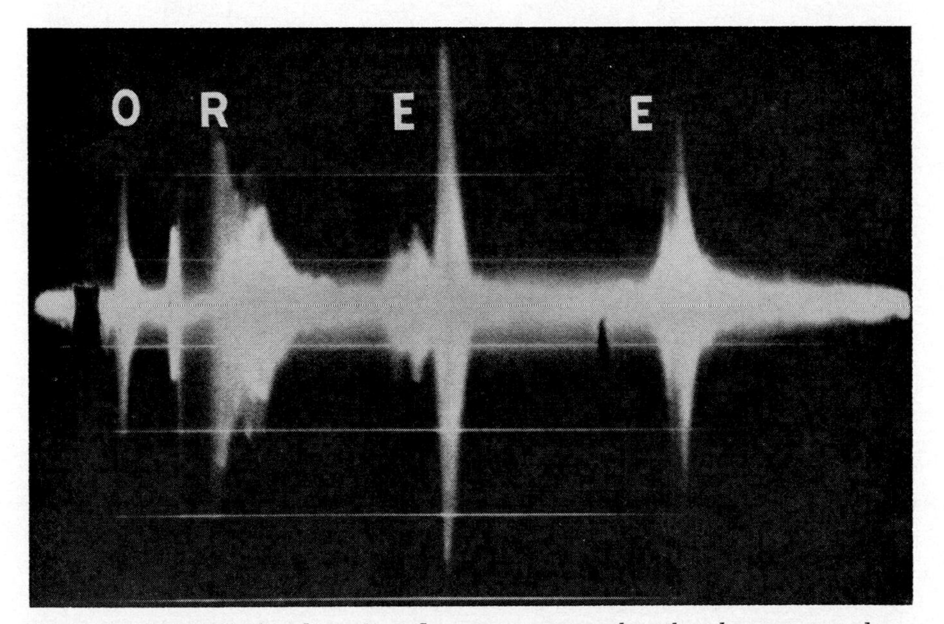

FIGURE 1. Pattern displayed on the reflectoscope screen when the ultrasonic transducer is placed on the thorax of a patient so that the ultrasonic beam passes through the heart. O, zero marker; R, echo from chest wall; E, echoes from heart structures.

limited number of echoes can be recorded simultaneously in their correct position in relation to each other; its disadvantages are the relatively poor appearance of the curves and the time-consuming developing of the film. In spite of the latter, most of the curves recorded at the University of Lund are obtained by this method.

In modern ECG recording, the direct-writing, high-speed "Mingograph" oscillograph has been used for the past 10 years. This oscillograph uses an ink jet ejected under high pressure from a fine nozzle instead of the light beam in the conventional oscillograph. Since this nozzle is connected to a

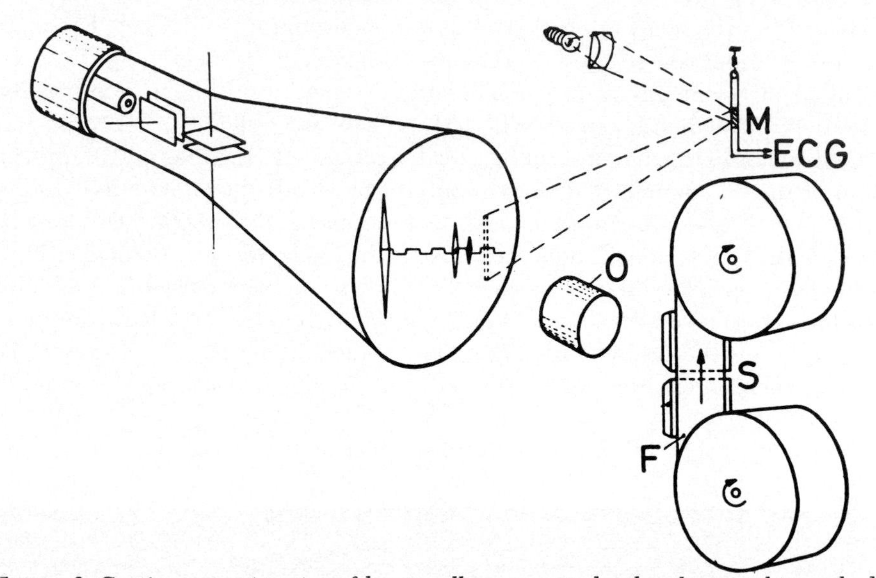

FIGURE 2. Continuous registration of heart wall movements by the photographic method. The film, F, moves with constant velocity behind a slit, S, on which the echo signals are projected by the lens, O. The electrocardiogram is simultaneously reflected on the CRT screen by the sling oscillograph, M, and thus also recorded on the film.

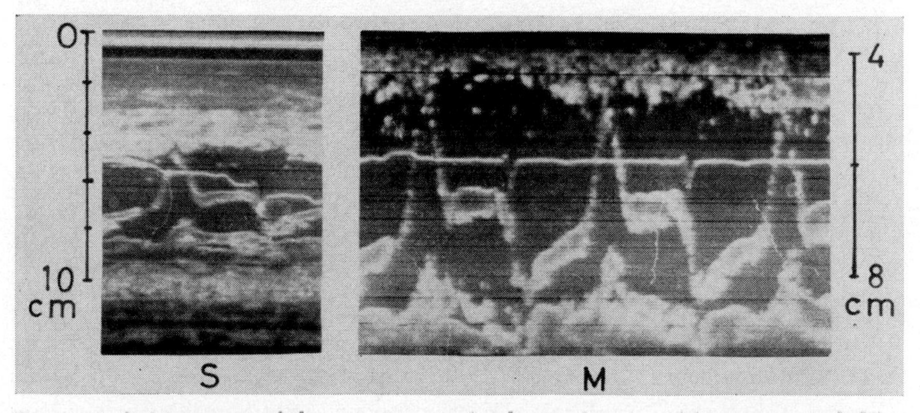

FIGURE 3. S. Movement of the anterior mitral valve in the normal heart as recorded by the photographic method. M. Ultrasound cardiograph shown in Figure 3S with the axis of the reflectoscope expanded by a factor of approximately three.

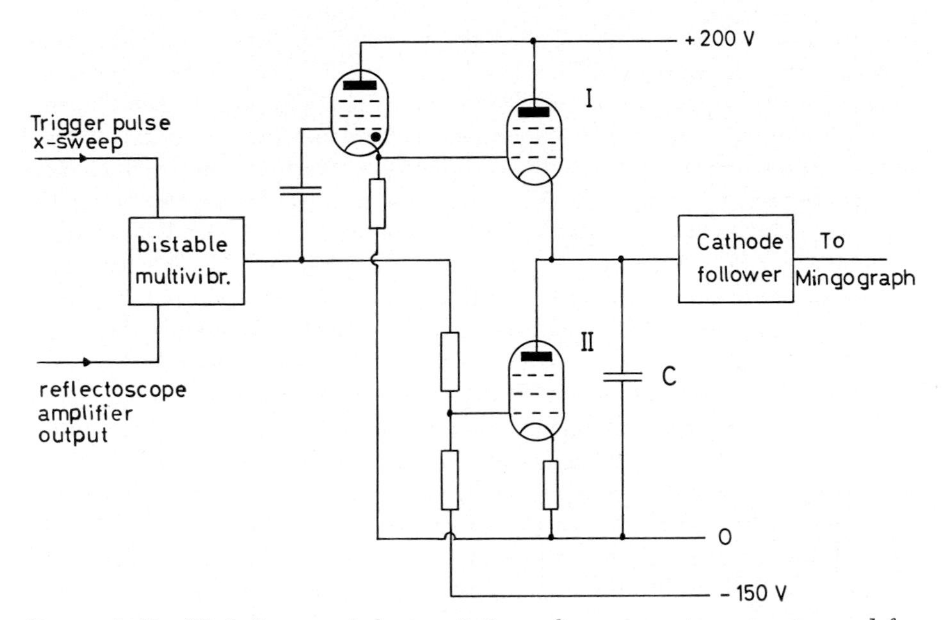

FIGURE 4. Simplified diagram of the transit-time voltage conversion apparatus used for the direct-recording method.

conventional oscillograph system, the ink jet produces a curve on moving recording paper comparable to those produced in the light beam oscillograph, but this method has the advantage that no developing is necessary. The upper frequency limit of this type of the oscillograph lies somewhat above 1000 cy/sec. Since the pulse frequency of the present reflectoscope is 200 cy/sec, the Mingograph recorder can be used to record separately each measurement of the time used by the sound to travel to and from the echo-giving structure (transit time), thereby creating the same UCG-curve as obtained by the photographic method. To achieve this, the transit time must be converted into a voltage signal which can be recorded by the Mingograph recorder. This conversion can be made by employing a condenser discharge for the measurement of the transit time as shown in Figure 4 (Effert, Hertz, and Böhme, 1959). The condenser, C, previously charged by pentode I to a predetermined level, is made to discharge through pentode II during the transit time required for the sound pulse to reach the echo-giving structure and return to the transducer. At this point the discharge is stopped. The residual charge on the condenser is measured by a cathode follower of high-input impedance and recorded by the Mingograph recorder during the 0.005 sec available until the next ultrasound pulse is generated. A UCG recorded in this way is shown in Figure 5. The synchronous recording of other variables may also be accomplished by this method.

The direct method outlined above permits the recording of one echo-giving structure only. Since several echoes are usually obtained simultaneously (cf. Fig. 1), it is necessary to select the echo to be recorded. This is done by using the built-in X-axis magnification of the reflectoscope. At a selectable time interval after the emission of the sound pulse, the X-sweep of the oscilloscope is actuated by a pulse from the reflectoscope. This pulse is also applied to a bistable multivibrator (cf. the simplified circuit in Fig. 4) which is flipped over. This creates a positive pulse at the grid of the thyratron which charges the condenser, C, in about 1 μs. At the same time the grid potential of the pentode II is raised to such a value that the condenser, C, is slowly discharged at a constant rate. Since the output of the Y-amplifier of the reflectoscope is connected to the other grid of the multivibrator, the next echo arriving at the transducer after the beginning of the X-sweep and the charging of the amplifier, throws the multivibrator back into its original position, which in turn makes the grid of pentode II negative, thereby stopping the discharge of the condenser, C. The remaining voltage of the condenser is then transmitted to and recorded by the Mingograph recorder as described above until the beginning of the next X-sweep. Thus, the movements of the first echo following the beginning of the X-sweep are recorded. While this method makes the record directly available for inspection and is more accurate than the photographic method, its disadvantage is that the movements of only one structure can be recorded at a time.

The reflectoscope used for these investigations is the Ultraschall-Impulsgerät II produced by the Siemens Reiniger Werke, Erlangen, Germany. An ultrasound frequency of 2.5 Mc/sec is most frequently used because it ensures a good compromise between the demands for a well-defined beam, short pulse duration, and an absorption coefficient which is not too large. For children, 5 Mc/sec can be used; for obese patients the frequency must be lowered to 1 Mc/sec. The specially designed transducer crystals are of the

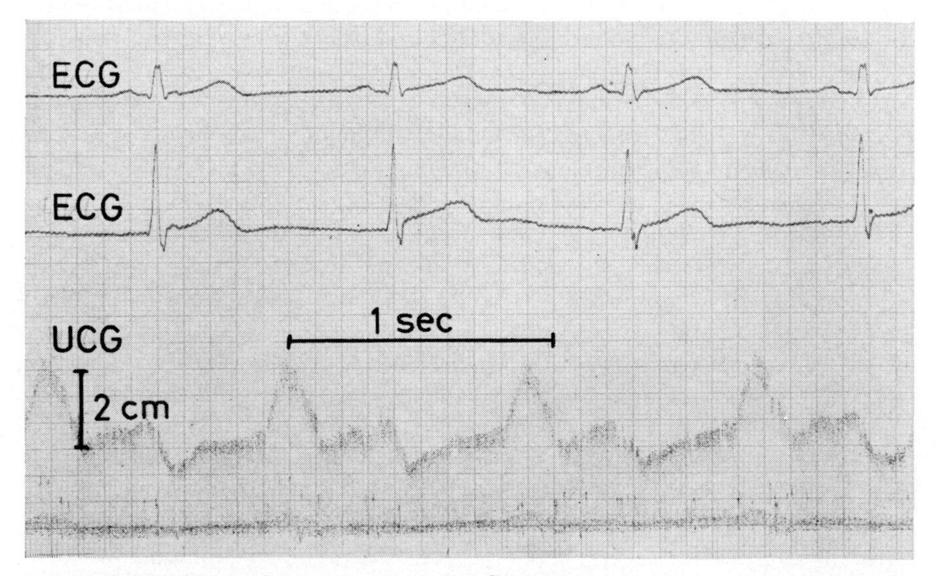

FIGURE 5. Movement of the anterior mitral valve in the normal heart as recorded by the direct-recording method. Two ECG curves appear above the UCG.

barium titanate type and have a diameter of 12 mm. A small HF-transformer is incorporated in the transducer head directly behind the crystal mounting, thereby increasing the maximum pulse intensity and sensitivity of the transducer. These latter features are very important for the success of the method. The maximum pulse intensity at 1 Mc/sec is about 80 w/cm^2 and at 2.5 Mc/sec it is 40 w/cm^2, while the pulse length varies from about 3 to 10 μs. A pulse repetition rate of 200 pulses per second is used.

REFERENCES

Edler, I. (1961). Ultrasoundcardiography. Acta Med. Scand. Suppl. 170.

Edler, I., and C. H. Hertz (1954). The use of ultrasonic reflectoscope for the continuous recording of the movements of heart walls. Kungl. Fysiogr. Sällsk. Förhandl. *24*, *5*.

Effert, S., C. H. Hertz, and W. Böhme (1959). Direkte Registrierung des Ultraschall-Kardiogrammes mit dem Elektrokardiographen. Z. Kreislaufforsch. *48*, 230.

Hertz, C. H., and I. Edler (1956). Die Registrierung von Herzwandbewegungen mit Hilfe des Ultraschall-Impulsverfahrens. Acustica *6*, 361.

Additional References to Ultrasound Cardiography

Braun, H., and W. Schmitt (1961). Ultraschalldiagnostik von Herzfehlern. Fortschr. Med. *79*, 475.

Edler, I., and A. Gustafson (1957). Ultrasonic cardiogram in mitral stenosis. Acta Med. Scand. *159*, II, 85.

Effert, S. (1959). Der derzeitige Stand der Ultraschallkardiographie. Arch. Kreislaufforsch. *30*, 213.

Effert, S. (1960). Diagnostische Anwendungen des Ultraschalles in der Medizin. Umschau *60*, 686.

Effert, S., and E. Domanig (1959). Diagnostik intraaurikulärer Tumoren und grosser Thromben mit dem Ultraschall-Echoverfahren. Dtsch. Med. Wschr. *84*, 1.

Effert, S., E. Domanig, and H. Erkens (1959). Möglichkeiten des Ultraschall-Echoverfahren in der Herzdiagnostik. Cardiologia *34*, 73.

Effert, S., H. Erkens, and F. Grosse-Brockhoff (1957). The ultrasonic echo method in cardiological diagnosis. Germ. Med. Month. (Engl. ed.) *2*, 325.

Gässler, R., and H. Samlert (1958). Zur Beurteilung des Ultraschall-Kardiogrammes bei Mitralstenosen. Z. Kreislaufforsch. *47*, 291.

Grosse-Brockhoff, F. (1961). Ultrasonic cardiography. Am. Heart J. *61*, 843.

Schmitt, W., and H. Braun (1960). Ergebnisse der Ultraschall-untersuchungen bei Herzgesunden und Mitralstenosen. Med. Welt *12*, 640.

Schmitt, W., and H. Braun (1960). Mitteilung der mittels Ultraschall-Kardiographie gewonnenen Ergebnisse bei Mitralvitien und Herzgesunden. Z. Kreislaufforsch. *49*, 214.

Schmitt, W., and H. Braun (1961). Ultraschallkardiographie bei angeborenen und erworbenen Herzfehlern. Münch. Med. Wschr. *103*, 523.

Schwan, H. P., and J. M. Reid (1961). Heart wall motion studies with ultrasound. El. Med. Lab., Univ. of Pennsylvania, Progress Rept. 1.

DISCUSSION

Dr. F. J. Fry: Have measurements been made of the ultrasonic absorption coefficients at these frequencies of excised heart tissue, such as the mitral valve tissue of experimental animals?

DR. HERTZ: No, but we are very interested in this question. We suspect that there is a big difference between the absorption coefficient of mitral valve and of muscle tissues.

DR. W. J. FRY: Do most of the valvular components of mitral, bicuspid, aortic, etc. tissue have the same general physical properties?

DR. HERTZ: Yes.

DR. W. J. FRY: I think someone was asking a question about the possibility of being able to detect major blood vessels and perhaps detect the presence of plaques. Has this ever been attempted by you?

DR. HERTZ: In the heart?

DR. W. J. FRY: No, in the aorta as such.

DR. HERTZ: It is difficult to get echoes from the aorta. Some work was attempted on this but not very much. You are likely to get a double line behind the heart due to echoes from the descending aorta pulsating a little.

DR. KUMMEROW: Is there a different result for a patient who is twenty and one who is sixty? Since the composition of the heart changes somewhat with age, I wonder if this has any effect on the sound?

DR. HERTZ: We have not observed it.

DR. KIKUCHI: I would like to comment that we did some work on a phase of the research that Dr. Reid presented this morning and our results were reported in the Journal of the Acoustical Society of America in 1957. I appreciate, of course, Dr. Reid's further development of this technique and his improvement in the resolution, but I thought it might be of some interest to refer to this earlier work.

DR. REID: We knew that you had reported on this work, but the echoes you obtained were not correlated with any particular structure in the heart. I believe the first person who really observed these phenomena was Ivan Greenwood, who made a short movie 13 or 14 years ago.

DR. GREENWOOD: That movie was shown at a Gordon's Research Conference on Instrumentation in New Hampshire in 1949. There were no proceedings or records; it was considered an off-the-record conference so we cannot claim a publication at that time. However, it was clear enough from this early work that there was an observed response, but it was a big job finding out precisely what it meant.

DR. KIKUCHI: Dr. Edler, you said that in a few cases out of 400 mitral stenosis patients you were not successful in recording the echo. What was the reason?

DR. EDLER: In five cases, emphysema was present; in two cases obesity; and in one case there was advanced displacement of the heart to the right, a sequel of right-sided lung changes.

DR. KELLY: Is there a problem in differentiating the structures that give strong echoes and those that give weak echoes?

DR. GREENWOOD: First of all, in dealing with the ocular tissues we are dealing with tissues which invariably produce weak echoes so we don't have the extremely strong echoes that tend to obscure the weaker echoes behind them. The strongest echo of importance in most areas is typically weaker than, let's say, —35 or —40 db. In regard to the question of how close to a relatively strong echo can you detect a weak echo, we can certainly see weak echoes behind echoes of normal physiological significance, certainly within a millimeter. Now, if it gets much closer than that then, with the present equipment, one hesitates to assign quantitative significance to the data.

DR. REID: Were you recording all of the five or six records on one scan of the patient—the 5 db per step material?

DR. GREENWOOD: We are recording on one scan at a time. Each sector scan is one frame of the 35-mm film. Thus, the intensities of all echoes on that film within the roughly 70-db physiological range lie within the region of the film density curve where there is still a little bit of slope left. Hence, you can go back and recover some absolute reflection coefficients from all the echoes on the film.

DR. REID: How long does the sector scan take?

DR. GREENWOOD: A sector scan is 1 sec across; the whole cycle between sector scans is about the order of 2 sec. It is an automatic process.

DR. MACKAY: Can you amplify Dr. Baum's remark about testing six things simultaneously?

DR. GREENWOOD: He stated that these different things can be interpreted from one picture, that is, it is possible for these different types of data to exist in a single picture.

DR. HOWRY: What possible information can be obtained from a differentiated vs undifferentiated ultrasonogram, and how significant is it?

DR. GREENWOOD: We have looked at the same structure with the differentiated and the undifferentiated shot. There is no appreciable difference, so far as the eye can discern, in terms of information content. However, I am certain there are instances where this will not be true, but in the average interpretation this is not of clinical significance.

DR. HERTZ: I believe we have reached the same conclusion.

DR. MACKAY: I believe the question of differentiated vs undifferentiated is dependent upon another factor, namely, the information content of the original image. There may be some types of images in which the detail is not fine enough to warrant differentiation, while in other cases differentiation is valuable.

DR. REID: One thing that hasn't been discussed is the question of the ultrasonic ray vs the x ray. Our pictures are composed of the echoes from regions where the impedance changes. In a sense, the picture itself is the first derivative of impedance throughout the tissue. Since this is a discontinuous function, we do not build up large blocks of echoes (the type of solid echo that would turn only into a leading or trailing edge on further differentiation) except in cases where there are distributions of interfaces. Therefore, our solid blocks in themselves are rather discontinuous functions and further video-differentiation yields a very similar result. If we could detect the sign of this first derivative, we could then integrate and present solid pictures of the impedance level throughout the tissues.

DR. HOWRY: My question referred to where you expected a drop in the receiver. You can take first and second derivatives and go on from there and each one is a little different. The essential question is: If you have a receiver which is over-loading and blocking, then you will get an entirely different appearing picture, figuratively blocked by 40- or 60-db signals so that the small microvolt signals are not discernible. You can carry this one step further and analyze what type of echo you would expect at various frequencies, that is, how far apart can these small structures be and their signals still be received. We published in the Proceedings of the Society of Nondestructive Testing, Vol. 2, some quantitative studies on this aspect in the metallurgy field which included methods by which one can at least begin to determine what the magnitude of these various objects might be and still be seen at a given frequency and, in addition, how rough the objects are. We have not seen the extremely fine echoes which Dr. Baum showed this morning. However, we are operating at 2 Mc so we wouldn't anticipate discernment of these small discrete particles. At 15 Mc it would be much more likely that detection is possible. Therefore, any varying results are probably due to a very logical difference between two pieces of equipment operating at two different frequencies rather than an error on the part of an investigator in regard to interpretation of pictures. The point I was really trying to make is that a number of parameters have to be defined in this type of work in order to establish correlated results between various investigators.

DR. HUETER: How about the MTI techniques? Would that unclutter your picture?

DR. REID: The MTI techniques are very nice but require extensive equipment and a large expenditure of money. I think there are more fundamental questions which need answering about the properties of the tissue. The present technique seems to be perfectly adequate for routine clinical application, just as it is now.

DR. HUETER: Are there other techniques available for testing of mitral stenosis? I know that probes are inserted inside the heart for diagnosis of certain heart ailments. Do you have to use the ultrasound techniques?

DR. REID: No. You can differentiate these mitral valve conditions with cardiac catheters, which is an operative procedure. However, such a procedure can not be applied to badly damaged hearts and would be totally useless in a survey of populations.

20

The Diagnostic Use of Ultrasound in Heart Disease

INGE EDLER, M.D.
University Hospital, Lund, Sweden

By means of ultrasound, echoes can be obtained from a variety of heart structures so that the actions of these structures are recorded as a tracing, the UCG (ultrasound cardiogram) (Edler and Hertz, 1954). The appearance of these tracings depends partly on where the crystal is placed on the precordium and partly on the incident angle of the beam.

I. ULTRASOUND CARDIOGRAM OF THE ANTERIOR MITRAL LEAFLET. THE CURVE AM.

Figure 1 shows tracings taken from various parts of the left second, third, and fourth interspaces. Tracing 1 is taken from the medial part of the second left interspace. Tracings 5, 8 and 9 are taken from the third left interspace with the beam directed anteroposteriorly. A completely different type of tracing is obtained, however, if the sound beam is directed 10 to 15° medially from the medial part of the third left interspace, as can be seen in tracings 2 and 4. Tracing 6 is taken from the medial part of the fourth left interspace, with the beam directed anteroposteriorly. This tracing shows the same characteristics as do tracings 5, 8, and 9 from the third interspace. This type of tracing, that is, 5, 8, 9, and 6, henceforth referred to as AM, is easy to record since the echo signal, with its quick and typical motion, is easy to identify on the oscilloscope screen.

In order to identify the heart structure from which a given echo emanates, it is necessary: (1) to analyze the tracing's movement pattern and correlate this with simultaneously recorded ECGs and intracardiac pressure recordings; (2) to determine the echo's localization within the heart, that is to say, to determine the distance between the transducer on the precordium and the echo source; and (3) to consider the heart in situ.

A. Relation Between UCG and Heart Activity

By making simultaneous recordings of the ECG and the characteristic ultrasound tracing AM, the latter has been correlated to atrial activity (see

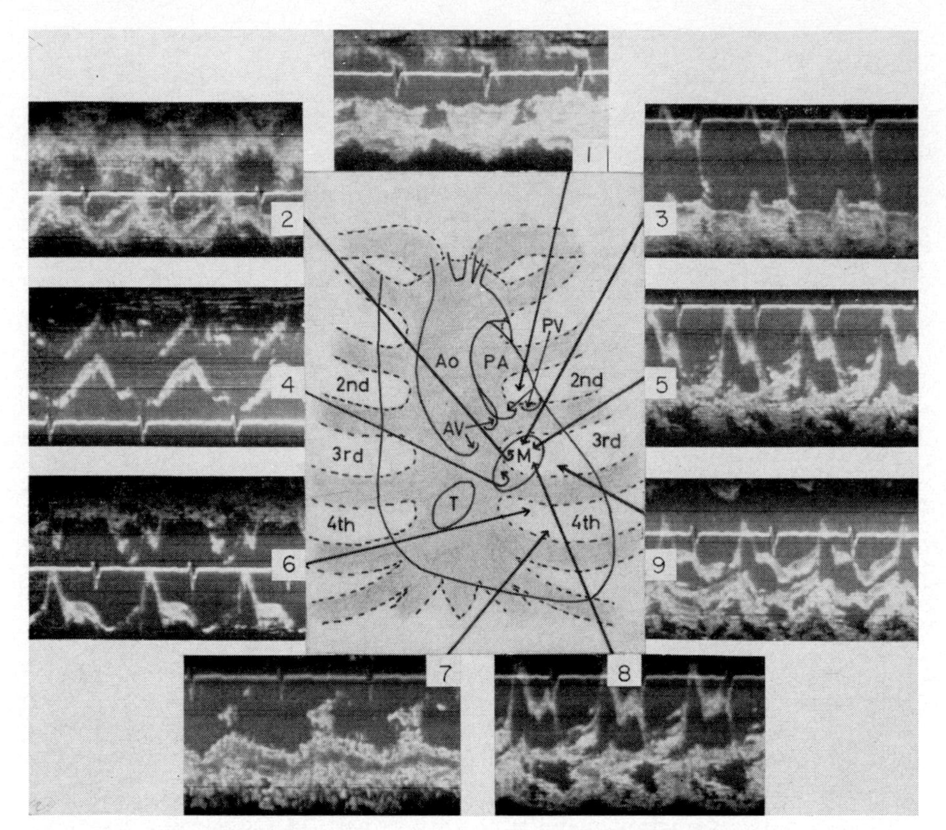

FIGURE 1. Ultrasound cardiograms obtained from different parts of the precordium. The picture shows the topographic relation among heart, sternum, and ribs. Ao, aorta; AV, aortic valve; PA, pulmonary artery; PV, pulmonary valve; M, mitral ostium; T, tricuspid ostium. 2nd, 3rd, and 4th indicate the interspaces. The arrows on the diagram indicate the situation of the crystal on the precordium. Curve 1 shows recording from the second left interspace over the pulmonary artery. Curves 3, 5, 8, and 9 show recordings from the third left interspace with the beam directed anteroposteriorly. Curves 2 and 4 show recordings from medial part of third left interspace and the fourth rib with the beam directed medially and upwards. Curves 6 and 7 show recordings from the fourth left interspace.

Figs. 2, 3) (Edler and Hertz, 1954; Edler, 1955, 1956; Hertz and Edler, 1956; Edler and Gustafson, 1957, 1961; Effert, 1959). Normally the peak A begins 0.08 to 0.12 sec after the start of the P-wave in the ECG (Edler and Gustafson, 1957). The same time relationship between the A-wave in the UCG and the P-wave in the ECG is seen in atrioventricular block, both partial and complete (Edler, 1955; Edler and Gustafson, 1957; Effert, 1959). In atrial flutter, the tracing displays multiple peaks corresponding in number to the flutter waves during ventricular diastole (Edler, 1955; Edler and Gustafson, 1957; Effert, 1959). In atrial fibrillation, no A-waves are seen in the UCG tracing (Edler, 1955). Figure 3 shows simultaneous recordings of the UCG, phonocardiogram, and intracardiac pressure changes. Atrial systole, indicated by the letter A in the pressure curve is synchronous with peak A in the UCG (Edler,

1961). Thus the A-waves in UCG are associated with atrial systole and are consequently absent in atrial fibrillation. Point E in UCG represents the instant at which the echo-giving structure is closest to the crystal. This instant coincides with early ventricular diastole (Edler, 1961). At the beginning of ventricular systole, the echo-giving structure has reached its most distant point from the crystal on the anterior chest wall (see Fig. 3).

B. Localization of the Echo Source

In a series of 86 healthy men aged between nineteen and fifty-four years, a characteristic type of tracing, namely AM, was obtained in 79 cases when the beam was directed anteroposteriorly from the medial end of the third or fourth left interspace. (In 38 cases the record was obtained from both the third and the fourth interspace. In 22 cases it could be recorded only from

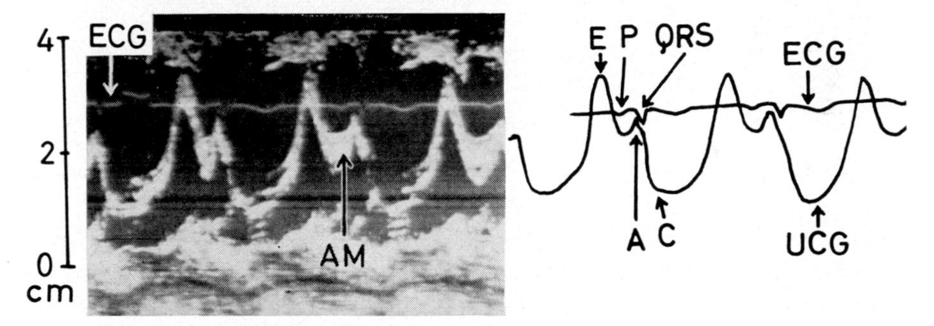

FIGURE 2. Ultrasound cardiogram obtained from the third left interspace in a normal case. Left: tracing AM produced by the photographic method. Right: schematic representation of tracing AM. The rising curve represents the movement of the echo source toward the crystal on the anterior chest wall. The falling curve represents the movement of the echo source away from the crystal. E represents the most ventral position attained by the echo source, and C the most dorsal position. The P-wave in the ECG is followed by a peak A in the UCG record.

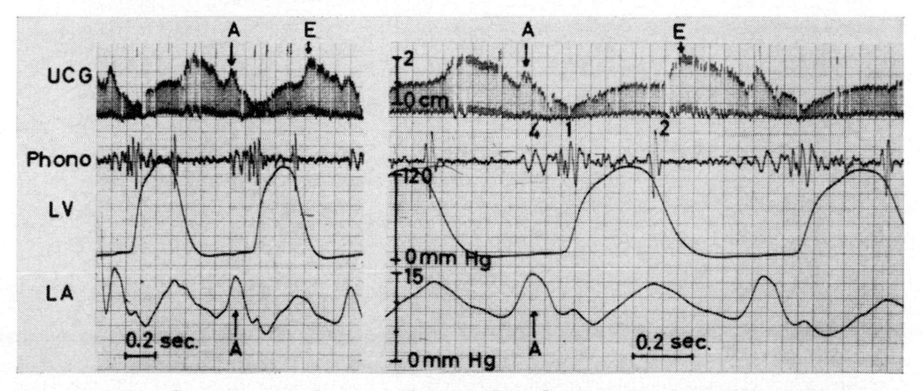

FIGURE 3. Simultaneous recordings of ultrasound cardiogram (tracing AM), phonocardiogram, left ventricular pressure (LV), and left atrial pressure (LA). Direct-writing method. Left: paper speed 50 mm/sec. Right: paper speed 100 mm/sec. The lowest point in the UCG curve is reached at the beginning of ventricular systole. After second heart sound (2 in phonogram), the UCG tracing rises steeply to peak E which is the highest point reached in the record. E is reached 0.10 sec after the second heart sound.

the third interspace, and in 19 cases only from the fourth [Edler, 1961].) In two cases the characteristic tracing AM was obtained in the fifth left interspace. In five cases no tracing at all was obtained (see Table I). For the same group of subjects a curve was obtained in sixty cases with the crystal placed over an area of the third left interspace between 2.5 and 4 cm from the midline. In 57 cases a tracing was obtained from the fourth left interspace in an area 2.5 to 4 cm from the sternal midline.

TABLE I. LOCATION OF CRYSTAL ON PRECORDIUM IN 86 HEALTHY MALES.

Subject	*Area from which echo signal AM received*	*Number of cases*
Healthy males	Both third and fourth left interspace	38
" "	Only third left interspace	22
" "	Only fourth left interspace	19
" "	Only fifth left interspace	2
" "	No trace obtained	5

Point E (Fig. 2) on the tracing represents the instant at which the echo source is closest to the crystal on the anterior chest wall; C represents the same echo source at the opposite end of its travel. As indicated in Table II (same series of 86 healthy men), the minimum crystal-echo-source distance was found to be 58 mm when measured from the third left interspace and 59 mm when measured from the fourth left interspace. The maximum crystal-echo-source distance was 82 mm when measured from the third left interspace and 83 mm when measured from the fourth left interspace.

TABLE II. THE DISTANCE BETWEEN CRYSTAL AND ECHO SOURCE IN SUBJECTS OF TABLE I.

Crystal applied to	*Number of cases*	*Distance in each cardiac cycle*	
		Maximum	*Minimum*
Third left interspace	60	82 mm	58 mm
Fourth left interspace	57	83 mm	59 mm
Fifth left interspace	2	96 mm	68 mm

C. The Heart Considered in Situ

Considering the heart in situ, we find that the heart structures which normally project onto the medial 3 to 4 cm of the third left interspace are the following: the anterior wall of the right ventricle, the conus pulmonalis, the interventricular septum, the left ventricular outflow tract, the mitral ostium, and the left atrium (see Fig. 4). Of those heart structures which project onto the medial part of the left third interspace, only the left atrium and the mitral valve are affected by atrial activity. Since in the adult the sagittal diameter of the heart is normally 85 to 90 mm and the echo source moves along the sagittal line through the heart at a distance of 58 to 82 mm from the anterior chest wall (Table II), this source must be situated, at least during part of the cardiac cycle, reasonably centrally within the heart. Thus, the posterior wall of the atrium is excluded as a possible source of this echo. With regard to movement pattern and localization, therefore, the echo-giving structure must be assigned to the anterior region of the atrium in the vicinity of the mitral ostium. The characteristic ultrasound tracing, AM, is recorded from the region of the sternal margin and approximately 2 cm lateral thereto, in the third left interspace and/or the fourth left interspace. This region, as pointed out previously, represents the surface projection of the anterior mitral leaflet (Edler, 1961).

The anterior wall of the left atrium is proximal and to the right of the mitral ostium. Normally the anterior wall of the left atrium does not reach so far downward as to project onto the fourth left interspace where the tracing can often, in fact, be recorded. The anterior wall of the left atrium and the anterior limit of the left auricular appendage can subsequently be disregarded as possible sources of this characteristic echo tracing (Edler, 1961). In experiments on the isolated heart we have found it possible to record ultrasound tracings from the anterior cusp of the mitral valve (Edler, Gustafson, Karlefors, and Christensson, 1960b, 1961). (The results of these investigations will be shown in a movie film following this lecture.) Consequently, the tracing AM must represent the movements of the anterior leaflet of the mitral valve during the various phases of the cardiac cycle (Edler, 1961; Edler, Gustafson, Karlefors, and Christensson, 1960a, 1960b; Edler, Hertz, Gustafson, Karlefors, and Christensson, 1960).

II. ULTRASOUND CARDIOGRAM OF THE ANTERIOR MITRAL LEAFLET IN MITRAL STENOSIS

In mitral stenosis the appearance of the tracing AM is entirely different (Figs. 5, 6, 7) (Edler, 1956). The quick component, E-F, in early diastole is lacking, and the tracing shows a slow fall, as a rule continuing during the whole diastole. Peak A is usually absent in mitral stenosis. In normal cases and in other cases of heart disease without mitral involvement this movement of the mitral valve in early diastole (E-F) occurs at a speed of more than 80 mm/sec (Edler and Gustafson, 1957; Effert, 1959). In mitral stenosis, with or without an element of incompetence, this movement is much slower, max. 40 mm/sec (Edler and Gustafson, 1957; Edler, 1961). This figure accords with that reported by Effert (1959).

As a measure of the rate of dorsalward movement of the anterior mitral cusp during ventricular diastole, Edler (1956) and Hertz and Edler (1956) used the angle formed by the horizontal and tracing AM during its fall from peak E (horizontal line is time axis) (see Fig. 5). In normal cases, the angle α is more than 70 to 80°, while in all cases of mitral stenosis it is less than 40°. The angle α is a measure of the mitral block, and in severe mitral stenosis it has a value of 5 to 10°. If the angle is less than 25° (a movement of the anterior mitral leaflet at a speed of less than 20 mm/sec), this is an indication for the

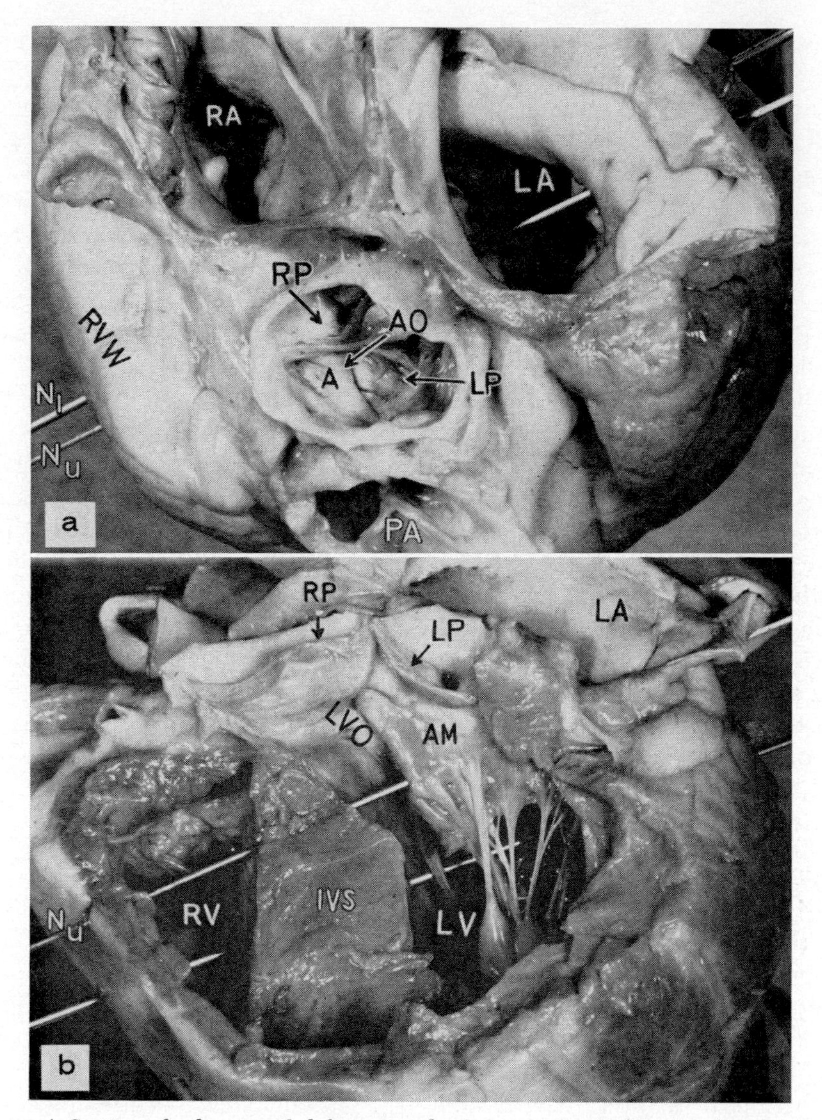

FIGURE 4. Section of a heart with left ventricular hypertrophy. Before the thoracic cavity had been opened, the needles which transect the preparation had been inserted in an anteroposterior direction from the third left interspace (upper needle) and fourth left interspace (lower needle) at the sternal margin. Due to advanced hypertrophy and the continued presence of rigor mortis, the ventricular muscle was rigid and the heart retained its original shape during manipulation. A. Picture taken from above. RA, right atrial cavity; LA, left atrial cavity; AO, aortic ostium; A, anterior aortic cusp; RP, right posterior aortic cusp; LP, left posterior aortic cusp; PA, pulmonary artery; RVW, anterior wall of right ventricle; N_u, upper needle; N_l, lower needle. The upper needle passes left atrial cavity. B. Picture taken from obliquely upward. The left and upper part of the ventricular wall and the interventricular septum has been cut away. RV, right ventricular

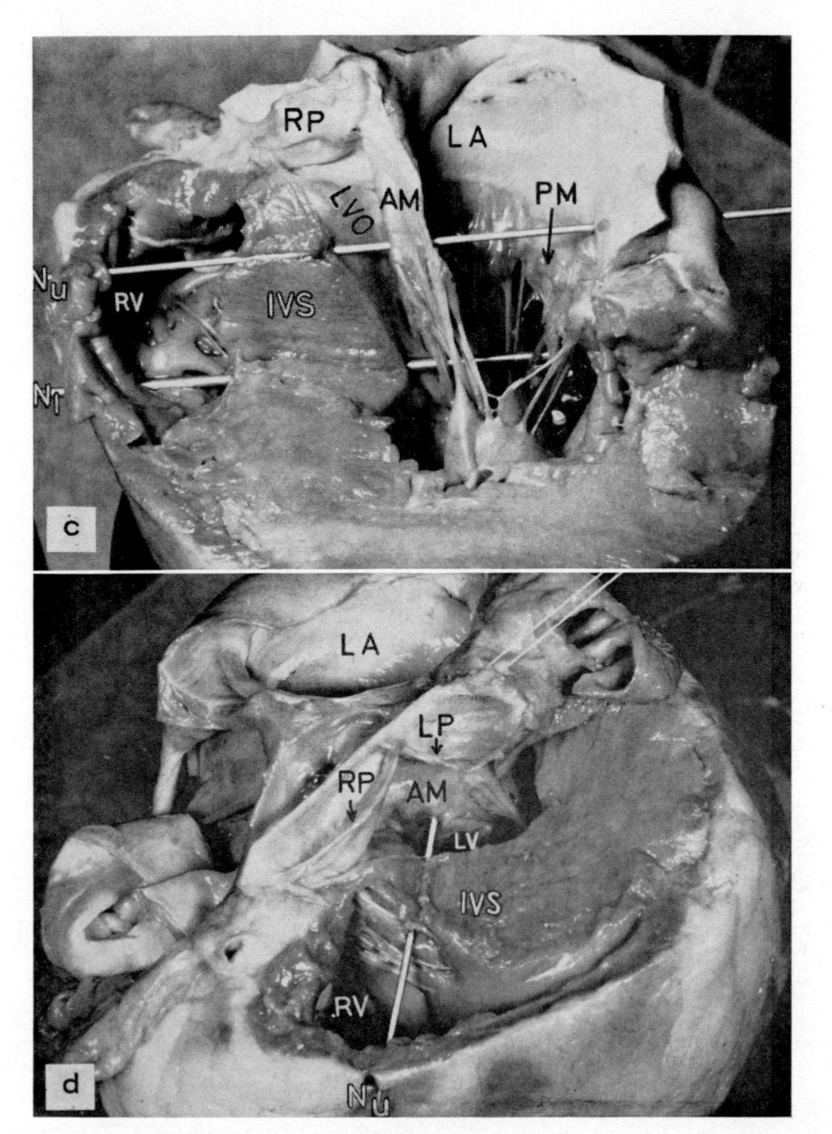

cavity; LV, left ventricular cavity; IVS, interventricular septum; AM, anterior mitral leaflet; LP, left posterior aortic cusp; RP, right posterior aortic cusp; LA, left atrial cavity. The upper needle (inserted in anteroposterior direction from third left interspace) passes anterior wall of the right ventricle, right ventricular cavity, interventricular septum, left ventricular outflow tract, and anterior mitral leaflet. C. The lateral or left part of the mitral funnel has been cut away. The anterior leaflet of the mitral valve, AM, hangs like a curtain in the central part of the left ventricle. LVO, left ventricular outflow tract; PM, posterior mitral leaflet. The upper needle passes left atrial cavity and the base or attachment of posterior mitral leaflet, PM. D. Same preparation as in Figure 4B. Depicted as seen from in front and somewhat above. The needle passes the anterior mitral leaflet, AM, just below the left posterior aortic cusp, LP.

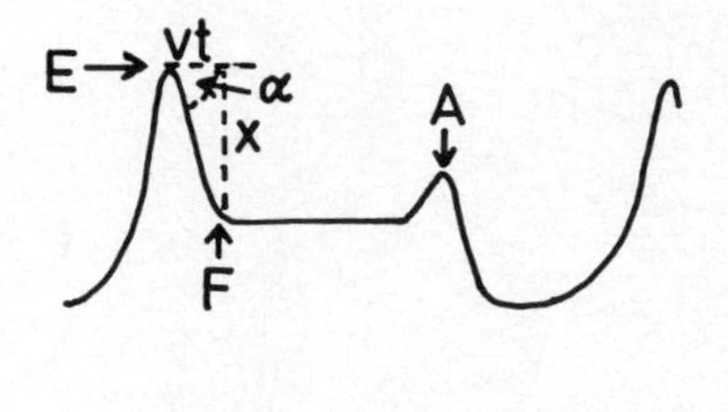

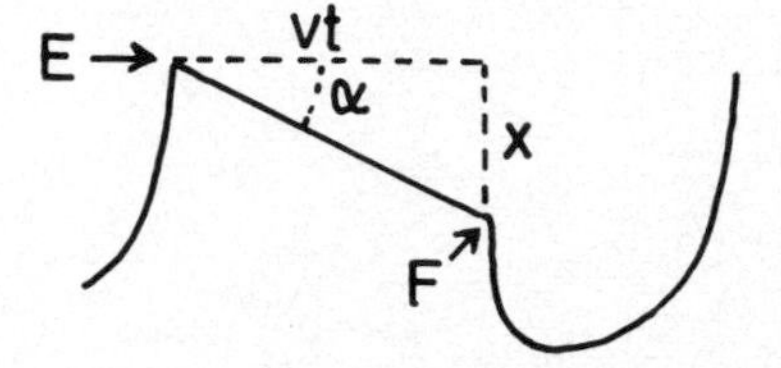

FIGURE 5. Schematization of tracing AM. Above: normal case. The curve falls rapidly from peak E to point F. Below: mitral stenosis. The normal fairly steep fall E–F is replaced by a slow declining line throughout or during major part of diastole. The angle α is a measure of the rate of dorsalward movement of the anterior mitral cusp during ventricular diastole. x, the movement of the mitral leaflet during time t; v, velocity of the film or ECG paper. The angle is determined by the equation $tg\alpha = \frac{x}{vt}$.

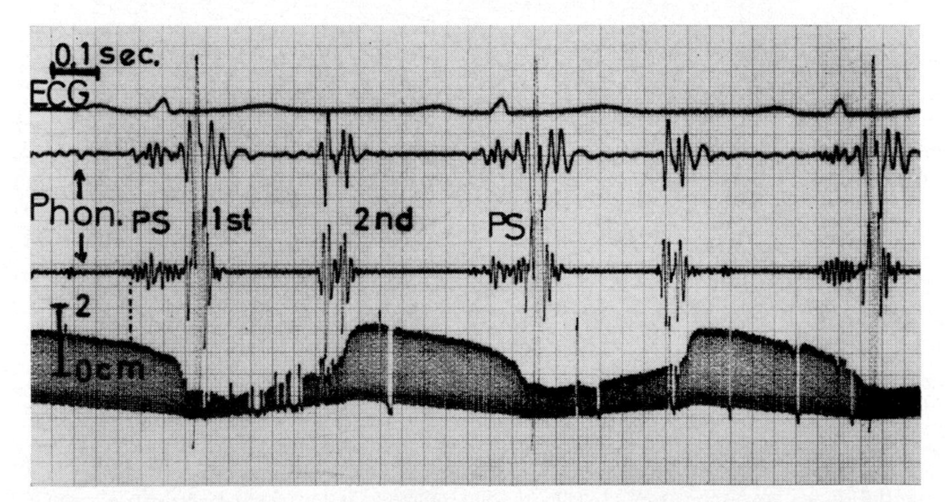

FIGURE 6. Tracing AM in a case of mitral stenosis. Simultaneous recording of ECG, phonocardiogram, and UCG by direct-writing method. PS, presystolic murmur, first and second heart sounds are labeled accordingly. After the second heart sound, tracing AM rises steeply. After the highest point is reached it falls again slowly. Later, at the time of the presystolic murmur (PS) the tracing falls more steeply.

necessity of surgery (commissurotomy) as has been shown by Edler and Gustafson (1957). The immediate postoperative result can be studied (see Fig. 7). Effert (1959) reports the same result. We have carried out follow-up studies of the mitral stenosis cases treated by surgery since 1955. Recurrence of the mitral stenosis can be diagnosed early and consequently reoperation can be carried out in time to insure a successful result (Fig. 8) (Edler, 1961; Edler, Gustafson, Karlefors, and Christensson, 1960a, 1960b; Edler, Hertz, Gustafson, Karlefors, and Christensson, 1960). In Lund we have been able to obtain these typical records in more than 400 cases of mitral stenosis with only eight cases of mitral stenosis for which it was impossible to record the typical tracing from the anterior mitral leaflet.

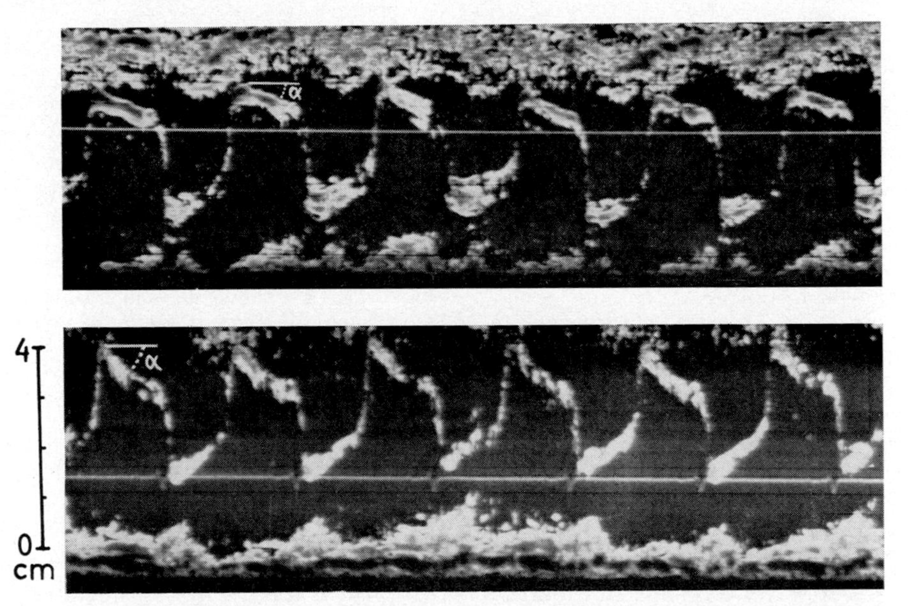

FIGURE 7. Tracing AM in a case of mitral stenosis. Recording by photographic method. Above: before commissurotomy. Below: after commissurotomy. α indicates the angle between the horizontal line and that portion of the tracing which represents AM:s movement during ventricular diastole. The smaller the movement of the echo source the smaller becomes this angle.

III. ULTRASOUND CARDIOGRAM OF THE MITRAL FUNNEL

Inspection of Figure 4 indicates that if the needle were directed somewhat more laterally and caudally, the posterior mitral cusp could also be pierced. This suggests that it may be possible to record movements of this cusp by means of ultrasound echo-ranging from the third or the fourth left interspace. In practice it has been possible to record an echo signal from behind the anterior mitral cusp when recording from a zone 2 to 4 cm lateral to the left margin of the sternum (Edler, Gustafson, Karlefors, and Christensson, 1960a, 1960b). This new echo signal has a motion sequence which is partially a mirror image of that from the anterior cusp (see Figs. 9, 10). To obtain such

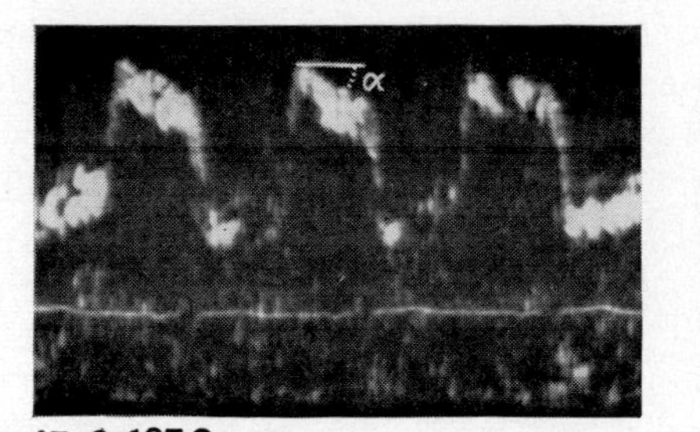

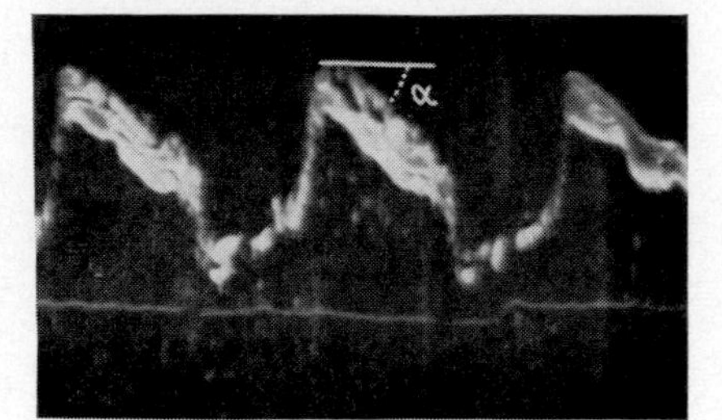

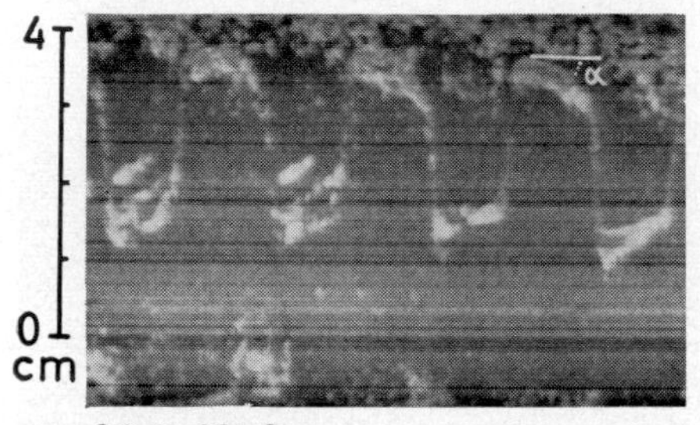

FIGURE 8. Tracing AM in a case of mitral stenosis which has undergone commissurotomy twice. Above left: tracing taken on 2/15/56 before commissurotomy. Above right: tracing taken on 3/9/56 after commissurotomy. Below left: tracing taken on 5/29/59 before reoperation. Below right: tracing taken on 6/17/59 after reoperation. At the first operation the mitral ostium admitted the tip of the index finger prior to commissurotomy. After commissurotomy the ostium was widened to about 1½ fingers. At reoperation 3 years later the ostium was very narrow and was widened to permit the passage of 2½ to 3 fingers. Below left: the angle α is less than after the first operation = restenosis. After reoperation a bigger angle again.

recordings, the beam must be directed 15° laterally with reference to the anteroposterior plane. In Figures 9 and 10, AM is the tracing of the anterior mitral valve movement and PM is the tracing resulting from this new echo signal. During ventricular systole, VS, when the mitral ostium is closed, AM and PM are confluent. Early in diastole, and during atrial systole, A (that is, during the phase of the heart cycle in which the flow of blood through the mitral ostium is at its greatest), the distance between AM and PM is maximal. It must be borne in mind that the separation between the two tracings represents a cross-section at an unknown level in the mitral funnel and is not an absolute measurement as regards the mitral ostium.

IV. ULTRASOUND CARDIOGRAM OF THE LEFT VENTRICULAR OUTFLOW TRACT

When the action of the anterior mitral valve cusp is recorded, a tracing of entirely different character suddenly appears if the incident angle of the sound beam is shifted 5 to 10° medially toward the midline (Edler, Gustafson, Karlefors, and Christensson, 1960a, 1960b; Edler, Hertz, Gustafson, Karlefors, and Christensson, 1960). This is illustrated by Figure 11. These tracings represent a structure with distinctly reduced movement amplitude,

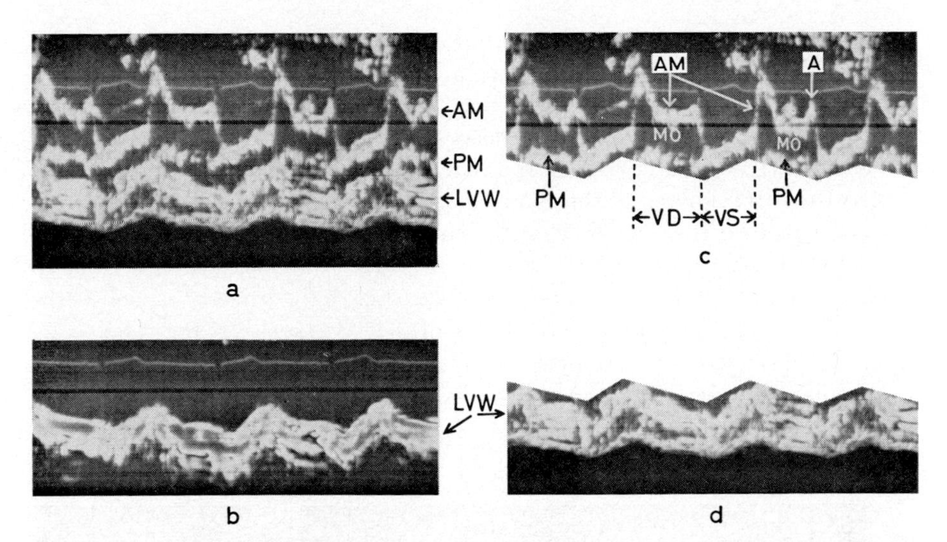

FIGURE 9. Ultrasound cardiogram of the mitral funnel and the posterior wall of the left ventricle. A. When the movements of the anterior mitral leaflet are recorded, the complicated curve (multiple echoes) can be obtained by slight laterocaudal change in the direction of the beam. AM, anterior mitral leaflet; PM, posterior mitral leaflet; LVW, posterior wall of left ventricle. B. Normal curve of the movements of the posterior wall of the left ventricle. The echogram is obtained from the fourth left interspace. C, D. Section of Figure 9A divided horizontally and separated. By this bisecting of the figure, the tracings of the multiple echo signals are identified. AM, tracing of the anterior mitral leaflet; PM, tracing of the posterior mitral leaflet. AM and PM separate markedly from one another in the beginning of diastole, VD, and then run parallel until atrial systole, A, when they again separate, though less markedly. During ventricular systole (VS) AM and PM coincide. The distance between AM and PM during ventricular diastole is a measure of the size of the mitral funnel in the section passed by the impulses. MO, mitral ostium. Figure 9D shows the recording of the posterior echo signal and is identified as tracing of the posterior wall of the heart (see Fig. 9B).

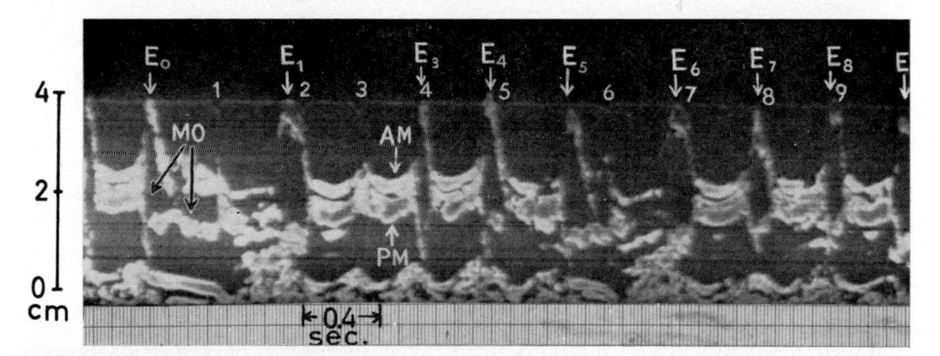

FIGURE 10. Ultrasound cardiogram of the mitral funnel in a case of atrial fibrillation. The A-waves are absent. In ECG record (reproduction is poor), QRS complexes are indicated by numbers 1 through 9. Between QRS complexes 2 and 3 the time interval is only 0.3 sec and peak E is absent. AM, anterior mitral leaflet; PM, posterior mitral leaflet; MO, mitral ostium. AM and PM are confluent during ventricular systole.

in fact only 3 to 6 mm. This altered type of tracing found when the beam is directed medially can be obtained regardless of whether mitral valve action is being recorded from the third or from the fourth left interspace. Figure 4 indicates how the anterior mitral cusp constitutes the dorsal boundary of the left ventricular outflow tract and reaches from the posterior region of the root of the aorta down into the central part of the left ventricle. It is apparent from the picture that on altering the incident angle, the beam strikes the basal part of the anterior mitral cusp near its attachment to the root of the aorta. This explains the altered characteristics of the tracing, as well as the reduction in movement amplitude. In Figure 11, M represents the echo signal from the basal part of the mitral valve, and IVS the signal from the interventricular septum. The intervening area corresponds to the left ventricular outflow tract.

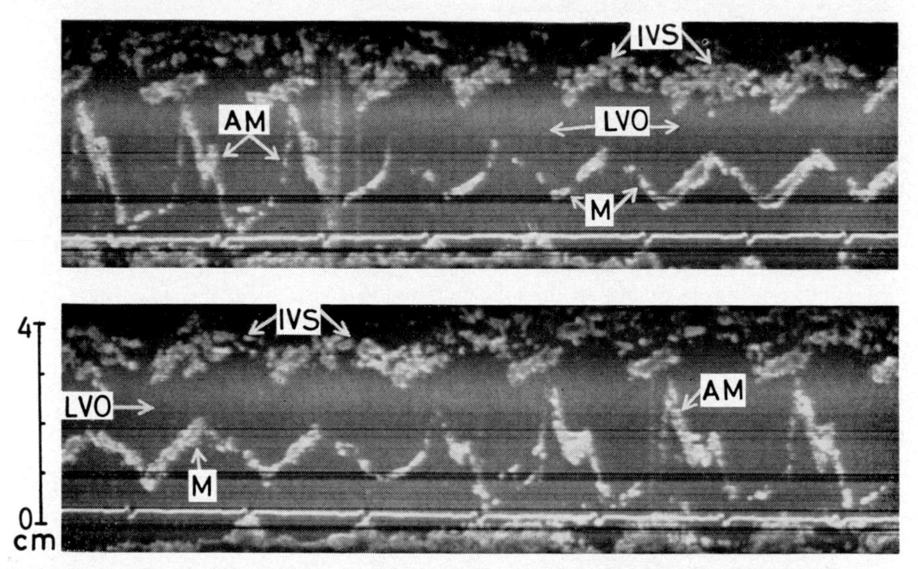

FIGURE 11. Ultrasound cardiogram of the left ventricular outflow tract. AM represents the action of the anterior mitral leaflet. M represents the movements of basal part of the anterior mitral leaflet near its attachment to the root of aorta (see Figs. 4B, C, D). IVS, interventricular septum; LVO, left ventricular outflow tract. The crystal was placed in the third intercostal space 1 to 3 cm from the left sternal border. Above: the characteristic tracing AM is replaced by tracing M when the direction of the sound beam is shifted 5 to 10° medially. Below: tracing M converted into AM when the sound beam was altered to the anteroposterior direction.

Figure 12 demonstrates the ventricular outflow tract: (a) in a normal subject, (b) in aortic valvular incompetence, and (c) in advanced aortic stenosis. It follows from the UCG record that the left ventricular outflow tract is dilated in aortic valvular incompetence and stenosed in aortic stenosis (in the latter case, autopsy revealed that the left ventricular outflow tract was stenosed as the result of advanced hypertrophy of the interventricular septum).

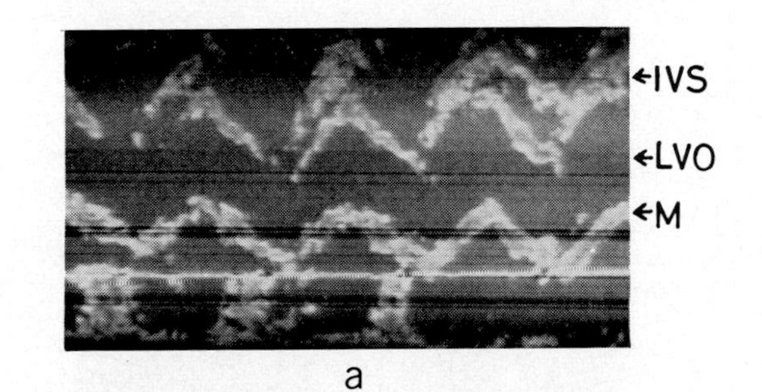

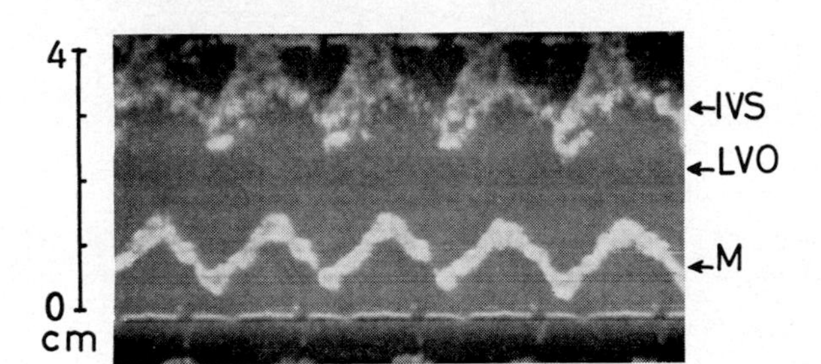

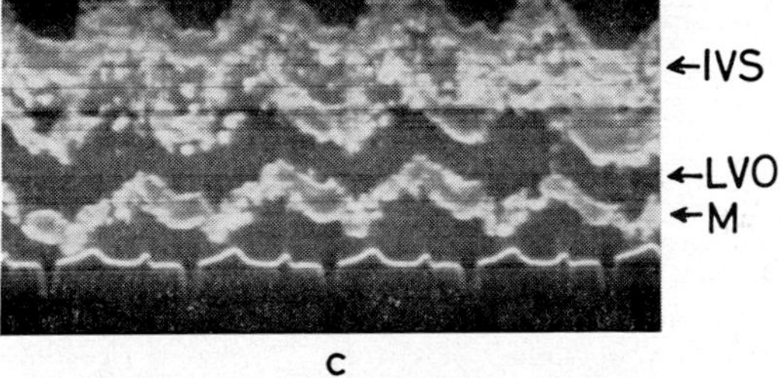

FIGURE 12. Ultrasound cardiogram of the left ventricular outflow tract. M, tracing of the movements of the basal part of the mitral leaflet; IVS, tracing of the echo signal from the interventricular septum; LVO, left ventricular outflow tract. A. Normal case. The distance between M and IVS is about 1.5 cm. B. Aortic valvular insufficiency. The distance between M and IVS is 2 cm. C. Aortic valvular stenosis. The distance between M and IVS is 1 cm. The left ventricular outflow tract was stenosed as the result of advanced hypertrophy of the interventricular septum.

V. ULTRASOUND CARDIOGRAM OF THE AORTIC VALVE

By experiments on isolated heart preparations we have been able to show that from the epicardial surface of the right ventricle it is possible to obtain recordings, first, of mitral valve-cusp activity, and second, of aortic valve-cusp activity (Edler, Gustafson, Karlefors, and Christensson, 1961). The beam angles required for these recordings differ by about 15°. When recordings from the left ventricular outflow tract in a live human subject are made, it is possible, by altering the beam 10 to 15° medially with reference to the antero-posterior plane, to obtain echo signals from structures situated within this tract (Fig. 13). These signals emanate from the aortic valve cusps (Edler,

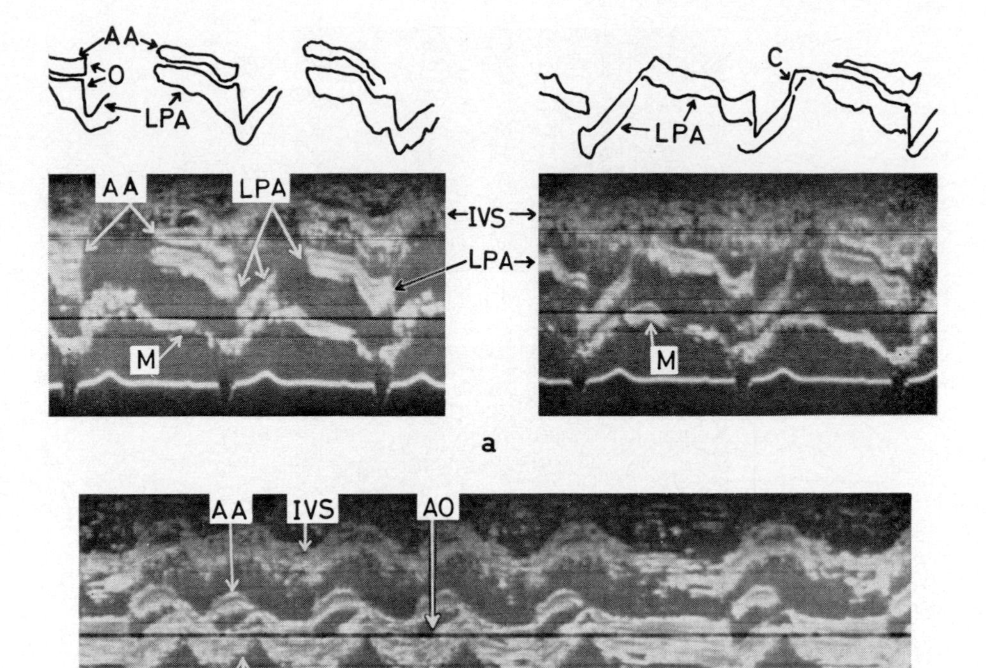

FIGURE 13. Ultrasound cardiograms showing the movements of the aortic valve cusps. The sound beam directed from the third left interspace toward the aortic ostium. IVS, interventricular septum; M, the basal part of the anterior mitral leaflet or the posterior wall of the root of the aorta; LPA, left posterior aortic cusp; AA, anterior aortic cusp. A. Normal case. Above: a schematic representation of aortic cusp movements. O, rapid opening of aortic valves in beginning of systole; C, rapid movements of the aortic cusp on change from systole to diastole. During early ventricular systole the curves LPA and AA separate. During ventricular diastole the curves LPA and AA are close to one another and parallel. B. Case of aortic valvular stenosis. Curves LPA and AA separate slower than in normal cases. The distance between LPA and AA during ventricular systole indicates opening of aortic ostium. AO, aortic ostium during ventricular systole.

Gustafson, Karlefors, and Christensson, 1960a, 1960b). Figure 13 shows how tracings LPA and AA separate during ventricular systole and converge during ventricular diastole. Figure 13B shows the action of the aortic valve in a case of aortic valvular stenosis.

VI. ULTRASOUND CARDIOGRAM OF THE ANTERIOR LEAFLET OF THE TRICUSPID AND PULMONARY VALVES

In a number of patients with right ventricular dilation, tracings representing the anterior cusp of the tricuspid valve have been recorded (Edler, 1961). The crystal in these cases was placed over the fourth left interspace, 4 to 5 cm from the midsternal line, with the beam directed 10 to 20° medially toward the midline (Fig. 14). The record is similar to the mitral valve tracings, but in this case it represents a structure lying anteromedially and caudally with

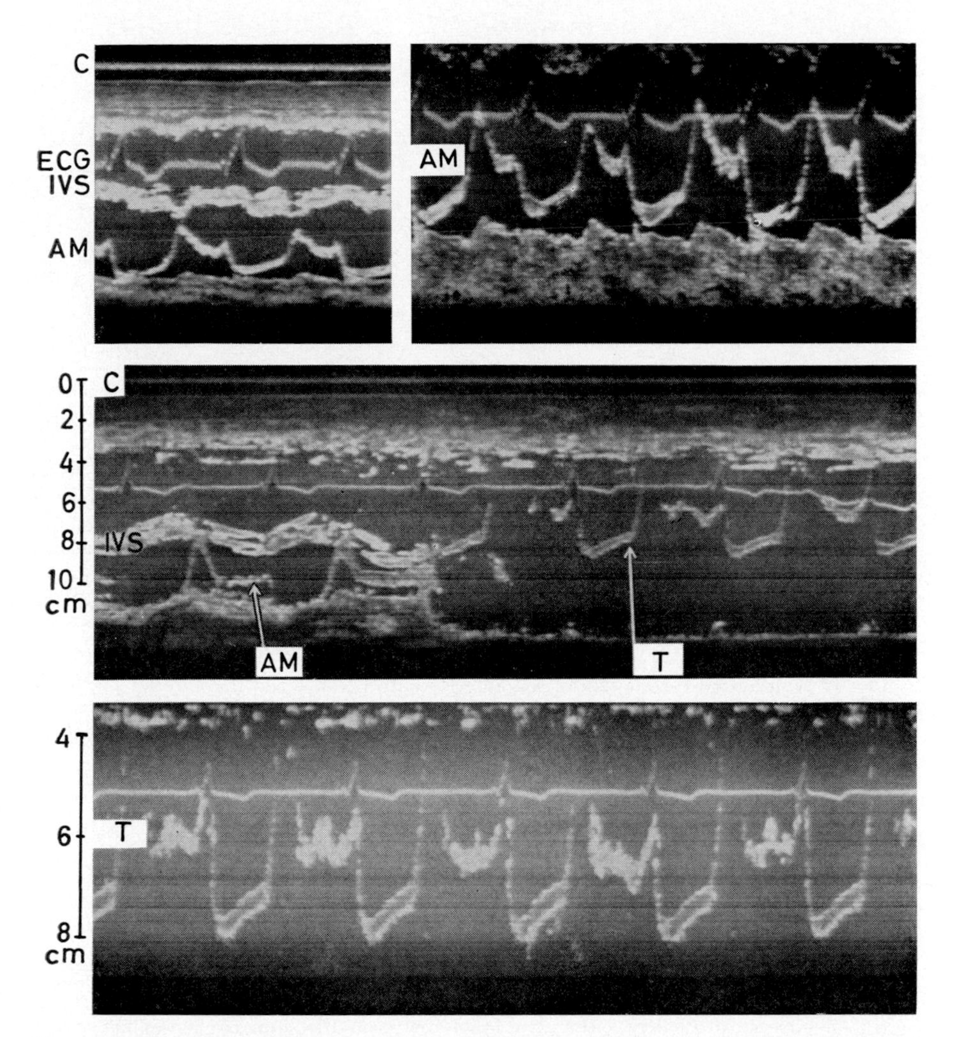

FIGURE 14. Tracings representing the action of the mitral and tricuspid valves in a case of atrial septal defect. The crystal was applied to the fourth left interspace 5 cm from the midsternal line. Above: anteroposterior beam direction. Left: small-scale picture. AM represents the anterior cusp of the mitral valve. The minimum and maximum distances between AM and C (representing the crystal on the anterior chest wall) are 8.0 and 10.3 cm, respectively. IVS, interventricular septum. Right: tracing AM to bigger scale. Middle: while recording of tracing AM is in progress, the direction of the beam is altered so as to diverge 15 to 20° medially from the anteroposterior line. Hereupon, tracing AM disappears, to be replaced by tracing T representing the anterior leaflet of the tricuspid valve. The minimum and maximum distance between T and C are 4.5 and 8 cm, respectively. Below: tracing T to greater scale.

reference to the mitral valve. In a case of complete right bundle branch block we have been able to demonstrate asynchrony (Fig. 15) between the mitral and tricuspid valve movements (Edler, 1961). In several cases of dilatation of the pulmonary trunk we have obtained echo signals from the second interspace corresponding to the pulmonary valve cusps (tracing 1, Figs. 1, 16).

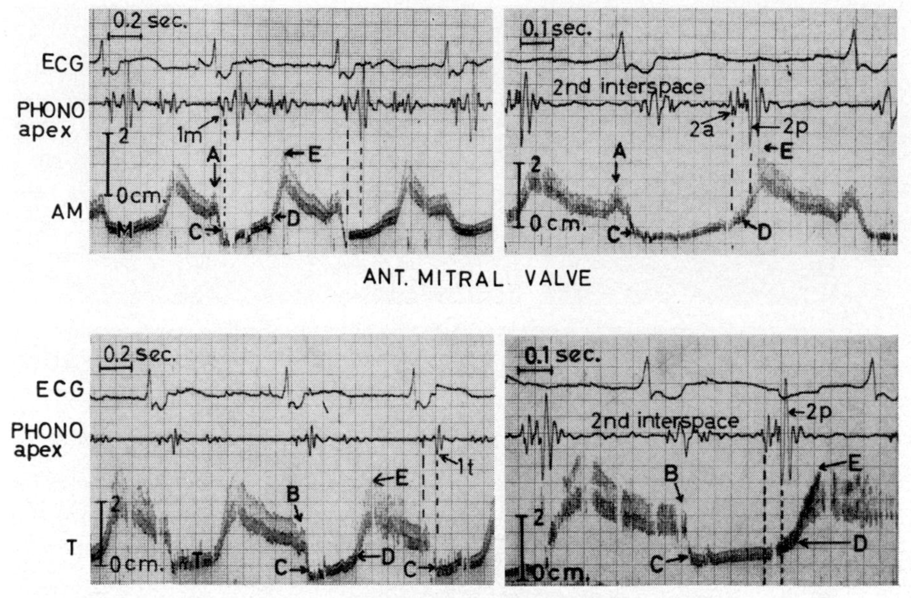

FIGURE 15. Ultrasound cardiogram of the anterior mitral leaflet and the anterior tricuspid leaflet in a case of atrial septal defect with complete right bundle branch block. There is wide splitting of the first and second heart sounds. Above left: action of anterior mitral leaflet (curve AM) recorded synchronously with ECG and apical phonogram. Paper speed 50 mm/sec. Point C is synchronous with the first component (1m) of the split first sound. Above right: action of anterior mitral leaflet recorded simultaneously with ECG and phonogram from second left interspace. Paper speed 100 mm/sec. Rise D–E begins after the aortic component (2a) of the split second sound, but before the pulmonary component (2p). Below left: action of anterior tricuspid leaflet (curve T) recorded synchronously with ECG and apical phonogram. Paper speed 50 mm/sec. Point C is here synchronous with the second component (1t) of the split first sound. Compare above left Below right: action of anterior tricuspid leaflet recorded simultaneously with ECG and phonogram from second left interspace. Paper speed 100 mm/sec. Rise D–E begins when the pulmonary component of the second sound (2p) is maximal. Compare above right. The curves demonstrate the correlation between the components of the heart sounds and the action of the mitral and the tricuspid valves.

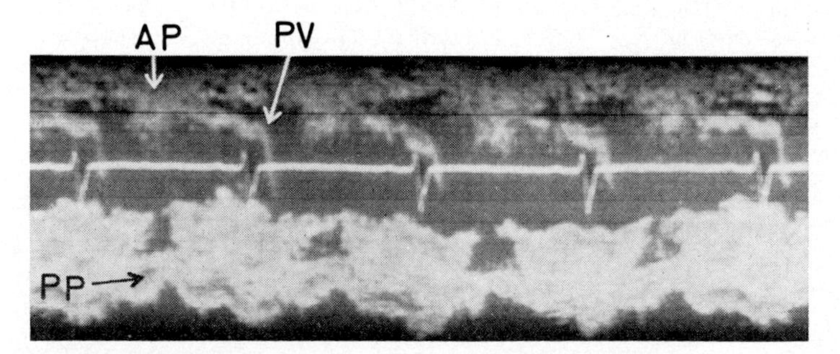

FIGURE 16. Ultrasound cardiogram showing movements of the posterior pulmonary valve cusp. AP, anterior wall of the pulmonary artery; PP, posterior wall of the pulmonary artery; PV, tracing representing the posterior pulmonary valve cusp. In early ventricular systole the echo-giving structure moves rapidly dorsalward.

VII. THE DIAGNOSIS OF PERICARDIAL EFFUSIONS

In twelve cases we have been able to demonstrate the presence of pericardial effusions. Normally, the echo signals from the chest wall, from the pericardium, and from the anterior wall of the right ventricle merge into one. In the presence of pericardial effusions, the ultrasound echo method reveals that the anterior wall of the right ventricle lies on a deeper plane than normal and that it fails to merge with pericardial echo (Edler, 1955). The intervening interval is a measure of the amount of fluid in the pericardium. Figure 17 shows the fluid layer before and after pericardial puncture. The method has proved to be of value in the detection of pericardial effusions and in subsequently following the course of the disease.

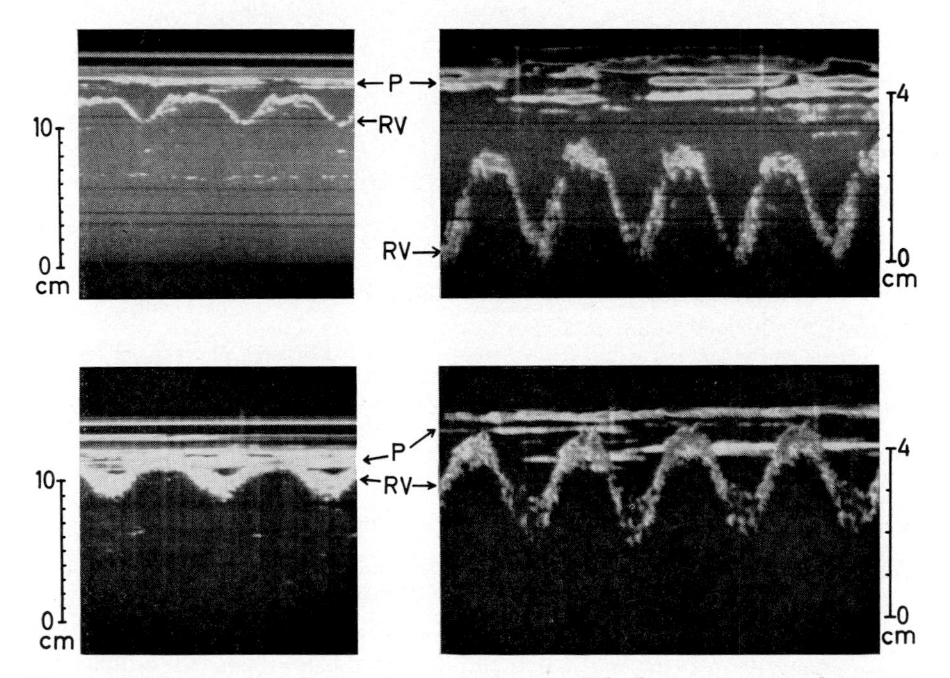

FIGURE 17. Ultrasound cardiogram in a case of pericardial effusions. P, pericardium; RV, anterior wall of the right ventricle. Distance between P and RV is duc to accumulation of fluid. Above: before pericardial puncture. Left: small-scale picture. Right: tracing to greater scale. Below: after pericardial puncture. Distance between P and RV is reduced. P and RV confluent during ventricular systole. Left: small-scale picture. Right: tracing to greater scale.

VIII. THE DIAGNOSIS OF THROMBI AND TUMORS IN THE LEFT ATRIUM

Thrombi in the left atrium cause multiple echo signals to appear in the record in a position corresponding to the interior of the left atrium (Edler, 1955). Tumors in the left atrium similarly give rise to multiple echo signals (see Fig. 18) (Effert, 1959; Edler, Gustafson, Karlefors, and Christensson, 1960b).

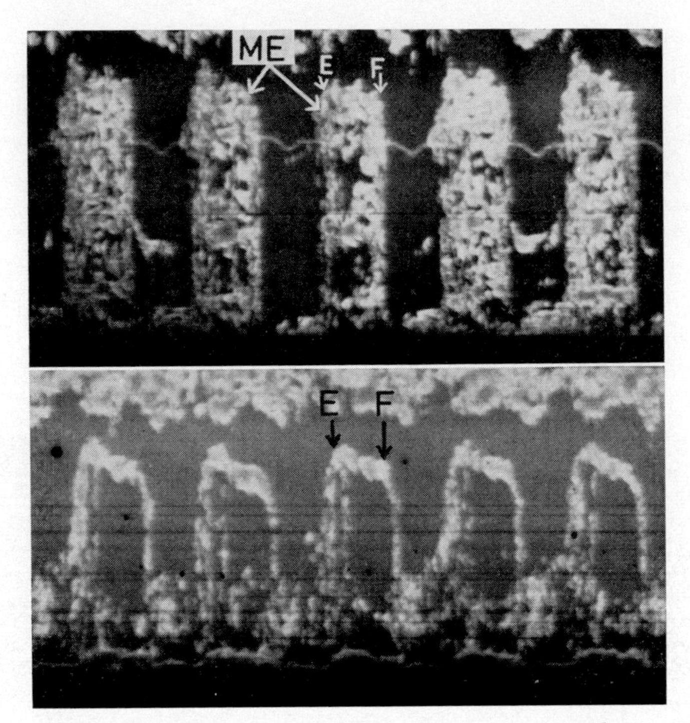

FIGURE 18. Ultrasound cardiogram in a case of left atrial tumor. Above: UCG of the movements of the anterior mitral leaflet completely masked by multiple echo signals from the inner of the left atrium which operation revealed to be an atrial myxoma adherent to the mitral leaflet. ME, multiple echoes. Below: UCG after subtotal removal of tumor. The E–F segment of the curve is of the same type as seen in mitral stenosis. The multiple echo signals are absent.

SUMMARY

A. The ultrasound echo method enables the following recordings to be made:
  1. The action of the heart valves. The movement sequence of the anterior mitral cusp is particularly easy to record. In some cases, aortic, pulmonary, and tricuspid valve action can also be recorded. Similarly, it is sometimes possible to record the actions of the anterior and posterior mitral cusps simultaneously, resulting in a composite picture of the dynamics of the mitral funnel.
  2. Movements of the left ventricular outflow tract.

B. In clinical work the ultrasound cardiogram has the following main applications:
  1. In the diagnosis of mitral stenosis.
  2. In estimating the degree of stenosis and thus in deciding whether operation (commissurotomy) is indicated.
  3. In judging the immediate postoperative result after surgery for mitral stenosis.
  4. In follow-up studies after surgery for mitral stenosis. Restenosis can be diagnosed early and reoperation carried out in good time.

5. In detecting pericardial effusions.
6. In detecting the presence of thrombi and tumors in the left atrium.

C. Ultrasound can be used for physiological and pathophysiological studies of valve action and its correlation with the heart sounds and intracardiac pressure variations.

REFERENCES

Edler, I. (1955). The diagnostic use of ultrasound in heart disease. Acta Med. Scand. Suppl. 308, 32.

Edler, I. (1956). Ultrasoundcardiogram in mitral valvular diseases. Acta Chir. Scand. *111*, 230.

Edler, I. (1961). Ultrasoundcardiography. Part III. Atrioventricular valve motility in the living human heart recorded by ultrasound. Acta Med. Scand. Suppl. 370, 83.

Edler, I., and A. Gustafson (1957). Ultrasonic cardiogram in mitral stenosis. Acta Med. Scand. *159*, 85.

Edler, I., A. Gustafson, T. Karlefors, and B. Christensson (1960a). A dynamic study of the heart valves and ventricular outflow tracts using an ultrasound echo method. Paper read at 27th Nord. Kongr. f. Inre Med. (Oslo, June 29–July 2).

Edler, I., A. Gustafson, T. Karlefors, and B. Christensson (1960b). The movements of aortic and mitral valves recorded with ultrasonic echo techniques. Scientific film at 3rd European Cong. of Cardiol. (Rome, Sept. 18–24).

Edler, I., A. Gustafson, T. Karlefors, and B. Christensson (1961). Ultrasoundcardiography. Part II. Mitral and aortic valve movements recorded by an ultrasonic echo method. An experimental study. Acta Med. Scand. Suppl. 370, 67.

Edler, I., and C. H. Hertz (1954). The use of ultrasonic reflectoscope for the continuous recording of the movements of heart walls. Kungl. Fysiogr. Sällsk. Förhandl. *24*, *5*.

Edler, I., C. H. Hertz, A. Gustafson, T. Karlefors, and B. Christensson (1960). The movements of the heart valves recorded by means of ultrasound. Nord. Medic. *64*, 1178.

Effert, S. (1959). Der derzeitige Stand der Ultraschallkardiographie. Arch. Kreislaufforsch. *30*, 213.

Hertz, C. H., and I. Edler (1956). Die Registrierung von Herzwandbewegungen mit Hilfe des Ultraschall-Impulsverfahrens. Acustica *6*, 361.

21

A Mirror System for Ultrasonic Visualization of Soft Tissues

CARL HELLMUTH HERTZ and SVEN OLOFSSON
University of Lund, Lund, Sweden

During the past 10 years two-dimensional cross-sections of biological objects have been successfully produced with the ultrasonic reflectoscope technique by several investigators. During these investigations it was found that it was necessary to move the ultrasonic transducer by some means around the object to be visualized in order to obtain good quality pictures (Howry, 1957; Donald *et al.*, 1958; Baum *et al.*, 1960). This necessity exists partly because of the fact that the irregular surfaces of biological objects often do not reflect the sound back to the transducer and partly because so-called ghosts, caused by double reflections of the sound, may be present. Further, the transverse resolution of the system may be somewhat increased by the scanning technique.

However, some biological structures cannot be visualized in this way, since they can be approached by ultrasound from one direction only. An example of such a structure is the human heart, which is surrounded almost entirely by lung tissue which has a very high ultrasound absorption coefficient. There is, however, a relatively small "window" in the thoracic wall through which ultrasound can be passed into the heart (Edler and Hertz, 1954). Thus, if a two-dimensional cross-section of the heart is to be produced by ultrasound, the beam has to be swept back and forth through a sector with its apex relatively near the above mentioned "window." Furthermore, in the case of the heart, a minimum of about ten pictures per second has to be produced in order to follow its motion, necessitating a simple sweeping arrangement. To circumvent the difficulties described above, which arise with such a sweeping arrangement, it might seem advantageous to use a small transducer for the transmission of the ultrasound with a large-area receiver crystal of suitable shape to ensure the reception of echoes which are not reflected back exactly in the direction of the incoming beam. Unfortunately, for various reasons, such an arrangement is not practical. However, it is possible to devise an ultrasonic mirror system which has important advantages (Fig. 1). This

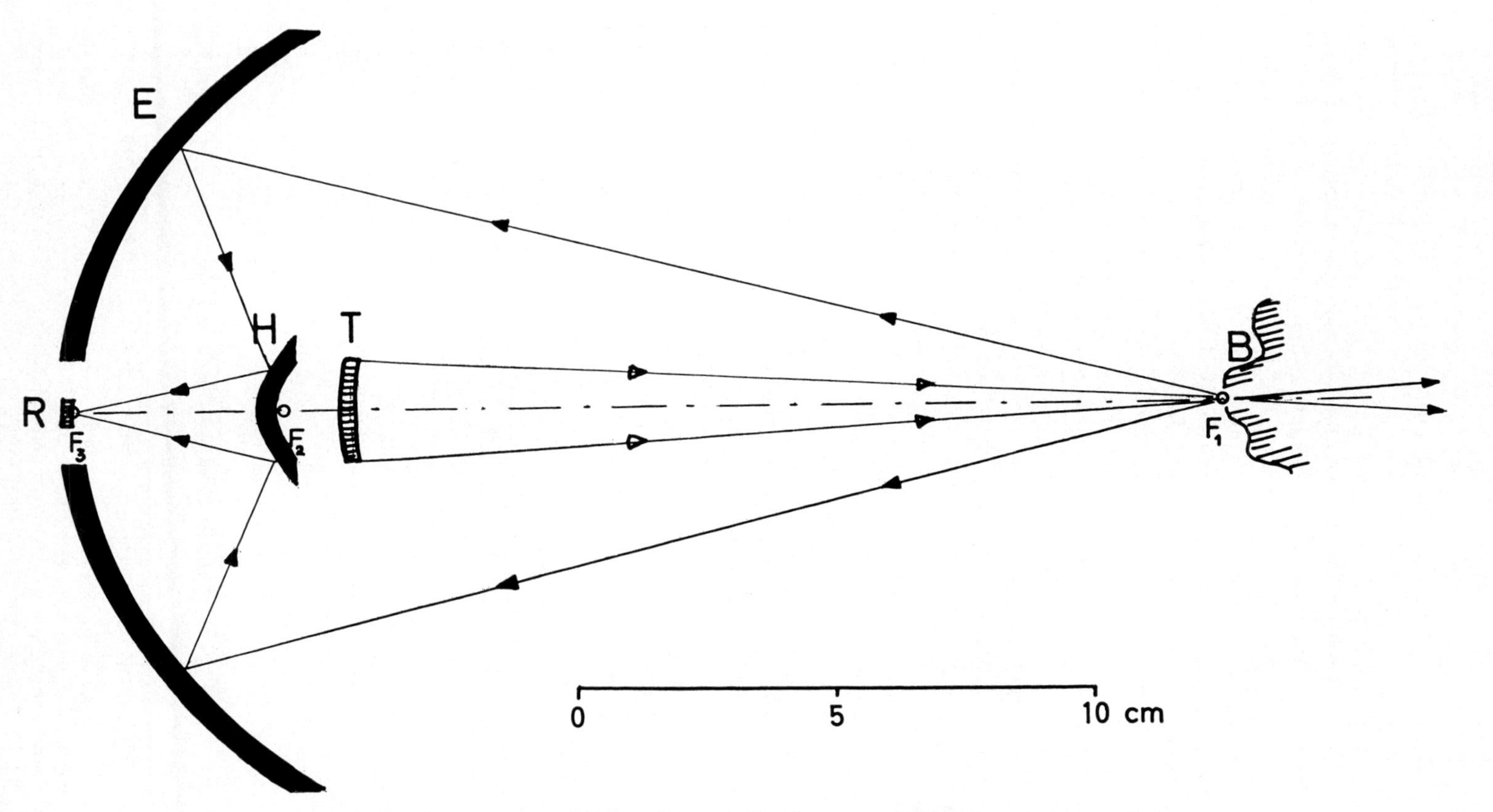

FIGURE 1. Ultrasonic mirror system. The sound pulse generated by the transmitter, T, is reflected from the boundary, B, and collected by the ellipsoidal mirror, E, and the hyperboloidal mirror, H, onto the receiving crystal, R.

system consists of a large ellipsoidal mirror surface, E, which collects all radiation coming from the farther focus, F_1, into its second focus, F_2. Before arriving at F_2 the radiation is again reflected at the hyperboloid, H, the focus of which coincides with F_2. By this second reflection the radiation is focused into F_3, the second focus of the hyperboloid, where the sound is detected by a small receiving crystal, R. In front of the hyperboloid, H, the spherical transmitting crystal, T, generating the pulsed ultrasound, is attached in such a way that its focus coincides with the focus of the mirror system.

Two-dimensional cross-sections of a biological object can be produced by this system by rotating the entire system back and forth around an axis vertical to the beam direction in such a way that the outgoing ultrasonic beam sweeps over the object to be investigated. Although the system is immersed in water, this can be accomplished easily with a motor operating at the required speed. The present system produces five pictures per second.

It is clear from this arrangement that because of the wide aperture of the mirror system, a large part of the ultrasound that is not directly reflected back to the transmitter will be collected on the receiving crystal. At the same time the appearance of ghosts will be greatly decreased. Moreover, because of its large diameter relative to the wavelength of the ultrasound, the resolution of the system transverse to the beam is much increased at F_1 (Fig. 2). This is also true, although to a lesser extent, along the axis at a distance of some centimeters from F_1. Furthermore, the sensitivity of the system varies along the beam axis and is largest at F_1 (Fig. 3).

The actual appearance of such a mirror system is shown in Figure 4. In this system the maximum diameter of the ellipsoid is 14 cm, its eccentricity 0.692 (distance between foci divided by largest diameter of ellipse) and the distance between F_1 and F_2 is 18 cm. The accuracy of the surfaces of

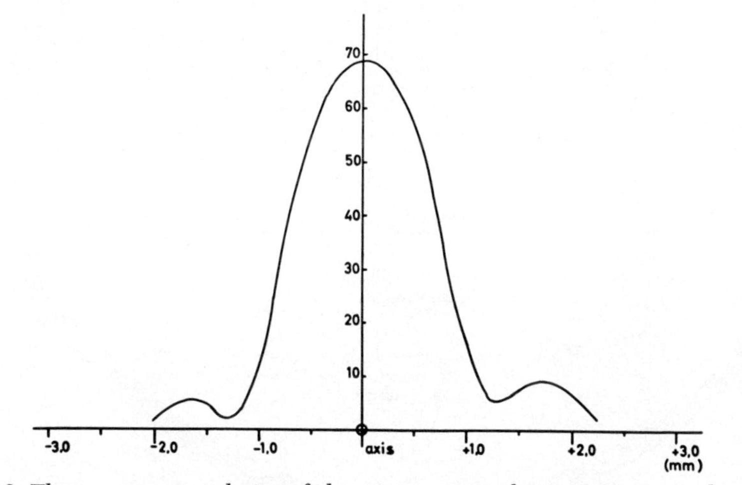

FIGURE 2. The transverse resolution of the mirror system shown in Figure 1 obtained by moving a small glass sphere (1 mm diameter) across the axis of the system at the focus, F_1. Abscissa: distance from F_1 of sphere moved perpendicular to the axis of the mirror system; ordinate: echo amplitude (scale proportional to pressure amplitude).

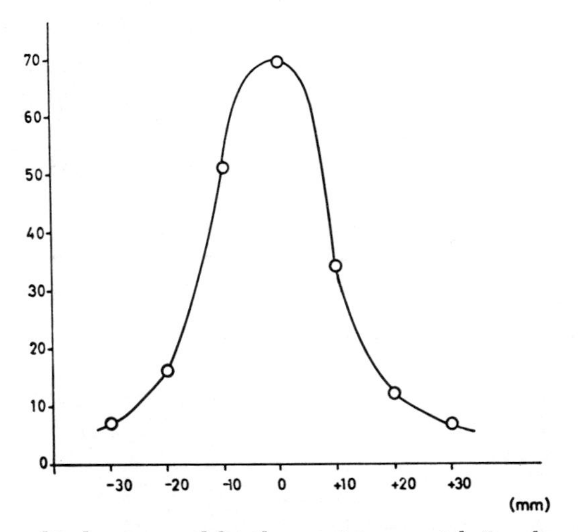

FIGURE 3. Echo amplitude measured by the receiving crystal, R, when the sound is reflected by a small sphere at different distances from F_1 along the axis of the mirror system. Abscissa: distance from focus F_1 along the axis of the system; ordinate: echo amplitude (scale proportional to pressure amplitude).

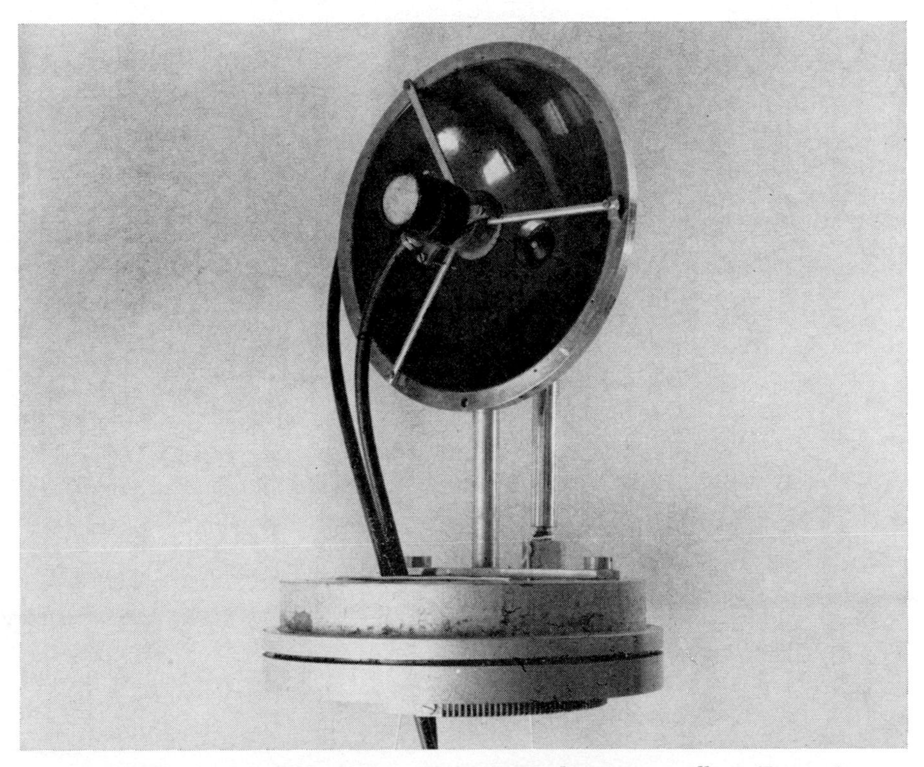

FIGURE 4. A photograph of the mirror system shown diagrammatically in Figure 1.

the mirror system is ± 0.01 mm, which proved sufficient for our purposes. The transmitter is a bowl of lead-zirconate-titanate with a resonance frequency of 2.5 Mc/sec and a diameter of 2 cm. Lead-zirconate-titanate is also used for the receiver, which is made of a disk of 3.5 mm diameter. The mirror system itself is made of fine tungsten powder held together by Araldite, a resin. During the construction of the system, care has to be taken to avoid a residual echo which may arise due to secondary reflections between the receiver crystal, R, and the hyperboloid, H. This can be achieved by a suitable form of that part of the hyperboloid which lies directly opposite R. A cross-section of a heart in vitro as obtained with this system is shown in Figure 5.

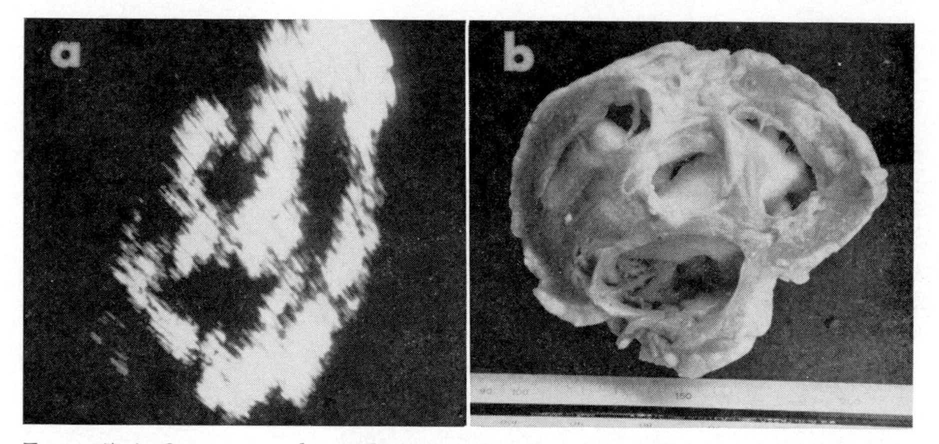

FIGURE 5. A. Cross-sectional recording of the heart in vitro obtained with the ultrasonic mirror system shown in Figure 4. B. Photograph of the heart cut (following the experiment depicted in 5A) in the same plane as the ultrasonic visualization path.

REFERENCES

Baum, G., and I. Greenwood (1960). Ultrasound in ophthalmology. Am. J. Ophthal. *42*, 249.

Donald, I., J. MacVicar, and T. G. Brown (1958). Investigation of abdominal masses by pulsed ultrasound. Lancet *I*, 1188.

Edler, I., and C. H. Hertz (1954). The use of the ultrasonic reflectoscope for the continuous recording of the movements of heart walls. Kungl. Fysiogr. Sällsk. Förhandl. *24*, *5*.

Howry, D. H. (1957). Techniques used in ultrasonic visualization of soft tissues, *in* "Ultrasound in Biology and Medicine," E. Kelly, ed. (American Institute of Biological Sciences, Washington, D.C.).

22

Registration of Movement of Cardiac Walls Using an Ultrasonic Reflection Procedure

SVEN EFFERT, M.D., F. J. DEUPMANN, and J. KARYTSIOTIS
I. Medizinische Klinik der Medizinischen Akademie, Duesseldorf, Germany

Introduction by Dr. Hueter

The increasing interest in ultrasonic research on a worldwide basis has been made quite evident these past several days by the papers presented at this symposium by the scientific representatives of the countries of England, Japan, Germany, Italy, and Sweden. This afternoon's session will continue the discussions initiated this morning on the application of ultrasonic reflection techniques for the diagnosis of medical problems. Dr. Sven Effert of Germany will present a paper on the use of ultrasonic reflection procedures for the diagnosis of heart ailments, Dr. Toshio Wagai of Japan will discuss the use of ultrasound for the diagnosis of intracranial diseases, breast tumors, and abdominal diseases, and finally, Dr. George Kossoff of Australia will tell us about his work on the application of ultrasound to problems associated with pregnancy.

From 1956 until the end of April, 1962, we employed the ultrasonic reflection procedure to examine 3270 patients, of whom 2156 were suffering from mitral valve disease. Since Drs. Hertz and Edler have previously described in detail the reflection procedures, I will not specifically discuss such techniques. Figure 1 illustrates our most recent instrument for ultrasound cardiography. This instrument is intended for clinical use and was designed so that its operation would be simple. Frequencies of 1 or 2 Mc are the most satisfactory choice for cardiac diagnosis. The transducers are 1 cm in diameter. The curve is registered either by an electrocardiograph using a converter or photographically by means of a second cathode ray tube. Following clinical trial this instrument will be produced on a commercial basis.

The principal application of the ultrasound cardiography is the functional grading of degree of mitral stenosis. Figures 2B, C, and D illustrate the

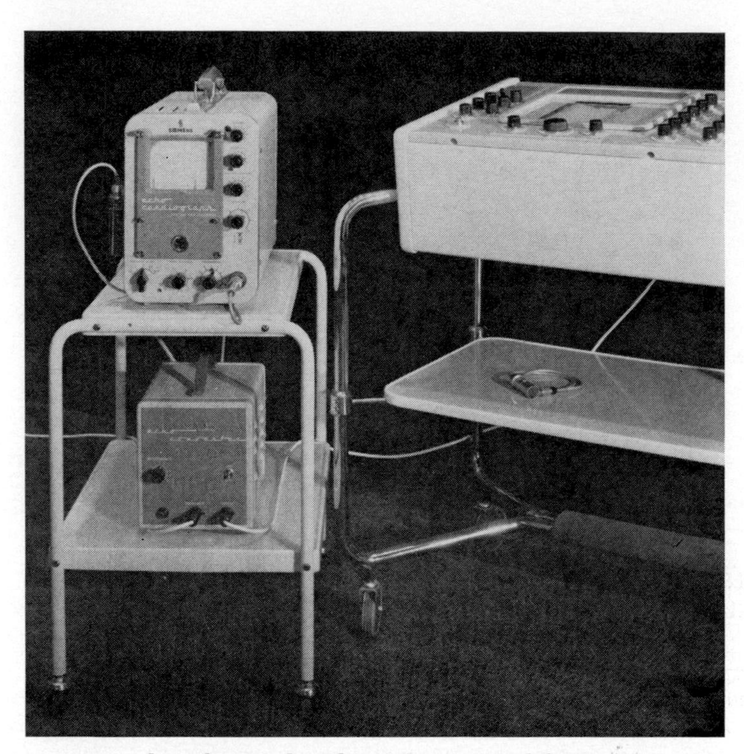

FIGURE 1. Device used in ultrasound cardiography. Bottom left: the converter. Right: the electrocardiograph used for registration of the curves.

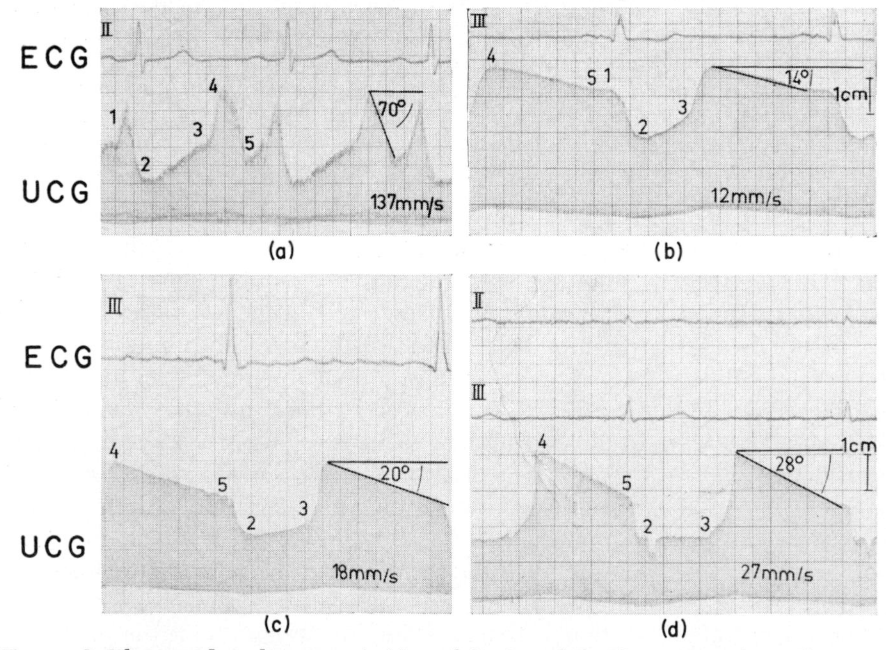

FIGURE 2. Ultrasound cardiograms. A. Normal. B, C, and D. Three cases of mitral stenosis of differing degree. 1, atrial systole; 2, low point, valve closed; 3, end of the ventricular systole; 4, high point, valve open; 5, end of ventricular filling.

type of curves registered for varying degrees of mitral stenosis. These may be compared with a curve (Fig. 2A) recorded from a healthy individual. As Dr. Edler pointed out, the index of degree of stenosis is the angle between time-axis and the curve registered during the emptying phase of the auricles, that is, during ventricular diastole. Instead of this angular measurement, the curve may be described in terms of its gradient, that is, the rate of motion in millimeters per second; thus, one may obtain values which are independent of the calibration of the particular apparatus.

The more slowly the reflecting cardiac wall withdraws from the anterior chest wall, the higher is the degree of mitral stenosis. We have investigated this phenomenon on all of the mitral stenosis patients investigated with ultrasonic reflection procedures. Comparisons with the clinical picture, wedged pressure or left auricular pressure, the phonocardiogram, and the operative findings revealed the following correlations between ultrasound cardiogram and grade of mitral stenosis: In controls of normal hearts or patients with isolated mitral insufficiency, the average rate of motion during the emptying phase of the left auricle is 125 mm/sec, with a range of 75 to 200 mm/sec. In cases of extreme mitral stenosis, in which the surgeon can just dip his fingertip into the valvular orifice, the rate is reduced below 10 mm/sec. In high-grade stenosis, in which the surgeon's fingertip can just pass the mitral orifice, rates between 10 and 25 mm/sec are found. A rate exceeding 40 mm/sec indicates that the stenosis bears no hemodynamic significance. The range between 25 and 40 mm/sec includes borderline cases. The highest rate found in a case of mitral stenosis, clinically diagnosed by auscultation and phonocardiogram, was 72 mm/sec.

The practical value of the reflection method is particularly obvious in cases in which the other findings are equivocal. Figure 3 shows a phonocardiogram and ultrasound cardiogram of a patient presenting a loud systolic murmur over the apex. The ultrasound cardiogram registered a rate of motion of 20 mm/sec and suggested a high-degree stenosis. On operation, the mitral orifice just permitted the insertion of a fingertip. The reflection procedure also permits quantitative evaluation of the result of the operation as illustrated in Figure 4B which indicates normalization of the ultrasound cardiogram following operation. Following surgery, the rate of motion showed an increase from 12 to 112 mm/sec.

The circular diagrams in Figure 5 demonstrate changes in the rate of motion following operation in 279 patients. Each radius represents one individual case and its length is proportional to the difference between the preoperative and postoperative rates. The difference is 10 mm/sec from one of these concentrical circles to the next. The cases were entered in these different sectors according to preoperative rate: sector 1 includes the range from 0 to 15 mm/sec, sector 2 from 16 to 25 mm/sec, sector 3 from 26 to 35 mm/sec, and sector 4 exceeding 35 mm/sec. The diagram at top left shows those cases operated on in 1960; top right, January to June, 1961; bottom left, July through December, 1961; and bottom right, through April, 1962. In isolated functionally unfavorable cases in which the valve, because of calcification or rigidity, does not open in spite of commissurotomy, the rate

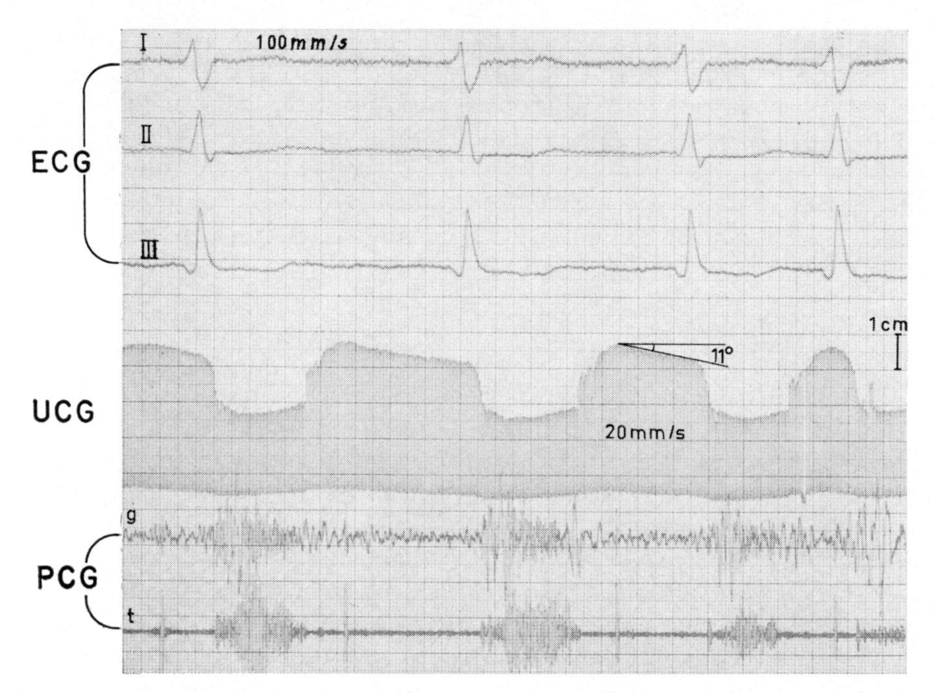

FIGURE 3. Patient, twenty-seven-year-old male. UCG shows high-grade mitral stenosis; PCG shows loud systolic murmur over the apex. Operative findings indicate residual mitral orifice of fingertip size, PCG with stethoscopic characteristic (g) and with a rated frequency from 35 Hz (t).

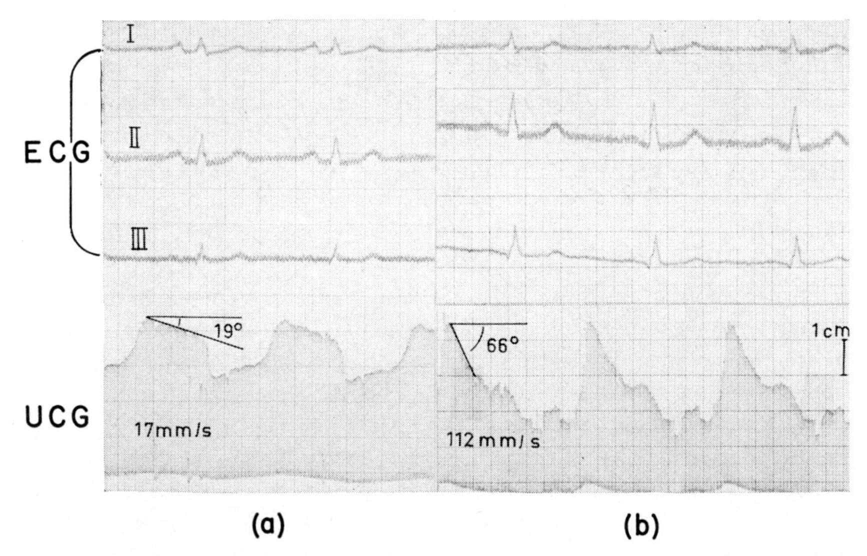

FIGURE 4. UCG in mitral stenosis. A. Before operation. B. Complete normalization following commissurotomy.

of motion remains practically unchanged. The average increase for 279 patients is 24.5 mm/sec. In the majority of cases an increase of 10 to 30 mm/sec is observed. In a few cases the velocity reaches rates exceeding 70 mm/sec, that is, it attains the normal range. The degree of improvement obtained by operation is independent of the preoperative rate.

The question of true or pseudo-recurrence of mitral stenosis, at present a controversial topic among cardiologists, can be answered reliably by the ultrasound cardiogram. The curves in Figure 6 demonstrate a true recurrence of mitral stenosis. The patient whose cardiogram is illustrated in Figure 6 underwent surgery in October, 1959, at which time a high-grade mitral stenosis with partial valvular calcification was found. The mitral orifice was enlarged in such a way that two fingers could pass through. Six weeks prior to operation the UCG had revealed a rate of motion of 13 mm/sec. Postoperatively, an increase to 50 mm/sec was observed and the patient felt well. Following uncomplicated pregnancy, the patient was delivered of a healthy baby in March, 1961, with delivery being entirely uneventful. Two weeks postpartum, a recurrent carditis with involvement of joints set in. The results of our examination of this patient, which did not take place until 8 months later, suggested an appreciable mitral stenosis. For example, the UCG once again showed a reduction of the rate of motion to 21 mm/sec. Our observation periods are, as yet, too short to permit detailed statistical evaluation of the cases of recurrent stenosis, but our experiences indicate that true recurrent stenosis is rare. In the majority of so-called recurrences, the mitral orifice could not be sufficiently dilated at the first operation.

The practical significance of the ultrasonic reflection procedure is revealed by the fact that at the Duesseldorf Surgical Hospital, intracardiac pressure recordings by cardiac catheterization and auricular puncture are carried out in only 3% of cases with mitral valve disease. In approximately 97% of all cases, the usual clinical examination, in conjunction with the UCG, enables one to differentiate between mitral insufficiency and mitral stenosis, to determine the grade of stenosis, and to decide whether surgery is indicated. The degree of mitral insufficiency cannot be determined from UCG curves. If surgery for mitral insufficiency is performed more frequently in the future, then a greater number of direct pressure recordings will be required.

There can be no doubt regarding the diagnostic significance of the UCG, but one may ask the question what structure or motion is actually registered? On the basis of his experiments with the cadaver and the isolated heart, Dr. Edler has expressed the opinion (Edler, Gustafson, Karlefors, and Christensson, 1961) that the curve represents the motion of the anterior mitral cusp. We have investigated this problem by conducting experiments during cardiac surgery. A transducer was applied directly to the heart. When the transducer was located 2 cm below the atrioventricular groove and approximately 1.5 cm to the right of the interventricular groove, the typical curve was recorded (Fig. 7), that is, the curve normally obtained when the transducer is placed over the third or fourth intercostal space. The site of the transducer was

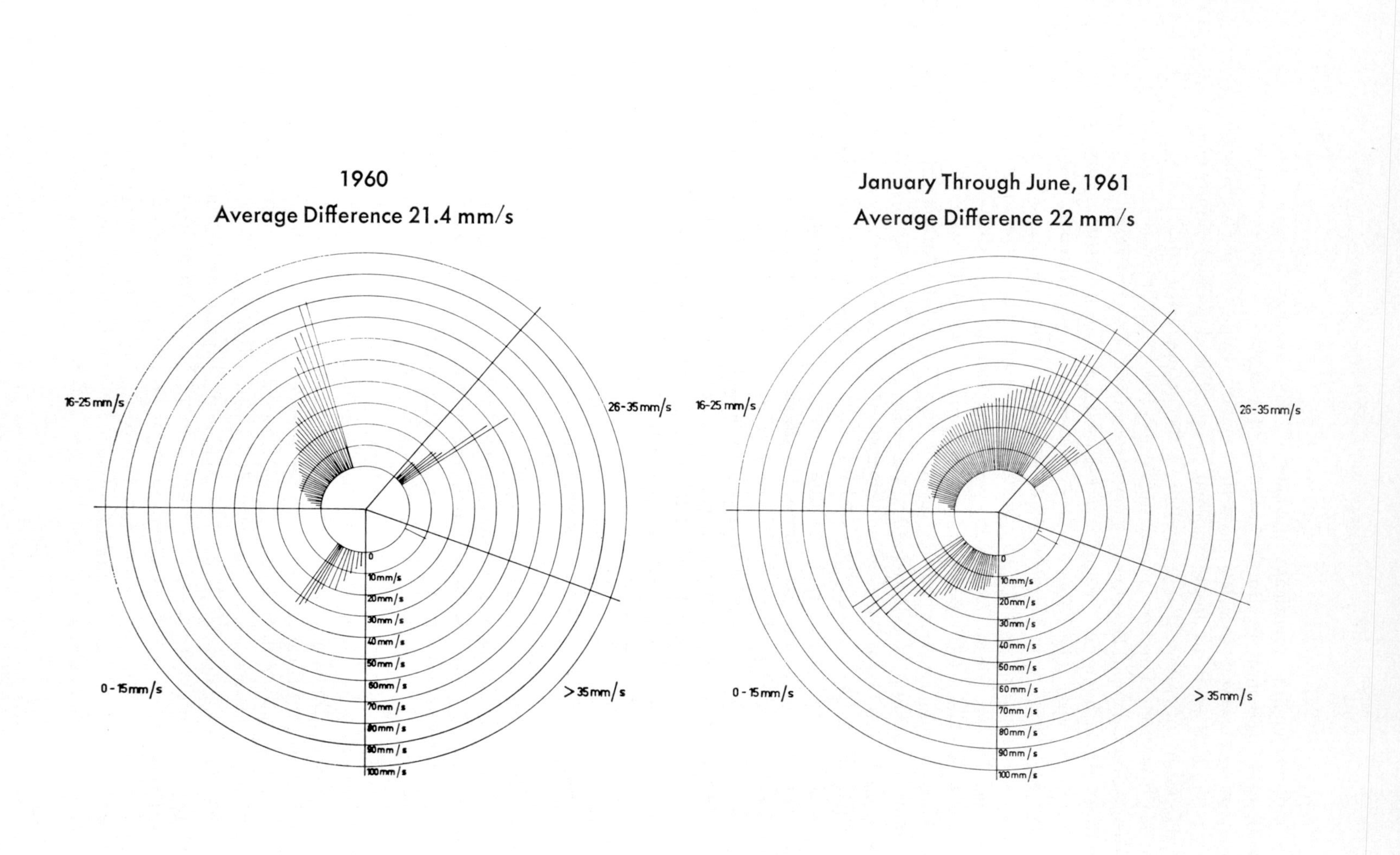
1960
Average Difference 21.4 mm/s
16-25 mm/s
26-35 mm/s
0-15 mm/s
> 35 mm/s
0
10 mm/s
20 mm/s
30 mm/s
40 mm/s
50 mm/s
60 mm/s
70 mm/s
80 mm/s
90 mm/s
100 mm/s
January Through June, 1961
Average Difference 22 mm/s
16-25 mm/s
26-35 mm/s
0-15 mm/s
> 35 mm/s
0
10 mm/s
20 mm/s
30 mm/s
40 mm/s
50 mm/s
60 mm/s
70 mm/s
80 mm/s
90 mm/s
100 mm/s

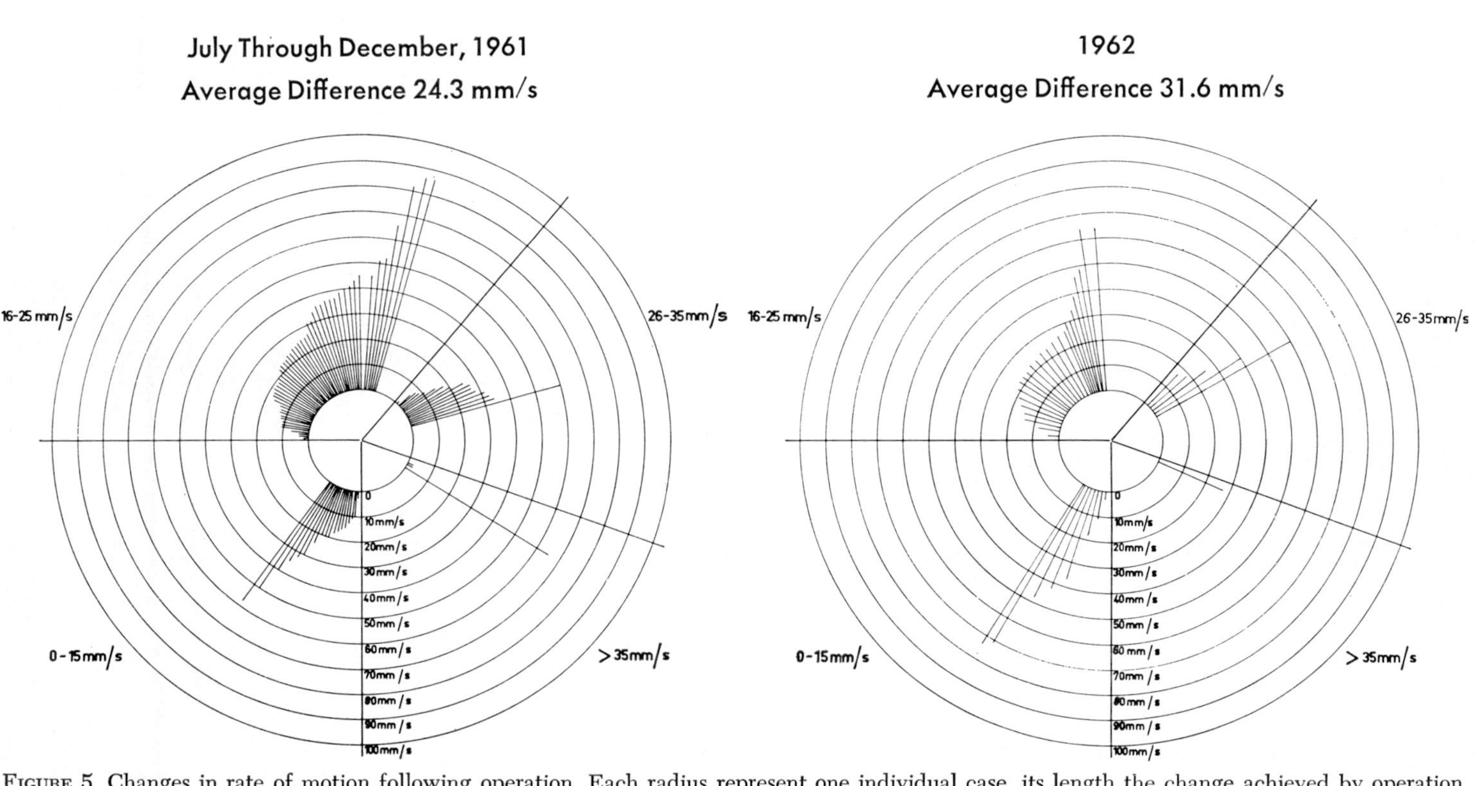

FIGURE 5. Changes in rate of motion following operation. Each radius represent one individual case, its length the change achieved by operation.

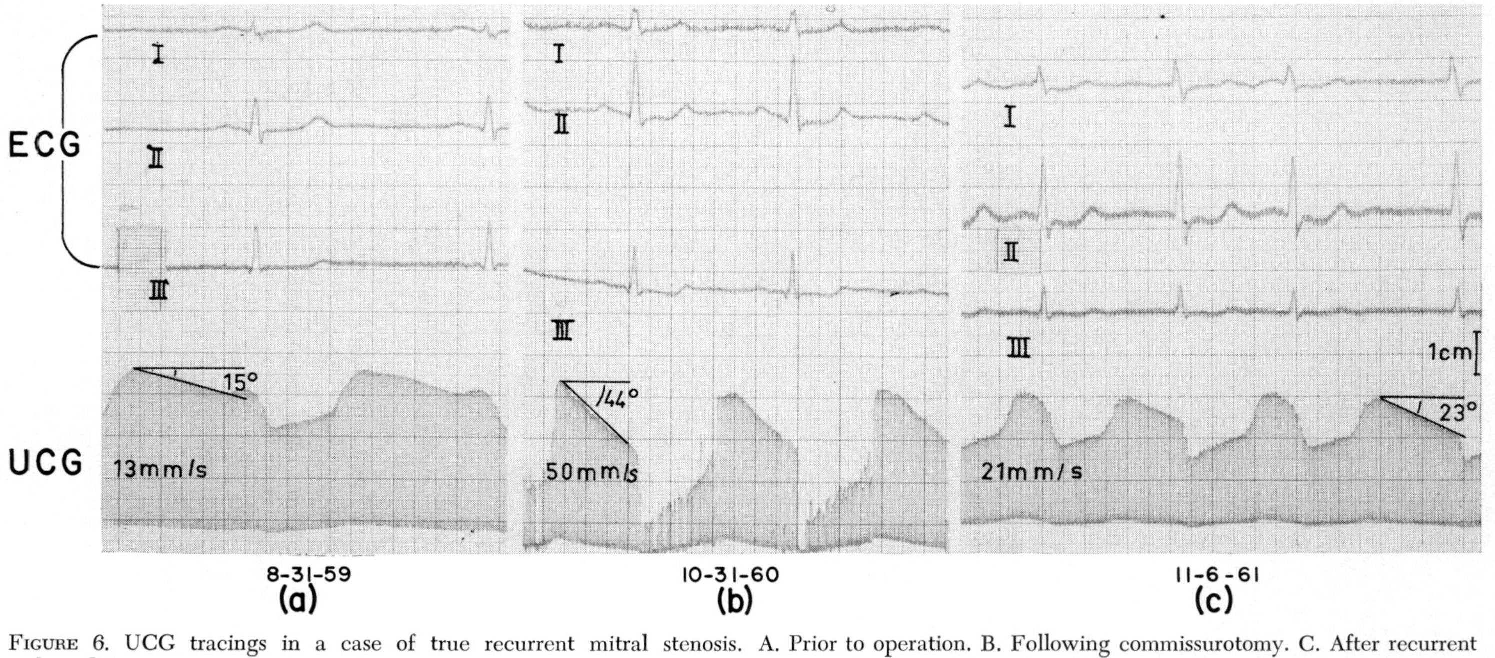

FIGURE 6. UCG tracings in a case of true recurrent mitral stenosis. A. Prior to operation. B. Following commissurotomy. C. After recurrent endocarditis.

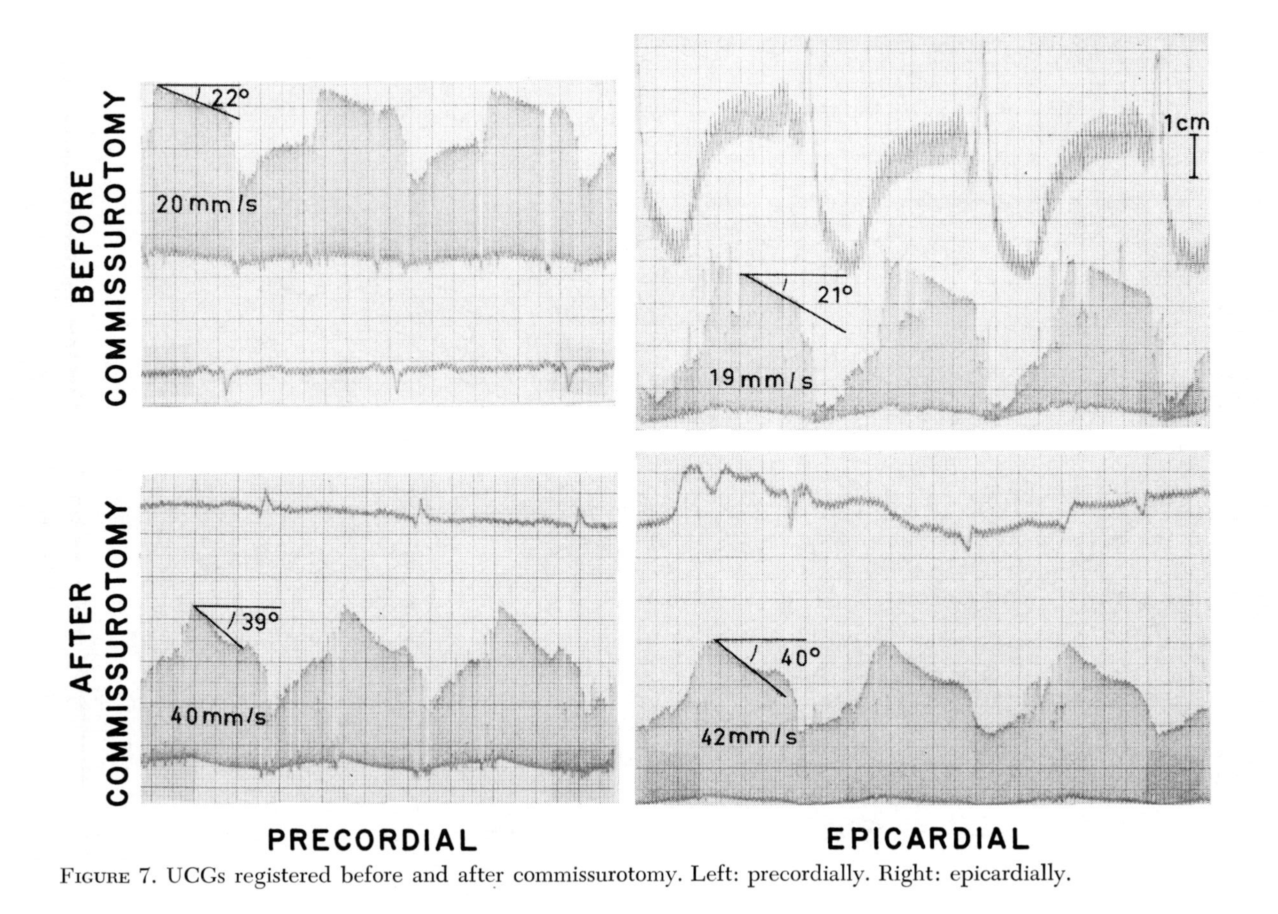

Figure 7. UCGs registered before and after commissurotomy. Left: precordially. Right: epicardially.

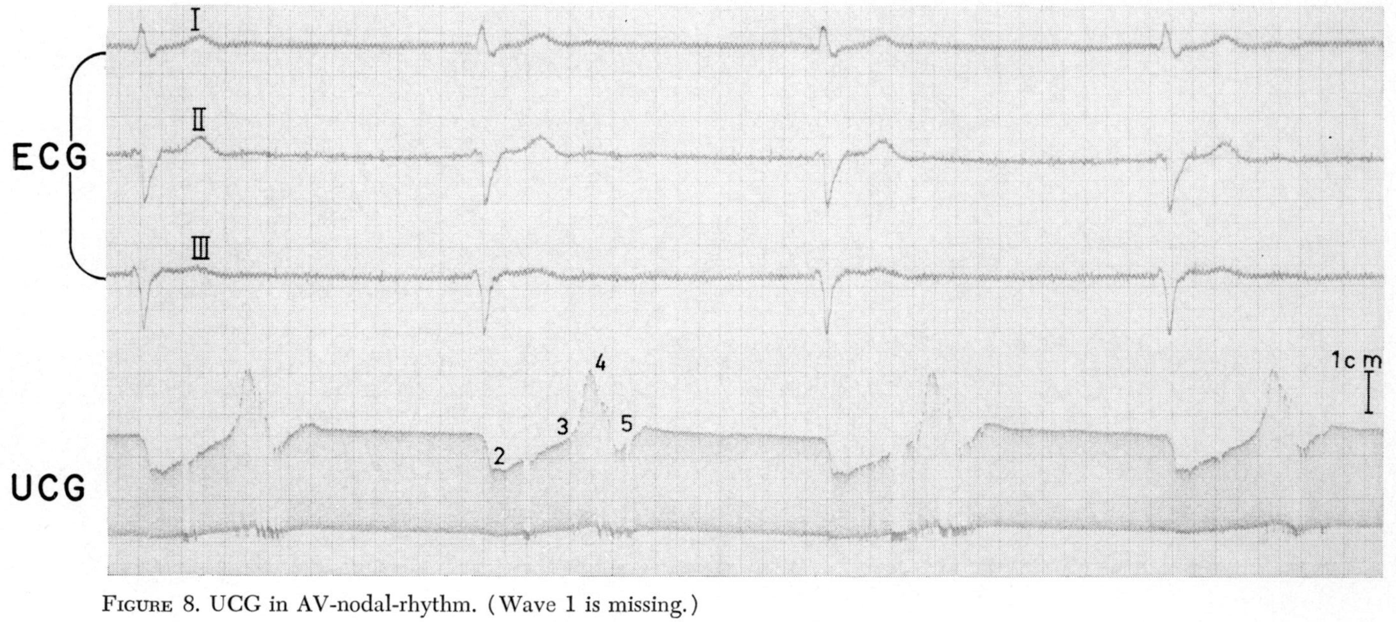

FIGURE 8. UCG in AV-nodal-rhythm. (Wave 1 is missing.)

directly over the anterior mitral cusp. Our present concept of the UCG is that we are dealing with the ultrasonic echo return curve from the anterior mitral cusp. Contraction of the auricle causes the cusp to approach the anterior chest wall. The succeeding precipitate downward movement results from valvular closure. During ventricular systole, the cusp bulges anteriorly. This produces a slight rise of the curve. Next, the valve opens and jerks toward the anterior chest wall. Following the phase of rapid blood influx into the ventricle, the mitral valve returns to an intermediate position and remains in this position until the next auricular systole sets in. This interpretation of the UCG curve is confirmed by studies in cases of cardiac arrhythmia. When, in an AV-nodal-rhythm, auricular and ventricular systoles coincide, wave no. 1 is missing (Fig. 8). It is also always absent in auricular fibrillation. In AV-block, wave no. 1 appears about 0.07 sec after the onset of the P-wave. In auricular flutter, the mechanical flutter waves appear in the UCG with an amplitude of about 0.5 cm so there is no doubt that it is caused by the systole of the auricle. The first sound at the moment of mitral valve closure begins slightly before the minimum 2, representing the definitive closing position of the cusps, that is, it coincides with this point. In 36 cases we recorded synchronously PCG and UCG. The first sound preceded point 2 by a mean interval of 0.025 sec (the range was 0 to 0.08 sec). The second sound, the closing sound of the aortic and the pulmonary valves, begins about 0.02 sec before the steep rise to peak 4. It follows point 3 by a mean interval of 0.026 sec. Point 4, representing maximal opening of the valve, coincides in mitral stenosis with the middle of the mitral opening snap (Fig. 9). The maximal difference between peak 4 and the middle of the opening snap was found to be 0.03 sec in 33 cases with synchronous registration. Measurement is difficult when peak 4 of the UCG is not sharp but rounded.

Relations between UCG curves and the motion of the posterior wall of

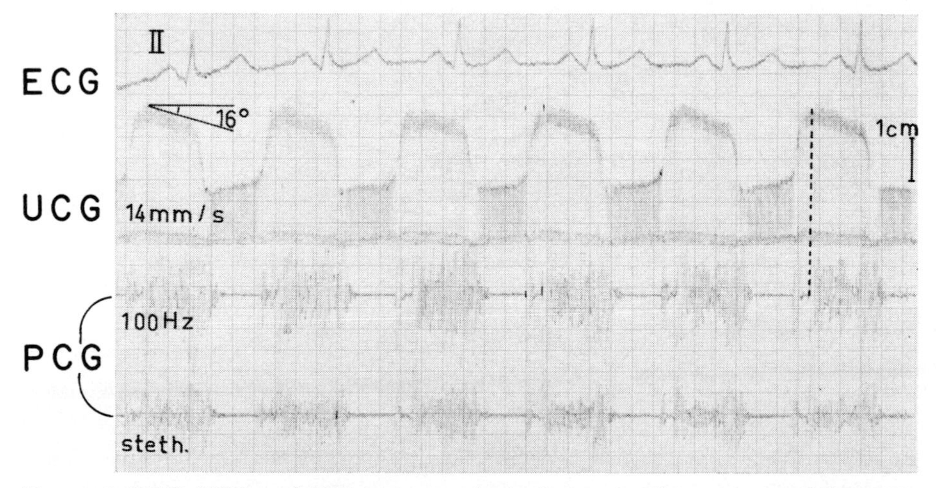

FIGURE 9. ECG, UCG, and PCG in a case of mitral stenosis. The maximum of the UCG curve coincides with the mitral opening snap. PCG with a rated frequency of 100 Hz and stethoscopic characteristic (steth.).

the left auricle also seem to be unequivocal (Effert and Sachs, in preparation). In Figure 10 we see synchronous registration of UCG and the so-called esophago-atriogram (Friese, 1955). Under fluoroscopic control a condenser attached to a gastric tube is inserted in the esophagus and placed directly posterior to the left auricle. By converting changes of capacity into voltage fluctuations, one can register the movement of the posterior wall of the left auricle. In these two curves the waves representing atrial systole coincide. In the esophago-atriogram the closure of the mitral valve appears as a distinct second wave. When the left auricle fills during ventricular systole, there is a steep rise in the esophago-atriogram which reaches a maximum at the very moment when, in the UCG, the rapid ascent to wave no. 4 begins. Then the esophago-atriogram drops abruptly, the UCG leaps upward. In other words, when the mitral valve opens during the interval 3–4, blood flows from the left atrium into the left ventricle. The posterior wall of the left atrium moves in an anterior direction. In mitral stenosis (Fig. 11) the esophago-atriogram also falls steeply during the interval 3–4. Simultaneously with point 4 (the moment of maximal valve opening and of the

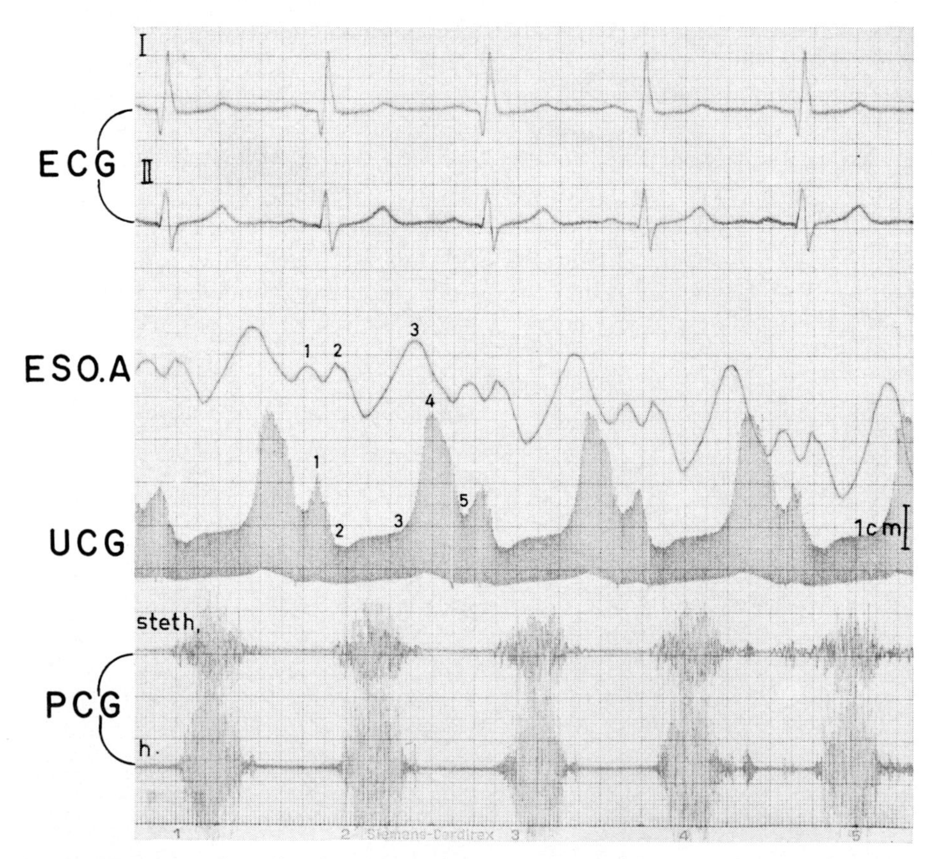

FIGURE 10. UCG and esophago-atriogram (ESO. A) recorded in a case of ventricular septal defect. PCG with stethoscopic characteristic (steth.) and with a rated frequency from 250 Hz (h.).

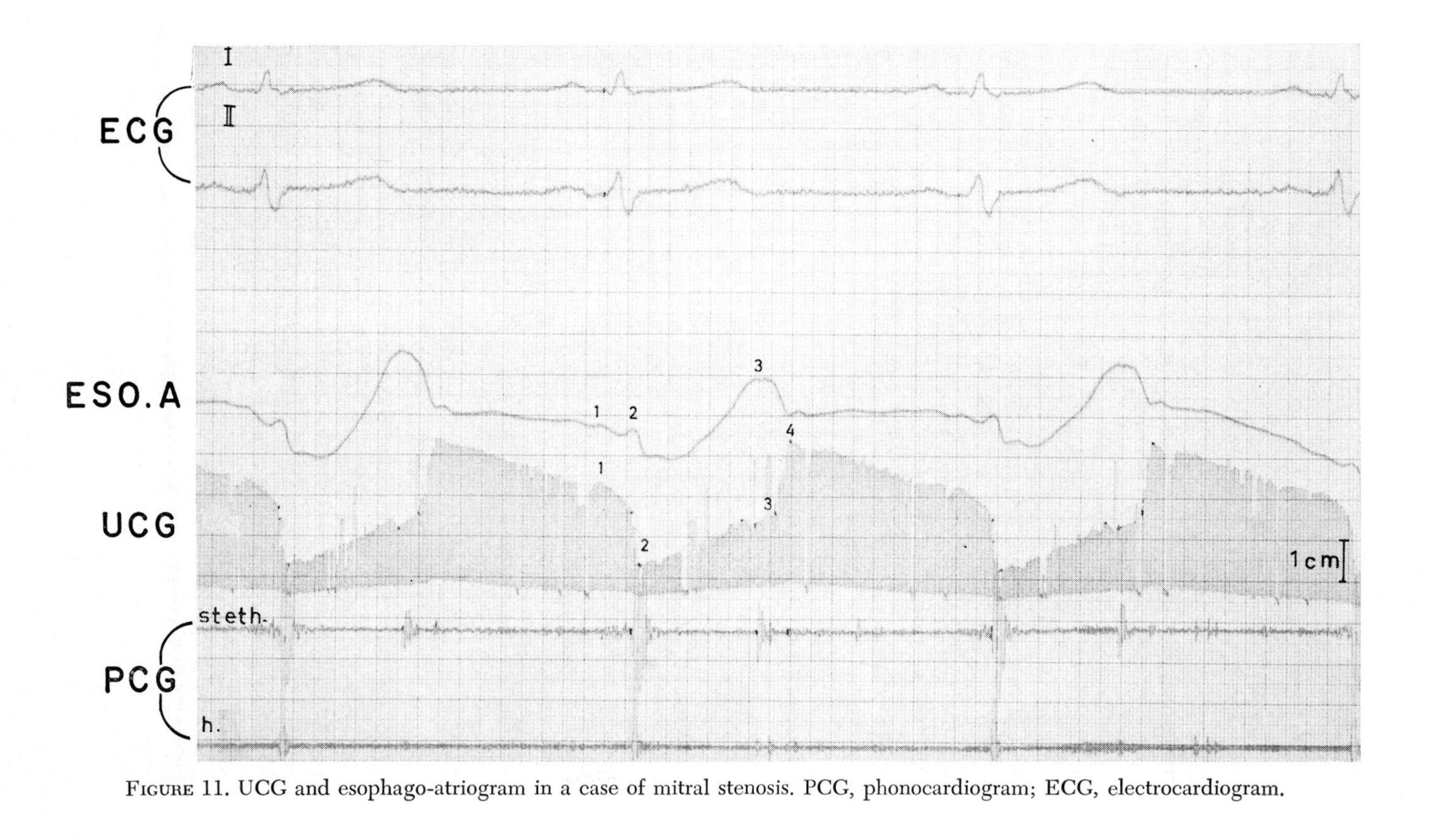

FIGURE 11. UCG and esophago-atriogram in a case of mitral stenosis. PCG, phonocardiogram; ECG, electrocardiogram.

opening snap), the curve kinks and then falls less steeply. On the basis of our observations, this type of curve encountered in mitral stenosis may be interpreted as follows: By fusion of the mitral cusps the valvular apparatus becomes funnel shaped. During atrial systole this conical structure bulges. The ensuing steep descent of the curve is caused by closure of the cusps. After the end of the ventricular systole, when ventricular pressure drops below atrial pressure, the mitral "funnel" is blown out in all directions. The ultrasonic echo-return curve rises. At the very moment when the cusps reach their final position in this phase, the UCG curve reaches its maximum. This maximum coincides with the opening snap. Next, emptying of the left atrium and consequent filling of the left ventricle begins. During this phase the reflecting portion of the mitral "funnel" again withdraws from the anterior chest wall and the transducer. The higher the degree of mitral stenosis the more slowly this happens. The correlation between epicardial UCG and hemodynamic events supports such an interpretation. Still, there remain obstacles to a comprehensive understanding of the tracings. The unvarying curve pattern contrasts with the great anatomical diversity of mitral stenosis. One does not always find the funnel-shaped stenosis that we postulated in the above interpretation. In cases with totally calcified, rigid cusps we also recorded rates of about 20 mm/sec. We assume that in these cases the motion registered was the passive motion of the entire AV-ring, brought about by ventricular systole and diastole, as well as by emptying of the atrium. There is no doubt that the rate of motion of the AV-ring depends upon the size of the residual mitral orifice. The significance of the movement of the AV-ring is demonstrated by the following case: In a patient with extensive destruction of the mitral valve, Dr. Loehr of the Duesseldorf Surgical Hospital implanted an artificial ball valve. After surgery, we registered the same type of curve as that indicated by Dr. Joyner this morning. We believe this is not an indication of the movement of the ball, but of the movement of the metal basket in which the ball moves up and down. The same type of curve pattern was obtained as is found in mitral stenosis.

Finally, I should like to discuss some additional diagnostic applications of our technique. When there is pericardial effusion, the echoes from the cardiac walls do not closely follow the wide echo band from the anterior chest wall. The fluid layer produces an echo-free zone. Characteristic echograms are registered photographically. Figure 12 shows x-ray films of a patient with hemorrhagic pericarditis – before pericardial aspiration (Fig. 12A) and after withdrawal of 1250 ml of exudate (Fig. 12B). With the transducer applied to the fourth intercostal space, 5 cm to the left of the midsternal line (prior to treatment), the UCG of the patient reveals the distance between the chest entry echo and the motion curve of the anterior ventricular wall (Fig. 13). After pericardial aspiration, this distance is reduced by about 2 cm. Three weeks later, another 2000 ml were withdrawn. Then the pericardium was partially inflated with air. When the transducer is applied to the third ICS (intercostal space), the layer of air totally reflects the beam (Fig. 14). During expiration the fluid level in the pericardium rises and the beam contacts the fluid

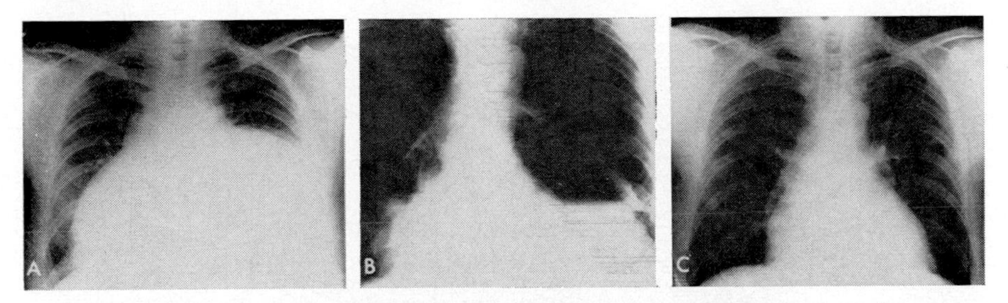

FIGURE 12. Patient, forty-seven-year-old male. Hemorrhagic pericarditis. A. Before treatment. B. After withdrawal of 1250 ml of exudate and inflation of air. C. 3 months later.

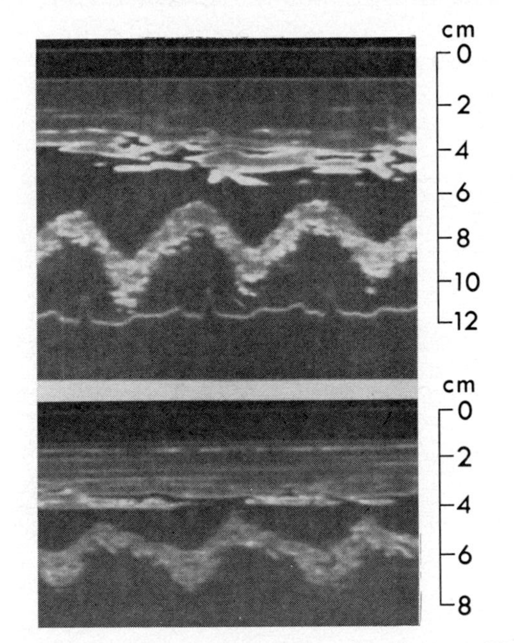

FIGURE 13. UCGs from the same patient whose record is shown in Figure 12. Top: prior to withdrawal of the exudate. Bottom: after withdrawal of the exudate.

level. This partial reflection from the rippling fluid surface disappears again after inspiration. Under adequate therapy the effusion was finally absorbed. Figure 12C shows the x-ray film 3 months later. The UCG in Figure 15 from the fourth and fifth ICS again shows the usual echogram; over the fourth ICS, the reflection curve of the anterior mitral cusp is recorded. The diagnostic reliability of the UCG in pericardial effusion cannot be assessed until further investigations are completed. We have succeeded in recording aortic valve movements by means of the UCG only in isolated cases. On the other hand, the outflow tract of the left ventricle can easily be registered. To what extent the UCG might enable one to differentiate between various aortic valve conditions cannot be predicted at this time.

A particular application of the ultrasonic reflection method is the detec-

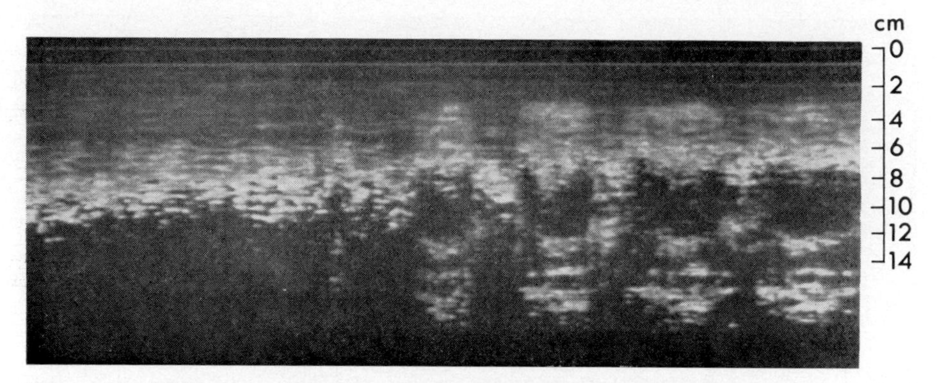

FIGURE 14. UCGs after inflation of air in the pericardium. Partial reflection from the fluid surface during aspiration. The left-hand area of the figure records inspiration; the area at the right, expiration. Same patient as indicated in Figure 12 (see text).

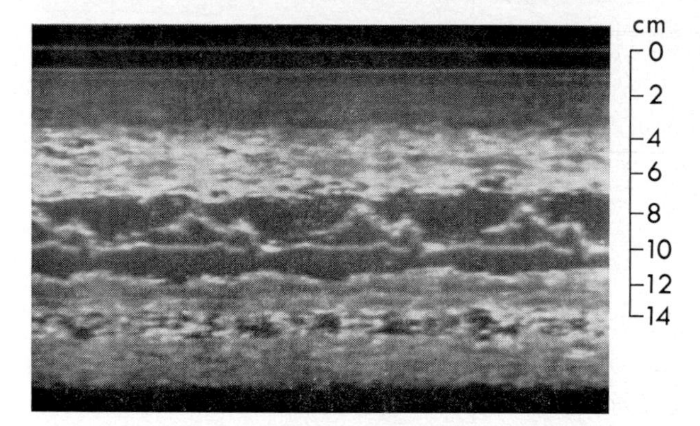

FIGURE 15. UCG from the same patient indicated in Figure 12, 3 months later. Fourth ICS, left parasternal.

tion of tumors or great thrombi in the left atrium. Acting as a valve, such a tumor can simulate mitral stenosis. Judging from the envelope, the tracing shows the same curve pattern as does mitral stenosis. In contrast to the curve found in uncomplicated mitral stenosis, however, this tracing is filled with echoes in a certain layer-order. Following operative removal, a perfectly normal UCG curve can be registered. Only in rare instances have we been able to register echograms from the tricuspid valve.

The present situation is as follows: The UCG permits highly accurate grading of mitral stenosis with or without coexistent insufficiency. There are, at present, no other means for registering the movement of the mitral cusps. Further progress can be expected in the diagnosis of aortic valve disease, particularly in distinguishing valvular from subvalvular stenosis, and also in the detection of pericardial effusions. Tricuspid valve action can be registered only in a few cases. Atrial tumors are rarities, but by no other technique can they be demonstrated so directly. Small atrial thrombi cannot be reliably identified. It is to be hoped that more extensive use of the technique will reveal further diagnostic possibilities.

REFERENCES

Edler, J., A. Gustafson, T. Karlefors, and B. Christensson (1961). Ultrasound cardiography. Acta Med. Scand. Suppl. 370.

Effert, S., and H. Sachs (in preparation). Die Beziehungen zwischen dem Osophagoatriogramm und dem Ultraschallkardiogramm. Z. Kreislaufforsch.

Friese, G. (1955). Über das Osophagoatriogramm des Herzgesunden und Herzkranken. Arch. Kreislaufforsch. *22*, 288.

Additional References to Ultrasound Cardiography

Edler, J., and A. Gustafson (1957). Ultrasonic cardiogram in mitral stenosis. Acta Med. Scand. *154*, 85.

Edler, J., and C. H. Hertz (1954). The use of the ultrasonic reflectoscope for the continuous recording of the movements of heart walls. Kungl. Fysiogr. Sällsk. Förhandl. *24*, *5*.

Effert, S. (1959). Der derzeitige Stand der Ultraschallkardiographie. Arch. Kreislaufforsch. *30*, 297.

Effert, S., and E. Domanig (1959). The diagnosis of intra-atrial tumours and thrombi by the ultrasonic echo method. Germ. Med. Month. (Engl. ed.) *4*, 1.

Effert, S., H. Erkens, and F. Grosse-Brockhoff (1957). The ultrasonic echo method in cardiological diagnosis. Germ. Med. Month. (Engl. ed.) *2*, 325.

Effert, S., C. H. Hertz, and W. Böhme (1959). Direkte Registrierung des Ultraschallkardiogrammes mit dem Elektrokardiographen. Z. Kreislaufforsch. *48*, 230.

Gässler, R., and H. Samlert (1958). Zur Beurteilung des Ultraschall-kardiogrammes bei Mitralstenosen. Z. Kreislaufforsch. *47*, 291.

Jacobi, J., R. Gässler, and H. Samlert (1958). Neue Ergebnisse mit der Ultraschallkardiographie. Verh. Dtsch. Ges. Kreislaufforsch. *24*, 295.

Schmidt, W., and H. Braun (1960). Mitteilung der mittels Ultraschallkardiographie gewonnenen Ergebnisse bei Mitralvitien und Herzgesunden. Arch. Kreislaufforsch. *49*, 214.

Schmitt, W., and H. Braun (1961). Ultraschallkardiographie bei angeborenen und erworbenen Herzfehlern. Munch. Med. Wschr. *103*, 523.

Strick, W. D. (1961). Die diagnostische Anwendung des Ultraschalls. Med. Klinik *43*, 1817.

DISCUSSION

DR. HUETER: Dr. Effert's paper is now open for discussion. I would like to use my privilege as chairman to start with a question. You showed in a very interesting manner that these curves could be interpreted as reflections from the valves. Why don't you obtain a double trace since you did record a double trace in one case in which you had the artificial valve installed?

DR. EFFERT: As Dr. Edler pointed out in referring to his experiment on the isolated heart, the echo source is the anterior mitral leaflet. Normally, the posterior leaflet does not contribute to the echo. You may get reflections from the posterior leaflet if the position of the heart is abnormal, but in most cases you do not.

DR. REID: We have seen a number of posterior cusp curves which are not a mirror image of the upper curve, but instead a double-peak lower curve. In stenosis the space between the leaflets was held to a constant width during the emptying phase, showing that the valve does indeed open to a maximum extent and stays there. However, the motion of the mitral ring must be carrying the valve as a whole forward with the same motion as the leaflets. We saw some of the Starr valves in angiocardiograms, and saw that as the heart beats, the whole cage moves toward the chest wall and back, and the ball, of course, being loose can move perhaps a centimeter more than the cage, but both of them are executing an almost identical movement.

DR. EFFERT: I agree. It is not only the movement of the valves, it is the movement of the whole heart, and of the anterioventral plane.

DR. HOWRY: I had the dubious pleasure of doing some very early work on these false echo displacement studies. Prior to the 1950 period, we were able to detect the valves, but we abandoned the work completely because of the complexity of the problem. At the time I started working in this field it had been conclusively proven that the heart is a very dynamic organ and that in the process of emptying itself, it wrings itself out like a sock and goes through some fantastic gyrations. It doesn't just collapse; instead of the left ventricular wall simply moving in during ventricular systole, it moves outward for nearly the first half of the ventricular systole and then goes in some other direction. In addition, it is undergoing a rotational motion in three different directions. Therefore, the use of a single measure of displacement as a measure of such complex motions appeared an oversimplification. It would be most amazing if the motion were exactly correct because it would not appear possible to even measure to the same point on the valve at all times. The point that I completely missed, however, was the practical application. I did not use this technique on normal and abnormal cases as these gentlemen did. They have, therefore, come up with a very practical instrument. It is really immaterial whether or not the posterior surface appears to be moving. I personally suspect the annulus moves forward and that they are both moving in equal amounts, but I don't think it matters particularly. This instrument is of value as a diagnostic tool even though the basic operation may not be thoroughly understood. This is also true of other diagnostic tools such as the EKG and the EEG.

DR. HUETER: I would like to know the statistics on the number of operations, that is, how often in per cent in a normal population does this defect occur? Is this in an area where mass surveys are indicated? Jack Reid mentioned the use of such a method for surveying a large part of the population.

DR. EFFERT: I don't know the exact number of cases in the population. I believe it is essential that facilities and staff be available for this type of operation in a cardiological center since there probably would be a number of patients with mitral stenosis in this type of hospital. However, in a nonspecialized hospital, mitral stenosis cases may be present only at the rate of one a month or one every two months.

DR. HUETER: In determining whether a patient has mitral stenosis, do you use the machine first, or do you first employ other methods for detecting mitral stenosis?

DR. EFFERT: We first perform a clinical examination with x-ray and electrocardiogram and then take the ultrasonic cardiogram. We no longer use cardiac catheterization in these cases as we did from 1956 to 1959. We have compared the results with this procedure to those of other techniques.

DR. REID: Dr. Joyner had to leave and requested that I ask the following question: There appears to be some difference of opinion concerning the significance of the so-called Austin-Flint murmur in cases of aortic insufficiency. As you know, after the ventricle has contracted, the blood spurts back into the heart because of the elasticity of the aorta. It has been observed in angiocardiograms that this blood spurts back against the mitral valve leaflet, tending to close it a little. The question has been raised, therefore, is this an Austin-Flint murmur, a false mitral murmur, or is it a true mitral murmur? In the few cases we encountered we have found that patients with an Austin-Flint murmur also had low normal velocities when there was no stenosis. Those without the Austin-Flint murmur and no stenosis had the highest normal velocity. Have you made similar correlations of the velocities for patients with and without Austin-Flint murmur?

DR. EFFERT: I am not certain. For the patients with a high degree of mitral stenosis and aortic insufficiency who underwent an operation, the results were about the same as indicated here. But in such cases the velocities were in the range of 50 or 60 mm/sec if unoperated. I cannot say if this is true mitral stenosis or not, but I think that Dr. Joyner is correct, that the direction of the jet toward the mitral valve may produce the Austin-Flint murmur and then diminish the velocity as indicated by the acoustical curves.

23

Ultrasonic Diagnosis of Intracranial Disease, Breast Tumors, and Abdominal Diseases

TOSHIO WAGAI, M.D., RYOICHI MIYAZAWA, and KAZUBUMI ITO
Department of Surgery, School of Medicine, Juntendo University, Tokyo, Japan

YOSHIMITSU KIKUCHI
Research Institute of Electrical Communication, Tohoku University, Sendai, Japan

As already reported at the second and third International Congress of Acoustics, we have been studying methods of ultrasonic diagnosis, especially in early cancer diagnosis, chiefly by means of the echo method (1, 2). In this paper, recent clinical results of the application of ultrasonic diagnostic techniques to intracranial disease, breast tumor, and abdominal tumor are presented.

In these studies, the echoes are displayed on the cathode ray screen both by an A-scope and B-scope. Figure 1 shows our new portable-type ultrasonic diagnostic apparatus used with the A-scope. This equipment is designed so that frequencies of 1, 2.25, 5, or 10 Mc may be used.

Various types of medical transducers are used with either barium titanate or quartz crystal employed as the transducer element. A complete view of the B-scope apparatus with a patient in position is pictured in Figure 2. This apparatus, which we have designated as an ultrasonotomograph, has been improved over previous models by the addition of such devices as a sensitivity time control (1). The equipment on the left is a scanning device which moves a transducer horizontally, and on the right is the observation device. Ultrasonic waves are transmitted into the patient through degassed water contained in a vinyl bag.

Currently, brain tumors are diagnosed by routine neurosurgical examination without too much difficulty. However, some of these examinations are painful and even dangerous for the patient. For this reason we have introduced the ultrasonic method into this field of diagnosis. This method of examination is also very useful for patients who are seriously ill and for children.

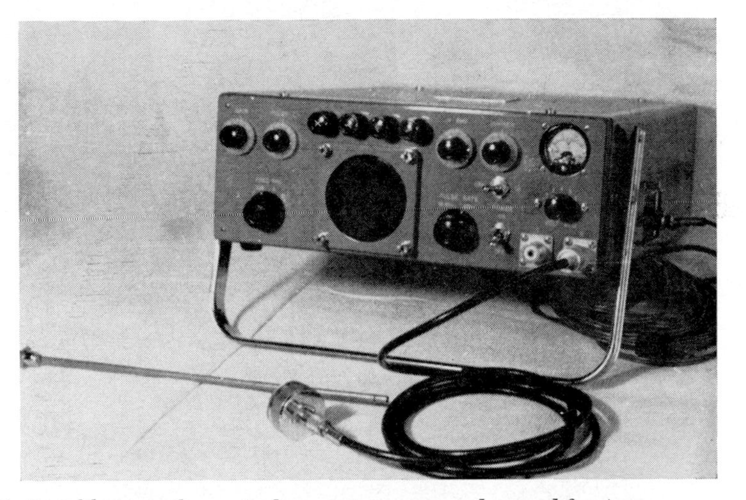

FIGURE 1. Portable-type ultrasonic diagnostic apparatus designed for A-scope use.

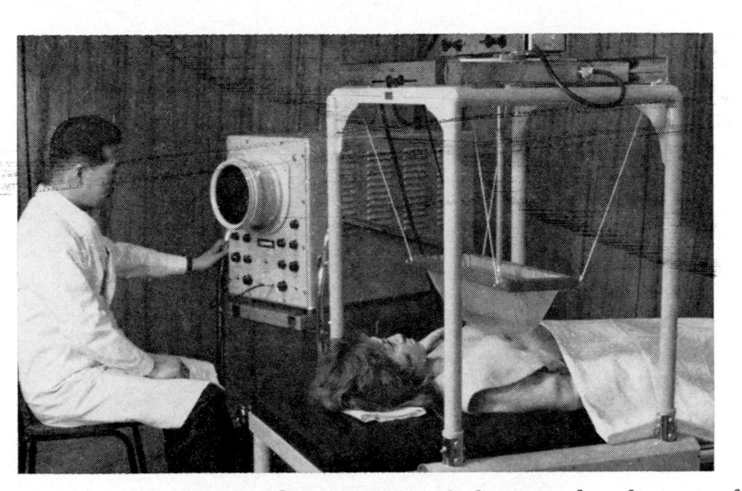

FIGURE 2. B-scope apparatus, the ultrasonotomograph, being used in diagnosis of breast tumor.

Ultrasonic diagnosis of brain injury in the frontal region using the A-scope is demonstrated in Figure 3. A frequency of 1 to 2.25 Mc is used. Frontal tumor, tumor of the pituitary gland, cerebellar tumor, etc., can be diagnosed with this type of examination. Figure 4 shows the ultrasonic echo pattern of a frontal tumor (fibrillary astrocytoma) in a schematic presentation. The tumor can easily be diagnosed by the irregular echoes following the transmitted pulse. Examination of the brain by ultrasound is also done by application of the transducer to the temporal region. Figure 5 shows the midline echo which is easily detectable at the temporal region. We have reported that this midline echo, if detected at the temporal region just above the ear, is that of the third ventricle wall (2, 3). If the midline echo is displaced, it can be suspected that a space-occupying lesion of the cerebral hemisphere exists.

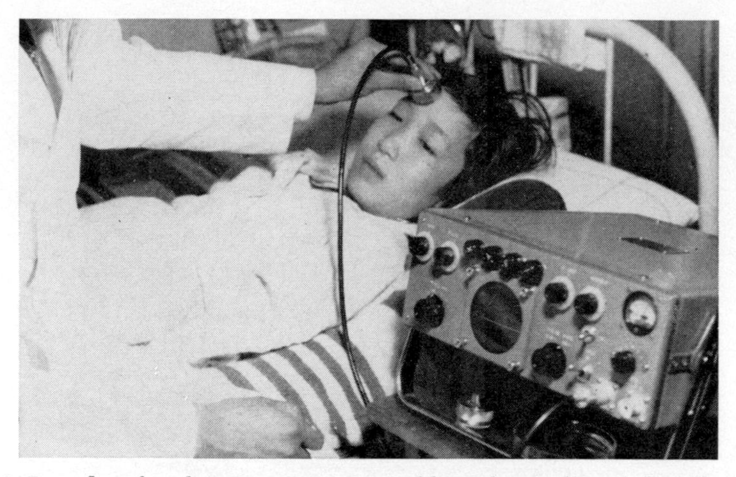

FIGURE 3. Procedure for ultrasonic examination of brain lesion through frontal region by A-scope.

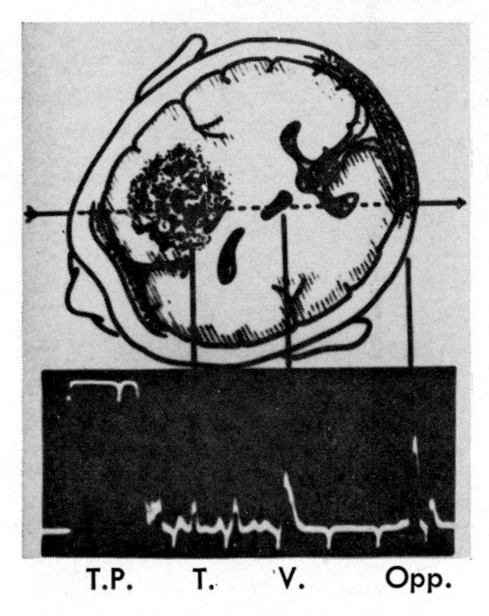

FIGURE 4. Schematic presentation of ultrasonic echo pattern of frontal tumor (fibrillary astrocytoma). T.P., transmitted pulse; T., tumor echo; V., ventricle echo; Opp., opposite side of head.

Figure 6 shows the ultrasonic echo of a brain tumor at the temporal region. The displacement of the third ventricle echo and the tumor bottom echo can be detected. The interior of the tumor is acoustically homogeneous.

Four hundred and seventy-one suspected cases of brain disease were examined by the ultrasonic method (Table I), and recent results of our ultrasonic diagnosis of brain tumor are charted in Table II. Sixty-nine cases of brain tumor were examined and were later confirmed by operation or autopsy. In 52 cases of supratentorial tumor, 43 cases were diagnosed by the ultrasonic method (83%). In 17 cases of subtentorial tumor, 4 cases were diagnosed

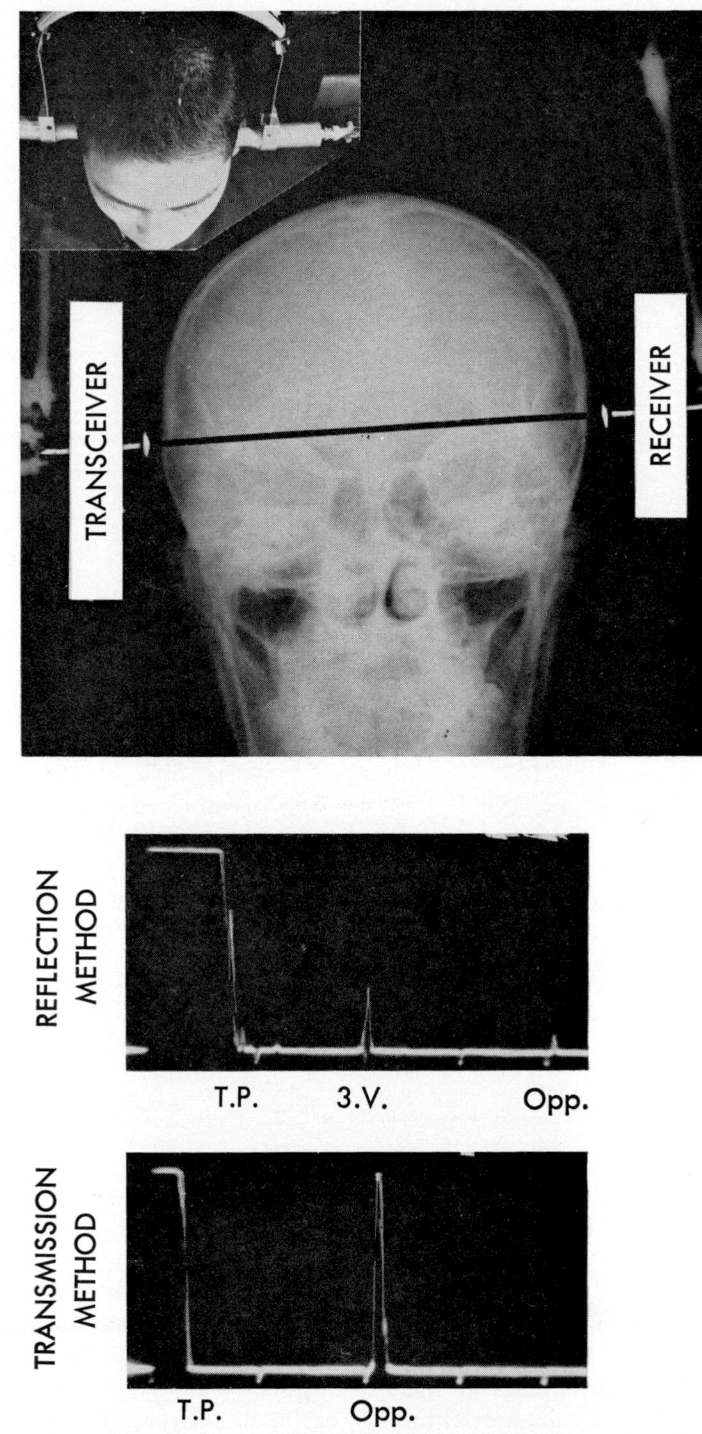

FIGURE 5. The midline echo at the temporal region which is confirmed as the echo of the third ventricle wall. T.P., transmitted pulse; 3.V., third ventricle echo; Opp., opposite side of head.

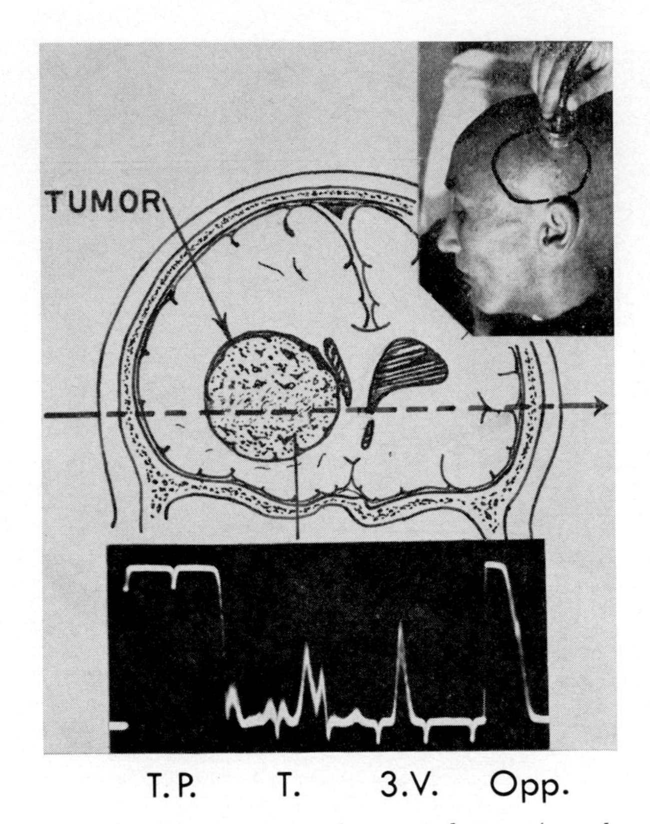

FIGURE 6. Ultrasonic echo of brain tumor at the temporal region (reticulosarcoma). T.P., transmitted pulse; T., tumor echo; 3V., third ventricle echo; Opp., opposite side of head.

TABLE I. TYPES AND NUMBERS OF SUSPECTED INTRACRANIAL CASES EXAMINED ULTRASONICALLY.

Type of disease	*Total number of patients examined*	*Patients 0 to15 years of age*
Brain tumor	160	22
Head injury	181	40
Epilepsy	21	14
Hydrocephalus	30	10
Brain abscess	5	0
Others	74	11
Total	471	97

(24%). The low percentage of successful diagnosis in subtentorial tumors is caused by the fact that it is difficult to propagate the ultrasonic beam through this region by our usual method. In an effort to find a more successful method, the examination for subtentorial tumors was made transorally. A transducer of 2.25 Mc was used, and ultrasonic waves were directed through the pharingeal region of the oral cavity (Fig. 7). Tumors in the subtentorial region

TABLE II. RECENT RESULTS OF ULTRASONIC DIAGNOSIS OF BRAIN TUMOR.

Location of tumor	*Number of cases examined*	*Number of correct diagnoses*
Cerebral hemispheres	33	31
Chiasmal region	10	8
Rostral brain stem	9	4
Caudal brain stem	3	0
Fourth ventricle	1	0
Cerebello-pontine angle	7	1
Cerebellum	6	3
Total	69	47

were successfully detected by this method. The transoral method (Fig. 8) is used in cases of neurinoma and cerebellar tumors.

Rapid diagnosis of extradural or subdural hematoma resulting from head injury is very important in deciding the operative indication. We were able to diagnose hematoma by detecting the bottom echo and the displacement of the midline echo. A follow-up observation of midline echo after operation for subdural hematoma showed that it took from 2 weeks to 1 month for the recovery of the displaced midline echo. The graph in Figure 9 shows this postoperative displacement. A continuous observation of midline echo is useful for the postoperative management of brain disease. Results of our ultrasonic diagnosis of hematoma are shown in Table III. Successful diagnoses of fifteen out of sixteen cases of hematoma were made.

It is very important to differentiate intracerebral hemorrhage from other conditions such as stroke for the purpose of surgical treatment of this disease. Displacement of midline echo was observed in clinical examination of intracerebral hemorrhage. It was possible to confirm experimentally that intracerebral hematomas made by injecting only 0.1 ml of blood into cat

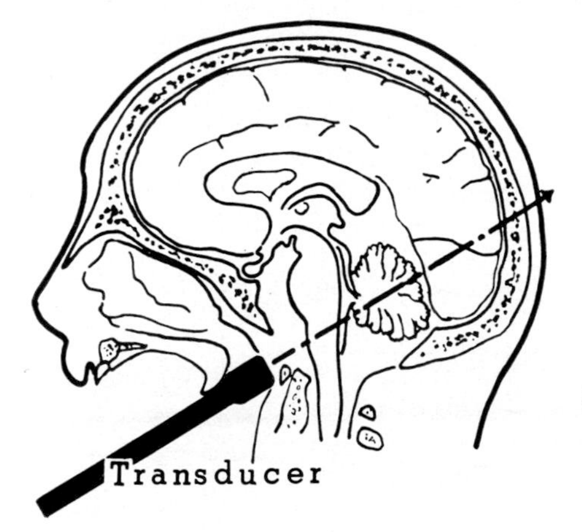

FIGURE 7. Schematic presentation of transoral ultrasonic examination for subtentorial tumors.

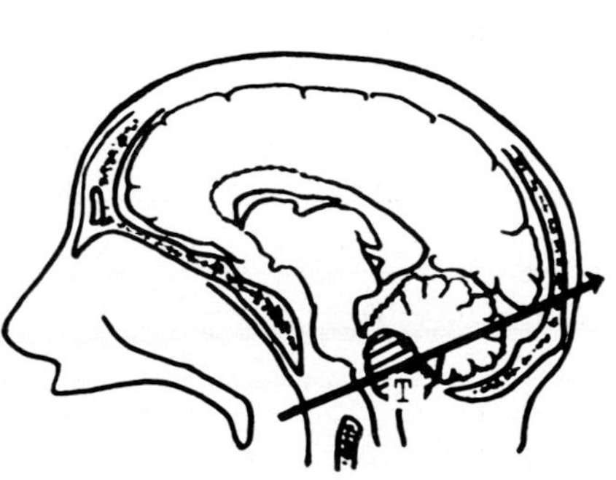

FIGURE 8. Transoral ultrasonic examination.

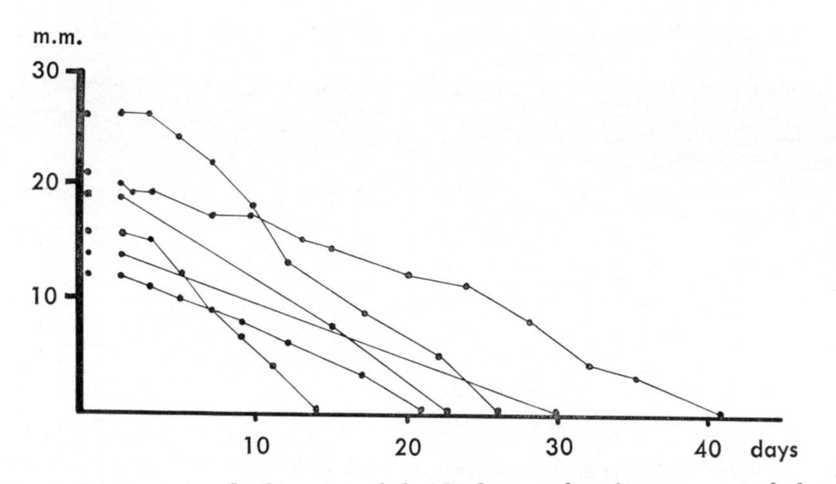

FIGURE 9. Postoperative displacement of the third ventricle echo in a case of chronic subdural hematoma.

brain could be detected. Figure 10 illustrates the clinical echo pattern obtained. However, as seen in Figure 11, we were unable to detect hematoma echo or displacement of midline echo in the case of subarachnoidal hemorrhage. It was observed that the recovery of midline echo took a relatively short period of time in the survival case of intracerebral hemorrhage. With further studies, it is hoped that the ultrasonic diagnosis of apoplexy may become possible.

Our ultrasonic examination of the brain was carried out by three methods: (1) through the scalp and skull, (2) through the dura mater following osteoplastic operation, and (3) directly on brain tissue after opening the dura mater. Figure 12 shows the latter procedure. A frequency of 10 Mc is ordinarily used. With this technique, it is possible to diagnose clearly an oligodendroglioma through the dura mater, which would be difficult with direct palpation and inspection of the brain.

Dr. Wild and his associates have used ultrasound in the diagnosis of breast tumor (4–6). In our studies with the ultrasonotomograph, the whole breast is examined using a frequency of 10 Mc. Several components are found in the tomograms of various kinds of breast tumors. For example, a linear pat-

TABLE III. RESULTS OF ULTRASONIC DIAGNOSIS OF SUBDURAL AND EXTRADURAL HEMATOMA.

Types of hematoma examined	*Number of cases examined*	*Correctly diagnosed cases*
Subdural	14	13
Subdural hygroma	1	1
Extradural	1	1
Total	16	15

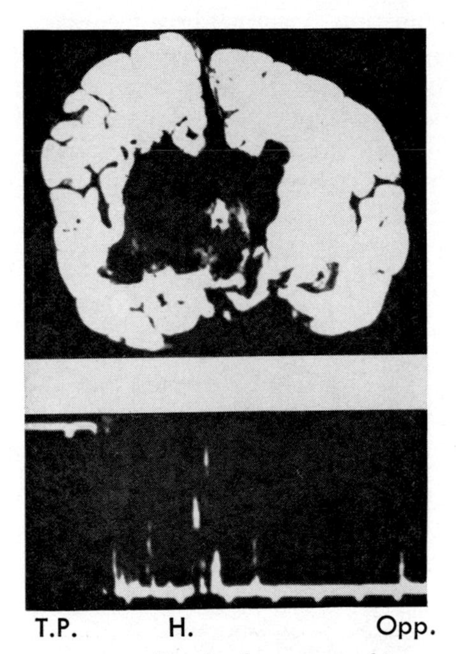

FIGURE 10. Clinical echo pattern of intracerebral hematoma. T.P., transmitted pulse; H., hematoma echo; Opp., opposite side of head.

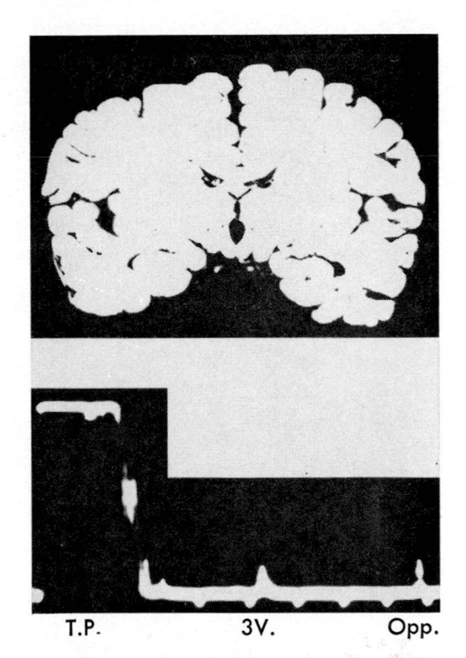

FIGURE 11. Ultrasonic examination of subarachnoid hemorrhage. T.P., transmitted pulse; 3V., third ventricle echo; Opp., opposite side of head.

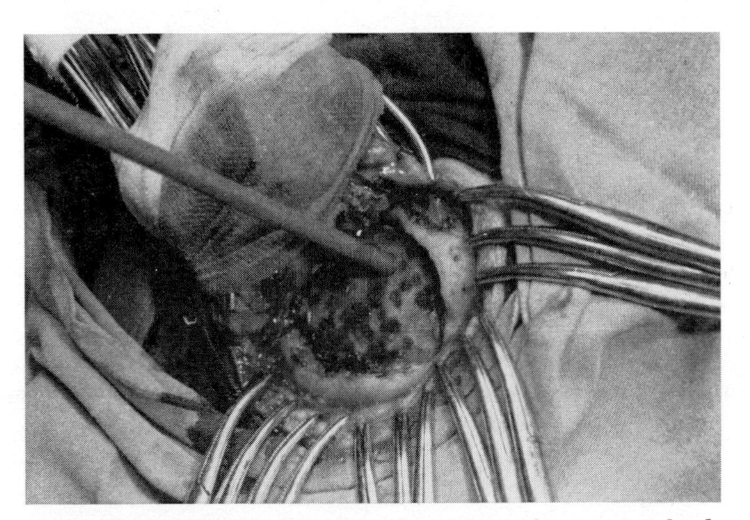

FIGURE 12. Ultrasonic examination directly on brain tissue after opening the dura mater.

tern, small spotted pattern, or irregularly continuous pattern can be observed. Such patterns appeared singly or in combination. A normal breast produces an acoustically homogeneous tomogram; this is shown in Figure 13. Figure 14 shows the linear and small spotted pattern which is generally observed in mastopathia. These component echo patterns can be detected whether the tumor is palpable or not. The tomogram of a fibroadenoma (Fig. 15) shows a circular pattern, the inside of which is almost homogeneous. Similar patterns are observed in the case of cysts or abscesses. In the case of malignant tumors, an irregular continuous pattern of intense brightness is observed. Tomograms

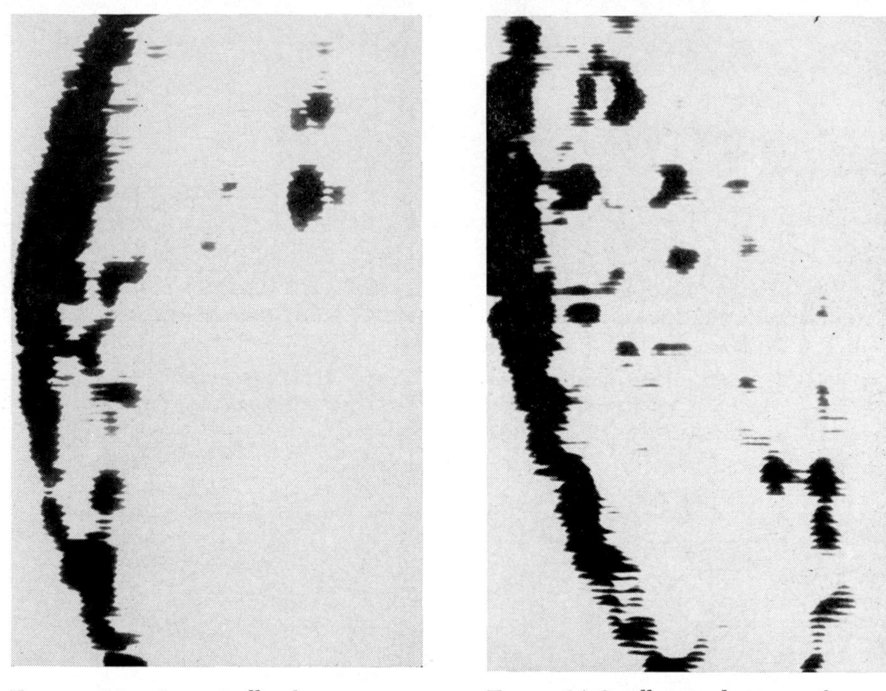

FIGURE 13. Acoustically homogeneous tomogram of normal breast.

FIGURE 14. Small spotted pattern of mastopathia.

of a certain type of abnormal secretion of the nipple show only a simple pattern like that of mastopathia; another type shows a specific pattern in the homogeneous area just under the nipple. The former pattern is observed in the case of mastopathia and the latter in intraductal papilloma. One hundred and forty cases of breast tumor were examined by the ultrasonic method. All of these cases were also examined histologically. In 66 cases which were diagnosed as malignant by the ultrasonic method, 57 cases were found to be histologically malignant. However, in 74 cases which were diagnosed as nonmalignant by the ultrasonic method, 2 cases proved to be histologically malignant. The question arises at this stage whether the ultrasonic method can differentiate between malignancy and nonmalignancy of breast tumors in those cases for which diagnosis is difficult by the usual methods. In one

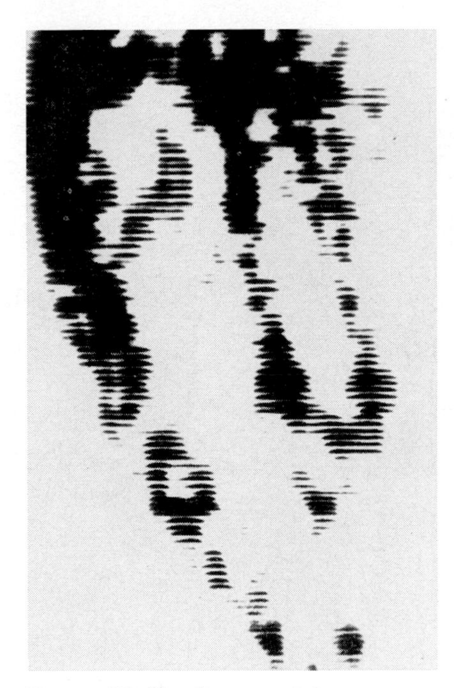

FIGURE 15. Circular pattern in tomogram of fibroadenoma.

case in which our ultrasonic tomogram showed a simple pattern, the clinical findings and radioisotope tests indicated a diagnosis of malignant tumor but the histological examination showed a change of nonmalignant senile involution. Figure 16 shows the histological picture of senile involution. Forty-two cases of mastopathia have been followed using the ultrasonic method for a period of 2 to 7 years. Among this group, early breast cancer was detected in one case which had been observed for 4 years. The tomogram in Figure 17 shows the malignant pattern in this case. We are encouraged, therefore, to hope for further success in the ultrasonic diagnosis of early breast cancer.

While x-ray study is routinely used for the diagnosis of gallstones, the results of this method are not satisfactory in Japan. We have been using the ultrasonic method for diagnosis of gallstones and various diseases in the bile duct and have found the results to be encouraging. A frequency of 2.25 to 5 Mc is used for the ultrasonic diagnosis of gallstones. A sharp echo reflected from a large gallstone is shown in Figure 18. It was possible to detect not only gallstones which were in the gallbladder but also those in the bile duct which were not revealed by x-ray examination. We examined 1231 cases of epigastralgia and in 162 of these cases, gallstone echoes were detected. Gallstone echo was detected in 78 of 94 confirmed cases (Table IV). In all of these cases x-ray examination had not clearly demonstrated gallstone figures. Ultrasonic diagnosis of cancer in the region of the common bile duct

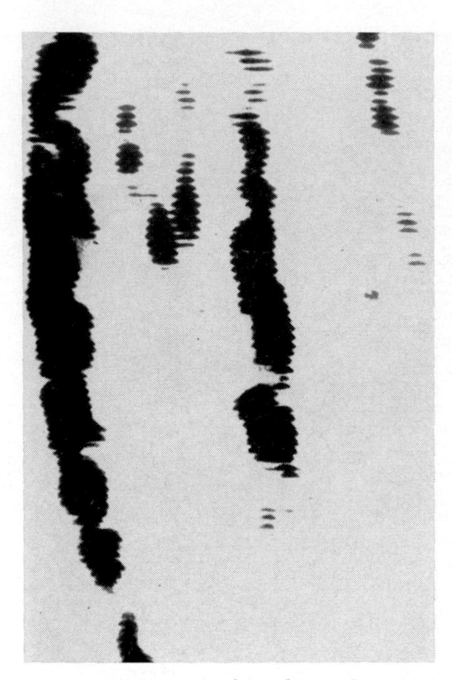

FIGURE 16. Pattern of senile involution of breast.

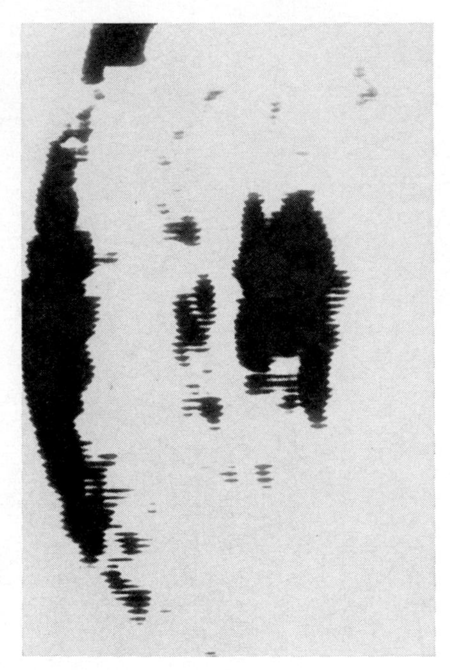

FIGURE 17. Pattern of breast cancer detected during the observation of benign mastopathia.

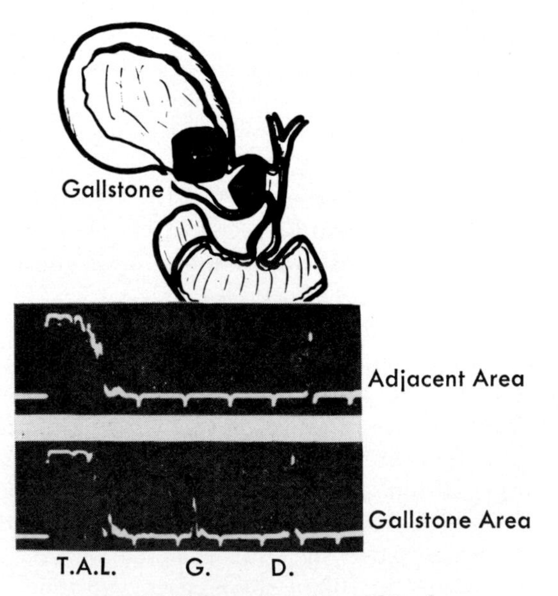

FIGURE 18. Sharp echo reflected from large gallstone in gallbladder. T., transmitted pulse; A., echo from abdominal wall; L., echo from liver; G., echo from gallstone; D., diaphragm echo.

Table IV. Operative Findings of Cholelithiasis in Cases Previously Examined by Ultrasound. (X-ray examination had not clearly demonstrated gallstones.)

Ultrasonic echo from gallstone	*Number of cases*	*Operative findings*	
Positive	78	Gallstones in gallbladder and cystic duct	50
		Gallstones in common bile duct	12
		Gallstones in gallbladder and common bile duct	16
Negative	16	Gallstones in gallbladder and cystic duct	12
		Gallstones in common bile duct	2
		Gallstones in gallbladder and common bile duct	2
Total	94		94

(Fig. 19) makes possible the differential diagnosis of extrahepatic obstructive jaundice. The cancerous echo is generally observed as an irregular and stable echo compared with the sharp gallstone echo. It was possible to detect a cancerous echo in 20 out of 26 cases of cancer at the region of the bile duct. These findings were confirmed by operation or autopsy. Ultrasonic diagnosis of liver disease using both A-scope and B-scope indication at a frequency of 2.25 or 5 Mc has been attempted. Figure 20 shows the procedure of the ultrasonic examination of liver disease diagrammatically, and Figure 21 illustrates echo patterns of four types of liver diseases. An ultrasonotomogram of normal liver is shown in Figure 22. The tomogram produced by hepatitis is demonstrated in Figure 23. Many linear patterns are observable in the case of liver cirrhosis shown in Figure 24. Figure 25 reproduces a tomogram of metastatic cancer of the liver. Thus, the ultrasonic diagnosis of liver disease can be interpreted as being characterized by the specific acoustical structure of pathological liver tissue.

In addition to the procedures described above, we applied the ultrasonic

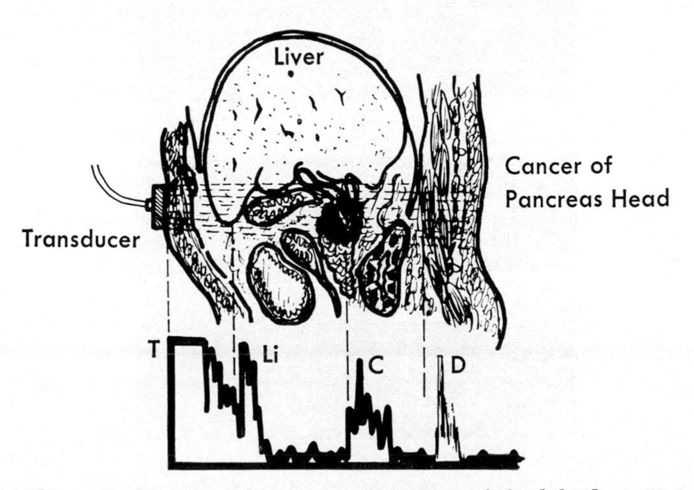

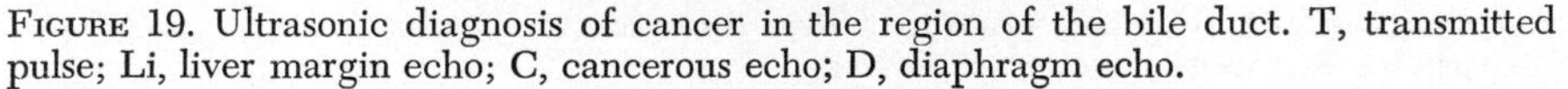
Figure 19. Ultrasonic diagnosis of cancer in the region of the bile duct. T, transmitted pulse; Li, liver margin echo; C, cancerous echo; D, diaphragm echo.

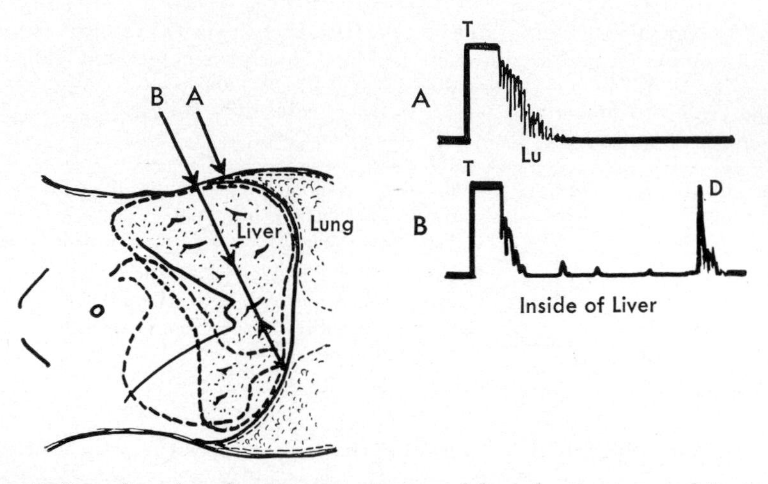

FIGURE 20. Procedure for ultrasonic examination of liver by A-scope and B-scope. T, transmitted pulse; Lu, lung echo; D, diaphragm echo.

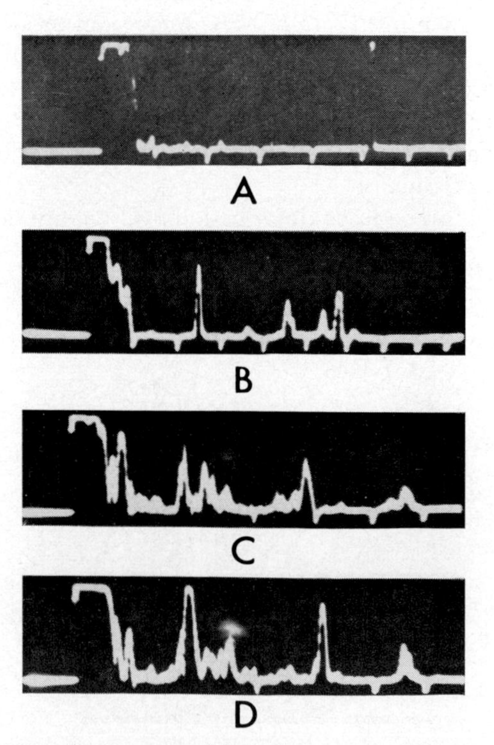

FIGURE 21. Intrahepatic echo patterns of liver diseases. A. Hepatitis. B. Liver cirrhosis. C. Hepatoma. D. Metastatic cancer of liver.

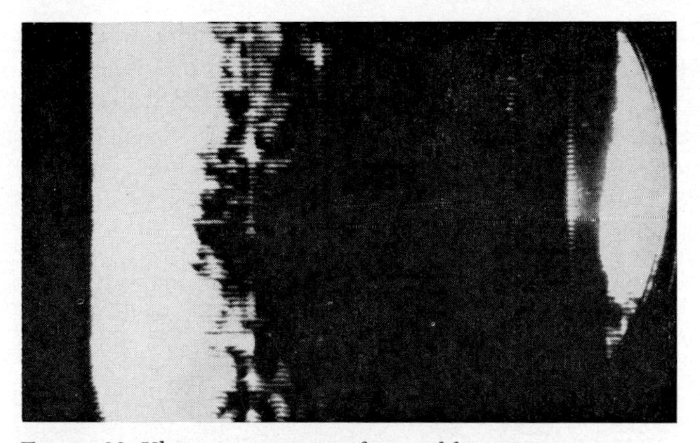

FIGURE 22. Ultrasonotomogram of normal liver.

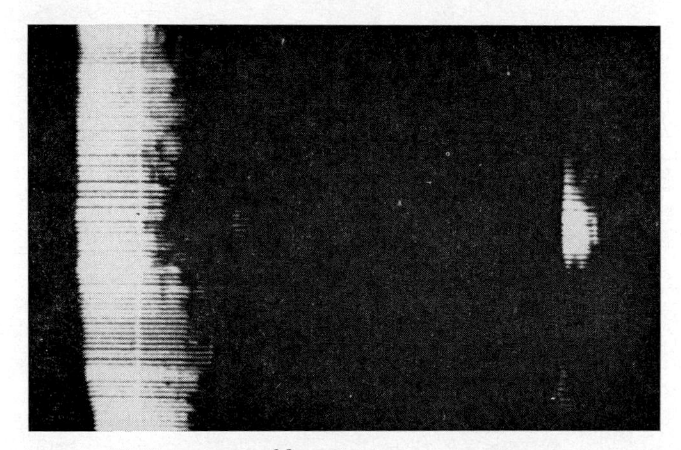

FIGURE 23. Tomogram of hepatitis.

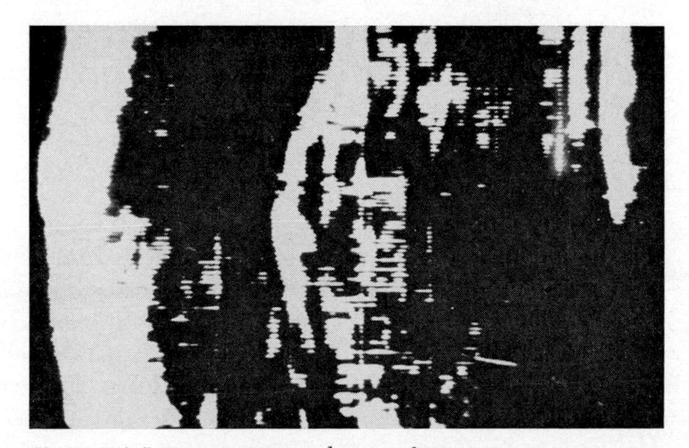

FIGURE 24. Linear patterns in liver cirrhosis.

method to laparoscopy. A specially designed slender transducer was used, on the top of which is fixed a small quartz crystal 3 mm in diameter, at a frequency of 10 Mc. This transducer was inserted into the abdominal cavity and placed directly on various organs under laparoscopic observation. In this manner, diagnosis of gallstones, liver diseases, stomach cancer, and other pathological conditions was made possible. These procedures will be shown in the following film.

FIGURE 25. Tomogram of metastatic cancer of liver.

REFERENCES

1. Kikuchi, Y. (1956). Early cancer diagnosis through ultrasonics. Lecture, 2nd ICA Cong. HD-9 (Cambridge, Mass.).
2. Kikuchi, Y. (1959). Recent results of research and industrial development in the field of ultrasonics in Japan. 3rd ICA Cong., Invited papers L-13 (Stuttgart, Germany).
3. Tanaka, K. (1959). Ultrasonic diagnosis of brain tumor. Lecture, 3rd ICA Cong. 1-L-6 (Stuttgart, Germany), Proc. 3rd ICA Congress, 1291 (1960).
4. Wild, J. J., and J. M. Reid (1952). Further pilot echographic studies on histologic structure of tumours of living intact human breast. Am. J. Pathol. 28, 839.
5. Wild, J. J., and J. M. Reid (1952). Application of echo-ranging techniques to determination of structure of biological tissues. Science *115*, 226.
6. Wild, J. J., and J. M. Reid (1954). Echographic visualization of the living intact human breast. Can. Res. *14*, 277.

DISCUSSION

DR. HUETER: Thank you, Dr. Wagai and colleagues, for your interesting paper. I think you demonstrated in a very clear fashion that there are indeed situations where ultrasound can detect abnormalities in the brain and other organs. Your presentation, particularly your film demonstration, also illustrates how difficult the whole situation is, that is, how much careful checking is required in order to determine whether a trace is significant or not significant.

DR. GORDON: I should like to congratulate Dr. Wagai on the excellent work that they have been doing in Japan. This sort of work was discussed in

London earlier this month, and the work on the displacements of the brain is now becoming fairly well established as a technique in Europe. Two English investigators reported 1000 neurosurgical cases at two hospitals, investigated ultrasonically, of which 867 cases had been confirmed radiologically. Evidently the remaining 133 cases were not checked radiologically because these investigators felt that surgery could proceed in a certain proportion of cases without the loss of time involved by x-ray examination. Such cases, of course, were usually those of acute head injury and intracranial hemorrhage. Some work has also been done in Britain on examining the gallbladder at operation. Quite frankly, the detection of gallstones through the abdominal wall seems rather an act of faith because although one can get a good echo from a gallstone, such an echo could be produced by gas in the intestine and one can't be certain as to the original source of the echo obtained. Investigation of the breast has not been pursued, as far as I know, in Europe. But the work on the liver and on the brain is now becoming accepted technique.

Dr. Howry: I would like to ask Dr. Gordon: In this 1000 cases, aren't you mainly referring to displacement of the midline echo, rather than an absolute diagnosis, that is, the exact position of the tumor as indicated by Dr. Wagai? We would certainly confirm the displacement of the midline echo, but as far as locating subcortical tumors or locating tumors anteriorly and posteriorly, I think this is a good deal more subjective than the midline echo.

Dr. Gordon: They were detecting more than midline echoes, that is, they were getting echoes from various boundaries of the ventricular system. In certain cases, if no shift of the midline of the ventricles was detected ultrasonically, they would accept this as a reason for not investigating brain shifting further.

Dr. Howry: Getting echoes out of the skull is a formidable job. We tried it. Perhaps the Japanese are much more patient about the wave forms they see on their oscilloscopes than we are.

Dr. Hertz: I am of the same opinion as Dr. Howry. There was a group at Lund working quite a long time to determine if the ultrasonic method could be employed to detect tumors inside the head. They studied this problem very carefully and concluded that there is no echo except the midline one that gives "certain" results, that is, that could be considered reliable.

Dr. Hueter: Would Dr. Kikuchi like to make a comment on this part of the discussion? The concensus seems to be that the most important value of this method is to identify the midline echo and draw conclusions from it, whereas localizing the tumor itself may still be problematical.

Dr. Kikuchi: With regard to the midline shift, we found that in 3 to 4% of the cases with tumors inside the brain no midline shift was evident. So, from the standpoint of a physician, Dr. Wagai suggests that other diagnostic methods be used in addition to the ultrasonic midline detection procedure. Dr. Wagai uses the ultrasonic method first because it is not a dangerous procedure and is very easily handled. Therefore, ultrasonic diagnostic procedures should be employed first in any case of brain disease.

Dr. Baum: I want to indicate that we did a study in which we tried to evaluate the use of the A-scope in the eye, and we concluded that it is hazardous. I think you never really know the site of origin of your echo, and I just wanted to make it part of the record that I think the A-scope should not be used in ocular work unless you have a scanning system so that the site of the echoes is known.

DR. HUETER: I think this is a very cogent comment. Some of the problems which Dr. Howry mentioned might be cleared up to some extent even in the brain work if one uses a B-scope, that is, a scanning technique in a different way. Offhand, I don't know how you would do it, but one could set up a program scanning procedure to include integrating over a large number of echoes, rather than presenting the information from only one echo at a time.

DR. KIKUCHI: In the early investigations, I thought that the B-scope was very much preferable to the A-scope. However, in certain cases a quick examination is required and for this type of case Dr. Wagai, after considerable experimentation, was able to establish an A-scope diagnostic technique. From the standpoint of a physicist, I feel that, at present, the B-scope is preferable, but in some cases the B-scope fails to detect a symptom which can be detected by an A-scope. For this reason, at present, I would like to insist that both methods be applied in diagnostic determinations. From the standpoint of the surgeon, Dr. Wagai would like to recommend that both A- and B-scopes should be used, not only at present, but in the future. The A-type instrument is a probe that the physician can use in an emergency—for example, in the case of a traffic accident where the physician attends the victim at the site of the accident. On the other hand, the B-scope has very superior characteristics because it exhibits cross-sectional views of the anatomic structures.

DR. HEIMBURGER: I think the same reasoning applies here as Dr. Howry mentioned in regard to the use of ultrasound for the diagnosis of heart disease. If one has sufficient experience, then it is possible to interpret this type of information just as one interprets electrocardiograms, electroencephalograms, etc. I believe that what Dr. Wagai is demonstrating this afternoon is that he has sufficient experience to interpret this A-scope information.

DR. HOWRY: We started with this type of research about 16 years ago—in 1947. At that time we made an A-scope and succeeded in producing echoes from the liver. However, in the presence of gallstones (these were gallstones introduced into a piece of liver and placed in a tank of saline), the echo pattern was ambiguous. We changed over to a B-scan, but we felt at that time that neither of these techniques gave us a diagnosis. Now, there are some very excellent exceptions. We have seen the research of the Japanese scientists and of the European scientists who have shown us their work on the heart. The A-scan, I think, has excellent application if you are approaching the gallbladder either by a laparotomy or by peritoneoscopy. I certainly agree that under such circumstances one can tell whether there is a gallstone in the gallbladder or in the common duct. However, if you don't know where the gallbladder is, I fail to see how in the world you are going to tell whether there are gallstones in it. As a radiologist, I can indicate that in certain conditions, I observed cases where the gallbladder was clear down in the pelvis. Therefore, I would have a very difficult time determining where to place an A-scope in order to determine what organ I was viewing, knowing full well that I would see all kinds of miscellaneous gas shadows and echoes. To continue, there are a few other places where an A-scope is probably of value. You can most assuredly make the AP dimension of the pelvis which is of interest in pregnancy. There are two or three other specific applications where it also has beneficial application, but insofar as its use as a general tool is concerned, then we are talking about memorizing an infinite number of arbitrary wave forms and attaching significance to them. This is going to require a computer of such size that you will need a very large building to house it.

The B-scan material is perfectly all right; you can see certain specific areas and, as was pointed out by Dr. Wild a great many years ago, it happens that for this method the breast is unique to some extent. Most assuredly, in certain spreading carcinomas of the breast, one obtains with this technique a fan-shaped pattern and echoes throughout. Therefore, in this regard, our work, in which we have been using focusing techniques, correlates with the results just presented. This is the point at which I began my investigations. If you continue along these lines, however, if you wish to really tell where a carcinoma is, you've got to see the normal structure with it. And if you can't see the chest wall in relation to the anatomy of the chest, that is, with the associated arteries and other structures in order to establish where something is located, how in the world can you tell what it is? I have no idea. This is the weak point. It is necessary to have much more elaborate equipment in order to obtain an adequate diagnosis. Dr. Baum, I think, has found the same thing to be true in the eye. Frankly, we wouldn't have had the need to do our last 10 years' work if this type of difference had not been very authentic.

Dr. Hueter: This is an interesting question, namely, how elaborate must your equipment be in order to get accurate results? Obviously, if the elaboration is too great, then this technique is restricted to a very small circle.

Dr. Carlin: As you know, there have been a number of government projects on evaluation of various types of scanning equipment. In my experience, the A-scan gives the most information but is also the most difficult to interpret. If you are very skilled in using the A-scan, you can very often get additional information which may not be present in the B- or C-scan.

Dr. Gianturco: Why apply this new tool to the diagnosis of gallstones when with standard techniques one may diagnose this condition with 95% accuracy? Why use the ultrasonic method? I agree that ultrasound is very useful and very helpful for detecting stones in the common duct, but if I have a choice between having pictures of my gallbladder and having two instruments inserted in me, I would prefer the picture.

Dr. Kikuchi: Our present situation in Japan is as follows: X-rays can detect 30% of gallstones, but the ultrasonic technique can detect 70 to 80% of gallstones, as you have seen in our slide (Table IV). I don't know whether the nature of the gallstones found in Japanese clinics is somehow different from that of gallstones found in the United States.

DR. GORDON: Are you talking about gallstones which are not opaque to x rays, and the stones in the common duct?

DR. KIKUCHI: The gallstones found in Japan are very transparent to x rays.

DR. GIANTURCO: Perhaps we don't understand each other. We determine gallstones by means of a gallstone dye. If you are talking about stones that don't show up in a plain film, I agree with you. Very few of them show up in the film, but we seldom examine a gallbladder without the use of a dye. Ultrasound is a wonderful tool which I would hate to see wasted on gallstones.

DR. WAGAI: (The following statement was inserted during editing process.) The x-ray diagnosis in Japan is about 30% effective in spite of the use of several kinds of dye.

DR. HUETER: Perhaps we had better relegate this part of the discussion to a strictly medical circle on gallstone detection techniques. One more question.

DR. MACKAY: There is a much simpler procedure in connection with localizing stones in the bladder by ultrasonic techniques. Many years ago, we used small sound transducers at the end of wires which were set in oscillation and passed up the urethra into the bladder. When the wire contacted a stone, one would suddenly notice a change in electrical input impedance of the transducer. It is a very convenient way of finding the position of a stone.

DR. HUETER: Is it convenient for the patient?

DR. MACKAY: It is a lot more convenient than the alternative which consists of placing a lump of wax on the end of a catheter and passing it up the urethra to the bladder and then pulling it out to see if there is a dent in the wax. If not, you stick it up a little further. So I would say that this application of ultrasound is better than others.

DR. HUETER: I would like to thank our Japanese colleagues for a very interesting paper which certainly has provoked a lot of comments and interest here. Also, we would like to encourage you to continue in the future to put an occasional pretty geisha girl and a Japanese landscape in your slides.

24

An Ultrasonic Echoscope for Visualizing the Pregnant Uterus

G. KOSSOFF, W. J. GARRETT,[1] and D. E. ROBINSON
Commonwealth Acoustic Laboratories, Sydney, Australia

Ultrasonic mapping of the internal structures of the human body has attracted the attention of numerous investigators. The returned echoes are generally displayed on the oscilloscope either as deflections of the trace or as intensity-modulated spots on the otherwise blanked trace. The first method is called A-scope and requires simpler instrumentation as the transducer is normally hand held. It provides useful clinical information, such as the detection of the midline in the brain and the registration of movements of heart structures. In general, however, the applications of A-scope are quite limited as the echo pattern is drastically altered by slight changes of the position or direction of the transducer, making any clinical interpretation a matter of guesswork unless used in conjunction with two-dimensional visualization (Baum and Greenwood, 1961).

For two-dimensional visualization, the instrumentation becomes necessarily more complex as the transducer is mechanically swept and its position and direction are monitored in some way. Sometimes useful data can be obtained by means of a B-scan, where structures are scanned once only, but such echograms have very poor azimuthal resolution and structures and interfaces not normal to the ultrasonic beam fail to register on the screen. Because the structures are scanned once only, great laxity can be placed on the mechanical and electronic stability of such equipment. For accurate anatomical visualization, a "compound-scanning" technique must be adopted (Howry, 1957). In "compound scanning," the transducer moves in such a way so as to be normal to each structure at some stage of the scanning period. Since some structures are scanned from more than one position and one angle, great stringency must be placed on the accuracy and stability of the mechanical scanner and associated electronic equipment, so that a single target registers as a single spot on the screen of the display unit.

The pregnant uterus is ideal for ultrasonic visualization as it consists es-

[1]Queen Elizabeth II Research Institute for Mothers and Infants, University of Sydney.

sentially of soft tissues and liquids, media in which ultrasound is readily propagated, and whose structure it then differentiates, giving the possibility of obtaining echograms comparable to true anatomical cross-sections. The fetus, having a complicated geometrical shape, acts as a very stringent test object showing the inadequacies of the ultrasonic visualization technique. The equipment to be described has been specifically designed for the visualization of the pregnant uterus, but it can also be used to scan various other abdominal organs such as the liver or kidneys.

THE SCANNER

Method of Scanning

To scan the pregnant uterus, the transducer may be placed directly on the skin (Donald and Brown, 1961) or used with a water delay path. The first method has several disadvantages. The scanning period is necessarily much longer and the patient's breathing can then spoil the resolution of the echogram. The transducer must maintain a certain pressure on the skin to ensure good coupling. The underlying structures are displaced, but they return to their original position when the pressure is removed. When these structures are then scanned from a different angle their detail becomes blurred. Compound scanning ensures that all structures in the horizontal plane normal to the beam are registered on the screen. Any vertically inclined structures are not registered, and the direct contact method does not lend itself to placement of offset receiving transducers to pick up these deflected echoes. The advantage of the method is that it dispenses with the water delay path, allowing patients to be scanned in bed. As accurate anatomical visualization was the main requirement, the water delay path method was adopted in the present work.

The degree of compound scanning must be carefully watched so that errors due to refraction do not spoil the resolution of the echograms. One of the sources of refraction is the impedance mismatch between water and skin which can be eliminated by changing the impedance of the water with chemicals. The mismatch between various internal structures cannot be avoided, and the scanned path must be such as to keep the beam normal to the skin as far as practicable. For the pregnant uterus a circular path achieves this object. During the scanning period, the transducer rides on a semicircular track pointing inward (30 sec for the horizontal sweep) while undergoing oscillations of $\pm 20°$ (1 sec for the horizontal scan), thus giving the desired compound scan. Vertical scanning on the linear rack (15 sec for the vertical sweep) with oscillation of $\pm 40°$ (2 sec for the vertical scan) is also employed as shown in Figure 1. These vertical echograms show up any vertically inclined structures which are not shown on the horizontal echograms.

Positioning of the Patient

The water delay path consists of a perspex tank with one side made of latex rubber 0.6-mm thick. The rubber membrane molds to the shape of the abdomen, giving support and preventing movement due to breathing of the patient. A mixture of 60% castor oil and 40% alcohol is used as a coupling agent. With the patients standing upright, the best horizontal echograms are usually obtained when the scanning direction is normal to the skin line, usually a couple of centimeters below the umbilicus. In our later studies we intend to tilt the patients to bring the skin line and anterior uterine wall more normal to the beam.

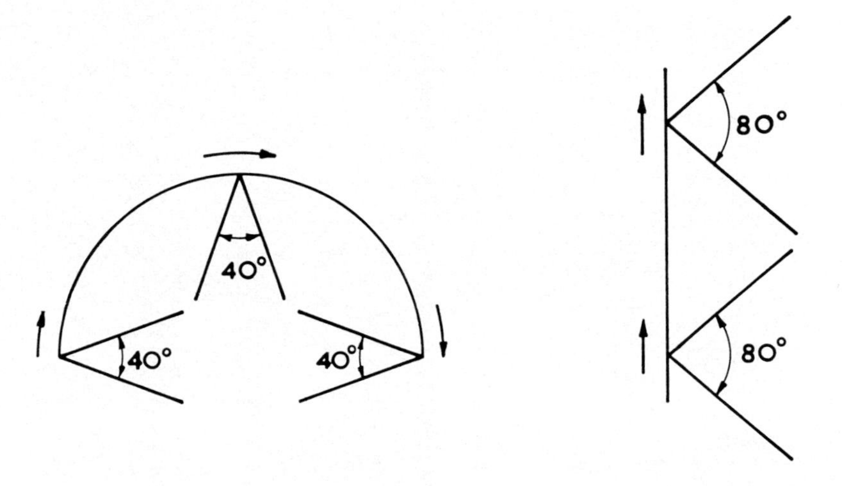

FIGURE 1. Transducer compound-scanning path for horizontal and vertical echograms.

Scanner

Figure 2 shows the scanner and the associated electronic equipment. All the mechanical components are rigid and machined accurately to the required dimensions, and the gears are spring loaded to avoid backlash. The design criterion is the spot size of the display unit, a typical value in this case being between 0.5 and 1 mm. The reduction ratio from actual size to displayed picture is 2.5:1, allowing the whole pregnant uterus to be visualized on the 4-in screen diameter of the display tube. The spot size corresponds to 2 mm in the patient.

The necessity for a high degree of accuracy and stability can be understood by considering the main semicircular track. The radius of the track is 60 cm and the wavelength of the beam at 2 Mc/sec is only 0.75 mm. For a target at the center of the circle to remain a spot on the display screen, the accuracy of the track to the true circle should be better than 1 mm. Twisting of the track under load or on installation is more serious, as the error is magnified by the lever arm to the transducer. A maximum twist of 0.1 mm across the track can be tolerated as it will result in an error of under 1 mm on the display tube. Alignment posts are provided along the track to remove any such twist.

Sine-cosine potentiometers of 0.5% conformity are used to determine the position and direction of the transducer. The potentiometer which determines the direction of the trace rides on the main carriage and its casing is geared to retain a constant angular reference. These wire-wound potentiometers have been one of the major sources of resolution error and of great inconvenience due to persistent mechanical breakdowns. These will shortly be replaced by film potentiometers of 0.15% conformity and it is hoped that these will give the required accuracy and reliability.

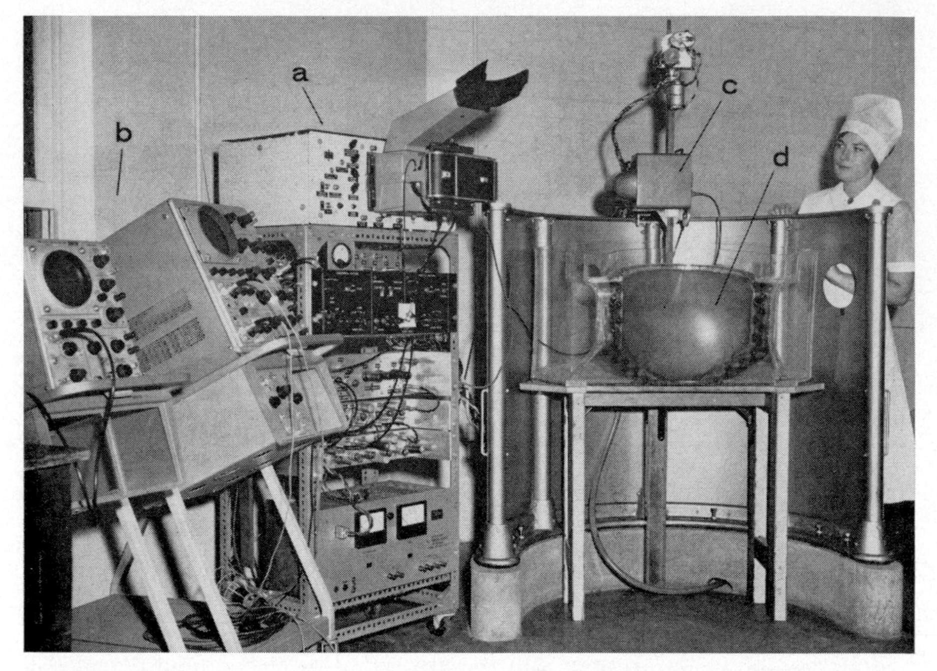

FIGURE 2. The prototype echoscope installed in the Royal Hospital for Women. A. The electronic equipment rack with a display storage tube and camera, a scanner control panel, a transmitter, a receiver, a STC generator, and the power supply. B. Monitoring oscilloscopes. C. Mechanical scanner. D. Water coupling tank.

THE TRANSDUCER

The design of the transducer largely determines the resolution of the echograms. The transducer resolution can be divided into two components – axial and azimuthal. The first is determined by the electrical properties and the second by the geometry of the transducer.

Axial Resolution

The axial resolution is determined by the bandwidth. In order to achieve optimum resolution, short pulses are employed. Unless the bandwidth is sufficiently wide, the returned echoes will be distorted by ringing. The development of ceramic materials has made available transducers with large coefficients of coupling. Even these materials have insufficient bandwidth so that some form of absorbing backing is necessary. However, the use of backing materials has two disadvantages. The transmitted power must be proportionately increased with use of such materials and they are physically bulky, making the overall transducer dimensions fairly large. This is a distinct disadvantage in internal scanning.

Another way to widen the bandwidth is to employ a quarter-wave seal whose impedance is the geometrical mean of the load and transducer impedances (Arm, Lambert, and Silverberg, 1962). This impedance lies between those of plastics and metals and can be achieved by doping epoxy resins with aluminum or tungsten powders or by building sandwich layers of aluminum and araldite (McSkimin, 1959). The latter method was attempted but abandoned due to manufacturing difficulties. The echograms presented in this paper were obtained by using a barium titanate ceramic (80% $BaTiO_3$, 12% $PbTiO_3$, 8% $CaTiO_3$) with a polyester backing material.

Azimuthal Resolution

To preserve azimuthal resolution, scanning is carried out in the near field region of the transducer. For a plane transducer the optimum diameter is given by:

$$\text{Diameter} = 2\ (\text{Wavelength} \times \text{Penetration})^{1/2}.$$

For an operating frequency of 2 Mc/sec and 20-cm penetration, this diameter is 2.5 cm. The beamwidth over the required penetration can be improved by weakly focusing the transducer either by means of a lens or by shaping the actual transducer. Geometrical optics are not adequate for the calculation of the dimensions of the transducer and diffraction theory must be applied. It can be shown (Kossoff, 1963) that, for the above conditions, a transducer of 2.5-cm diameter and 18-cm radius of curvature gives optimum resolution. Good reduction in beamwidth is obtained in the focal region, but, for deeper penetration, there is little improvement as compared with the plane transducer. By combining compound scanning and the integrating properties of either a film or storage tube, further improvement can be obtained as illustrated in Figure 3, in which the transducer is assumed to have

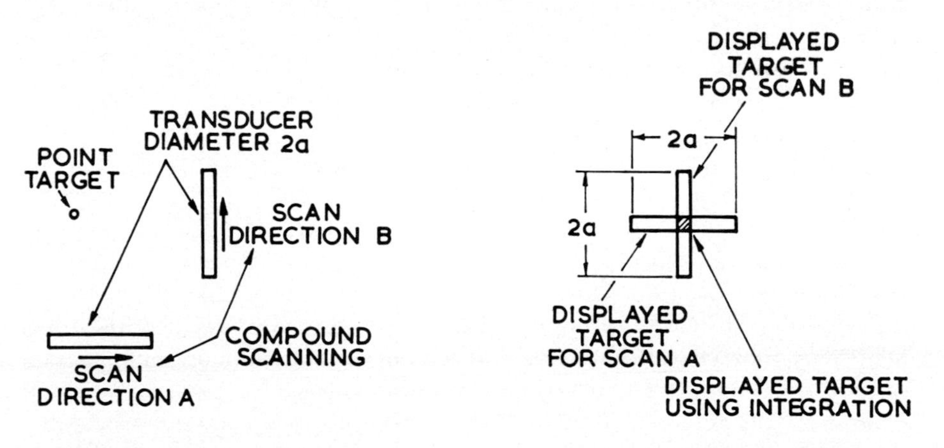

FIGURE 3. Compound scanning of a point target combined with display integration being used to improve the azimuthal resolution.

a uniform field intensity distribution. This technique is difficult to apply, and the lack of azimuthal resolution is one of the main problems in ultrasonic visualization work.

THE ELECTRONIC EQUIPMENT

The electronic equipment consists of a transmitter, a receiver, a display unit, a monitoring oscilloscope, and associated power supplies.

Transmitter

The shape of the transmitted pulse is relatively unimportant. However, it cannot be made too narrow (Kossoff, 1963) since for a plane transducer of the size of interest here, the first 0.25 μ sec are used to set up the steady state conditions. With a focusing transducer, this transient period is reduced but is still significant. The master trigger for the transmitter is a free-running blocking oscillator of 1 kc/sec repetition rate, and a clamped oscillator tube is used to provide one sine wave of 0.5 μ sec duration which drives the transducer. The r.m.s. electrical power of the pulse is 2 w. For a repetition rate of 1 kc, the average power is 1 mw. The voltage and current of the transducer are measured on an externally triggered oscilloscope, and the r.m.s. pulse power is calculated by graphical multiplication. The acoustic conversion efficiency is measured at resonant frequency and used to compute the peak and average acoustic power outputs. This technique is suitable with ceramic transducers due to the associated low impedances and high capacities. High-impedance transducers do not lend themselves to this technique due to loading by the measuring equipment. Some direct method of obtaining the acoustic output is preferable and the radiation pressure float (Kossoff, 1962) is being modified to measure average output power of the order of 1 mw. The voltage waveform usually shows considerable ringing but the current waveform is only in phase over the first cycle, as shown in Figure 4. The transducer must be tuned to obtain maximum bandwidth. Three adjustments are used as shown in Figure 5. The component values can be computed for optimum bandwidth (Thurston, 1959; Baerwald, 1961), but in practice they are experimentally adjusted to minimize the length of the returned echoes. A piece of glass is used for a target, as the scanned structures usually present plane interfaces rather than point discontinuities.

Receiver

A low noise twin-triode is used in the first stage to optimize the signal to noise ratio. As the transducer is a source of low impedance, the noise received at the output of the amplifier is primarily produced by the input tube. Sensitivity time control (STC) makes the output voltage more uniform and consists of a circuit which develops a variable voltage for two remote cutoff pentodes. This voltage is triggered by the first returned echo, increasing the gain of the receiver to compensate for the absorption of energy as the beam penetrates into the patient. The receiver consists of a 50-db low noise preamplifier, a 40-db STC amplifier and a 30-db video amplifier. This type of

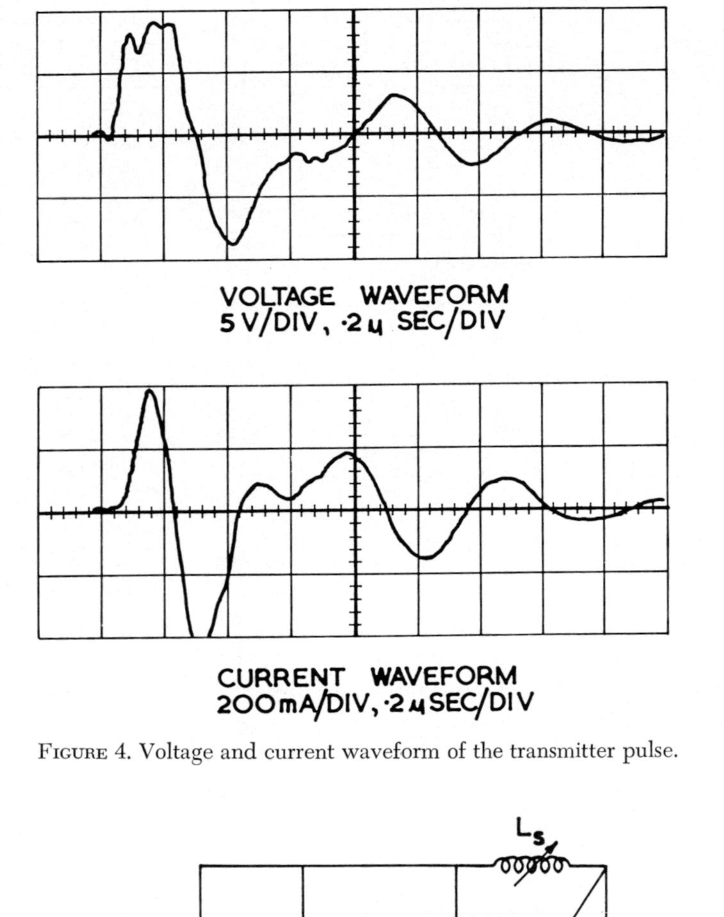

FIGURE 4. Voltage and current waveform of the transmitter pulse.

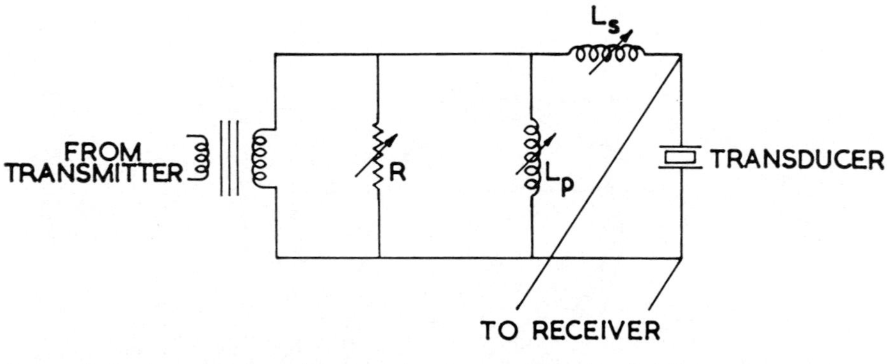

FROM TRANSMITTER
R
L_p
L_s
TRANSDUCER
TO RECEIVER

FIGURE 5. Tuning controls used to optimize the transducer bandwidth.

receiver works well with tissues which show uniform absorption. The pregnant uterus does not show a uniform absorption as the beam sometimes goes through the fetus which has a high and nonuniform absorption and sometimes only through the amniotic fluid which has no absorption. Structures behind the fetus are then shadowed whereas others tend to bloom. Strong echoes can drive the receiver into grid current, giving long recovery times. Adjustment of the STC controls drastically changes the quality, information

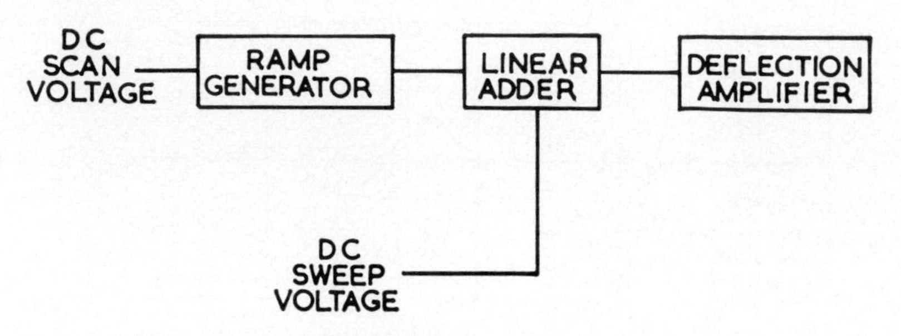

FIGURE 6. Deflection circuit block diagram.

content, and general appearance of the echograms. It is felt that consistent clinical interpretations can be made only if the quality of the echograms is not affected by such variables, and logarithmic receivers are now being investigated in order to overcome this problem.

Display Unit

A direct-viewing storage tube is used for display purposes. Some of the advantages of a storage tube are: (1) The integrating properties of the tube are used to improve the signal to noise ratio. (2) Small changes in electrode voltage are equivalent to changing the aperture and film speed of a photographic plate. (3) The echogram is available immediately for diagnostic work and, if found suitable, can be photographed for permanent records; this corresponds to fluoroscopy with x rays. (4) It is very useful for setting-up purposes, especially with compound scanning, as the adjustments of the

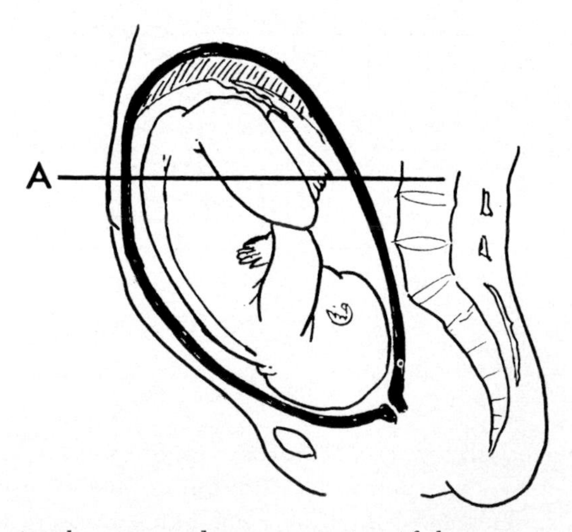

FIGURE 7. Ultrasonic echograms produce cross-sections of the part examined. The normal attitude of the fetus in advanced pregnancy is one of complete flexion. The head is bent forward, the arms crossed upon the chest, and the legs are drawn up with the feet crossed in front of the abdomen. An echogram, such as one at the level of line A, will therefore show the fetal trunk and limbs. As the arms and legs are flexed, the plane of section may cut any individual limb more than once. The uterus, though a distinct muscular structure, does not appear as a definite entity in the echograms obtained so far.

controls are critical and otherwise time-consuming. Since the trace is off the screen for most of the time, an electrostatically deflected display tube was chosen to simplify the power supply problem. The storage tube is a "Tonotron" manufactured by the Hughes Aircraft Co. on which the pattern can be stored and viewed for at least 30 min by modulating the flood gun.

Conventional storage tube circuitry is used to establish the DC conditions for the tube. The deflection circuit deserves a mention. Two sine-cosine potentiometers provide deflection information for the horizontal echograms, and a linear and a sine-cosine potentiometer for the vertical echograms. The sweep potentiometer provides the position, and the scan, the direction information. The sweep voltages are fed to the deflection amplifiers to

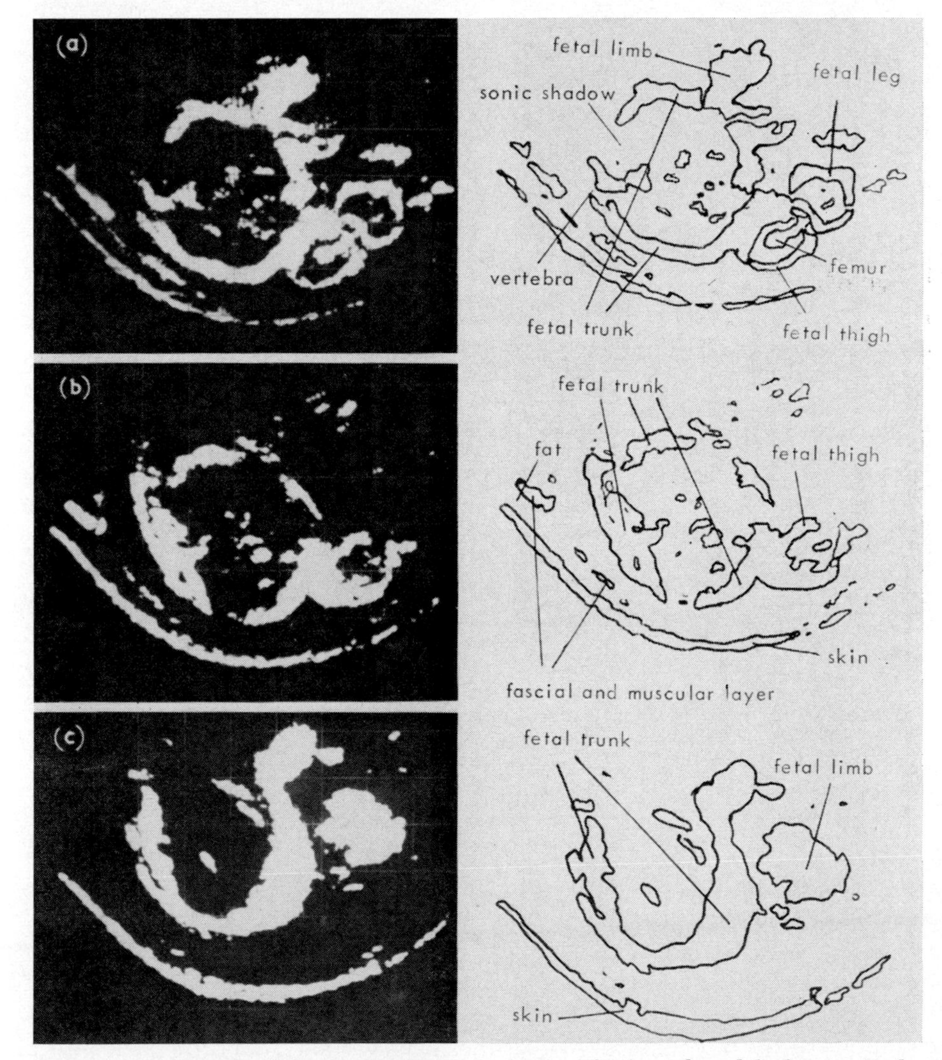

FIGURE 8. Echogram of the pregnant uterus showing fetal trunk and limbs. A. At the level of the umbilicus. B. 2.5 cm below the umbilicus. C. 5 cm below the umbilicus. The identified structures have been confirmed by x-ray examination.

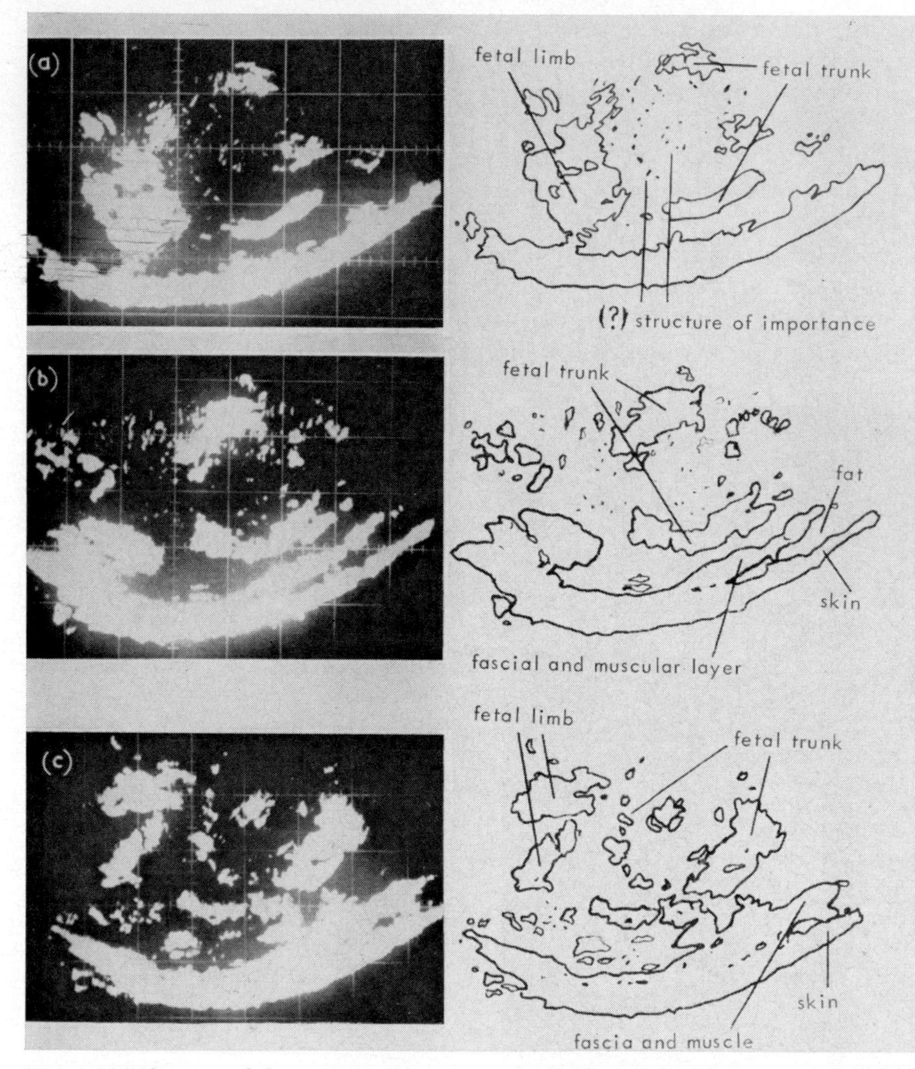

FIGURE 9. Echogram of the pregnant uterus with details of the fetus shown. A. 2 cm above umbilicus. B. At the level of the umbilicus. C. 4 cm below the umbilicus. In the fetal trunk concentric circles of dots appear at level A and similarly a heavier echo is seen at level C. These probably represent anatomical structures but owing to the plane of section, it is at present difficult to interpret them accurately. The fascial and muscular layers of the anterior abdominal wall are clearly shown.

determine the starting position of the trace. The scan DC voltages determine the direction of the trace and are converted to ramp voltages before being fed into the deflection amplifiers. The circuit block diagram is shown in Figure 6. A simple RC network is used in the ramp generator, and it can be shown that, provided the circuit charges to only 5% of the total voltage, the resolution of the display is as good as the spot size. The adder linearity must be of the order of 0.1%. The deflection amplifiers need not be very linear as

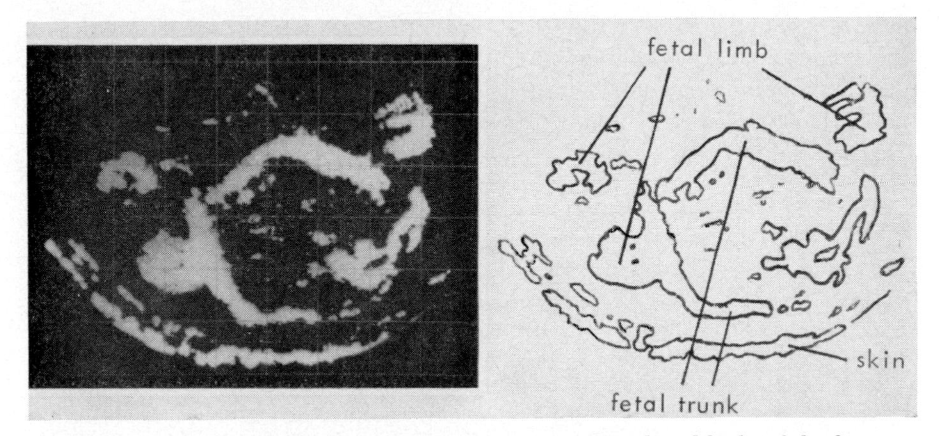

FIGURE 10. Echogram of the pregnant uterus showing the trunk and limbs of the fetus.

there is a single valued relationship between the voltages at their inputs and the position of the spot on the screen. Their nonlinearity only distorts the echogram but does not affect its resolution, and up to 5% distortion can be readily tolerated.

DOSAGE STUDY

On the question of safety, we have done a series of experiments on approximately 100 pregnant mice which were irradiated for 2 min using continuous 1 Mc/sec ultrasound. The mice were apparently unharmed after irradiation at the full output of the machine (approximately 15 w total output) as long as the water-coupling technique was used. Lethal effects could be produced at the full output by placing the applicator in direct contact with the mice, but such dosages are far in excess of those normally used with this equipment. Thermocouples were inserted in the mice, and it was found that the increased temperature was responsible for the lethal effect. As a matter of interest, the difference in the temperature increase between the direct and water-coupling techniques (for the same power level) was more than 12°C. The time rate of rise of temperature was quite different in the two cases. Further experimental work on pregnant mice is being carried out and will be reported elsewhere.

CLINICAL RESULTS

The echograms show transverse sections of the part as if examined looking down from above as illustrated in Figure 7. The skin gives a strong echo as also does the fascial and muscular layer of the anterior abdominal wall. Few, if any, echoes are received from fat, and it is apparently not possible to identify the muscular wall of the uterus with the present equipment. The fetal trunk and limbs are quite well seen. Structures within the abdominal and thoracic cavities of the fetus send echoes which, at present, are difficult to interpret because of the plane of section, but this may be simplified in the future by better positioning of the patient. The power levels used to date have been too low to outline the posterior abdominal wall. Examples of echograms are shown in Figures 8, 9, and 10. The identification of structures was assisted by a knowledge of the position and presentation of the fetus obtained by detailed palpation, by auscultation of the fetal heart, and by x-ray examination of the mother's abdomen.

REFERENCES

Arm, M., L. B. Lambert, and B. Silverberg (1962). IRE Trans. Ultrasonic Eng. *10*.

Baerwald, H. G. (1961). A limit theorem on passive reactance two-ports with constraints. Trans. Nat. Conv. IRE, Circuit Theory, 244–250.

Baum, G., and I. Greenwood (1961). A critique of time-amplitude ultrasonography. A.M.A. Arch. Ophthal. *65*, 353–365.

Donald, I., and T. G. Brown (1961). Demonstration of tissue interfaces within the body by ultrasonic echo sounding. Brit. J. of Radiology *34*, 539–546.

Howry, D. H. (1957). Techniques used in ultrasonic visualization of soft tissues, *in* "Ultrasound in Biology and Medicine," E. Kelly, ed. (American Institute of Biological Sciences, Washington, D.C.), 49–65.

Kossoff, G. (1962). Calibration of ultrasonic therapeutic equipment. Acustica *12*, 84–90.

Kossoff, G. (1963). Design of narrow beamwidth transducers. J. Acoust. Soc. Am. *35* (6).

McSkimin, H. J. (1959). Performance of high frequency barium titanate transducers for generating ultrasonic waves in liquids. J. Acoust. Soc. Am. *31*, 1519–22.

Thurston, R. N. (1959). Effect of electrical and mechanical terminating resistances on loss and bandwidth according to the conventional equivalent circuit of a piezoelectric transducer. IRE Nat. Conv. Record, Part 6, 260–278.

DISCUSSION

DR. HEUTER: Thank you, Dr. Kossoff. I sort of missed a picture here of a wattle tree or kangaroo.

DR. KOSSOFF: Well, somebody did suggest that we use ultrasound to find out if the kangaroo had anything in her pouch.

DR. HEUTER: Are there any questions on this paper?

DR. GORDON: What's the earliest stage of pregnancy in your program?

DR. KOSSOFF: We have done only twelve patients. All of our patients have been in the last stages of pregnancy.

DR. KIKUCHI: Have you discovered anything unusual in pregnancy?

DR. KOSSOFF: No, since the instrumentation requires critical adjustment, our major effort to date has been in maintaining properly operating equipment.

25

The Ultrasonic Tomograph and Its Use in Medical Diagnosis[1]

DOUGLAS GORDON, M.D.
Willesden General Hospital, London, England

The use of ultrasonic pulses and their echoes as a method of measuring distances and direction has been well known in marine work since World War I. The use of ultrahigh-frequency pulses of radio waves and their echoes has been well known since World War II. For the latter, a system of two-dimensional display on the screen of a cathode ray tube became common practice. It was not surprising, therefore, that the two techniques were "married" so that the plane of a moving ultrasonic beam was reported in proportion on the screen of a cathode ray tube.

Until the first ultrasonic tomograph was reported by Wild and co-workers (1–10), the use of ultrasound in medical diagnosis had been confined to the transmission technique of Dussik *et al.* (11–15). Wild employed a simple linear movement of the probe at right angles to the emergent beam. This was used for the investigation of carcinoma of the female breast (Fig. 1A). Later, Wild (16) employed a small probe within the rectum which was rotated through 360° or even more as it was withdrawn (Fig. 1B).

Wild's two techniques, though geometrically very different, had a common limiting feature, namely, the beam reached any one point in the tissues from a single probe position. This was the crucial defect which hampered a large proportion of the work in this field. Where the information required is the measurement of a distance, as with displacements of the brain within the skull, the measurement of the foetal skull, or the movements of the walls of the heart, a stationary probe is adequate although considerable dexterity is demanded in eliciting good echo signals and considerable difference of opinion is possible as to which structure within the patient is producing

[1]Due to a change in program, Dr. Gordon's talk, originally scheduled to follow Dr. Kossoff's paper, was presented earlier in the symposium.

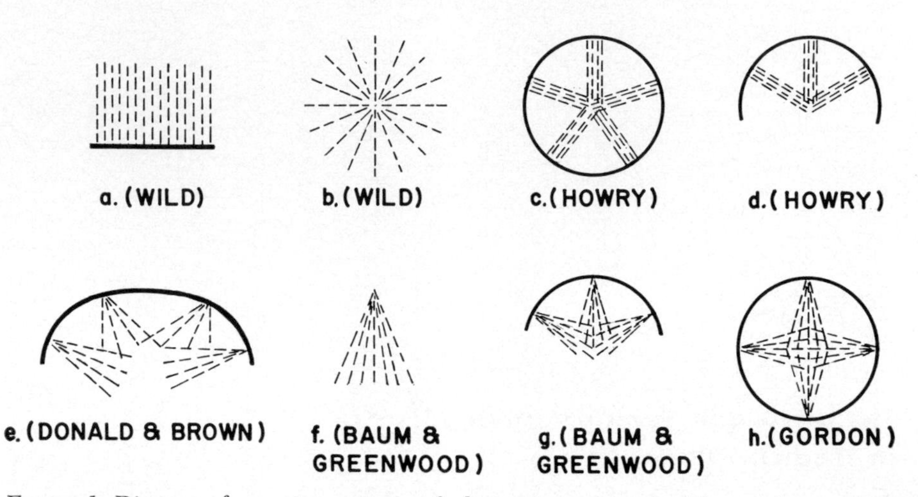

FIGURE 1. Diagram of scanning patterns of ultrasonic tomographs. The continuous lines represent the probe course; the interrupted lines, the paths of the ultrasonic beams.

which echo. In order to identify accurately the source of an echo, it is necessary to employ a scanning system.

Although it is tempting to regard the production of echoes by surfaces as identical with the reflection of light, this is very misleading. All workers with ultrasound discover at a very early stage that the overriding factor in the production of echoes is the angulation of the rays to the surface that produces the echo. As the speaker reported to the Second International Conference of Medical Electronics in Paris in 1959, the geometry of the reflecting object is much more important in determining the amplitude of the returning echo than the size, the distance, or the nature of the reflecting surface.

The difference of reflected sound from the behavior of reflected light can best be brought out by an analogy. Suppose an observer with a searchlight is investigating the countryside on a pitch dark night. His searchlight can illuminate at any time only one spot corresponding to an angle of 1° from his searchlight. By gradually scanning the countryside with his beam and measuring the reflected light at each point he could build up a fairly accurate picture of the countryside that would not differ, except in sharpness, from a picture taken in daylight. In fact, exactly this technique was used in one of the earliest systems of television.

If an exactly similar procedure were employed using ultrasound, the resulting picture would be grossly misleading. The highlights would consist of a random series of dots of varying size which would be found to correspond to convex surfaces — the larger the radius of curvature, the brighter the spot produced. Other highlights would be recorded or ignored in what would appear to be a most arbitrary manner. A large mansion would be represented by some vertical lines from the pillars of its portico, but its vast frontage would be completely lost as it was inclined at an angle to the light beam. On the other hand, the doghouse in front of the mansion would appear as the most important feature of the landscape because it happened to receive and reflect the light at right angles. In fact, a better comparison would be with a heliograph which is visible at a distance of many miles when correctly adjusted while all other detail is completely lost.

The only way in which the arbitrary distortion occasioned by this phenomenon can be overcome is to ensure that any one point in the field being examined is scanned from a multiplicity of points of observation. If the searchlight referred to earlier is mounted on a truck and driven past the mansion, at some point in its journey the whole facade will be normal to the light and the doghouse will cease to be the most important feature of the landscape.

The magnitude of this effect, reported in 1959 (17), was that a flat surface, normal to the rays, gave an echo signal that was attenuated by 27 db if the surface were tilted by 4° in any direction.

The first practical tomograph to employ a compound scan (Fig. 1C) was that of Howry and co-workers (18–25). The probe mounting was arranged to travel around a cylindrical bath for the full 360°. As it turned around the center of the bath, the probe moved relative to its mounting so that the beam scanned a strip on either side of the radius. The oscillating movement was through a comparatively small path, compared with the radius, so that only the central area of the patient was able to receive beams from a multiplicity of directions.

The inconvenience of immersing the patient in water, often as high as the chin, militated against the use of this technique with seriously ill patients. Howry's (26) later tomograph (Fig. 1D) employed the same scanning system but restricted the probe travel to a semicircle. It was then possible to surround the patient with a crescentic bath applied to the area to be examined, but the water was separated from the patient by a thin sheet of plastic and a film of jelly was applied to the skin to ensure that no air was retained between water and tissue.

Donald and Brown (27–29) of Glasgow, Scotland, developed a tomograph (Fig. 1E) particularly for gynecology and obstetrics. Taking advantage of the pliability of the female abdominal wall in the presence of pregnancy or tumor, they were able to eliminate the water bath and to apply a probe directly to the oiled skin without losing coupling. The probe was able to move in any path dictated by the shape and size of the patient and these movements were ingeniously reproduced on the screen. As the probe moved around the abdomen, it was tilted backward and forward manually in the plane of its movement and these movements were also reproduced on the screen. The Donald and Brown tomograph had the additional advantage that it could be used for longitudinal planes, and the absence of the water bath enabled it to be used with the most gravely ill patients. A later tomograph provided an automatic movement of the probe by a servo system sensing the abdominal contour.

Baum and Greenwood (30–33) in New York developed a tomograph (Fig. 1F) for ophthalmology. The first machine involved a single probe position and an angular scan. Owing to the high frequency employed, the directionality effect was less serious, but in a later model now marketed in the U.S.A. (Fig. 1G), the probe has a compound scan traveling through an arc and tilting through an angle, giving a compound scan very similar to that of Donald and Brown. Owing to the high frequency, the range is limited but the discrimination in distance is much improved. This is of particular value in ophthalmology or breast examination but is a disadvantage in other areas. As with Howry's later machine, a water bath is applied to the target area only.

All of the machines described that have a compound scan depend upon the use of radar techniques for the display. Photographic integration is used to build up a satisfactory picture, and, by the way, the resulting picture gives a cross-sectional view that looks as if the patient had been cut through with a guillotine. As the absorption of ultrasound by bone is very high, no detail is recorded within bone, but tissue interfaces which are impossible to demonstrate by x rays without contrast materials show up very well. In general, ultrasonic diagnostic radiology is complementary to diagnostic x radiology.

Compared with the simple ultrasonic flaw detector of industry, these radar-type ultrasonic tomographs are much more complicated, are much more expensive, and demand a much higher standard of operator skill. The speaker, therefore, set about obtaining the same type of result with a mechanical system capable of operation by an x-ray technician. It seemed inherently more reasonable to reproduce the physical movement of a probe by the physical movement of a cathode ray tube than to convert the probe movement into an electric analog and reproduce it in the form of a movement of the trace in a cathode ray tube screen. It was also obvious that, whereas with the passage of time and with temperature variations, electrical devices would show considerable variation, a mechanical system would retain its exact dimensions indefinitely.

Going back beyond the work of Sir Robert Watson-Watt to that of Leonardo da Vinci, we decided to employ the pantograph principle. With suitable alterations to meet the requirements of a compound scan, it was rapidly discovered and proved on a model that it was possible by means of six members and two wires to reproduce by the physical movement of the cathode ray tube an exact analog of the movement of the probe and its emergent beam.

Since the new tomograph (Figs. 1H, 2) patent application (34–35) was made as recently as January 5, 1962, and its full realization involves the construction of a special ruggedized cathode ray tube capable of withstanding lateral accelerations and decelerations, it is not yet possible to record in detail the clinical results obtained with the prototype. It is, however, designed to give the type of scan provided by the later Baum and Greenwood system, but it will also give a probe movement of 360° for the examination of parts of the body such as the neck, forearm, or leg. The results are recorded on a continuous roll film 5-in wide in an aircraft-type camera with automatic interlock so that the film is moved to the next frame before the next scan is possible.

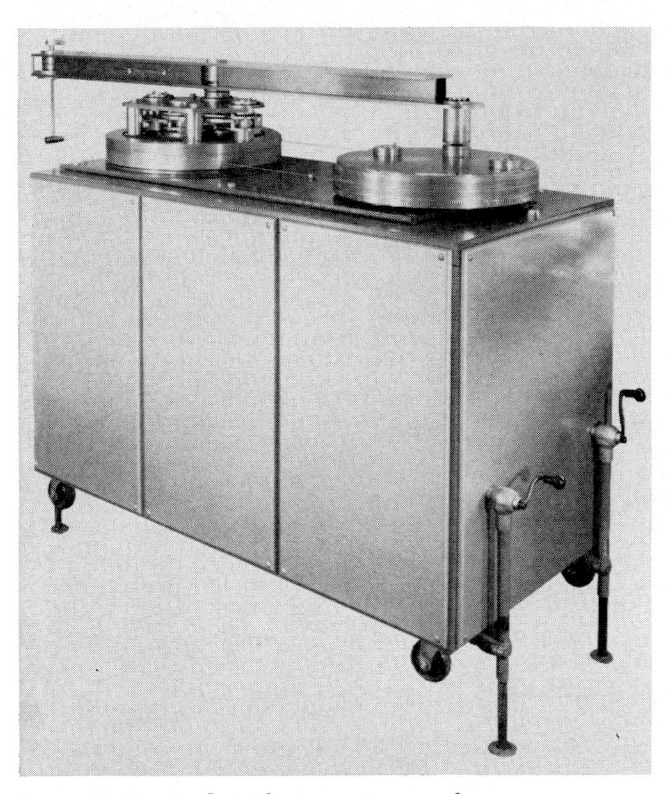

FIGURE 2. The Gordon Ultrasonic Tomograph.

The patient's details are printed in the corners of the frame. At the end of an examination, the used section of the film is cut off and processed on a spiral former.

It is not for the speaker to assess the value of the new device at this stage. It is merely a simplification of the existing devices of proven value in their own fields, but it also has the merit that the same instrument can be used to examine any part of the body with probes of any size working at any frequency. The prototype is planned to provide radii of probe movement of 4 in for use in ophthalmology, of 6 in for use for the neck, and of 8 in for the trunk. The angle of scan may be varied from 0 to 360°.

Howry's work in showing cirrhosis, abscess, and metastases in the liver, kidney tumors, soft tissue detail in the limbs and neck, and elsewhere; Donald and Brown's work in diagnosing uterine and ovarian cysts and tumors with and without pregnancy, hydatidiform moles, and carcinomatosis of the peritoneum; and Baum and Greenwood's work in showing retinal and choroid detachments and retro-ocular tumors of the orbit can now all be applied on an extensive scale with an apparatus of moderate cost. Clearly, the aspect likely to attract the attention of a large number of clinicians, whether surgeons or physicians, will be the possibility of demonstrating metastases in the liver. Donald has achieved such a high standard of accuracy of diagnosis in ovarian and uterine masses that it is reasonable to expect that in the course of time the differential diagnosis of different types of hepatic lesions may be placed on a reliable basis.

REFERENCES

1. French, L. A., J. J. Wild, and D. Neal (1950). Detection of cerebral tumors by ultrasonic pulses: pilot studies on postmortem material. Cancer *3*, 705–708.
2. Wild, J. J. (1950). The use of ultrasonic pulses for the measurement of biologic tissues and the detection of tissue density changes. Surgery *47*, 183–188.
3. French, L. A., J. J. Wild, and D. Neal (1951). Attempts to determine harmful effects of pulsed ultrasonic vibrations. Cancer *4*, 342–344.
4. French, L. A., J. J. Wild, and D. Neal (1951). The experimental application of ultrasonics to the localization of brain tumors. Preliminary rept., J. Neurosurg. *8*, 198–203.
5. Wild, J. J., and D. Neal (1951). Use of high-frequency ultrasonic waves for detecting changes of texture in living tissues. Lancet I, 655–657.
6. Wild, J. J., and J. M. Reid (1952). Further pilot echographic studies on the histological structure of tumors of the living intact human breast. Am. J. Pathol. *28*, 839–861.
7. Wild, J. J., and J. M. Reid (1952). Ultrasonic ranging for cancer diagnosis. Electronics *25*, 136.
8. Wild, J. J., and J. M. Reid (1952). Application of echo-ranging techniques to the determination of structure of biological tissues. Science *115*, 226–230.
9. Wild, J. J., and J. M. Reid (1954). Echographic visualization of lesions of the living intact human breast, Can. Res. *14*, 277–283.
10. Wild, J. J., and J. M. Reid (1956). Diagnostic uses of ultrasound. Brit. J. Phys. Med. *19*, 248–257.
11. Dussik, K. T. (1942). Über die Möglichkeit Lochfrequente mechanische Schwingungen ab diagnostiches Hilfsmittel zu verwierten. Z. Neurol. Psychiat. *174*, 153–168.
12. Dussik, K. T., F. Dussik, and L. Wyt (1947). Auf dem Wege zur Hyperphonographie des Gehirnes. Wien. Med. Wschr. *97*, 425–429.
13. Dussik, K. T. (1948). Ultraschall Diagnostik, insbesondere bei Gehirnerkrankungen, mittels Hyperphonographie. Z. Phys. Ther. *1*, 140–145.
14. Dussik, K. T. (1949). "Kongressbericht der Erlanger Ultraschall-Tagung" (S. Hirzel Verlag, Zurich).
15. Dussik, K. T. (1952). Weitere Ergebnisse der Ultraschalluntersuchung bei Gehirnerkrankungen. Acta Neurochir. *2*, 379–401.
16. Wild, J. J., and J. M. Reid (1957). Progress in the techniques of soft tissue examination by 15 mc pulsed ultrasound, *in* "Ultrasound in Biology and Medicine," E. Kelly, ed. (American Institute of Biological Sciences, Washington, D.C.), 30–48.
17. Gordon, D. (1960). Echo-encephalography, *in* "Medical Electronics," C. N. Smyth, ed., Proc. 2nd Internat. Conf. Med. Electron., Paris, 1959 (Iliffe, London), 380–390.
18. Howry, D. H., and W. R. Bliss (1952). Ultrasonic visualization of soft tissue structures of body. J. Lab. Clin. Med. *40*, 579–592.
19. Howry, D. H., J. J. Holmes, R. R. Lanier, and G. J. Posakony (1954). J. Proc. 3rd Ann. Conf. Ultrasonic Ther. 1–17.
20. Howry, D. H., D. A. Stott, and W. R. Bliss (1954). Ultrasonic visualization of carcinoma of breast and other soft tissue structures. Cancer 7, 354–358.

21. Holmes, J. J., D. H. Howry, G. J. Posakony, and C. R. Cushman (1955). Ultrasonic visualization of soft tissue structures in human body. Trans. Amer. Clin. Climat. Assn. *66*, 208–225.
22. Howry, D. H. (1955). IRE Nat. Conv. Record, 75–88.
23. Howry, D. H., J. J. Holmes, C. R. Cushman, and G. J. Posakony (1955). Ultrasonic visualization of living organs and tissues with observations on some disease processes. Geriatrics *10*, 123–128.
24. Howry, D. H., G. J. Posakony, C. R. Cushman, and J. J. Holmes (1956). 3-dimensional and stereoscopic observation of body structures by ultrasound. J. Appl. Physiol. *9*, 304–306.
25. Howry, D. H. (1957). Techniques used in ultrasonic visualization of soft tissues, *in* "Ultrasound in Biology and Medicine," E. Kelly, ed. (American Institute of Biological Sciences, Washington, D.C.), 49–64.
26. Howry, D. H. (1960). Personal communication.
27. Donald, I., J. MacVicar, and T. G. Brown (1958). Investigation of abdominal masses by pulsed ultrasound. Lancet *I*, 1188–95.
28. Brown, T. G. (1960). Direct contact ultrasonic scanning techniques for the visualization of abdominal masses, *in* "Medical Electronics," C. N. Smyth, ed., Proc. 2nd Internat. Conf. Med. Electron., Paris, 1959 (Iliffe, London), 258–366.
29. Donald, I., and T. G. Brown (1961). Demonstration of tissue interfaces within the body by ultrasonic echo sounding. Brit. J. Radiol. *34*, 539–546.
30. Baum, G. (1958). The application of ultrasonic locating techniques to ophthalmology. II. Ultrasonic slit lamp in the ultrasonic visualization of soft tissue. A.M.A. Arch. Ophthal. *60*, 263–279.
31. Baum, G., and I. Greenwood (1958). The application of ultrasonic locating techniques to ophthalmology: theoretical considerations and acoustic properties of ocular media. I. Reflective properties. Am. J. Ophthal. *46*, 319–329.
32. Baum, G., and I. Greenwood (1960). Ultrasonography – an aid in orbital tumor diagnosis. A.M.A. Arch. Ophthal. *64*, 180–194.
33. Baum, G., and I. Greenwood (1960). Ultrasound in ophthalmology. Am. J. Ophthal. *49*, 249–261.
34. Gordon, G. A. D. (1964). A new or improved tomograph. Brit. Pat. No. 956/56.
35. Gordon, D. (1962). San Diego Symposium for Biomedical Engineering. An Ultrasonic Tomograph for Medical Diagnosis, 20–22.

DISCUSSION

Dr. Baum: What is the time required for a single scan in this device? What is its speed or rate of scan?

Dr. Gordon: Not having actually done this, I am only speculating. Obviously, the system will work better mechanically and electrically if it is done slowly, but from the patient's point of view, the shorter the time, the better. I believe it is reasonable to expect that we will be able to do a complete scan of, shall we say, a liver in something like 5 to 10 sec – something that the patient can hold his breath for, but this is a pious hope, not a practical experience. We are, of course, using an appropriate type of sensitive screen to get the best image and special films to get the best photographic conditions.

Dr. Howry: In relation to Dr. Donald's work in Great Britain, there is one advantage in technique in that they could travel in a linear motion down the patient, still obtaining a compound scan and thereby achieving a cross-section in another direction. Everyone is restricted by the current state of the art of television tubes which is about 1000 lines per inch. These are quite expensive tubes, to put it mildly, and when you start getting 16-in tubes that will print 1000 lines, you have really bought yourself a piece of equipment. You must have automatic focusing, that is, dynamic focusing of the system which in itself requires sufficient equipment to fill three relay racks. The advantage that Dr. Gordon would have is that with a single tube, the pantograph motion will literally travel clear down the abdomen. You are making use of the techniques we formerly used in this planographic scan in radiography, a type of traveling grid that would allow you a great many lines without the necessary restrictions on the overall system. I'm not sure that your fast sweep axis is as good as moving the overall tube with the slow scan axis. It is possible that it might offer more potentialities. There are two problems with high rep-rate systems, particularly at low frequencies. If you use something of water tank size in conjunction with ultrasound frequencies of 1 or 2 Mc, you run into a very wicked "sing-around" signal, as we call it. In other words, the signals from the previous pulses are still traveling in the tank of water, going around like a billiard ball on the table, at the time one is attempting to receive the new train of signals back out of the abdomen. This brings all kinds of wild ghost signals. To some extent you can get rid of this by wobulating your repetition rate and blurring them out. The only other thing that one might do is to reduce the repetition rate, which is what Brown usually did. Instead of having a rep-rate of approximately 2000 pulses per second, his equipment was down to 50 pulses per second. The other point in regard to high repetition rates is that patients get a little unhappy when things start flying around at several miles per second in front of them and pinball machines run in and out and down the line, so that approximately a 10-sec examination of the abdomen is about as fast as we, at least, are currently trying to accomplish. We feel most patients can hold their breath for 10 to 15 sec and give us a compound scan of the complete abdomen. This is our present objective.

DR. BELL: All the factors are the same for his mechanical scan except one. It's very possible by moving a whole tube that you will get better resolving power, or you will get the same resolving power from a compound scan that you would otherwise get from a noncompound scan. The recordings will tend to fall on top of each other, except for certain refractions.

DR. HOWRY: You would have the same old problem of mechanical backlash which has been one of the greatest of all the problems. If you have only 2° backlash in the coupling between your patient and your transducer or anywhere in your system, it produces a large error at some point 20 cm away.

DR. MACKAY: At least with the eye work that some of us are interested in, you can eliminate the parallelogram, and you just have a shaft running from the transducer up to the small cathode ray tube, that is, the tube is rigidly fixed to the top of the transducer.

DR. HOWRY: I'll buy it, but I think it is going to be an awfully big washing machine when it goes around that pregnant woman.

DR. CARLIN: I don't quite see, if you are going to move the source of light, why you need a cathode ray tube. You might just as well move a neon bulb or any other source of light.

DR. GORDON: To begin with, the linear time base on the cathode ray tube has to be of a very high order, when you're working at 4 in of water; that's the equivalent of only a short sweep.

DR. HOWRY: Transparent materials such as Sylvania is marketing will do the job. In fact, they recently came out with a three-dimensional tube, but it is nothing but a series of arms that rotate very rapidly in apogee.

DR. REID: I think it might be possible to eliminate the cathode ray tube in that these subminiature galvanometers used in high-speed recorders have resonant frequencies in the order of 10 kc and can be equalized, such that you would only have to move the magnet block of the galvanometer by some very clever optical arrangement that you could no doubt work out.

DR. HOWRY: Does this have to work in one constant direction?

DR. GORDON: No, this is a reversible motor.

DR. HOWRY: If you were on the outside of the patient and you kept going in one direction, you would solve your inertia problems.

DR. GORDON: On the contrary, you would tear off the connections to the cathode ray tube.

DR. HOWRY: Then you would blank it out if you tried to do the whole 360°.

DR. GORDON: We don't expect to do the whole 360° in more than a small proportion of cases. That will apply to the neck and to the arms protruding through the bottom of the tank, but for most areas, 270° would be the practical limit, but then this is a matter for experiment. This is a preliminary communication, only presented because it seemed such an opportunity to present this new approach to an audience such as this.

DR. KIKUCHI: We have found that if we want to use this kind of equipment in the clinical laboratory that in order to obtain a clear photograph we must adjust some amplification factors or other parameters to match each patient's situation. Therefore, in your case, you must have some arrangements before you reach the optimum adjustment.

DR. GORDON: Well, we have in fact a monitor, that is, you have a second tube in parallel with the first, with a conventional A-scan so that you know whether you have set your probes to give you the optimum amplitude of echoes.

DR. MACKAY: Since part of this discussion seems to be devoted to unorthodox scan methods, I would like to mention one more possibility—something that I always mean to try, but haven't as yet. This concerns moving the subject rather than the transducer, for scanning purposes. In the case of eye work, you might fix the crystal, take electrooculography signals from the patient's temple, and tell the subject merely to look from one side to the other. Since the eyeball does not rotate exactly around a fixed point, this would give a distorted view, but for some purposes it would probably be adequate. Gross movement in the liquid would be minimized.

DR. GORDON: In ophthalmology it is what you see behind the eye that is of value clinically, not what you can see with an ophthalmoscope.

Dr. Mackay: In case of a detached retina in the presence of a cataract—

Dr. Gordon: The technique of treating detached retinas was not a problem to my colleagues. They were interested in tumors behind the eye but not in detached retinas because they feel they can take care of that with an ophthalmoscope.

Dr. Mackay: Perhaps not with a cataract present, as in one case sent to us at Berkeley.

Dr. Baum: I think I can answer that. The first thing is that in ophthalmology, if you have a retina detached immediately behind a cataract of any magnitude whatsoever, you just do a simple light projection test and you probably would have a field beam test in the area of light projection. And then in terms of actual ultrasonic retina examination I think the kind of picture you would get using ocular motion to control your scan would be so poor that you would not be able to interpret it accurately.

Dr. Mackay: From distortion the eyeball might look more elliptical than round.

Dr. Baum: If your patient moves while you are doing an ultrasonograph, you will get bulging and waves at the back of the eye that may be uninterpretable. You get actual superimposition of structure.

Dr. Mackay: Remember, you monitor motion here to correct the display. I would think that in general the major action or motion of the eye is rather smooth, and when people are asked to move their eyes I think the movement would not be of a ripply nature.

Dr. Howry: I think there is another point with considerably more than academic interest in terms of mechanical scan. Everybody is looking at this in terms of the mechanical scan. I would like to point out that a sonar head does not move, but the sonar beam goes around. But by using a phase discrimination and/or simple delay line techniques and running serial segments of the transducer, you can achieve either focusing or scan. Now, this turns out to be a very bearcat of a problem, particularly if you pick the wrong kind of crystal, let's say a titanate or zirconate. One might try to make a flat delay line or a variable delay line to do this, since it offers some real possibilities in that your transducer does not have to move at all. In fact, you could very easily place a mosaic of transducers around a tank, let's say, with nothing moving. Let the whole thing be electronic and nothing move at all.

Dr. Mackay: Well, in principle, you can do something even more than is indicated by this method. In principle, with a single ping and receiving all those echoes, you can get the entire structure of the eye and thus minimize "dose" as well as the effect of subject motion. But if you look at it rather carefully, there are some difficulties which have to do with the fact that the eyeball or the liver or whatever biological material you are using is not at infinity as submarines often are—therefore, there is an added source of confusion here that does not exist in ocean-going sonar.

Dr. Howry: Well, at least your fast scanning or focusing could be done by some such system.

Dr. Mackay: Oh, it's a very interesting possibility, but it is a little more complicated than one might think on first consideration — as I am sure you are well aware.

DR. REID: In partial answer to that last question, some years ago we built phase delay lines that were flat in their transmission characteristics to beyond 15 Mc for the electrically focused transducer. But the problem in applying these sonar techniques, as far as our own evaluation has been concerned, is that the practical bandwidth is much larger because of our lower set of frequencies and that many of the sonar techniques which are simply single frequency devices don't have the bandwidths to maintain the pulses.

Low-Intensity Ultrasound Research as Applied in Clinical Medicine[1]

JOHN H. ALDES, M.D.
Ben R. Meyer Rehabilitation Center, Cedars of Lebanon Hospital, Los Angeles California

This study covers a period of 10 years of application of low-intensity ultrasound in clinical medicine. Progress in this field was made possible only by combining laboratory and clinical investigations. During the early years of this study, experimental animals (pigs) were subjected to this form of energy in order to determine the appropriate choices of frequency and intensity and to determine the direct and side effects of this new type of radiation. The results obtained by European and other American investigators were considered and utilized in this study. Ultrasonic radiation was applied therapeutically in many pathologic conditions of the human, and in some cases the results were better than in others. Indications and contraindications were compiled and compared and some of these that were considered in the early studies are now found to be irrelevant to the present-day use of low-intensity ultrasound in clinical medicine.

Over 15,000 patients were subjected to low-intensity ultrasonic radiation during the course of this study. This report includes statistical data on the results first reported in 1952 and on the data obtained since that time. The original 1952 study reported 237 cases in which ultrasonic therapy was used for arthritic and discogenic diseases of the spine, and it was found that 75% showed improvement. In the 1962 report, 79.2% of a total of 5387 cases of arthritic and discogenic diseases of the spine showed improvement following ultrasonic therapy. It is concluded that low-intensity ultrasonic radiation is not indicated for cancer or tuberculosis or a myriad of other disorders, but ultrasonic energy is an important adjunct in clinical medicine for the relief of pain in traumatic, neuromuscular, and arthritic disorders.

[1] This is an abstract of the paper which Dr. Aldes was scheduled to present at this symposium. Unfortunately, he was unable to attend.